DATE DUE

OC 14 97			
AP 1 99			
JE 7 01			
MY 24 05			
JY 25 05			
MY 2 5 06			
DE 18 07			
9 10 09			

Handbook of Adolescent
Health Risk Behavior

Issues in Clinical Child Psychology

Series Editors: **Michael C. Roberts,** *University of Kansas–Lawrence, Kansas*
Lizette Peterson, *University of Missouri–Columbia, Missouri*

A Continuation Order Plan is available for this series. A continuation order will bring
delivery of each new volume immediately upon publication. Volumes are billed only
upon actual shipment. For further information please contact the publisher.

Handbook of Adolescent Health Risk Behavior

Edited by

RALPH J. DiCLEMENTE

University of Alabama at Birmingham
Birmingham, Alabama

WILLIAM B. HANSEN

Bowman Gray School of Medicine
Winston-Salem, North Carolina

and

LYNN E. PONTON

University of California, San Francisco
San Francisco, California

PLENUM PRESS • NEW YORK AND LONDON

...loging in Publication Data

... / edited by Ralph J. DiClemente, William B.

...ology)
...ex.

...taking in adolescence. 3. Health promotion. 4.
Health behavior in adolescence—United States. 5. Risk-taking in adolescence—United
States. I. DiClemente, Ralph J. II. Hansen, William B. (William Bunker), 1949–   . III.
Ponton, Lynn E. IV. Series.
RJ47.53.H36 1995   95-43464
616.89′022—dc20   CIP

ISBN 0-306-45147-6

© 1996 Plenum Press, New York
A Division of Plenum Publishing Corporation
233 Spring Street, New York, N. Y. 10013

10 9 8 7 6 5 4 3 2 1

Printed in the United States of America

Contributors

Robert Wm. Blum, M.D., Ph.D., Department of Pediatrics, University of Minnesota, Minneapolis, Minnesota

Larry K. Brown, M.D., Brown University School of Medicine and Department of Child and Family Psychiatry, Rhode Island Hospital, Providence, Rhode Island

Oscar Bukstein, M.P.H., M.D., University of Pittsburgh Medical Center, Western Psychiatric Institute and Clinic, Pittsburgh, Pennsylvania

Coleen Cantwell, Division of Social and Community Psychiatry, Department of Psychiatry, University of California, Los Angeles, Los Angeles, California

Yifat Cohen, M.D., Brown University School of Medicine and Department of Child and Family Psychiatry, Rhode Island Hospital, Providence, Rhode Island

Renee Cunningham, Ph.D., George Warren Brown School of Social Work, Washington University, St. Louis, Missouri

Lawrence J. D'Angelo, M.D., Department of Pediatrics, Adolescent/Young Adult Medicine, Children's National Medical Center, Washington, D.C.

Ralph J. DiClemente, Ph.D., Departments of Health Behavior and Pediatrics, University of Alabama, Birmingham, Alabama

Peter Dore, M.A., George Warren Brown School of Social Work, Washington University, St. Louis, Missouri

Felton Earls, M.D., Department of Behavioral Science, Harvard University School of Public Health, Boston, Massachusetts

Sharon Farber, M.S.W., George Warren Brown School of Social Work, Washington University, St. Louis, Missouri

Susan Scavo Gallagher, Children's Safety Network, Education Development Center, Inc., Newton, Massachusetts

Denise C. Gottfredson, Ph.D., Department of Criminal Justice and Criminology, The University of Maryland, College Park, Maryland

Marya Gwadz, M.A., Division of Social and Community Psychiatry, Department of Psychiatry, University of California, Los Angeles, Los Angeles, California

William B. Hansen, Ph.D., Department of Public Health Sciences, Bowman Gray School of Medicine, Winston-Salem, North Carolina

Vivien Igra, M.D., Department of Pediatrics, University of California, San Francisco, San Francisco, California

Charles E. Irwin, Jr., M.D., Department of Pediatrics, University of California, San Francisco, San Francisco, California

Christopher S. Koper, Ph.D., Department of Criminal Justice and Criminology, The University of Maryland, College Park, Maryland; *present address:* Crime Control Institute, Washington, D.C.

Ilana Lescohier, Ph.D., Injury Control Center, Harvard School of Public Health, Boston, Massachusetts

Elizabeth R. McAnarney, M.D., Department of Pediatrics, University of Rochester Medical Center, Rochester, New York

Debra A. Murphy, Ph.D., Division of Social and Community Psychiatry, Department of Psychiatry, University of California, Los Angeles, Los Angeles, California

Patrick M. O'Malley, Ph.D., Survey Research Center, Institute for Social Research, The University of Michigan, Ann Arbor, Michigan

Michelle Parra, B.A., Division of Social and Community Psychiatry, Department of Psychiatry, University of California, Los Angeles, Los Angeles, California

Cheryl L. Perry, Ph.D., Division of Epidemiology, University of Minnesota School of Public Health, Minneapolis, Minnesota

Lynn E. Ponton, M.D., Langley Porter Psychiatric Institute, Division of Child and Adolescent Psychiatry, University of California, San Francisco, San Francisco, California

Mary Jane Rotheram-Borus, Ph.D., Division of Social and Community Psychiatry, Department of Psychiatry, University of California, Los Angeles, Los Angeles, California

Miriam D. Sealock, M.A., Department of Criminal Justice and Criminology, The University of Maryland, College Park, Maryland

C. Wayne Sells, M.D., M.P.H., Department of Pediatrics, University of Minnesota, Minneapolis, Minnesota

Jean Thatcher Shope, M.S.P.H., Ph.D., University of Michigan Transportation Research Institute, Ann Arbor, Michigan

John B. Sikorski, M.D., Child and Adolescent Psychiatry, University of California, San Francisco, San Francisco, California

Anthony Spirito, Ph.D., Brown University School of Medicine and Department of Child and Family Psychiatry, Rhode Island Hospital, Providence, Rhode Island

Michael J. Staufacker, M.P.H., Division of Epidemiology, University of Minnesota School of Public Health, Minneapolis, Minnesota; *current address:* StayWell Health Management Systems, Inc., St. Paul, Minnesota

Catherine Stevens-Simon, M.D., Division of Adolescent Medicine, University of Colorado Health Science Center, The Children's Hospital, Denver, Colorado

Arlene Rubin Stiffman, Ph.D., George Warren Brown School of Social Work, Washington University, St. Louis, Missouri

Michael Windle, Ph.D., Research Institute on Addictions, Buffalo, New York

Preface

Adolescence is a developmental period of accelerating physical, psychological, social/ cultural, and cognitive development, often characterized by confronting and surmounting a myriad of challenges and establishing a sense of self-identity and autonomy. It is also, unfortunately, a period fraught with many threats to the health and well-being of adolescents and with substantial consequent impairment and disability. Many of the adverse health consequences experienced by adolescents are, to a large extent, the result of their risk behaviors.

Many adolescents today, and perhaps an increasing number in the future, are at risk for death, disease, and other adverse health outcomes that are not primarily biomedical in origin. In general, there has been a marked change in the causes of morbidity and mortality among adolescents. Previously, infectious diseases accounted for a disproportionate share of adolescent morbidity and mortality. At present, however, the overwhelming toll of adolescent morbidity and mortality is the result of lifestyle practices. Contemporary threats to adolescent health are primarily the consequence of social, environmental, and behavioral factors, the so-called "social morbidities."

Social morbidities include a broad spectrum of behaviors and related outcomes such as substance use and abuse, violence, suicide, unintentional injury, eating disorders, teenage pregnancy, and sexually transmitted diseases, to name but a few. More recently, the emergence of human immunodeficiency virus infection and its related outcome, AIDS, poses yet another serious health threat for adolescents. In addition to the morbidity and mortality associated with adolescent risk-taking, often underemphasized is the high proportion of adolescents who are school dropouts or homeless. As a consequence, many youth do not attain their full potential and do not become productive members of society. Clearly, the cost to adolescents and society, in general, is staggering, in terms of disease, premature mortality, wasted human potential, and economic expenditures for health care, rehabilitation, and incarceration in juvenile detention facilities.

This *Handbook of Adolescent Health Risk Behavior* attempts to describe the epidemiologic trends associated with specific risk behaviors, assess a broad array of preventive strategies, and evaluate the efficacy of treatment modalities. To accomplish this goal, a multidisciplinary group of researchers and clinicians, all with extensive experience working with adolescents, offer a variety of perspectives with direct relevance, implications, and practical strategies for promoting the health and well-being of adolescents. Specifically, this volume serves to highlight the epidemiologic data describing the socio-demographic correlates and trends in adolescent risk behavior. Further, it examines a variety of prevention strategies and evaluates their effectiveness. And, finally, treatment modalities are evaluated and recommendations offered regarding their efficacy for specific adolescent subpopulations.

In the introductory chapter, DiClemente, Hansen, and Ponton provide an overview of the impact of adolescent risk behaviors on health and well-being and assess the role of prevention and treatment interventions for reducing these behaviors. Sells and Blum follow with a careful analysis of temporal trends in adolescent morbidity and mortality. In the next chapter, Igra and Irwin describe a biopsychosocial model for understanding the factors influencing adolescent risk-taking behaviors.

The next group of chapters address specific adolescent risk behaviors. Each chapter follows a similar template; that is, they describe the scope of the problem, the epidemiology associated with a particular risk behavior, assess prevention strategies, and describe and evaluate treatment modalities. First, Perry and Staufacker address tobacco use, a critical risk factor for a host of subsequent disease conditions. Ponton follows with a discussion of disordered eating. Next, Windle, Shope, and Bukstein describe the epidemiology of alcohol use among adolescents and evaluate prevention and treatment approaches. In a related chapter, Hansen and O'Malley examine drug use as a risk behavior associated with a myriad of adverse health and social outcomes. Cohen, Spirito, and Brown examine suicide and suicidal behavior among adolescents, what influences these self-destructive thoughts and behaviors, and how best to prevent and treat them. Lescohier and Gallagher describe factors associated with unintentional injury among adolescents. Gottfredson, Sealock, and Koper describe the causes and consequences of delinquency among adolescents. Stiffman, Earls, Dore, Cunningham, and Farber address an issue that has emerged as critically important for adolescents, particularly inner-city youth: violence among adolescents. Switching to sexual risk-taking, Stevens-Simon and McAnarney address the continuing problem of teen pregnancy. In a similar vein, D'Angelo and DiClemente describe the epidemic of sexually transmitted diseases, including HIV infection, as an emerging health threat for adolescents and offer prevention and treatment recommendations. Rotheram-Borus, Parra, Cantwell, Gwadz, and Murphy address homelessness as a risk behavior among adolescents and its association with other risk behaviors and adverse health outcomes. Finally, Sikorski addresses the problem of academic underachievement and school refusal among adolescents and how this translates into risk behavior and poor health outcomes. The closing chapter by DiClemente, Hansen, and Ponton provides an overarching synthesis of key findings from risk behavior-specific chapters and offers recommendations for the design of future adolescent risk prevention and health promotion research and interventions.

The chapters in this handbook provide a wealth of information about the epidemiology, prevention, and treatment of adolescent risk behaviors. Only by understanding the myriad of psychological, sociological, and cultural influences on adolescent risk behavior can we begin to meet the challenges posed by these risk behaviors and design the necessary programs to prevent and reduce risk behaviors and, consequently, their adverse social and health sequelae. The issues confronting us are complex, however, and simple answers will only yield illusory solutions. Real progress will come grudgingly, through the tireless efforts of the many individuals, both professional and lay, concerned with adolescent health and well-being. The clock is ticking. How many more of our young people must become statistics before we acknowledge the threat risk behaviors pose for our youth, before we as a society effectively address these issues with the necessary fiscal and intellectual resources? Without prompt attention to identifying the causes of adolescent risk behaviors and developing effective prevention and treatment modalities, the future of many adolescents will be in jeopardy.

Ralph J. DiClemente
William B. Hansen
Lynn E. Ponton

Acknowledgments

We would like to thank our families for their love, support, patience, and encouragement.

We would not have been able to produce this important volume without our contributors, their determination to understand the behavior of the adolescents with whom they work, and their dedication to improving the quality of life for adolescents. All of the contributors spent a great deal of time, effort, and careful thought in organizing and clearly presenting their respective subjects.

We extend our thanks to Gina Wingood for her helpful reviews and suggestions, to Robert Pack for his careful reviews, comments, and editing, and to Amy Wilner for her superb editorial acumen.

We acknowledge the Series editors, Michael Roberts and Lizette Peterson, for their careful review of the proposal for this volume and their constructive recommendations.

We also acknowledge our Plenum editor, Mariclaire Cloutier, who has been instrumental in producing this volume. She has been diligent in guiding its preparation, thoughtful in conceptualization of the format, understanding of our needs, and helpful in many other ways. She has become a dear friend and a valued resource.

And, finally, we acknowledge all of those involved in helping adolescents navigate a safe course to a healthy and fulfilling future.

Contents

Chapter 7.   Drug Use **161**

William B. Hansen and Patrick M. O'Malley

Chapter 10.   Delinquency **259**

Denise C. Gottfredson, Miriam D. Sealock, and Christopher S. Koper

Chapter 11.   Adolescent Violence **289**

*Arlene Rubin Stiffman, Felton Earls, Peter Dore, Renee Cunningham,
    and Sharon Farber*

Chapter 12.   Adolescent Pregnancy **313**

Catherine Stevens-Simon and Elizabeth R. McAnarney

Chapter 13.   Sexually Transmitted Diseases Including Human Immunodeficiency Virus Infection **333**

Lawrence J. D'Angelo and Ralph J. DiClemente

Chapter 15.   Academic Underachievement and School Refusal 393

John B. Sikorski

Chapter 16.   New Directions for Adolescent Risk Prevention and Health Promotion Research and Interventions 413

Ralph J. DiClemente, Lynn E. Ponton, and William B. Hansen

1

Adolescents at Risk
A Generation in Jeopardy

RALPH J. DiCLEMENTE, WILLIAM B. HANSEN, and LYNN E. PONTON

INTRODUCTION

Adolescence is a developmental period of rapid physical, psychological, sociocultural, and cognitive changes characterized by efforts to confront and surmount challenges and to establish a sense of identity and autonomy. While many adolescents navigate the sometimes turbulent course from childhood to adulthood to become productive and healthy adults, there is growing concern that far too many others may not achieve their full potential as workers, parents, and individuals. Unfortunately, adolescence is also a period fraught with many threats to the health and well-being of adolescents, many of whom suffer substantial impairment and disability. Much of the adverse health consequences experienced by adolescents are, to a large extent, the result of risk behaviors (Ginzberg, 1991). As such, they are preventable.

ADOLESCENT MORBIDITY AND MORTALITY IS OFTEN THE RESULT OF LIFE-STYLE PRACTICES

There has been a marked change in the causes of morbidity and mortality among adolescents. Adolescents today are increasingly at risk for adverse health outcomes, even

RALPH J. DiCLEMENTE • Departments of Health Behavior and Pediatrics, University of Alabama, Birmingham, Alabama 35294.   WILLIAM B. HANSEN • Department of Public Health Sciences, Bowman Gray School of Medicine, Winston-Salem, North Carolina 27157.   LYNN E. PONTON • Langley Porter Psychiatric Institute, Division of Child and Adolescent Psychiatry, University of California, San Francisco, San Francisco, California 94117.
Handbook of Adolescent Health Risk Behavior, edited by Ralph J. DiClemente, William B. Hansen, and Lynn E. Ponton. Plenum Press, New York, 1996.

1

death, that are not primarily biomedical in origin. Whereas infections previously accounted for a disproportionate share of disease and mortality, at present the overwhelming toll of adolescent morbidity and mortality is the result of life-style practices. The majority of current threats to adolescent health are the consequence of social, environmental, and behavioral factors, the so-called "social morbidities." These social morbidities include a broad spectrum of behaviors and related outcomes such as substance use and abuse, violence, suicide, eating disorders, teenage pregnancy, and sexually transmitted diseases, to name but a few. More recently, the emergence of human immunodeficiency virus infection and its related outcome, AIDS, poses yet another serious health threat to adolescents.

TRENDS IN ADOLESCENT RISK BEHAVIORS

Trends indicate that adolescent risk behaviors may become increasingly problematic in the future. The initiation of risky behaviors is occurring at progressively younger ages. For example, youth start using alcohol, tobacco, and other drugs at markedly earlier ages. Furthermore, the proportion of younger adolescents who are from socioeconomically disadvantaged groups, and therefore at higher risk for risk behaviors, is also increasing. As a result of these trends, many more young adults may be vulnerable to experiment and initiate risk behaviors that have deleterious consequences during adolescence and, moreover, some of these behaviors have consequences that are not readily manifest until early adulthood, as is the case with HIV infection acquired during adolescence progressing to AIDS or smoking which may significantly contribute to morbidity and mortality in later life (Office of Disease Prevention and Health Promotion, 1993).

Potentially preventable causes (i.e., accidents, homicide, and suicide) account for approximately two-thirds of adolescent deaths in the United States. Furthermore, adolescent morbidity is significantly associated with preventable behaviors and socioenvironmental conditions. These include, for example, the consequences of unprotected sexual intercourse, which may result in unplanned pregnancy and sexually transmitted diseases, including HIV infection; substance use, which is strongly associated with vehicular accidents and unintentional injuries; and, often neglected, homelessness, which may make the adolescent vulnerable to a host of risk behaviors such as unintended pregnancy, STD/HIV, and substance use.

ADOLESCENT RISK BEHAVIORS AND QUALITY OF LATER LIFE

To a large extent, we as a society have tended to focus on morbidity and mortality as the more tangible outcomes and more readily quantifiable consequences of risk behaviors. Although it is abundantly clear that adolescent risk behaviors pose serious threats to health during adolescence, in early adulthood and in later life, it is also important to note that these risk behaviors are strongly linked to significant indicators of social and psychological well-being, including educational and job performance, quality of family and social relationships, and economic stability. All too often the outcomes of risk behaviors on adolescents' ability to effectively function in traditional social and occupational domains have been underemphasized. Understanding the pervasiveness of these behaviors as they influence a spectrum of social, economic, and health indices is valuable both for capturing the "true" magnitude of the seriousness of adolescent risk behaviors from a societal perspective, and in assisting in the design of effective interventions.

ESTIMATING THE COST OF ADOLESCENT RISK BEHAVIORS

While accurately assessing the impact of adolescent risk behaviors is difficult, the cost associated with preventable morbidity and mortality is equally difficult to calculate. Estimates vary markedly; however, it is apparent that the cost is extremely high. For example, the cost for confining adolescents in juvenile detention facilities in the United States is estimated at $2 billion a year. This is clearly a small fraction of the total costs for providing care and services to those adolescents experiencing adverse health consequences as a result of their risk behavior. Further, future costs as a result of chronic injuries sustained during adolescence, or the loss in later productivity attributable to adolescent risk behaviors are extremely difficult to estimate with any degree of accuracy. So although the true cost of adolescent risk behaviors may be undetermined, the limited data available suggest that it may be staggering in terms of medical, custodial expenditures, and lost future revenues.

ADOLESCENT RISK BEHAVIORS AS INTERRELATED

Singly, risk behaviors and their associated adverse health outcomes represent a serious threat to adolescents' health. Unfortunately, risk behaviors are likely to cluster, further exacerbating the health threat. There are considerable empirical data suggesting that adolescent risk behaviors are correlated; that is, engaging in one behavior may indicate an increased likelihood for engaging in other behaviors or patterns of risk behaviors (Dryfoos, 1990, 1991). The multicollinearity between risk behaviors not only poses an elevated risk for adolescents' health, but challenges our ability to develop and implement effective prevention and treatment programs. Clearly the issue of multitargeted interventions, primary, secondary, and tertiary, will receive increasing attention as clinicians, health educators, and public health policymakers wrestle with designing effective interventions.

CONCLUSION

As a society we are now faced with what can appropriately be referred to as an adolescent "risk behavior epidemic." This epidemic has a myriad of root causes. Adolescents' willingness to tolerate, seek, and participate in risk behaviors represents the outcome of a multifactorial decision-making process in which many influences inform their eventual choices. Much more remains to be learned about factors motivating the adoption or reinforcement of risk behaviors, and future studies will need to define more precisely the interrelationship between determinants and their applicability for different adolescent populations. However, it is imperative that we as a society begin to address the cost, both financially and in terms of damaged lives that risk behaviors exact each and every year. Only by addressing this problem on the broadest of all possible levels will we meaningfully address the causes, antecedents, and adverse health outcomes associated with adolescent risk behaviors. Without prompt redirection of our resources, our commitment, and our concern, adolescents will face continued and perhaps even greater challenges to avoid behaviors that rob them of the opportunity to be healthy, fulfilled, and productive individuals.

REFERENCES

Dryfoos, J. G. (1990). *Adolescents at risk*. London: Oxford University Press.
Dryfoos, J. G. (1991). Preventing high-risk behavior. *American Journal of Public Health, 81,* 157–158.
Ginzberg, E. (1991). Adolescents at Risk Conference Overview. *Journal of Adolescent Health, 12,* 588–590.
Office of Disease Prevention and Health Promotion. (1993). Intervention for adolescents at risk. *Prevention Report, February/March* (pp. 1–2). Washington, DC: United States Department of Health and Human Services, U.S. Public Health Service.

2

Current Trends
in Adolescent Health

C. WAYNE SELLS and ROBERT Wm. BLUM

INTRODUCTION

Demography of Youth

Over the past three decades, there have been two major demographic shifts among those in the second decade of life. Since the adolescent population (10 to 19 years of age) peaked in 1976 as a consequence of the postwar "baby boom," the population of young people declined steadily at a rate of approximately 2% per year until 1985. However, in the years between 1985 and 1991, the decline slowed to only 2% over that entire period (U.S. Bureau of the Census, 1993; Hollmann, 1993). In 1992, there were over 35 million young people between the ages of 10 and 19 in the United States, representing 14% of the population (Hollmann, 1993). Over the past few years, the decline has reversed; and by 2020, there will be 43 million teenagers in the United States (Figure 1) (U.S. Bureau of the Census, 1993; Hollmann, 1993; Campbell, 1994).

Concurrent with the shift in numbers of 10- to 19-year-olds has been the increase in the proportion of young people of color. Specifically, between 1980 and 1991, there has been a nearly 28% increase in the proportion of youth of color. The largest increases were in Hispanic and Asian/Pacific Islander youth (U.S. Bureau of the Census, 1993; Hollmann, 1993). In 1992, African-American youth represented 14.8% of all 10- to 19-year-olds, Hispanics 12%, Asian or Pacific Islander 3.4%, and Native Americans, Eskimo, or Aleut 1% (Figure 2) (Hollmann, 1993).

C. WAYNE SELLS and ROBERT Wm. BLUM • Department of Pediatrics, University of Minnesota, Minneapolis, Minnesota 55455.

Handbook of Adolescent Health Risk Behavior, edited by Ralph J. DiClemente, William B. Hansen, and Lynn E. Ponton. Plenum Press, New York, 1996.

C. WAYNE SELLS and ROBERT Wm. BLUM

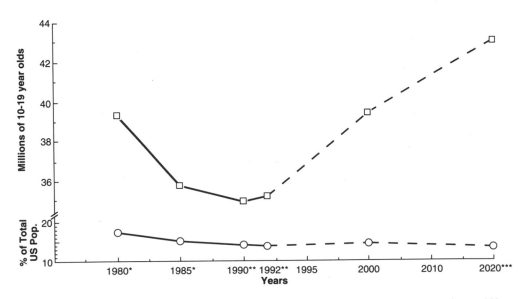

Figure 1. Number of adolescents and percentage of U.S. population among youth 10–19 years of age, 1980–2020. *Data from Current Population Reports. *U.S. population estimates by age, sex, race, and hispanic origin: 1980–1991.* U.S. Bureau of the Census, 1993. **Data from Hollmann, F. W.. *U.S. population estimates by age, sex, race and hispanic origin: 1990–1992.* U.S. Bureau of the Census, 1993. ***Data from Campbell P. R.. *Population projections for states, by age, race, and sex: 1993–2020.* U.S. Bureau of the Census, 1994.

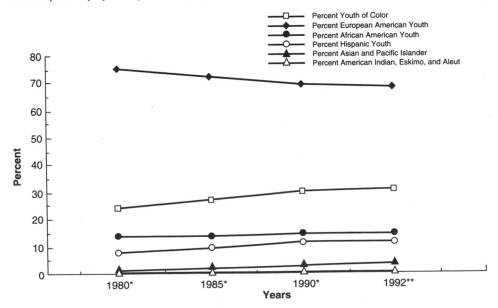

Figure 2. Percentage of adolescents (10–19 years of age) by race across time. *Data from Current Population Reports. *U.S. population estimates by age, sex, race and hispanic origin: 1980–1991.* U.S. Bureau of the Census, 1993. **Data from Hollmann, F. W.. *U.S. population estimates, by age, sex, race and hispanic origin: 1990–1992.* U.S. Bureau of the Census, 1993.

Poverty

As the number of young people increases, especially youth of color, so too will poverty. It is well known that poverty is closely related to health, education, emotional well-being, and delinquency (The Annie E. Casey Foundation, 1994). So, too, is ethnicity. In 1992, 14.6 million children (21.9% of all children) under the age of 18 lived in poverty (Children's Defense Fund, 1994). While alarmingly high, when one looks at the discrepancy by race, the differences are even more stark. Specifically, 17% of European-American children, 47% of African-American children, and 40% of Hispanic children lived in poverty in 1992 (U.S. Department of Commerce, 1993).

As race is associated with poverty, so, too, is family structure. The percentage of children growing up in single-parent households increased over 10% between 1985 and 1991. Holding race constant, the poverty rate for single-parent families is 42%, compared to 8% for two-parent families (The Annie E. Casey Foundation, 1994). The proportion of young families with a head of household under 25 years of age has increased by 17% between 1986 and 1991, to 38% of all families. While young families are more likely to live in poverty, this is especially true for families of color. Specifically, while 31% of young European-American families lived in poverty, the proportions were more than double (67.4%) for African-Americans and 50% higher for young Hispanic families (46%) (Current Population Reports, U.S. Bureau of the Census, 1993).

Insurance Status of Youth

Not only are youth the largest segment of America's poor, but a growing proportion of young people are uninsured or underinsured. One in eight (8.3 million) children under the age of 18 had no health insurance at any time in 1992 (Children's Defense Fund, 1994). Approximately 4.7 million (15.5%) adolescents aged 10–18 were uninsured in 1989; this represents an increase of 10% between 1984 and 1989. Poor, near-poor, and youth of color were at the highest risk for being uninsured. Twenty percent of youth under the age of 18 and 42% of those between the ages of 18 and 24 with family income below the poverty level were without medical insurance of any kind in 1992 (Newacheck, McManus, & Gephart, 1992). Not surprising, then, is the finding that Hispanic youth were three times (34%) and African-American youth twice as likely (20%) as European-American youth (11%) to be uninsured. Even after poverty status, living arrangement, and place of residence were controlled for, Hispanic youth were still more likely to be uninsured than other ethnic groups (Newacheck, McManus, & Gephart, 1992). Of those youth with insurance, 86% had private insurance, 12% public insurance (Medicaid, Medicare, military, or other), and 2% had both. Again, youth of color were significantly more dependent on public assistance than their European-American peers with 6% of European-American youth, 23% of African-American teenagers, and 16% of Hispanic youth reporting having public insurance (Newacheck et al., 1992).

Adolescents who were described by their family as having fair or poor health were 69% more likely to be uninsured than those in excellent health. Nearly one-third of youth (31%) who reported fair or poor health and lived below the poverty level were uninsured. In contrast, only 9% of young people with excellent health and living above the poverty level were uninsured. In addition, those without insurance were more than twice as likely to have gone without seeing a physician in the past 2 years as those with insurance (Newacheck *et al.*, 1992). Clearly, poor health, poverty, lack of health insurance, and limited access to services are intercorrelated for adolescents.

MAJOR MORTALITIES OF YOUTH

Over the past 30 years, there have been dramatic shifts in the leading causes of death for young people from natural to violent etiologies. Marked reductions in communicable diseases have been mostly offset by large increases in violent deaths (unintentional injuries, homicide, and suicide) (Figure 3). In 1991, violent deaths accounted for nearly 77% of all deaths in youth ages 15 to 24. Overall, between 1979 and 1991, the national death rate for youth between the ages of 15 and 24 decreased 13% (National Center for Health Statistics, 1993). While the reductions in the national death rate (between 1979 and 1987) for European-American males and females (17 and 12%, respectively) were significant, there have been only modest reductions for African-American females (2%). The death rates for African-American males increased 11% during the same time period (U.S. Department of Health and Human Services, 1993a).

Unintentional Injuries

Unintentional injuries are the leading cause of death for youth (15 to 24 years of age), accounting for over 42% of all deaths (National Center for Health Statistics, 1993).

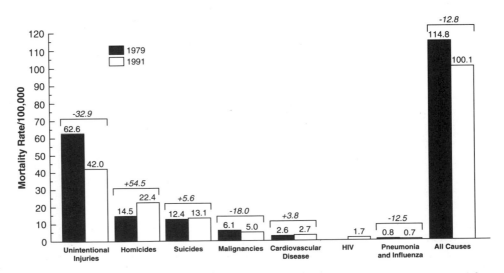

Figure 3. Mortality among youth ages 15 to 24 in the United States, 1979 and 1991. Data obtained from Monthly Vital Statistics Report (1993). *Advance report of final natality statistics, 1991.* Hyattsville, MD: Public Health Services; *42*(3) (Suppl.).

Between 1979 and 1991, there has been a 33% reduction in accidental deaths, with a remarkable 10% reduction from 1991 to 1992 (National Center for Health Statistics, 1993; National Safety Council, 1993). Despite this improvement, the unintentional injury death rate for these youth remains higher than for any group under the age of 65 (National Center for Health Statistics, 1993).

Motor Vehicle Fatalities

Seventy-eight percent of all unintentional injuries among youth are attributable to motor vehicle accidents, with males accounting for three-fourths of these deaths (National Safety Council, 1993). A disproportionate percentage of fatal motor vehicle injuries occur at night (50%) while only 20% of adolescent driving occurs during evening hours (U.S. Department of Transportation, 1989). Almost two-thirds of all motor vehicle deaths in youth (ages 15 to 24) were in rural areas (National Safety Council, 1993). Between 1979 and 1992, motor vehicle death rates decreased 38%, with an 11% reduction between 1991 and 1992 (National Center for Health Statistics, 1993; National Safety Council, 1993). Despite this improvement, the motor vehicle death rate was higher in youth 19 and under than any other age group (National Safety Council, 1993).

Automobile safety does not always appear to be a priority for many young people as evidenced by the high percentage of youth who drink and drive or fail to wear safety belts. While safety belt use increases with age, it is still the minority of youth who wear seat belts consistently. Youth between the ages of 12 and 13 (32%) were significantly less likely than those 18–21 years old (36%) to report always using a safety belt (The Centers for Disease Control and Prevention [CDC], 1992b). Additionally, alcohol-related motor vehicle trauma remains a significant problem for adolescents. Drivers between the ages of 16 and 20 who were involved in fatal crashes were more likely than any other age group to be alcohol-impaired with blood alcohol levels between 0.01% and 0.1%. Twenty percent of drivers ages 16 to 20 and 34% ages 21 to 24 who were involved in fatal motor vehicle accidents had blood alcohol levels of 0.10% or higher (U.S. Department of Transportation, 1993).

Over the past 7 years, there has been a significant reduction in alcohol-related automotive fatalities among young people. The alcohol-related traffic fatality ratio decreased by more than one-third between 1987 and 1992 for persons between the ages of 15 and 24. This represents a reduction from 21.5 in 1987 to 14.1 per 100,000 persons in 1992—significantly below the year 2000 goal of 18.1 (CDC, 1994). While drinking and driving appears common for youth, equally startling is the proportion of youth who report riding with others who have been drinking. The percentage of youth who report that in the past 30 days they have been a passenger with a driver who has been drinking markedly increases with age (12 to 13-year-olds, 11%; 14- to 17-year-olds, 22%; 18- to 21-year-olds, 35%) (CDC, 1992c).

Drowning (6%), firearm injuries (3%), poisons (3%), and fires (2%) are currently other major causes of unintentional injuries. All unintentional injuries are much more common in males than females. In 1992, firearms were responsible for 500 accidental deaths in youth ages 15 to 24, more than in any other age group (National Safety Council, 1993).

Homicide and Violent Crimes

In the United States, 14 children and youth under the age of 20 die from gun-related accidents, homicides, and suicides every day (Fingerhut, 1993). Between 1979 and 1991, almost 40,000 youth ages 15 to 19 died as a result of firearms (The Annie E. Casey Foundation, 1994). In 1990, there were 9462 firearm deaths with nearly nine out of ten occurring in males. Of these deaths, 60% were homicides, 33% suicides, 5% unintentional injuries, and 1% undetermined (National Safety Council, 1993). A major concern is the easy availability of firearms to children and youth. Surveys suggest that a quarter of all U.S. homes contain a handgun (American Academy of Pediatrics and Center to Prevent Handgun Violence, 1994) and nearly half have some type of a gun (Children's Defense Fund, 1994). A 1990 survey of gun owners found that over half reported keeping their guns unlocked and nearly one in four always kept it loaded (Yankelovich, Clancy, & Shulman, 1990). In a national survey of 6th through 12th grade students, 59% reported knowing where they could get a gun, and one in three reported they could acquire a gun in less than an hour (American Academy of Pediatrics and Center to Prevent Handgun Violence, 1994).

Homicide

A child is murdered every two hours in the United States (Children's Defense Fund, 1994). We have the highest firearm-related homicide rate of any industrialized nation (Fingerhut & Kleinman, 1990). Homicides are the second leading cause of adolescent fatalities in the United States, accounting for 22% of all deaths for youth ages 14–25 in 1991 (National Center for Health Statistics, 1993). In 1991, there were over 8000 teenage homicides. The homicide rate in 1991 was 22.4 per 100,000 youth (ages 15 to 24), an increase of 54% since 1979, nearly quadrupling since 1960 (National Center for Health Statistics, 1993; U. S. Department of Health and Human Services, 1989). While there have been increases in homicides in all ages, the largest percentage increases were noted in youth ages 10 to 14 (U.S. Department of Health and Human Services, 1993a). The homicide rate for males is over 400% higher than for females (National Center for Health Statistics, 1993). African-American youth are disproportionately represented in national homicide rates (National Safety Council, 1993). Homicide is the leading cause of death for African-American males and females between the ages of 15 and 24. The homicide rate is over 700% higher for African-American youth than for European-American teenagers. While African-American females have a homicide rate slightly below the national average (21.6/100,000), it is still nearly 400% above that for European-American females (4.4/100,000). Among African-American males, the homicide rate is over 600% higher than the national average, at 158.9 per 100,000, and over 800% above the rates found in European-American males (16.9/100,000) (National Center for Health Statistics, 1993).

Victimization

Youth ages 12 to 19 are at highest risk for personal crime victimization for both violence and theft. However, less than one in four personal crimes are reported by youth ages 12 to 19, a lower percentage than for any other age group (U.S. Bureau of Justice Statistics, 1994). Violent victimization (female rape, robbery, assault) crime rates for teens have markedly increased, while personal crimes of theft have dramatically decreased between 1973 and 1992. Overall, there has been an increase in violent victimization of 36% for youth ages 12 to 15, and 27% for youth ages 16 to 19. On the other hand, personal crimes of theft have decreased 44% for youth ages 12 to 15 and 41% for youth 16 to 19 during this same period (U.S. Bureau of Justice Statistics, 1992, 1994). While African-American males between the ages of 12 and 19 have the highest violence victimization rates, European-American males report the highest personal theft victimization rates (Zawitz *et al.,* 1993). While victimization rates for young people are high, the fear of such events are even higher. A national *New York Times*/CBS News poll reported that over one-third of European-Americans (36%) and over one-half of African-American (54%) youths worry about being victimized (The *New York Times*/CBS News Poll, 1994).

While much is known about the victims, less is known about offenders. In general, teenage victims report that offenders tend to be adolescents of the same race, and are often under the influence of drugs and alcohol. It has been estimated that approximately 31% of all violent offenders are under the age of 21. Violent crimes committed against youth ages 12 to 19 by solo offenders were perceived to be committed by teens under the age of 21 in the majority of cases (68.9%). When more than one offender is involved, in nearly two-thirds (63%) of the cases, the offenders were perceived to be teenagers (U.S. Bureau of Justice Statistics, 1992). Over one-half (54%) of offenders were reported to be using drugs or alcohol. Crimes of violence (80%) and robbery (63%) tend to be committed by offenders of the same race as their victims (Zawitz *et al.,* 1993).

Interpersonal violence is common among youth. In a national *New York Times*/CBS News poll, both European- and African-American youth identified violence as the biggest problem encountered at their school (*The New York Times*/CBS News Poll, 1994). The 1992 national Youth Risk Behavior Survey (YRBS) reported that physical fighting during the previous 12 months was quite common and decreased with age (between ages 12 and 17). Nearly one-half (49%) of teens ages 12 to 13 and 44% ages 14 to 17 reported physical fights in the previous year. Approximately one in seven (14.8%) between the ages of 12 and 21 reported carrying a weapon (gun, knife, or club) in the past 30 days. Of even greater concern was the fact that 13% of young teenagers, ages 12–13, reported this activity (CDC, 1992c). The Centers for Disease Control reported that males were nearly four times as likely to carry a weapon as females (32 versus 8%). The percentages of African-American (39%) and Hispanic (41%) males who carried weapons were greater than for European-American males (29%). African-American females (17%) were over three times as likely to carry a weapon and Hispanic females (12%) over twice as likely to carry a weapon as European-American females (5%). Of those youth who carry a weapon, 54% of African-Americans report carrying a firearm, while 55% of European-American youth and 47% of Hispanic youth report carrying knives or razors (CDC, 1991c).

Interpersonal violence, prevalence of weapons in the junior and senior high school years, and highly publicized in-school violence have placed this issue on the national agenda. School safety has become a concern of students and parents alike. A poll conducted by the *New York Times*/CBS News reported that 31% of European-American and

70% of African-American teenagers between the ages of 13 and 17 knew someone who was shot in the past 5 years (The *New York Times*/CBS News Poll, 1994). A national survey reported that 9% of students were victimized during the previous 6 months with three-quarters (78%) reporting property crimes and one-fifth (22%) reporting violent crimes. Public school students were more likely than private school students to have reported being victimized. In addition, in that study students at public schools were significantly more likely to indicate fear of attack at school than private school students. They also indicated they were more likely to avoid specific places at school because of this fear than private school peers. Students reported the existence of gangs in 25% of central city schools and 8% of nonmetropolitan schools (Zawitz *et al.*, 1993). In a separate study, 18% of European-American youth and 33% of African-American teenagers reported that organized gangs were a problem in their school (The *New York Times*/CBS News Poll, 1994).

Juvenile Violent Arrest Rates

A minor is arrested for a violent crime every five minutes (Children's Defense Fund, 1994). The juvenile violent crime arrest rate (homicide, forcible rape, robbery, or aggravated assault) for youth ages 10 to 17 increased from 305 per 100,000 in 1985 to 457 per 100,000 in 1991, nearly a 50% increase. Between 1991 and 1992, the violent crime arrest rates for teens increased 2%. While the number of violent acts appear to be about the same as a decade ago, the number of arrests and the lethality of these acts have increased. Much of the lethality is believed to be secondary to the increasing use of handguns (The Annie E. Casey Foundation, 1994).

Suicide

Suicide is the third leading cause of death for young people. In 1991, suicide was responsible for 4751 deaths, accounting for 13.1% of all deaths for teens ages 15–24. Since 1960, suicide has increased more than 150% to the current level of 13.1 per 100,000 15- to 24-year-olds in 1991 (National Center for Health Statistics, 1993; Rosen, Xiangdong, & Blum, 1990). Between 1979 and 1988, the national suicide rates increased by 7.9%. While there were significant reductions in youth ages 20 to 24 (8.5%), there were marked increases in both youth 10 to 14 (75%) and 15 to 19 (34.5%) (U.S. Department of Health and Human Services, 1993a). Firearms are the most common method of suicide for both young men and women (National Institute of Mental Health, 1993). U.S. youth between the ages of 10 and 19 commit suicide with a handgun on average every six hours (Fingerhut, 1993).

Fortunately, only a fraction of youth who have attempted suicide are successful. It is estimated that less than one in 50 suicide attempts result in death (Bearinger & Blum, 1994). One survey found that 27% of high school students reported a history of suicidal ideation, while over 8% reported an attempted suicide in the past 12 months. Only 2% of those who attempted suicide actually came to medical attention. Females were more likely than their male counterparts to report suicidal ideation (34 versus 21%), or to have previously attempted suicide (10 versus 6%). Reports of suicidal ideation and attempted suicide were highest for Hispanic youth, followed by European-American youth, and lowest for African-American youth (CDC, 1991a).

MAJOR MORBIDITIES OF YOUTH

Alcohol and Substance Use

Alcohol Use

Alcohol is the most commonly used and abused substance by youth. Nearly all high school seniors report experience with alcohol. While not all youth who drink have a drinking problem, nearly one in three seniors reported being intoxicated in the past 30 days (Figure 4). As would be expected, drinking activity increases with increasing grade (8th, 10th, 12th). The percentage of seniors who engaged in daily drinking has declined over 60% from a peak of 7% in 1978 to less than 3% in 1993. Daily consumption of alcohol and drinking to intoxication is more common in males than in females. Regional differences are also present. The highest percentages of annual and 30-day alcohol use and intoxication in the previous 30 days are reported in the Northeast with the lowest rates in the West. Alcohol use in metropolitan regions and nonmetropolitan areas are reported to be similar among seniors. Racial differences in alcohol use are significant. European-American youth report the highest prevalence of lifetime, annual, 30-day, and daily alcohol use. African-American seniors report the lowest prevalence for all categories,

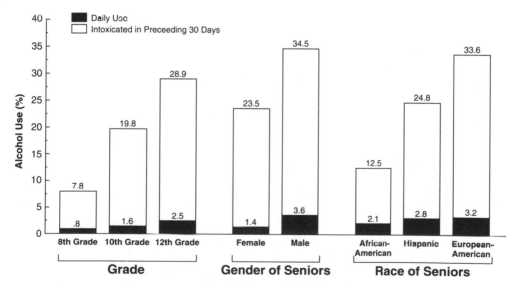

Figure 4. Percentage of students reporting alcohol use. Data obtained from Johnston, L. D., O'Malley, P. M., & Bachman, J. G. (1994). *National survey results on drug use from the Monitoring the Future Study, 1975–1993* (Vol. I). Rockville, MD: The National Institute on Drug Abuse.

while Hispanic youth report rates between those of European-American and African-American youth (Johnston, O'Malley, & Bachman, 1994).

Tobacco Use

The long-term deleterious effects of cigarette use have been well described. Smoking cigarettes has been linked to lung cancer, atherosclerosis, coronary heart disease, chronic obstructive pulmonary disease, and other malignancies. Passive smoke has been associated with lung cancer in nonsmokers. While few adolescents die of these complications, it is during their teen years that young people begin tobacco use that undoubtedly contributes to adult disease. First-time tobacco use is nearly always initiated before graduation from high school (U.S. Department of Health and Human Services, 1994b). Of those teenagers who are able to smoke two cigarettes to completion, 85% will become regular smokers (Silvis & Perry, 1987). Adolescent smokers are as addicted to nicotine as adults; and despite reporting wanting to quit, they have difficulty doing so. Teenage smokers experience withdrawal symptoms and relapse rates comparable to adults (U.S. Department of Health and Human Services, 1994b).

Those adolescents at highest risk for tobacco use include youth with low school achievement, with friends who use tobacco, and those with lower self-esteem. Of those young people who use marijuana, alcohol, or other drugs, tobacco is often their gateway drug. Studies suggest that cigarette advertising may be effective by changing young peoples' perceptions of how many people smoke and the type of people who smoke (U.S. Department of Health and Human Services, 1994b).

Despite the fact that 48 states and the District of Columbia prohibit the sale of tobacco products to minors, the majority of smokers between the ages of 12 and 17 report buying their own cigarettes (58%). Males were slightly more likely to report buying their own cigarettes than females. Racial differences also have been noted, as 59% of European-American youth, 44% of African-American youth, and 42% of Hispanic youth reported buying their own cigarettes (CDC, 1992b).

Cigarettes are the most commonly used daily substance by youth. Daily cigarette smoking among high school seniors has declined over a third from the peak of 29% in 1977 to the current levels of 19% in 1993. While cigarette use has declined for adults, the rates for high school seniors, until recently, has been steady for over a decade. Of special concern, however, is the reported increase in rates for daily smoking for 8th, 10th, and 12th grade students between 1992 and 1993. Although the percentages by gender are similar, males are slightly more likely to have reported smoking than females (Figure 5). As with alcohol use, regional differences are evident in reported daily cigarette use with the highest rates found in the Northeast (24%) and the lowest in the West (13%). Reported daily cigarette smoking rates are similar among youth residing in metropolitan and nonmetropolitan areas. The racial differences in daily cigarette use, however, are striking. European-American youth reported over five times the prevalence of daily smoking compared to African-American teens and almost twice the percentage as Hispanic youth. African-American youth have had long-term reductions in smoking while cigarette use among European-American and Hispanic teenagers has leveled off over the past decade (Johnston et al., 1994).

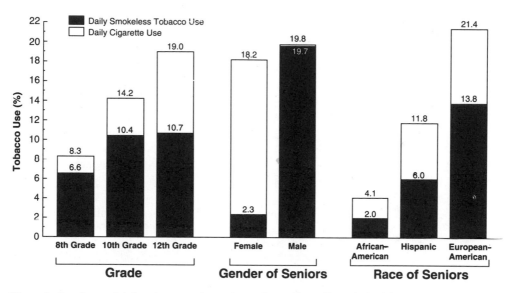

Figure 5. Prevalence of daily tobacco use by grade, gender, and race. Data obtained from Johnston, L. D., O'Malley, P. M., & Bachman, J. G. (1994). *National survey results on drug use from the Monitoring the Future Study, 1975–1993* (Vol. I). Rockville, MD: The National Institute on Drug Abuse.

It is well recognized that smokeless tobacco is associated with oral cancer, periodontal degeneration, and soft tissue lesions (U.S. Department of Health and Human Services, 1994b). However, many youth believe that smokeless tobacco is much less harmful than cigarettes (Guggenheimer, Zullo, Kruper, & Verbin, 1986). Currently, smokeless tobacco is second only to cigarettes in terms of the proportion of high school seniors reporting daily use. The use of chewing tobacco and snuff rose dramatically between 1970 and 1985 for youth between the ages of 17 and 19 (150 and over 800%, respectively) (U.S. Department of Health and Human Services, 1986). Over the last decade, the use of smokeless tobacco has been relatively constant. Smokeless tobacco use increased with age in terms of lifetime, 30-day, and daily use (Figure 5). Senior males report nearly nine times the daily prevalence rate of females. Daily smokeless tobacco use among high school seniors was most common in North central and South regions, and least common in the West. Nonmetropolitan youth reported nearly two times the 30-day prevalence of smokeless tobacco use than urban teens. European-American youth reported a 30-day prevalence nearly seven times greater than African-American teens and a threefold increase above Hispanic youth (Johnston *et al.*, 1994).

Drug Use

Nationwide, chemical use and abuse continues to be a significant problem for youth and families (Figure 6). Reported annual and 30-day prevalence of illicit drug use has declined since peaking in 1979. Overall, the reported 30-day prevalence of illicit drugs among high school seniors has been cut in half, from a peak of 39% in 1979 to 18% in

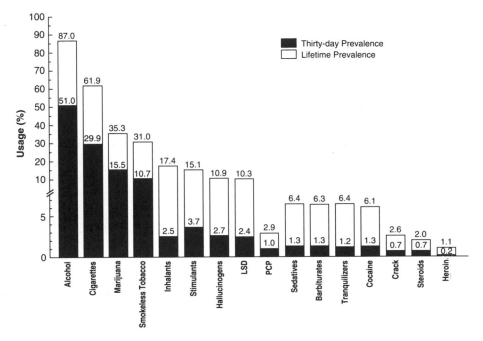

Figure 6. Percentage of high school seniors reporting substance use. Data obtained from Johnston, L. D., O'Malley, P. M., & Bachman, J. G. (1994). *National survey results on drug use from the Monitoring the Future Study, 1975–1993* (Vol. I). Rockville, MD: The National Institute on Drug Abuse.

1993 (Figure 7). Of concern is the recent increases in reported use of illicit substances in addition to changes in attitudes and beliefs associated with drug use. The 1993 annual survey of U.S. high school students reported a sharp rise in marijuana use in 8th, 10th, and 12th grade students. In addition, there were significant increases in stimulant, LSD, and inhalant use at all three grades. Of greatest concern, the survey noted decreased perceived dangers and decreased disapproval of individuals using illicit substances (Johnson *et al., 1994*).

Important gender, age, regional, race, and population density differences were noted among seniors. With the exception of stimulants and barbiturates, male high school seniors report higher 30-day prevalence rates for all substances when compared to females. In general, the proportion of youth who reported substance use in the previous 30 days increases by grade. The only exception appeared to be for inhalant use, which decreased with increasing grade. Regional differences in 30-day prevalence rates have been noted with these substances as with others. The highest proportion of youth who report use of marijuana, inhalants, hallucinogens, LSD, and heroin live in the Northeast. Highest cocaine and crack use are reported in high school seniors in the West. The greatest proportion of barbiturates, tranquilizers, and steroid users are found in the South. While it is commonly believed that illicit drug use is an urban problem, the 1993 Monitoring the Future Survey found similar rates among metropolitan and nonmetropolitan areas. Contrary to what has been portrayed in the media, the annual prevalence of illicit drug use

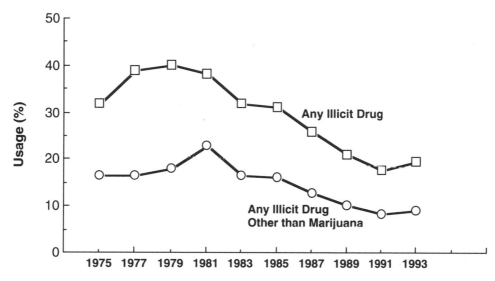

Figure 7. Thirty-day prevalence of illicit drug use, trends among twelfth graders, 1975–1993. Data obtained from Johnston, L. D., O'Malley, P. M., & Bachman, J. G. (1994). *National survey results on drug use from the Monitoring the Future Study, 1975–1993* (Vol. I). Rockville, MD: The National Institute on Drug Abuse.

among high school seniors is highest for European-American youth (31%), followed by Hispanic youth (29%), with the lowest rates for African-American teenagers (17%). African-American students reported the lowest rates for nearly all illicit and licit drugs (Johnston *et al.*, 1994).

Reproductive Health Issues

Sexual Intercourse

Once every 10 seconds, a teenager has sexual intercourse for the first time (Children's Defense Fund, 1994). Sexual activity among young men and women has increased dramatically since the 1970s. The proportion of females between the ages of 15 and 19 who have had premarital intercourse has doubled from approximately 25% in 1970 to over 50% in 1988 (CDC, 1991b). During this same period, teenagers have delayed marriage. Approximately 10% of youth are sexually active by age 13. One-third of males and one-fourth of females have had sexual intercourse by age 15. Over one-half of all males are sexually active by age 16–17, while the majority of females have had intercourse by age 17–18 (Seidman & Rieder, 1994). In 1992, approximately 54% of 9th- to 12th-graders reported sexual intercourse with almost 40% within the previous 3 months (CDC, 1992e). Of concern is the significant increase in the proportion of sexually active individuals under the age of 15 (CDC, 1992d). Gender differences among high school students are present, with males (61%) more likely than females (48%) to report previous sexual activity. African-American youth report the highest proportion of sexual activity (72%) followed by Hispanic (53%) and European-American youth (52%) (CDC, 1992e); however, the racial differences appear to be decreasing (Seidman & Rieder, 1994).

Contraceptive Use

A sexually active teenage female who does not use contraception has a 90% chance of becoming pregnant within a year (Harlap, Kost, & Forrest, 1991). Fortunately, two-thirds of young people report using some method of contraception at first sexual intercourse. For women ages 15–19, the percentage who report using condoms at sexual debut doubled between 1982 and 1988 (Forrest & Singh, 1990). Among sexually active high school students, 78% report the use of some form of contraception with the most recent intercourse (birth control pills, condoms, withdrawal, or another method). However, only 45% reported that condoms were used (40% of females and 49% of males) (CDC, 1992e). Somewhat surprisingly, condom use may decrease with age. The YRBS reported that the use of condoms during last intercourse was 59% for 14- to 17-year-olds compared to 37% for youth ages 18 to 21 (CDC, 1992c). Among both sexually active males and females, European-American youth reported the highest contraceptive use and Hispanic youth the lowest. Males of all races report greater condom use than females. Among males, African-American youth (55%) report the highest condom use, followed by European-American males (50%), with the lowest rates reported among Hispanic youth (47%). Among females, 42% of European-American youth reported condom use at last intercourse compared to 37% of African-American and 28% of Hispanic females (CDC, 1992e).

While efforts to improve condom use among adolescents continue, some authors estimate consistent and appropriate condom use to be as low as 10 to 20% (Seidman & Rider, 1994). Several studies have found little association between increased levels of STD knowledge and condom use (DiClemente, Brown, Beausoleil, & Lodico, 1993; DiClemente et al., 1992; Orr et al., 1992). Thus, while knowledge of STDs and condoms may be necessary and beneficial, it appears not to be sufficient to ensure condom use. A recent study found that teenagers who discuss AIDS with a health care provider were significantly more likely to consistently use condoms. Regrettably, in the same study, Hingson (1990) reported that, of the 80% of all adolescents who saw a health professional in the year preceding their study, only 13% had been counseled about AIDS.

Sexually Transmitted Diseases

The use of latex condoms with spermicides during each intercourse is reported to markedly reduce the risk of acquiring a sexually transmitted disease (STD), including HIV (Kestelman & Trussell, 1991). While significant improvements have been noted in condom use between 1982 and 1988, youth continue to be at increased risk for STDs (Forrest & Singh, 1990; Sonenstein, Pleck, & Ku, 1989). The YRBS reported that, between 1989 and 1992, there was a reduction of 21% in the proportion of youth who indicated having more than four partners (CDC, 1992d). Despite these trends, two-thirds of all STDs are acquired by youth under the age of 25 (U.S. Department of Health and Human Services, 1993b). In the United States, three million teens are diagnosed with STDs each year (Kolbe, 1992).

Human papilloma virus (HPV) and chlamydia appear to be the most common sexually transmitted infections among adolescents and young adults, although the exact prevalence is unknown (Cates, 1987; Martinez et al., 1988). The prevalence of cervicovaginal

HPV in sexually active female adolescents has been reported to range from 13 to 38% (Martinez *et al.*, 1988; Fisher, Rosenfeld, & Burk, 1991; Rosenfeld, Vermund, Wentz, & Burk, 1989). Independent risk factors for HPV include younger age and increased number of lifetime sexual partners (Moscicki, Palefsky, Gonzales, & Schoolnik, 1990; Ley *et al.*, 1991). While HPV is the cause of genital warts, it is the association with neoplasia (cervical and penile) that is most concerning (Wright & Richart, 1990). Chlamydia is a leading cause of nongonococcal urethritis in males and mucopurulent cervicitis in females (Cats, 1987). In addition, chlamydia is the leading cause of nongonococcal pelvic inflammatory disease (Washington, Arno, & Brooks, 1986). The reported infection rates among sexually active adolescents have been variable, ranging from 10 to 37% depending on the population studied (Shafer, 1992).

Gonorrhea infections continue to be a problem for teens and young adults. The infection rates among various populations of sexually active youth range from 3 to 18% (Shafer, 1992). Youth ages 10 to 24 were responsible for 63% of all cases of gonorrhea in 1992. The number of reported cases for youth ages 10–24 decreased 20% between 1990 and 1992. The smallest reductions were in youth ages 10–14. The reported cases were evenly distributed between male and female youth; however, African-American youth were disproportionately represented, accounting for over 82% of all cases of gonorrhea reported. European-American youth were responsible for 13%, Hispanic 4%, and Asian/Pacific Islanders and American Indian/Alaskan Natives combined were responsible for less than 1% of all gonorrhea cases (U.S. Department of Health and Human Services, 1993b).

Youth between the ages of 10 and 24 accounted for 34% of all (primary and secondary) syphilis infections. Males represented 43% of all reported cases. African-American youth accounted for over 88% of all reported cases of syphilis while European-American youth were responsible for 7%, Hispanic teens 5%, and Asian/Pacific Islander and American Indian/Alaskan teenagers less than 1%. Between 1990 and 1992, there has been a significant decrease in the reported number of syphilis infections in young people between the ages of 10 and 24 (31%). Specifically, significant reductions have been noted for youth ages 10–14 (22%), 15–19 (26%), and young adults between the ages of 20 and 24 (33%) (U. S. Department of Health and Human Services, 1993b).

Genital herpes may result from either herpes simplex virus type 1 (HSV-1) or herpes simplex virus type 2 (HSV-2); however, the vast majority of cases are from HSV-2. The prevalence of herpes among youth is not precisely known. Independent risk factors that have been reported to be associated with HSV-2 include: age, race (African-American), gender (female), previous STDs, and increased numbers of lifetime sexual partners (Ellen, Moscicki, & Shafer, 1994). A study of women attending family planning clinics in Pittsburgh found that 10% of the population ages 17–20 were HSV-2 seropositive (Breinig, Kingsley, Armstrong, Freeman, & Ho, 1990). It is estimated that by the conclusion of their teen years, 4% of European-Americans and 17% of African-Americans will have been exposed to HSV-2 (Cates, 1991).

Teenage Pregnancy

Once every 104 seconds, a teenage female becomes pregnant (Children's Defense Fund, 1994). The pregnancy, birth, and abortion rates for U.S. teenagers are among the highest in the world for industrialized countries even though the levels of sexual activity appear to be similar (The Alan Guttmacher Institute, 1994). Adolescent females wait, on average, 1 year after initiation of sexual intercourse before seeking family planning services (Lovick & Wesson, 1986). Unfortunately, 50% of all premarital teenage pregnancies occur within the first 6 months after initial intercourse (Zabin & Clark, 1983). Prior to their 20th birthday, four of ten adolescent females will have become pregnant (Stephenson, 1989). Five of six pregnancies between the ages of 15 and 19 are unintended (Kolbe, 1992). In 1989, 1,043,600 women under the age of 20 became pregnant (one in 8.5 adolescent females), of whom 27,810 were under the age of 15. Of those who became pregnant, nearly half gave birth, 37% had legal abortions, and an estimated 14% miscarried (Henshaw, 1994). Of those who give birth, very few will make adoption plans. With decreased stigmatization of childbearing among unmarried mothers, the chance that she will make adoption plans for her baby has declined dramatically from 19% (1965–1972) to 3% (1982–1988) in European-American women. During this same period, adoption plans among unmarried African-American women have decreased from 2% to 1% (Bachrach, Stolley, & London, 1992).

Pregnancy rates for women ages 15–19 have reached their highest level in nearly 20 years and have increased over 5% between 1985 and 1989, to a level of 114.9 per 1000. This increase reflects an increase in the proportion of sexually active youth. However, pregnancy rates among sexually experienced teens has actually declined 19% over the last two decades, suggesting that sexually experienced teens are using birth control more effectively than their counterparts in the past (The Alan Guttmacher Institute, 1994). On the other hand, birth rates increased by 22% between 1985 and 1991 to a rate of 62.1 per 1000. Pregnancy and birth rates for youth under the age of 15 represent a small, but rapidly growing, sector. For teens under the age of 15, the pregnancy rate increased 4% (1985–1989) while the birth rate increased 31% (Henshaw, 1994).

Marked differences in pregnancy and birth rates are present among different races. The pregnancy rate for non-European-American youth ages 15–19 was 184.3/1000 in 1992, almost twice as high for European-American teens at 93.4/1000 (Figure 8). The pregnancy rate for teens under the age of 15 was over 400% higher for non-European-American youth than for European-American youth (National Center for Health Statistics, 1992). Teenagers under the age of 20 accounted for 13% of all births, but the percentage of births accounted for within races varies dramatically: European-American 10%, Hispanic 17%, American Indian 20%, and African-American youth accounted for 23% of births by race. In 1991, the birth rates for European-American and Asian/Pacific Islander youth were significantly less than those of African-American, Hispanic, and American Indian teenagers for mothers under the age of 20 (Figure 9). While the birth rates are much higher for African-American than for European-American youth, the percent increase is greatest for European-American teenagers: for teens under the age of 15, birth rates increased 33% for European-American youth and 4% for African-American youth in the years between 1985 and 1991. During that same period, for youth ages 15–19, the birth rate for European-American youth increased 27% compared to 15% for African-Americans (Monthly Vital Statistics Report, 1993).

While the teen pregnancy rates may vary among race and ethnic groups, both mother and child are at risk for poor outcomes. For young mothers, poverty, parenting, and school failure are highly intercorrelated. Teenage mothers are more likely to drop out of

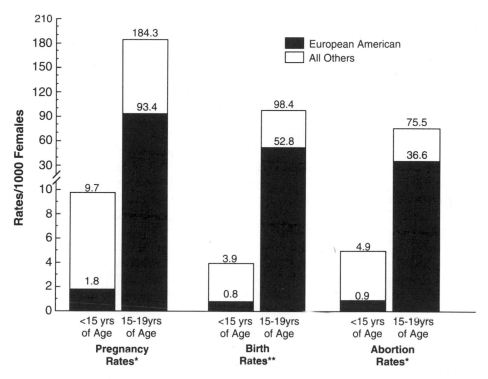

Figure 8. 1988 pregnancy, birth, and abortion rates in youth under 20 years of age by race. *Data obtained from Monthly Vital Statistics Report. (1993). *Trends in pregnancies and pregnancy rates, United States, 1980–1988.* Hyattsville, Maryland: Public Health Service, *43(3),* (Suppl.).

school and are less likely to go to college than other teens (The Alan Guttmacher Institute, 1994). On the other hand, those with sufficient support to stay in school are only slightly less likely to graduate than those who do not become mothers. In addition, approximately 30% of those who drop out of high school will eventually graduate (Upchurch & McCarthy, 1990). The increased risk of poor outcomes for both mother and child is not primarily related to the mothers' young age but, rather, secondary to her economic and social disadvantage prior to childbearing (Makinson, 1985).

In fact, almost 60% of those who become teenage mothers are living in poverty at the time they deliver. Infants born to teenage mothers are at increased risk of being low birth weight, more likely to have childhood health problems and to require hospitalization (The Alan Guttmacher Institute, 1994). This is especially true for children born to young teen mothers (under the age of 15) who account for 14% of all low birth weight neonates, while youth 15 to 19 years of age account for 9% (Monthly Vital Statistics Report, 1993). Children of teen mothers perform less well on cognitive tests than peers (Hofferth & Hayes, 1987). Additionally, children born to unmarried mothers have been reported to be at increased risk for adjustment problems including school failure, early childbearing themselves, divorce, and welfare dependence (Garfinkel & McLanahan, 1986). In addition to the social costs are the financial expenditures; approximately 60% of all first-time

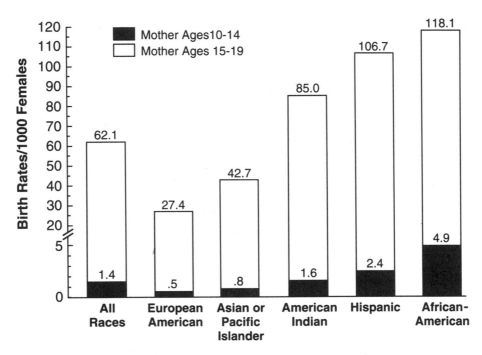

Figure 9. 1991 birth rates for mothers under the age of 20 by race. Data from Monthly Vital Statistics Report. (1993). *Advance report of final natality statistics, 1991.* Hyattsville, MD: Public Health Services; *42*(3) (Suppl.).

teenage births are supported by public funds (The Alan Guttmacher Institute, 1994). The public monetary cost associated with teenage pregnancy between 1985 and 1990 was over 120 billion dollars (CDC, 1993).

Much less is known about teenage fathers than about young mothers. The overall rate of teenage fatherhood (ages 15 to 19) increased by nearly 38% between 1986 and 1991. While the rate of teenage fatherhood for African-American youth is over three times that of their European-American counterparts, between 1986 and 1991 the percentage has increased more for European-American adolescent males (42%) than for African-Americans (35%) (Monthly Vital Statistics Report, 1993). Additionally, since men involved in teen pregnancy tend to be older than their female consorts, only 26% of the young men involved in teen pregnancy were under the age of 18 (The Alan Guttmacher Institute, 1994).

Teenage Abortion

Youth under the age of 20 were responsible for 24% of all abortions in 1989 (CDC, 1992a). While abortion rates increase with age for women under the age of 20, the proportion of pregnancies that result in abortions decreases with age. Thus, 46% of pregnancies for youth under the age of 15, 38% for women 15 to 17 years old, and 36% for women between the ages of 18 and 19 resulted in abortions in 1989. Abortion rates have decreased for all age groups over the past 5- and 10-year periods for women under the age of 20, with greatest decreases in youth under the age of 15 (Henshaw, 1994). In youth between the ages of 15 and 19, the majority of unintended pregnancies end in abortions (53%) (The Alan Guttmacher Institute, 1994). European-American teenagers were more likely to terminate unintended pregnancies than either African-American or Hispanic youth (The Alan Guttmacher Institute, 1994). Youth whose families were financially better off (Zabin, Hirsch, & Boscia, 1990) or where parental education is greater (Cooksey, 1990) are in general more likely to have terminated unintended pregnancies than teens from poorer or less educated homes. Developmentally, youth who choose abortion appear to have stronger future time perspective than parenting peers (Blum & Resnick, 1982).

Only three states and the District of Columbia have laws that explicitly allow a minor to consent for abortion without parental consent or notification. Twenty-one states require parental consent or notification prior to a minor obtaining an abortion. In most of these states, parental involvement can be avoided through a judicial bypass system (Donovan, 1992). In the remaining states, no laws currently exist. In states where parental notification is not required, the majority (61%) of unmarried teenagers reported telling at least one parent about their decision to terminate the pregnancy (Henshaw & Kost, 1992). Thus, some conclude that parental notification laws in fact have little impact on parental notification (Blum, Resnick, & Stark, 1987). In addition to speaking with parents, 75% of teens discussed their decision to have an abortion with their boyfriend. The majority consult with their boyfriend even when their parents are notified. Boyfriends provide at least some financial support for approximately half of the cases, the parents 40%, and approximately 25% of minor females pay for the abortion themselves (The Alan Guttmacher Institute, 1994).

HIV and AIDS

AIDS is the sixth leading cause of death in young adults ages 15 and 24 (National Center for Health Statistics, 1993). Once every 9 hours, a young person under the age of 25 dies of HIV (Children's Defense Fund, 1994). Twenty percent of all AIDS cases are individuals ages 20 to 29, most of whom acquired the disease during adolescence (Kolbe, 1992). With the increasing prevalence of HIV infection, there is an urgency to educate young people. The percentage of students who reported receiving HIV instruction between 1989 and 1991 increased from 54% to 83%. The percentage of students who reported discussing HIV and AIDS with their parents increased from 54% to 61%; and instruction appeared to increase the likelihood that a teenager would discuss HIV/AIDS with their parents (CDC, 1992d).

Through December of 1993, there were 1554 cases of AIDS among youth ages 13 to 19, with 69% of these cases in males. In this population of males, three causes accounted for 88% of cases: coagulation disorders, males having sex with males, and intravenous drug use. Among females ages 13–19, the leading cause of transmission was heterosexual contact, followed by intravenous drug use and blood transfusions. The leading causes of transmission for women ages 20–24 are similar to those of younger women. However, there are marked differences among men (ages 20–24) with 88% of all cases accounted for by: males who have sex with males, injecting drug use, or both (Figure 10) (U.S. Department of Health and Human Services, 1994c).

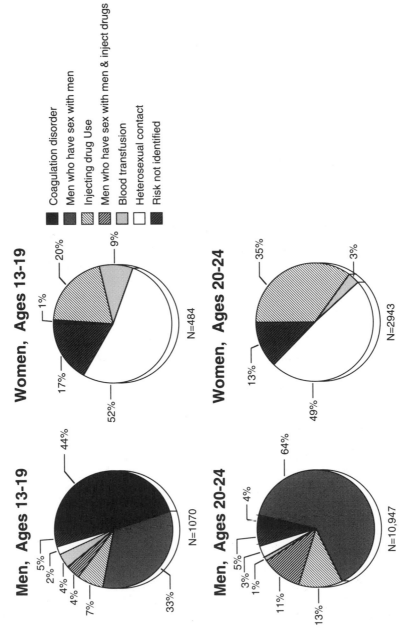

Figure 10. AIDS cases in youth under the age of 25 by sex and exposure. Data obtained from U.S. Department of Health and Human Services (1994). Public Health Service. Centers for Disease Control and Prevention. National Center for Infectious Diseases. Atlanta, *5*(4), 12–14.

Youth of color (African-American and Hispanic) are disproportionately represented in the number of AIDS cases in young people ages 13–24. African-Americans accounted for one-third of cases reported in males and over one-half (53%) of all cases among females. Likewise, Hispanic males represented 20%, and females 22%, of all reported cases by gender (U.S. Department of Health and Human Services, 1994c).

Physical and Sexual Abuse

In 1992, there were nearly 993,000 cases of child abuse and neglect that were substantiated or indicated, of which 49% were neglect, 23% physical abuse, and 14% sexual abuse. Approximately 35% of victims were between the ages of 10 and 18. Overall, victims were more likely to be female (53%). Females were more likely to be victims of physical abuse at ages 13 and above. At every age, females are more likely to be sexually abused than males (U.S. Department of Health and Human Services, 1994a).

While the exact number of young people who are neglected or abused is unknown, some believe the prevalence is higher in teenagers than younger children (Chadwick & Heaton, 1992; Randall, 1992). The associations between sexual victimization, adolescent sexual behavior, and teen pregnancy have only recently been explored (Boyer & Fine, 1992). The estimates of sexual victimization vary considerably for the general female population, from 6% to 62% (Finkelhor, 1986). In a survey of young women who had intercourse before the age of 14, 67% of European-American and 31% of African-American teens reported having had sex involuntarily (Moore, Nord, & Peterson, 1989). In another study of 535 young women who became pregnant as teens, two-thirds reported that they had been sexually abused, with 62% of the abuse episodes occurring prior to the first pregnancy (Boyer & Fine, 1992).

Runaway and Homeless Youth

Closely associated with abuse are runaway, homeless, and thrownaway youth. The exact number of runaway, homeless, and thrownaway teenagers is unknown. *Homeless-ness* is defined as having no place for shelter and in need of care, services, and supervision. *Runaway* youth are persons under 18 who leave home without permission of their parent/guardian and stay away at least one night (U.S. General Accounting Office, 1989b). *Thrownaway* youth are those who have been told to leave home, have been abandoned, or runaways whom the caretaker does not allow to return or makes no effort to recover (Finkelhor, Hotaling, & Sedlak, 1990).

The National Incidence Studies of Missing, Abducted, Runaway, and Thrownaway Children reported that in 1988 there were an estimated 446,700 runaways, with 12,800 children who ran from juvenile facilities. Most youth remained locally with only 10% going farther than 100 miles. The survey figures were comparable to the 1975 National Statistical Survey on Runaway Youth. The study also reported an estimated 127,100 thrownaway children and youth. Compared to runaways, thrownaways had been exposed to more family conflict and violence. The majority of thrownaway youth lived with friends or relatives, most staying within a 10-mile radius from their original home (Finkelhor et al., 1990). The American Youth Work Center and the National Network of

Runaway and Youth Services have estimated that there are 500,000 homeless youths each year (U.S. General Accounting Office, 1989b); others put the figure two to three times higher (U.S. Department of Health and Human Services, 1989). For every homeless young person in a shelter, it has been estimated that there are eight who are on the street (U.S. General Accounting Office, 1989b).

From a detailed analysis of youth who received services at federally funded shelters between 1985 and 1988, homeless youth are more commonly male (55%), older (60% 16 and over), and European-American (60%). African-American youth were disproportionately represented as they accounted for 28% of all homeless youth. Homeless youth were more likely to have dropped out of school (37%) compared to the national range of 14–29%. On the other hand, runaway youth were more likely to be female (65%), were younger (40% 16 and over), and the majority were European-American (70%). Seventeen percent of runaways were African-American, and 23% were not attending school (U.S. General Accounting Office, 1989a).

While one must be careful when generalizing, most homeless youth appear to be running from something. Sixty percent of homeless youth who lived in shelters or transitional living had been physically or sexually abused by parents, while 53% reported school problems. Many youth described problems in their home including: absence of father (45%), long-term economic problems (41%), reported violence from other family members (26%), and absence of a caretaker (23%). Homeless youth also reported previous mental health problems (26%), substance abuse (23%), alcohol abuse (19%), and previous suicide attempts (19%). While less is known about parents of runaway youth, the teens reported that 29% of parents abused alcohol, 24% abused drugs, and 18% had mental health problems (Bass, 1992).

The prognosis for homeless and runaway youth is uncertain. Many of these youth have long-term problems that may prevent them from returning home. In Bass's study (Bass, 1992), one in five youth who arrived at shelters were from foster or group homes, while 38% were in foster care during the previous year. An additional 11% of homeless youth came from runaway or crisis shelters; and 11% were on the street before entering the shelters. Overall, this study estimated that 50% of runaway and homeless youth would return to the parental or guardian home after leaving the shelter (Bass, 1992).

Mental Health Problems

Mental health problems are common in youth today. It has been estimated that between 12 and 22% (7.5–14 million) of youth under the age of 18 have at least one diagnosable mental disorder (U.S. Department of Health and Human Services, 1990). A study of Oregon students reported that, of those with a DSM-III-R diagnosable mental disorder, almost one-third experienced a second disorder during their lifetime (Lewinsohn, Hops, Roberts, Seeley, & Andrews, 1993).

While risk factors increase the likelihood of mental disorders, it is also clear that most young people exposed to those risk variables do not develop mental illness. The question then is what prevents some who are exposed to high-risk environments from developing negative outcomes. Recent research has focused on resiliency. Some of the protective factors for emotional and behavioral problems that have been identified include: good physical health, at least one supportive adult, ability to sustain good peer relationships, verbal proficiency, and social competency (Ellickson, Lara, Sherbourne, & Zina, 1993). Gender differences in mental health disorders have also been noted. Females were more likely to report unipolar depression, anxiety disorders, and adjustment disorders. Males are more than twice as likely to have attention-deficit hyperactivity disorder (ADHD), conduct, and oppositional defiant disorders than females (Lewinsohn *et al.*, 1993). Many risk factors for emotional and behavioral problems have been identified including: poverty, single-parent family, marital discord, divorce, parental mental illness and substance abuse, abuse and neglect, exposure to extreme violence, chronic physical illness, developmental delays, and mental retardation (Ellickson *et al.*, 1993).

Eating Disorders

The number of individuals who meet the criteria for anorexia or bulimia nervosa is small compared to the number of individuals with disordered eating. Dieting and binge eating with or without purging appears to be common behavior in female undergraduates (Yates, 1989). Many women experience symptoms of disordered eating such as: preoccupation with food and weight, body image distortion, restrictive and fad dieting, or purging through vomiting, laxative abuse, diuretic abuse, and exercise (Yager, 1988). While eating disorders were once thought only to affect higher social classes, it is now recognized that they affect the entire socioeconomic spectrum and all races (Gowers & McMahon, 1989). Athletes involved in sports that emphasize slimness to improve performance such as gymnastics, figure skating, and ballet may be at increased risk for eating disorders (Garner, 1993). Eating disorders may also be more common in gay males (Yager, Kurtzman, Landsverk, & Wiesmeier, 1988; Schneider & Agras, 1987).

The incidence of anorexia nervosa has been estimated at 1% among adolescent females. The age of onset has been reported to be bimodal in distribution with peaks at 13–14 and 17–18 years of age (Halmi, Casper, Eckert, Goldberg, & Davis, 1979). While anorexia is more common among females, it has been estimated that 5–10% of anorexics are males (Hoek, 1991; Lucas, Beard, O'Fallon, & Kurland, 1991). Despite long and intensive treatment, the prognosis for anorexia nervosa is often poor, resulting in a chronic illness (Yates, 1990). Long-term follow-up suggests that the mortality rate for individuals with anorexia nervosa has been between 3 and 18% (Patton, 1990).

Bulimia appears to be more common than anorexia. The incidence of bulimia is estimated to range from 1 to 10% in female adolescents and young adults (Fairburn & Beglin, 1990; Goldbloom & Garfinkel, 1989; Haller, 1992). That of bulimia in adolescent and young adult men in community-based studies has been estimated at 0.2%. Male bulimics may have a later onset of disease, increased premorbid obesity, and a higher prevalence of homosexuality compared with female bulimics (Carlat & Camargo, 1991). Of those youth with bulimia, 30–80% have a history of anorexia (Mitchell, Pyle, & Eckert, 1985). Recently, concern has been raised that some women who initially develop bulimia may later go on to develop anorexia (Kassett, Gwirtsman, Kaye, Brandt, & Jimerson, 1988). Much less is known about the long-term outcomes of bulimia. Bulimic patients appear less resistant to outpatient intervention and much less often require hospitalization than do those with anorexia. While the disease may fluctuate, the overall trend is toward improvement in disordered eating behavior (Mitchell, Davis, Goff, & Pyle, 1986; Yager, Landsverk, & Edelstein, 1987).

CONCLUSION

The data presented in this chapter should be cause for encouragement as well as alarm. After years of a downward spiral in adolescent health status, we see significant improvements. Overall, juvenile mortality has declined by 13% among 15- to 24-year-olds during the decade of the 1980s with dramatic improvements in motor vehicle deaths. Today, one-third fewer teenagers die of motor vehicle injuries than a decade ago. Alcohol-related vehicular deaths are markedly reduced. These data should stand as a constant refutation of the idea that "nothing can be done" to impact the major morbidities and causes of mortality of youth. Clearly, educational strategies coupled with technological improvements of cars and roads have all contributed to the improved outcomes.

But there is a warning in these data as well. The recent decline in motor vehicle deaths among juveniles is not the first time we have seen such trends. In the late 1970s and early 1980s a concerted antismoking campaign was accompanied by a dramatic decline in adolescent smoking on a daily basis from 29% in 1976 to 19% seven years later. We have seen little change over the past decade; and recently there is evidence of an increase in juvenile smoking despite the spate of reports reinforcing the data that smoking is harmful. When taken together, the warning is that information is insufficient to change behavior; without a comprehensive prevention strategy change does not occur; with it, we can make important advances and, once we diminish our efforts, the trends are most likely to reverse. We are seeing this pattern played out with cigarette smoking and drugs of abuse. The trend is early; and it is probably not too late to reverse it. If we choose to ignore it, however, we will be faced with another *crisis* in adolescent substance abuse 5 years from now. Likewise, unless we maintain our automobile safety campaigns, we will see a rise in vehicular mortality as well.

Another area where we have made significant, though not dramatic, gains over the last few years is with pregnancy prevention. Sexually active youth of today are better contraceptors than their predecessors; and as a consequence unwanted pregnancies have declined in this population. We have seen a significant increase in the use of contraception at sexual debut; likewise, we have seen a dramatic increase in the acceptability of condoms. As with vehicular safety, clear messages on the benefits of contraception for STD and pregnancy prevention, coupled with improved availability of contraceptive technology, have had an impact.

Not only is there cause for and the acknowledgment of warnings in these data; likewise, there is cause for alarm for we are faced with an epidemic of violence unparalleled in our history, and it is disproportionately impacting the youngest teenagers, males, and youth of color. Juvenile homicides have increased 54% over the last decade—in 1991 over 8000 teenagers were murdered. Males are four times more likely to die from violence than their female peers. Even more stunning is the homicide rate among African-American males which is 800% above that of their European-American counterparts with a mortality rate of 158.9 per 100,000.

If the etiology were infectious, there would be a national mobilization. However, we appear to be paralyzed despite the fact that we know some of the most salient contributors to this epidemic. We know that nearly half of all households in the United States have guns of which over one-half are unlocked and over one-quarter are always loaded. Access to firearms is easy for juveniles—sixty percent know where to get a gun; one-third can get a gun within an hour. One in seven youth have carried a knife, club, or gun to school in the last month, of which over one-fifth are firearms.

While easy access to firearms is not the underlying cause of the epidemic of violence (there are other societies, e.g., Israel, where there is comparable access to weapons without comparable homicide rates), it clearly is the most proximal cause. As access to contraception has increased its use (and decreased pregnancies), so too access to weapons has increased their use. Can we reduce this epidemic? There is every reason to believe we can. Do we have the national will to do so? That has yet to be seen.

But even if we choose to limit access to handguns and semiautomatic weapons, we must acknowledge that these data suggest an underlying cause for violence related to social disengagement. We see that alienation not only in the violence statistics but also in the rising rates of suicide (with a 75% increase among 10- to 14-year-olds in the last decade) and in the high rates (22%) of mental health problems; it is evident that a considerable minority of youth, and a large proportion of youth of color, feel increasingly alienated. Violence is the expression of that alienation and is turned outward or inward depending on culture, gender, and social class. It is not sufficient to interpret this angst as the "storm and stress" of adolescence; the social cost of doing so is too great. Likewise, it is not sufficient to explain the alienation of today's youth solely as the consequence of the stressful environments—abuse, poverty, family violence, alcoholism, and mental illness—within which so many of these young people live. For while we need to ameliorate such high-risk living situations, we also are aware that the majority of their neighbors reared in comparable environments are not participating in such destructive behaviors.

We have two decades of research and literature on those factors associated with positive outcomes among youth raised in high-risk social environments. If, over the next decade, we choose to build programs that enhance resilience among youth at highest risk for negative outcomes, then we have a chance when next these data are compiled to see trends in the social morbidities, homicide and suicide that are akin to what we see here for motor vehicle deaths—and dramatic reduction. If, on the other hand, we are paralyzed by the myth that "nothing can be done," then we stand a great likelihood of living out that self-fulfilling prophesy.

ACKNOWLEDGMENTS. This manuscript was supported in part by the Maternal and Child Health Bureau Adolescent Health Training Grant, MCJ000985-15.

REFERENCES

The Alan Guttmacher Institute. (1994). *Sex and America's teenagers.* New York.
American Academy of Pediatrics and Center to Prevent Handgun Violence. (1994). *STOP: Steps to prevent firearm injury.*
The Annie E. Casey Foundation. (1994). *Kids count data book. State profiles of child well-being.*

Bachrach, K. S., Stolley, K. S., & London, K. A (1992). Relinquishment of premarital births: Evidence from national survey data. *Family Planning Perspectives, 24*(1), 27–32.

Bass, D. (1992). *Helping vulnerable youths: Runaway and homeless adolescents in the United States.* Washington, DC: NASW Press.

Bearinger, L. H., & Blum, R. W. (1994). Adolescent health care. In H. Wallace, R. Nelson, & R. Sweeney (Eds.), *Maternal and child health practices* (4th ed.), pp. 573–584. California: Third Party Publishing Company.

Blum, R. W., & Resnick, M. D. (1982). Adolescent sexual decision-making: Contraception, pregnancy, abortion, motherhood. *Pediatric Annals, 11*(10), 797–805.

Blum, R. W., Resnick, M. D., & Stark, T. A. (1987). The impact of a parental notification law on adolescent abortion decision-making. *American Journal of Public Health, 77,* 619–620.

Boyer, D., & Fine, D. (1992). Sexual abuse as a factor in adolescent pregnancy and child maltreatment. *Family Planning Perspectives, 24,* 4–11.

Breinig, M. K., Kingsley, L. A., Armstrong, J. A., Freeman, D. J., & Ho, M. (1990). Epidemiology of genital herpes in Pittsburgh: Serologic, sexual, and racial correlates of apparent and inapparent herpes simplex infections. *Journal of Infectious Diseases, 162,* 299–305.

Campbell, P. R. (1994). *Population projections for states, by age, race, and sex: 1993 to 2020.* U.S. Bureau of the Census, Current Population Reports, P25-1111. Washington, DC: U.S. Government Printing Office.

Carlat, D. J., & Camargo, C. A (1991). Review of bulimia nervosa in males. *American Journal of Psychiatry, 148*(7), 831–843.

Cates, W. (1987). Epidemiology and control of sexually transmitted diseases: Strategic evolution. *Infectious Disease Clinics of North America, 1*(1), 1–23.

Cates, W. (1991). Teenagers and sexual risk taking: The best of times and the worst of times. *Journal of Adolescent Health, 12,* 84–94.

The Centers for Disease Control and Prevention. (1991a). Attempted suicide among high school students. *Morbidity and Mortality Weekly Report, 40*(37), 633–635.

The Centers for Disease Control and Prevention. (1991b). Premarital sexual experience among adolescent women—United States, 1970–1988. *Morbidity and Mortality Weekly Report, 39*(51), 929–932.

The Centers for Disease Control and Prevention. (1991c). Weapon-carrying among high school students—United States. *Morbidity and Mortality Weekly Report, 40*(40), 681–684.

The Centers for Disease Control and Prevention. (1992a). Abortion surveillance: Preliminary analysis—United States, 1989. *Morbidity and Mortality Weekly Report, 40*(47), 817–819.

The Centers for Disease Control and Prevention. (1992b). Accessibility of cigarettes to youths aged 12–17 years—United States, 1989. *Morbidity and Mortality Weekly Report, 41*(27), 485–488.

The Centers for Disease Control and Prevention. (1992c). Health-risk behaviors among persons aged 12–21 years—United States. *Morbidity and Mortality Weekly Report, 43*(13), 213–235.

The Centers for Disease Control and Prevention. (1992d). HIV instruction and selected HIV-risk behaviors among high school students—United States, 1989–1991. *Morbidity and Mortality Weekly Report, 41*(46), 866–868.

The Centers for Disease Control and Prevention. (1992e). Sexual behavior among high school students—United States, 1990. *Morbidity and Mortality Weekly Report, 40*(51–52), 885–888.

The Centers for Disease Control and Prevention. (1993). Teenage pregnancy and birth rates—United States, 1990. *Morbidity and Mortality Weekly Report, 42*(38), 733–738.

The Centers for Disease Control and Prevention. (1994). Reduction in alcohol-related traffic fatalities—United States, 1990–1992. *Journal of the American Medical Association, 271*(2), 100.

Chadwick, B. A., & Heaton, T. B. (Eds.) (1992). *Statistical handbook of the American family.* Phoenix: Oryn Press.

Children's Defense Fund (1994). *The state of America's children: Yearbook 1994.* Washington, DC.

Cooksey, E. C. (1990). Factors in the resolution of adolescent premarital pregnancies. *Demography, 27,* 207–218.

DiClemente, R. J., Brown, L. K. Beausoleil, N. I., & Lodico, M. (1993). Comparison of AIDS knowledge and HIV-related sexual risk behaviors among adolescents in low and high AIDS prevalence communities. *Journal of Adolescent Health, 14*(3), 231–236.

DiClemente, R. J., Durbin, M., Siegel, D., Krasnovsky, F., Lazarus, N., & Comacho, T. (1992). Determinants of condom use among junior high school students in a minority, inner-city school district. *Pediatrics, 89*(2), 197–202.

Donovan, P. (1992). *Our daughter's decision: The conflict in state law on abortion and other issues.* New York: The Alan Guttmacher Institute.

Ellen, J. M., Moscicki, A. B., & Shafer, M. B. (1994). Genital herpes simplex virus and human papillomavirus infection. *Advances in Pediatric Infectious Diseases, 19,* 97–124.

Ellickson, P. L., Lara, M. E., Sherbourne, C. D., & Zima, B. (1993). Forgotten ages, forgotten problems: Adolescents' health. *Rand,* 1–41.

Fairburn, C. G., & Beglin, S. J. (1990). Studies of the epidemiology of bulimia nervosa. *American Journal of Psychiatry, 147*(4), 401–408.

Fingerhut, L. A. (1993). *Firearm mortality among children and youth* (p. 231). Advance Data from Vital and Health Statistics of the National Center for Health Statistics. U.S. Department of Health and Human Services.

Fingerhut, L. A., & Kleinman, J. C. (1990). International and interstate comparisons of homicide among young males. *Journal of the American Medical Association, 263,* 3292–3295.

Finkelhor, D. A (1986). *Source book on child sexual abuse.* Newbury Park, CA: Sage.

Finkelhor, D., Hotaling, G., & Sedlak, A. (1990). U.S. Department of Justice, Office of Justice Programs, Office of Juvenile Justice & Delinquency Prevention. *Missing, abducted, runaway and thrownaway children in America* (pp. 1–19). First Report: Numbers and Characteristics. National Incidence Studies, Executive Summary.

Fisher, M., Rosenfeld, W. D., & Burk, R. D. (1991). Cervicovaginal human papillomavirus infection in suburban adolescents and young adults. *Journal of pediatrics, 119*(5), 821–825.

Forrest, J. D., & Singh, S. (1990). The sexual and reproductive behavior of American women, 1982–1988. *Family Planning Perspectives, 22,* 206–214.

Garfinkel, I., & McLanahan, S. S. (1986). *Single mothers and their children* (pp. 1–2). Washington, DC: The Urban Institute.

Garner, D. M. (1993). Pathogenesis of anorexia nervosa. *Science & Practice, 341,* 1361–1364.

Goldbloom, D. S., & Garfinkel, P. E. (1989). Anorexia nervosa and bulimia nervosa. In M. Hersen (Ed.), *Handbook of child psychiatric diagnosis* (pp. 407–426). New York: Wiley–Interscience.

Gowers, S., & McMahon, J. B. (1989). Social class and prognosis in anorexia nervosa. *International Journal of Eating Disorders, 8*(1), 105–110.

Guggenheimer, J. G., Zullo, T. G., Kruper, D. C., & Verbin, R. S. (1986). Changing trends of tobacco use in a teenage population in western Pennsylvania. *American Journal of Public Health, 76*(2), 196–197.

Haller, E. (1992). Eating disorders: A review and update. *Western Journal of Medicine, 157*(6), 658–662.

Halmi, K. A., Casper, R. C., Eckert, E. D., Goldberg, S. C., & Davis, J. M. (1979). Unique features associated with age of onset of anorexia nervosa. *Psychiatry Research, 1,* 209–215.

Harlap, S., Kost, K., & Forrest, J. D. (1991). *Preventing pregnancy, protecting health: A new look at birth control choices in the United States.* New York: The Alan Guttmacher Institute.

Henshaw, S. K. (1994). *U.S. teenage pregnancy statistics* (p. 1–7). New York: The Alan Guttmacher Institute.

Henshaw, S. K., & Kost, K. (1992). Parental involvement in minors' abortion decisions. *Family Planning Perspectives, 24*(5), 196–207.

Hingson, R. W., Strunin, L., & Berlin, B. M. (1990). Acquired immunodeficiency syndrome transmission: Changes in knowledge and behaviors among teenagers. Massachusetts Statewide Survey. 1986 to 1988. *Pediatrics 85(1),* 24–29.

Hoek, H. W. (1991). The incidence and prevalence of anorexia nervosa and bulimia nervosa in primary care. *Psychological Medicine, 21,* 455–460.

Hofferth, S. L., & Hayes, C. D. (Eds.). (1987). *Risking the future: Adolescent sexuality, pregnancy and childbearing* (Vol. II). Washington, DC: National Academy Press.

Hollmann, F. W. (1993). *U.S. population estimates, by age, sex, race and Hispanic origin: 1990 to 1992.* Population Projections Branch, Population Division, U.S. Bureau of the Census.

Johnston, L. D., O'Malley, P. M., & Bachman, J. G. (1994). *National survey results on drug use from the Monitoring the Future Study, 1975–1993* (Vol. I). Rockville, MD: The National Institute on Drug Abuse.

Kassett, J. A., Gwirtsman, H. E., Kaye, W. H., Brandt, H. A., & Jimerson, D. C. (1988). Pattern of onset of bulimic symptoms in anorexia nervosa. *American Journal of Psychiatry, 145*(10), 1287–1288.

Kestelman, P., & Trussell, J. (1991). Efficacy of simultaneous use of condoms and spermicides. *Family Planning Perspectives, 23*(5), 226–232.

Kolbe, L. J. (1992). The role of the federal government in promoting health through the schools: Report from the Division of Adolescent & School Health, Centers for Disease Control. *Journal of School Health, 62*(4), 135–137.

Lewinsohn, P. M., Hops, H., Roberts, R. E., Seeley, J. R., & Andrews, J. A. (1993). Adolescent psychopathology: I. Prevalence and incidence of depression and other DSM-III-R disorders in high school students. *Journal of Abnormal Psychology, 102*(1), 133–144.

Ley, C., Bauer, H. M., Reingold, A., Schiffman, M. H., Chambers, J. C., Tashiro, C. J., & Manos, M. M. (1991). Determinants of genital human papillomavirus infection in young women. *Journal of the National Cancer Institute, 83*, 997–1003.

Lovick, S., & Wesson, W. (1986). *School-based clinics: Update.* Washington, DC: Center for Population Options.

Lucas, A. R., Beard, C. M., O'Fallon, W. M., & Kurland, L. T. (1991). Fifty-year trends in the incidence of anorexia nervosa in Rochester, Minnesota: A population-based study. *American Journal of Psychiatry, 148*(7), 917–922.

Makinson, C. (1985). The health consequences of teenage fertility. *Family Planning Perspectives, 17*(3), 132–139.

Martinez, J., Smith, R., Farmer, M., Resau, J., Alger, L., Daniel, R., Gupta, J., Keerti, S., & Naghashfar, Z. (1988). High prevalence of genital tract papillomavirus infection in female adolescents. *Pediatrics, 82*, 604–608.

Mitchell, J. E., Davis, L., Goff, G., & Pyle, R. (1986). A follow-up study of patients with bulimia. *International Journal of Eating Disorders, 5*(3), 441–450.

Mitchell, J. E., Pyle, R. L., & Eckert, E. D. (1985). Bulimia. In R. E. Hales & A. J. Frances (Eds.), *Psychiatry update: American Psychiatric Association annual review* (Vol. 4). Washington, DC: American Psychiatric Association.

Monthly Vital Statistics Report. (1991). Hyattsville, Maryland: Public Health Service. *Advance report of final natality statistics, 42*(3) (Suppl.).

Moore, K. A., Nord, C. W., & Peterson, J. L. (1989). Nonvoluntary sexual activity among adolescents. *Family Planning Perspectives, 21*(3), 110–114.

Moscicki, A. B., Palefsky, J. M., Gonzales, J., & Schoolnik, G. K. (1990). Human papillomavirus infection in sexually active adolescent females: Prevalence and risk factors. *Pediatric Research, 28*, 507.

National Center for Health Statistics. (1992). Monthly Vital Statistics Report. Public Health Service. *Trends in pregnancies and pregnancy rates, United States, 1980–88, 41*(6) (Suppl.).

National Center for Health Statistics. (1993). Monthly Vital Statistics Report. *Advance report of final mortality statistics, 1991.* Hyattsville, MD: Public Health Service, *42*(2) (Suppl.).

National Institute of Mental Health. (1993). *Suicide facts.* Rockville, MD: Office of Scientific Information.

National Safety Council. (1993). *Accident facts.* National Safety Council: Itasca, IL.

Newacheck, P. W., McManus, M. A., & Gephart, J. (1992). Health insurance coverage of adolescents: A current profile and assessment of trends. *Pediatrics, 90*(4), 589–596.

The *New York Times*/CBS News Poll. (1994). Teenagers, in poll, speak of worry, and distrust that shuts out adults.

Orr, D. P., Langefeld, C. D., Katz, B. P., Caine, V. A., Dias, P., Blythe, M., & Jones, R. B. (1992). Factors associated with condom use among sexually active female adolescents. *Journal of Pediatrics, 120*(2), 311–317.

Patton, G. C. (1990). Mortality in eating disorders. *Psychological Medicine, 18*, 947–951.

Randall, T. (1992). Adolescents may experience home, school abuse: Their future draws researcher's concern. *Journal of the American Medical Association, 267*(23), 3127–3131.

Rosen, D., Xiangdong, M., & Blum, R. W. (1990). Adolescent health: Current trends and critical issues. *Adolescent Medicine: State of the Art Reviews, 1*(1), 15–31.

Rosenfeld, W. D., Vermund, S. H., Wentz, S. J., & Burk, R. D. (1989). High prevalence rate of human papillomavirus infection and association with abnormal Papanicolaou smears in sexually active adolescents. *American Journal of Diseases of Children, 143,* 1443–1447.

Schneider, J. A., & Agras, W. S. (1987). Bulimia in males: A matched comparison with females. *International Journal of Eating Disorders, 6*(2), 235–242.

Seidman, S. N., & Rieder, R. O. (1994). A review of sexual behavior in the United States. *American Journal of Psychiatry, 151*(3), 330–341.

Shafer, M. A. (1992). Sexually transmitted disease syndromes. In E. R. McAnarney, R. E. Kreipe, D. P. Orr, & G. D. Comerci (Eds.), *Textbook of adolescent medicine* (p. 696). Philadelphia: Saunders.

Silvis, G. L., & Perry, C. L. (1987). Understanding and deterring tobacco use among adolescents. *Pediatric Clinics of North America, 34*(2), 363–379.

Sonenstein, F. L., Pleck, J. H., & Ku, L. C. (1989). Sexual activity, condom use and AIDS awareness among adolescent males. *Family Planning Perspectives, 21*(4), 152–158.

Stephenson, J. N. (1989). Pregnancy testing and counseling. *Pediatric Clinics of North America, 36*(3), 681–696.

Upchurch, D. M., & McCarthy, J. (1990). The timing of first birth and high school completion. *American Sociology Reviews, 55,* 224–234.

U.S. Bureau of the Census. Current Population Reports, P25-1095. (1993). *U.S. population estimates by age, sex, race, and Hispanic origin: 1980 to 1991.* Washington, DC: U.S. Government Printing Office.

U.S. Bureau of Justice Statistics. (1992). *Criminal victimization in the United States, 1973–90 trends.* A National Crime Victimization Report: NCJ-139564.

U.S. Bureau of Justice Statistics. (1994). *Criminal victimization in the United States, 1992.* A National Crime Victimization Report: NCJ-145125.

U.S. Department of Commerce. (1993). Current Population Reports, Consumer Income Series P60-185. *Poverty in the United States: 1992.* Economics and Statistics Administration, Bureau of the Census, vii–171.

U.S. Department of Health and Human Services. (1986). *The health consequences of using smokeless tobacco:* A Report of the Advisory Committee to the Surgeon General. Public Health Service. NIH Publication 86-2874, Bethesda, MD.

U.S. Department of Health and Human Services. (1989). Prepared for the Office of the Assistant Secretary for Planning and Evaluation Systemetrics/McGraw–Hill. *A partial listing of problems facing American children, youth and families.* Lexington, MA: Author.

U.S. Department of Health and Human Services. (1990). National Plan for Research on Child and Adolescent Mental Disorders. National Institute of Mental Health. A Report Requested by the U.S. Congress. Submitted by the National Advisory Mental Health Council.

U.S. Department of Health and Human Services. (1993a). Adolescent Health: State of the nation monograph series, No. 1. CDC Publication 099-4112. *Mortality trends, causes of death, and related risk behaviors among U.S. adolescents.* Public Health Service, Centers for Disease Control & Prevention.

U.S. Department of Health and Human Services. (1993b). Division of STD-HIV Prevention. *Sexually transmitted disease surveillance, 1992.* Public Health Service, Centers for Disease Control & Prevention.

U.S. Department of Health and Human Services. (1994a). National Center on Child Abuse and Neglect. Child Maltreatment 1992: *Reports from the states to the National Center on Child Abuse and Neglect.* Washington, DC: U.S. Government Printing Office.

U.S. Department of Health and Human Services. (1994b). *Preventing tobacco use among young people: A report of the Surgeon General* (pp. 5–10). Public Health Service, Centers for Disease Control & Prevention.

U.S. Department of Health and Human Services. (1994c). *HIV/AIDS surveillance report,* Third Quarter Edition. Atlanta, 5(4), 12–14. Public Health Service, Centers for Disease Control & Prevention. National Center for Infectious Diseases.

U.S. Department of Transportation. (1989). *Fatal Accident Reporting System 1988: A review of information on fatal traffic crashes in the United States in 1988.* National Highway Traffic Safety Administration. Washington, DC.

U.S. Department of Transportation. (1993). *Fatal Accident Reporting System 1991: A review of information on fatal traffic crashes in the United States in 1988.* National Highway Traffic Safety Administration. Washington, DC.

U.S. General Accounting Office. (1989a). *Children and youths: About 68,000 homeless and 186,000 in shared housing at any given time* (Report No. GAO/PEMD-89-14). Washington, DC.

U.S. General Accounting Office. (1989b). *Homelessness: Homeless and runaway youth receiving services at federally funded shelters* (Report No. GAO/HRD-90-45). Washington, DC.

Washington, A. E., Arno, P. S., & Brooks, M. A. (1986). The economic cost of pelvic inflammatory disease. *Journal of the American Medical Association, 255,* 1735–1738.

Wright, T. C., & Richart, R. M. (1990). Role of human papillomavirus in the pathogenesis of genital tract warts and cancer. *Gynecologic Oncology, 37,* 151.

Yager, J. (1988). The treatment of eating disorders. *Journal of Clinical Psychiatry, 49*(9, Suppl.), 1825.

Yager, J., Kurtzman, F., Landsverk, J., & Wiesmeier, E. (1988). Behaviors and attitudes related to eating disorders in homosexual male college students. *American Journal of Psychiatry, 145,* 495–497.

Yager, J., Landsverk, J., & Edelstein, C. K. (1987). A 20-month follow-up of 628 women with eating disorders, I: Course and severity. *American Journal of Psychiatry, 144*(9), 1172–1177.

Yankelovich, Clancy, & Shulman. (1990, January 29). America and their guns. A Time/CNN telephone poll (pp. 20–21).

Yates, A. (1989). Current perspectives on the eating disorders: I. History, psychological and biological aspects. *Journal of the American Academy of Child and Adolescent Psychiatry, 28*(6), 813–828.

Yates, A. (1990). Current perspectives on the eating disorders: II. Treatment, outcome, and research directions. *Journal of the American Academy of Child and Adolescent Psychiatry, 29*(1), 1–9.

Zabin, L. S., & Clark, S. D. (1983). Institutional factors affecting teenager's choice and reasons for delay in attending a family planning clinic. *Family Planning Perspectives, 15*(1), 25–29.

Zabin, L. S., Hirsch, M. B., & Boscia, J. A. (1990). Differential characteristics of adolescent pregnancy test patients: Abortion, childbearing and negative test groups. *Journal of Adolescent Health Care, 11,* 107–113.

Zawitz, M. W., Klaus, P. A., Bachman, R., Bastian, L. D., Deberry, M. M., Rand, M. R., & Taylor, B. M. (1993). *Highlights from 20 years of surveying crime victims, the National Crime Victimization Survey, 1973–1992* (pp. 1–38). U.S. Department of Justice. Office of Justice Programs, Bureau of Justice Statistics.

3

Theories of Adolescent
Risk-Taking Behavior

VIVIEN IGRA and CHARLES E. IRWIN, JR.

INTRODUCTION

The study of adolescent risk-taking behavior gained prominence in the 1980s as it became increasingly evident that the majority of the morbidity and mortality during the second decade of life was behavioral in origin. The term *risk-taking behavior* has been used to link, conceptually, a number of potentially health-damaging behaviors including, among others, substance use, precocious or risky sexual behavior, reckless vehicle use, homicidal and suicidal behavior, eating disorders, and delinquency. The linkage of these behaviors under a single domain is theoretically useful because it allows for the investigation of particular behaviors in the context of other behaviors. The construct of risk-taking behavior also suggests a more parsimonious use of interventions, targeting groups of behaviors rather than applying multiple more narrowly targeted interventions.

With risk defined as the chance of loss, risky behaviors have been characterized as those behaviors that entail the possibility of subjective loss (Furby & Beyth-Maron, 1990). It follows that risk-taking is engaging in risky behavior. Inherent in the term *risk-taking behaviors* is the notion that the behaviors are volitional, that there is some conscious weighing of alternative courses of action. Irwin (1990) has defined adolescent risk-taking behaviors as those behaviors, undertaken volitionally, whose outcomes remain uncertain with the possibility of an identifiable negative health outcome.

Risk-taking behaviors are the most serious threats to adolescent health and well-being. In addition, once these behaviors are established during adolescence and young

VIVIEN IGRA and CHARLES E. IRWIN, Jr. • Department of Pediatrics, University of California, San Francisco, San Francisco, California 94143.

Handbook of Adolescent Health Risk Behavior, edited by Ralph J. DiClemente, William B. Hansen, and Lynn E. Ponton. Plenum Press, New York, 1996.

adulthood they often remain as major contributors to the health problems of adults (U.S. Preventive Services Task Force, 1989). Negative potential consequences of these behaviors include unwanted pregnancy, sexually transmitted diseases, severe disability, and death. The theories presented in this chapter have attempted to increase our understanding of why adolescents engage in risk-taking behaviors. Many of these theories have yet to be empirically verified.

Empirical evidence for the linkage of risk-taking behaviors as a conceptual entity comes from three sources. First, risk-taking behaviors generally display a developmental trajectory. For example, rates of sexual activity, substance use, reckless vehicle use, and delinquency have been found to increase with increasing age during adolescence. Second, these behaviors have been found to covary in predictable ways. Sexually active teens, for example, are more likely than their nonsexually active peers to be using alcohol and marijuana (Millstein *et al.*, 1992; Mott & Haurin, 1988). Finally, risk-taking behaviors often share similar psychological, environmental, and/or biological antecedents.

This chapter focuses, somewhat arbitrarily, on risk-taking behaviors that are considered "nonnormative"* because of their timing or extent. Behaviors considered risk-taking because of their timing include premature sexual behavior or alcohol use. Both behaviors become normative over time as adolescents approach adulthood. Behaviors considered risk-taking based on the relative level of the adolescents' involvement include delinquency and substance use. Most adolescents engage in some minor delinquent acts prior to adulthood (Elliot, 1993). Similarly, minor traffic infringements and experimentation with tobacco or alcohol are common in adolescence. However, true delinquency, reckless vehicle use, and illicit substance use are considered risk-taking behaviors because of the nonnormative degree of the adolescents' involvement in these behaviors. Given these caveats, we suggest that homicidal or suicidal behavior and eating disorders are never normative in degree or timing and, as a result, will not be considered in this chapter. For the purposes of this chapter, risk-taking behaviors will include risky sexual activity (at younger ages, with multiple partners, or in the absence of contraception), reckless vehicle use, substance abuse, and delinquency.

A variety of factors have been found to be associated with adolescent risk-taking behaviors. Theories of risk-taking behavior provide a framework for examining the range of factors thought to influence the likelihood of individuals engaging in risk-taking behavior. The remainder of the chapter looks at the developmental aspects and covariation of risk-taking behaviors, and reviews some of the biological, psychological, and environmental theories of adolescent risk-taking behavior. Wherever possible, empirical evidence for the various theoretical perspectives is presented.

RISK-TAKING BEHAVIOR AND DEVELOPMENT

Normal adolescent development encompasses increasing independence, autonomy from the family, greater peer affiliation and importance, sexual awareness, identity formation, and physiological and cognitive maturation. Risk-taking behaviors serve different

---

*"Normative" behaviors refer to those behaviors that we expect to see in the majority of individuals in a designated group. This is a population-based comparison as opposed to the concept of "normal" behaviors that presupposes an invariable standard of behavior.

functions and have different meanings at various developmental stages during adolescence.

Jessor's (1977) problem behavior theory is based on the premise that problem behaviors are part of normal adolescent development and play a major role in the process of transition to adulthood. According to Jessor (1982), behaviors such as smoking, drinking, illicit substance use, risky driving, or early sexual activity should be considered "purposeful, meaningful, goal oriented and functional rather than arbitrary or perverse." As such, problem behaviors in adolescence can be instrumental in gaining peer acceptance and respect; in establishing autonomy from parents, in repudiating the norms and values of conventional authority; in coping with anxiety, frustration, and the anticipation of failure; in confirming for self and significant others certain attributes of identity; or in affirming maturity and marking a transition out of childhood and toward a more adult status (Jessor, 1991).

Baumrind (1987) has also argued that risk-taking is a part of normal adolescence. According to Baumrind, a certain amount of "eustress" is necessary to build self-confidence, enhance competence, and provide reinforcement for taking initiatives. Baumrind distinguishes behaviors that are potentially developmentally adaptive from those that are "pathogenic"—dangerous with little or no chance for secondary gain. Irwin (1987) has used the term *exploratory behavior* to distinguish developmentally constructive risk-taking from negative behaviors traditionally associated with the term *risk-taking behavior*. The former refers to experimentation within a controlled or adaptive context; the latter refers to those behaviors that have the potential to jeopardize health and prosocial development.

Risk-taking behaviors may fulfill adolescents' evolving needs for autonomy, mastery, and intimacy (Irwin & Millstein, 1986). These changing attributes influence the trajectory of risk-taking behavior. Prevalence of sexual activity increases with increasing age; substance use and injury-related behavior peak in late adolescence and young adulthood. Behaviors such as sexual activity and alcohol use, which are considered risky, deviant, and problematic at age 12, are normative by age 18. Clearly the construct of risk-taking behavior is best defined within a developmental context.

COVARIATION OF RISK-TAKING BEHAVIORS

Risk-taking behaviors do not occur in isolation; rather they tend to cluster in somewhat predictable ways. In addition, over time, involvement in one type of risk behavior has also been found to increase the likelihood of becoming involved in other risk behaviors (Irwin & Shafer, 1992; Osgood, Johnston, O'Malley, & Bachman, 1988). Millstein *et al.* (1992) found co-occurrence of risk behaviors among early adolescents; those who were sexually active were more likely than their nonsexually active peers to report driving or riding in a car under the influence of substances. Mott and Haurin (1988) reported sequential involvement in risk-taking among adolescents; sexually active adolescents in their study were more likely than nonsexually active adolescents to use alcohol and marijuana during the following year. Conversely, adolescents who used marijuana or alcohol were more likely than nonusers to become sexually active within the year.

The term *covariation* has been used to describe the complex interrelationships among risk-taking behaviors. Three types of theories have been proposed to explain the covariation of risk-taking behaviors: (1) individual behaviors influence one another, (2) risk-taking behaviors can be seen as alternative manifestations of a general tendency toward deviance, and (3) a finite constellation of factors are responsible for multiple risk-taking behaviors.

Studies of adolescent substance use support covariation theories of individual behaviors precipitating one another. Adolescent substance use tends to follow a predictable progression with alcohol and tobacco use preceding marijuana and other illicit substances (Kandel & Logan, 1984). Furthermore, the earlier adolescents begin using marijuana, the more likely they are to use other illicit substances (Yamaguchi & Kandel, 1984a,b). Other behaviors that appear to influence one another include substance use, especially alcohol, and injury-related behavior.

In San Francisco, for example, Friedman (1985) found that half of the 12- to 24-year-old victims of fatal accidents of all kinds were alcohol-intoxicated. Despite recent declines in alcohol-related traffic fatalities, in 1992 more than a third of 15- to 20-year-old drivers dying in motor vehicle crashes were alcohol-impaired (CDC, 1993). Alcohol has been implicated in boating accidents and other adolescent drownings (Wintemute, 1990).

The observed relationship between alcohol use and crashes among adolescents may be the chemical effects of alcohol on the brain. Alcohol-related impaired mentation, judgment, and reaction time may make otherwise benign driving behavior risky. Alternatively, the associated disinhibition may increase the likelihood of adolescents driving recklessly (Rogers & Adger, 1993). A third possibility is that substance use and injury-related behavior co-occur because they have common antecedents or possibly because both types of behavior occur in individuals who have a tendency toward "deviant" behavior.

Donovan, Jessor, and Costa (1988, 1991) found that adolescent problem behaviors such as alcohol abuse, marijuana use, delinquency, and precocious sexual activity were associated with one another and were inversely related to conventional behaviors such as church attendance. They postulated that the covariation of problem behaviors is related to an underlying common factor that reflects "unconventionality," and represents a "syndrome" of problem behavior. Osgood et al. (1988), however, found that although much of the variance in these behaviors could be accounted for by a general tendency toward deviance, a significant proportion of the variance was unique to the individual behaviors.

A number of theoretical antecedents to risk-taking behavior have been postulated with varying support in the literature. Theories of risk-taking behavior have taken essentially three forms: biological, psychological/cognitive, and environmental/social. This distinction is somewhat arbitrary in many cases because features from more than one category play a role in several of the theoretical models.

Biologically based theories suggest that risk-taking behaviors result from hormonal effects, asynchronous pubertal timing, or genetic predispositions. Psychological/cognitive theories implicate deficits in self-esteem, cognitive immaturity, affective disequilibrium, or high sensation seeking. Social/environmental theories rely on family and peer interactions, or community and societal norms to explain adolescent participation in risk-taking behaviors. The biopsychosocial model (Irwin & Millstein, 1986) of adolescent risk-taking behavior incorporates all three theoretical perspectives. The model proposes that asynchronous pubertal maturation interacting with cognitive and social factors increases the likelihood of adolescents engaging in risk-taking behavior.

BIOLOGY AND RISK-TAKING BEHAVIOR

Biologically based theories attribute tendencies toward risk-taking behavior to genetic predispositions, "direct" hormonal influences, and the influence of hormonal changes mediated through pubertal timing. Risk-taking behaviors tend to cluster within families. Certain families have a greater propensity for injury-related behavior. In a study utilizing a socioeconomically and ethnically homogeneous prepaid health plan population, Schor (1987) found that a small number of families accounted for a disproportionately large number of visits for injuries. (This difference persisted even after adjusting for family size.) Individual members of these families had similar rates of unintentional injuries, and these rates tended to be stable over time.

The familial nature of certain risk behaviors has led to speculation about the role of genetic predispositions toward risk-taking behavior. Genetic models have been proposed to explain familial patterns of substance use. Children of alcoholics are more likely than children of nonalcoholics to abuse alcohol (Adger, 1991; Marlatt, Baer, Donovan, & Kivlahan, 1988). Clearly this could be the result of social/environmental influences; however, twin-adoption studies show a greater predisposition toward alcohol abuse among children of alcoholic biological parents even when raised by nonalcoholic parents, implicating a role for heredity (Cloninger, 1987).

Cloninger (1987) has suggested that a certain subtype of alcohol abuse is more likely to show a familial distribution. This subtype occurs primarily in males, has onset during adolescence, and is characterized by inability to abstain from drinking, involvement in fights, and legal intervention while drinking and engaging in "novelty seeking" behavior. Historically, the study of genetic influence on human behavior has been difficult and controversial. With the advent of more sophisticated gene mapping techniques, the opportunity to explore further the role of genetic predisposition to risk-taking behaviors may be on the horizon.

Hormones have been postulated to play a role in the onset of adolescent risk-taking behavior both directly and through their role in pubertal development. Udry, Billy, Morris, Groff, and Raj (1985), for example, found that male coital debut was related to the rise in testosterone levels during adolescence. Female initiation of coitus, on the other hand was more closely related to social controls and pubertal development (Udry, Talbert, & Morris, 1986). Recently, Udry (1990) has expanded his model to include "environmental" variables from Jessor's problem behavior theory, reflecting tendencies toward unconventionality. The combined effects of biological (hormonal) and environmental (social) factors explained more of the variation in problem behaviors (used cigarettes or marijuana, had been drunk, had had sex) than either of these factors alone.

The timing of pubertal maturation is related to both genetics and hormonal fluctuations. (Menarcheal age of mothers and daughters are typically correlated, and physical development is preceded by elevations in respective sex steroid levels.) Asynchronous pubertal maturation (that is, earlier or later than peers), in turn, is hypothesized to be a factor in risk-taking behavior (Irwin & Millstein, 1986). The societal expectation of a physically mature-appearing adolescent is that he or she will engage in "adult" behaviors, perhaps including drinking, smoking, and intercourse (Brooks-Gunn, 1988). In addition, the physically mature adolescent may have an older peer group in which these behaviors may be more normative. Early maturing females are more likely to initiate intercourse at younger ages (Phinney, Jensen, Olsen, & Cundick, 1990). Younger age at sexual debut is associated with less consistent contraception and increased numbers of sexual partners, resulting in an increased risk for pregnancy and sexually transmitted diseases (CDC, 1991; Mosher & McNaley, 1991).

Biological development during adolescence is accompanied by physiological changes in the ways in which adolescents perceive both themselves and the world around them. Cognitive development may occur in concert or asynchronously with physical development. When physical development precedes cognitive development, adolescents are at increased risk for behavioral morbidities. The social world may have unrealistic or unhealthy expectations of mature-appearing adolescents whose lack of experience and relative cognitive (im-)maturity may render them vulnerable.

PSYCHOLOGY, COGNITION, AND RISK-TAKING BEHAVIOR

Psychological theories of risk-taking behavior examine the roles of cognitive ability, personality traits, and dispositional characteristics, such as self-esteem, in risk-taking behavior. Cognitively based theories of risk-taking behavior look at the ways in which individuals perceive risk and make decisions about risk-taking. Adolescent risk perception theory has been influenced by the premise that adolescents are "optimistically biased" in their risk perception or that they feel that they are "invulnerable." Elkind's (1967) work on adolescent egocentrism posits that the adolescent has an exaggerated sense of uniqueness, creating a "personal fable" in which he/she is special and not susceptible to harm. The concept of invulnerability has been used to explain adolescent risk-taking behavior although there is little evidence to support this. People generally underestimate their likelihood of experiencing negative events. Adolescents do not appear to be more biased in that regard than adults.

Based on work in primarily adult populations, Fischoff (1992) identified five salient components of decision-making: (1) identify alternative options, (2) identify possible consequences, (3) evaluate the desirability of the potential consequences, (4) assess the likelihood of those consequences, and (5) combine the information to make a decision. According to Keating (1990), by middle adolescence, most individuals make decisions in similar ways to adults. Although the decision-making process may be similar for adults and adolescents, the content of the different components may differ substantially based on experience, biases, judgment, social pressure, situations, and so forth.

By age 14 or 15 adolescents have the ability to generate and evaluate a range of alternative options (Keating, 1990). There is no empirical evidence that adolescents generate options that are significantly different from those generated by adults given the same situational constraints. Similarly, given the same options there is no evidence that adolescents would choose differently from adults. Adults and adolescents may differ substantially, however, in the magnitude and types of social/environmental influences that they bring to bear on such decisions, and therefore may prefer different options.

Assumptions about how adolescents identify, evaluate, and assess the likelihood of potential consequences can be traced to Piagetian cognitive developmental theory. According to Piaget (1972), early adolescence marks the transition from the concrete operational thinking that characterizes late childhood to the formal operational thinking that characterizes adulthood. The latter confers the ability to think abstractly (and therefore anticipate or envision the potential negative consequences of risk-taking behavior). Based on Piaget's model, adolescent reasoning resembles adult reasoning. Yet as many as 50% of adults never obtain formal operations (Muuss, 1988). In addition, the practical significance of the transition from concrete to formal operations has been questioned as evidence suggests that the transition may not be a prerequisite for critical or logical thinking (Keating, 1990).

There is some evidence that adolescents give greater weight to proximal (less severe) rather than distal (and potentially more severe) possible consequences when making decisions. For example, Kegeles, Adler, and Irwin (1988) found that among a group of 14- to 16-year-olds, intentions to use condoms were not related to the adolescents' beliefs about the degree to which condoms prevent STDs or pregnancy. Rather, intentions to use condoms were correlated with the degree to which the adolescents perceived that condoms are easy to use, popular with peers, and facilitate spontaneous sex. Adolescent smokers and nonsmokers have similar perceptions of their risk for long-term morbidities such as cancer (Greening & Dollinger, 1991). On the other hand, adolescent smoking prevention programs have successfully emphasized the immediate physiologic consequences of smoking (Flay, 1985).

The relative influence of individual factors on adolescent decision-making may reflect a general tendency toward unconventional behavior. Jessor's problem behavior theory links "unconventionality" in personality (as well as perceived environment and behavioral systems) with an increased likelihood of engaging in problem behaviors such as precocious sexual activity, substance use, and delinquency (Jessor & Jessor, 1977). Unconventionality in the personality system is represented by a greater value placed on independence than achievement, lower expectations for academic achievement, lesser religiosity, and greater tolerance for deviance. These factors have been correlated with problem drinking, marijuana use, and precocious sexual debut (Jessor, Chase, & Donovan, 1980; Jessor, et al., 1983).

Sensation-seeking as a personality trait has been used to explain risk-taking behavior. According to Zuckerman (1979), sensation-seeking is a "trait defined by the need for varied, novel and complex sensations and experiences and willingness to take physical and social risks for the sake of such experiences." Zuckerman developed a Sensation Seeking Scale to assess individual differences in optimal levels of arousal. There is a tendency for high-sensation seekers to perceive less risk in many activities than low-sensation seekers. But even when the evaluation of the risk involved is equal between the two groups, high-sensation seekers are likely to anticipate more positive potential outcomes than low-sensation seekers. Sensation-seeking has been associated with risk-taking behaviors such as substance abuse, reckless motor vehicle use, and delinquency (Andrucci, Archer, Pancoast, & Gordon, 1989; Newcomb & McGee, 1991; Tonkin, 1987; Zuckerman, 1991). Interestingly, sensation-seeking has been linked to a number of biological markers including electrodermal and heart rate responses, cortical evoked potentials, and testosterone levels (Zuckerman, 1990).

The impulsivity seen among sensation-seekers may be seen in psychopathologic
states that have been linked to an increased likelihood of risk-taking behaviors, primarily
in male adolescents. Attention-deficit hyperactivity disorder (ADHD) in males has been
associated with an increased risk for delinquency. One study found that male youth with
ADHD had arrest rates more than twice those of controls (Farrington, Loeber, & Van
Kammen, 1990). Similarly, male youth with conduct disorders are an increased risk for
alcohol and substance abuse (Kazdin, 1989). Finally, neuropsychological testing reveals a
variety of cognitive differences between nonaggressive matched control adolescents on
the one hand, and aggressive, violent adolescents on the other (Moffitt, 1990).

Self-esteem, depression, and locus of control have often been cited as theoretical
predictors of risk-taking behavior. Lower self-esteem has been associated with sexual
debut in adolescent females (Orr, 1989). Depressive mood and stress are related to
initiation and intensity of adolescent tobacco use (Covey & Tam, 1990). Depression and
external locus of control have been implicated in substance use (Baumrind, 1987; Dielman, Campanelli, Shope, & Butchart, 1987). Research has not supported a consistent role
for any of these psychological factors, however (Dryfoos, 1990; McCord, 1990).

In summary, cognitive factors such as risk perception and decision-making contribute to adolescent risk-taking. Adolescents' decision-making processes appear to differ
little from their adult counterparts, although differences appear in the content of issues
they bring to bear on their decisions. Adolescents lack adult experience interacting with
the social/environmental world in general, and engaging in decision-making specifically.
Their judgments cannot reflect the influence of these experiences. Second, the influence
of peers peaks in early to middle adolescence, as reflected by the high levels of conformity
at this age. As a result, decisions during this period may rely more heavily on peer input.
Finally, adolescents appear to give greater weight to short-term, rather than long-term,
potential consequences.

The relative strength of the influences on adolescent risk-related decision-making
may reflect young people's tendencies toward unconventionality and/or sensation-
seeking. While the tendency toward sensation-seeking is clearly related to increased rates
of risk-taking behaviors, not all risk-taking behavior can be construed as sensation-
seeking. Psychological disequilibrium in the form of excessive aggressivity, impulsivity,
and attention-deficit and conduct disorders increase the likelihood of adolescents engaging
in risk-taking behavior. And although depression has been linked to substance abuse, the
role of depressive mood in other types of risk behavior has yet to be established. The
evidence for a causal role for self-esteem and locus of control is unclear.

Biological and psychological factors are themselves important determinants of risk-
taking behavior. They also are the personal filters through which social and environmental
stimuli are interpreted and translated into action.

SOCIAL/ENVIRONMENTAL FACTORS AND RISK-TAKING BEHAVIOR

Social or environmental models of risk-taking behavior look at the roles of peers,
parents, family structure and function, and institutions (school and church) in risk-taking

behaviors. These theories examine how social/environmental contexts provide models, opportunities, and reinforcements for adolescent participation in risk-taking behaviors.

Family

Adolescence is a time of emerging autonomy and individuation from the family. Recent evidence suggests that most adolescents maintain close relations with their parents despite the "minor perturbations" accompanying this transition (Steinberg, 1990). As a result, a model of transformation, realignment, and revision of roles and expectations has largely replaced traditional views of adolescent "storm and stress." Consistent with this view, parents continue to influence their offsprings' behavior throughout adolescence.

Parents play an important role in determining adolescent involvement in risk behaviors. Adolescents may "learn" to engage in risk-taking behavior from observing their parents' behavior. Parental modeling of and permissive attitudes toward substance use have been implicated in the initiation of substance use in early adolescence (Hawkins & Fitzgibbon, 1993; Werner, 1991). Adolescents are less likely to abuse substances and to initiate sexual activity when parents provide emotional support and acceptance, and have a close relationship with their children (Turner, Irwin, Tschann, & Millstein, 1993).

Family structure correlates fairly consistently with adolescent risk-taking behavior. Adolescents from single-parent families are more likely to use illicit substances (Flewelling & Bauman, 1990). Female adolescents from single-parent families are more likely to initiate intercourse and less likely to use contraception than their peers from intact families (Hayes, 1987; Mosher & McNally, 1991). The nature of the relationship between family structure and adolescent risk-taking behavior is unclear. Newcomer and Udry (1987), for example, found that male adolescent initiation of sexual intercourse was more closely related to disruption of the two-parent household rather than living in a single-parent household *per se*. The association of risk-taking behaviors with single-parent families may be related to lower levels of adolescent supervision. A recent study found a twofold increase in substance use among eighth graders who took care of themselves after school as compared to their supervised peers (Richardson *et al.*, 1989). Clearly the influence of family structure on adolescent risk-taking is related to characteristics of the parent–child relationship. In one study the effects of family structure on adolescent risk-taking were no longer significant when sociodemographic variables and emotional distancing between parents and adolescent children were taken into account (Forman, Irwin, & Turner, 1990).

Parental influence on adolescent behavior appears to vary with the quality of the relationship between the adolescent and the parent. High levels of familial conflict are associated with increased rates of adolescent risk-taking behaviors. Bijur, Kurzon, Hamelsky, and Power (1991) noted that compared to those from low-conflict families, British youth from families reporting a high degree of adolescent–parent conflict were almost three times as likely to report having injuries requiring hospitalization. Family cohesion, on the other hand, is associated with lower rates of sexual activity and substance use among early adolescents (Turner *et al.*, 1993).

Parental approaches to child rearing may influence the likelihood of adolescents engaging in risk-taking behaviors. Baumrind (1991) found an association between adolescent substance use and parenting styles. Adolescents whose parents were "authoritative" (demanding and responsive) were less likely to use substances than either those with "authoritarian" (demanding but unresponsive) or those with "permissive" (nondemanding but responsive) parents. Adolescents with "neglecting and rejecting" parents were the most likely to engage in substance abuse.

In summary, family approval and modeling of risk behavior has been linked to adolescent risk-taking behavior. Family structure is also related to adolescent risk-taking behavior; however, the relationship appears to be mediated by the nature of parent–child interactions. Parent–child relationships characterized by conflict, increased emotional distance, and nonresponsiveness increase the likelihood of adolescents engaging in risk behaviors.

Peers

One of the developmental tasks of adolescence involves individuation from the family and identification with a peer group. As a result, parental impact on risk-taking behavior may wane as peer influences increase throughout adolescence. According to Jessor & Jessor (1977) the relatively greater influence of peers compared to parents is associated with a greater tendency (or proneness) toward problem behaviors. Consistent with this theory, Jessor, Chase, & Donovan (1980); and Jessor, Costa, Jessor, & Donovan (1983) found that the relative dominance of peer influence over parental influence predicted marijuana use, problem drinking, and precocious sexual debut.

Peer influence has been cited as a factor in adolescent substance use (Kandel, 1985; Newcomb & Bentler, 1989), delinquency (McCord, 1990), and sexual behaviors. Billy and Udry (1985) found, for example, that a white virgin adolescent female whose best male and female friends were sexually active was almost certain to become sexually active within 2 years. Traditionally "peer pressure" has been viewed as an etiologic factor in adolescent risk-taking behavior. It is unclear, however, if risk behaviors are initiated in order to conform to an existing peer group or if those inclined to engage in risk-taking behaviors are drawn to those who are similarly inclined.

Society

Societal influences such as mass media and community norms may also influence risk-taking behavior. Role models for such behavior are regularly presented by the media (including unprotected sexual behavior and alcohol use), though evidence for the influence of these models on actual behavior is lacking. Clearly different communities and neighborhoods provide adolescents with opportunities and motivations to engage in risk-taking behavior. Local peer norms reflected in local rates of substance use and teen pregnancy create expectancies of "typical" adolescent behavior (Crockett & Petersen, 1993). Local ordinances permitting cigarette vending machines, or lower ages to purchase alcohol provide opportunities for engaging in risk-taking behavior. Johnston, O'Malley, and Bachman (1993) have shown, however, that the perceived availability of marijuana in a community is not necessarily related to prevalence of use by adolescents. Declines in marijuana use by high school seniors have been accompanied by unchanged or even increased perceived availability in recent years.

Cultural expectations may influence the onset of risk-taking behavior. For example, despite similar ages of sexual debut, the United States has the highest rates of adolescent childbearing and abortion in the developed world (Blum, 1991). This is thought to be related to differing cultural attitudes toward adolescent sexuality and contraception (Perry, Kelder, & Komro, 1993). Even within the United States, contraception rates vary significantly by ethnicity and religious affiliation (Mosher & McNally, 1991). Rates of adolescent substance use and early sexual debut also differ among different ethnic groups (Bachman, Wallace, O'Malley, Johnston, & Kurth, 1991; Sonenstein, Pleck, & Ku, 1991). (Ethnicity-associated differences may be confounded by factors related to socioeconomic status.)

The range of theories reflects the complexity of the interaction between adolescents and their social world. The biopsychosocial model provides a framework in which social environmental factors are brought to bear on existing biological and psychological predispositions to influence risk-taking behavior.

BIOPSYCHOSOCIAL MODEL OF RISK-TAKING

The biopsychosocial model proposes that the timing of biological maturation influences adolescents' cognitive scope, self-perceptions, perceptions of the social environment, and personal values (Irwin & Millstein, 1986). These factors in turn are hypothesized to predict adolescent risk-taking behavior through the mediating effects of risk perception and peer group characteristics (see Figure 1).

Support for this model comes from a number of sources. Early maturational timing is associated with a more negative self-image, and, among female adolescents, with earlier onset of sexual activity among female adolescents (Brooks-Gunn, 1988). Early maturation is a risk factor for the initiation of substance use in both male and female adolescents (Tschann et al., 1994). Studies by Jessor & Jessor (1977) support the role of perceived environment and personal values in the onset of adolescent risk-taking behavior; specifically the predominance of peer over parental influence, as well as the greater personal value placed on independence versus achievement resulted in a greater likelihood of adolescents engaging in risk-taking behavior.

Given the framework of the biopsychosocial perspective, Irwin and colleagues (Irwin, 1990; Irwin & Millstein, 1986; Irwin & Ryan, 1989) have elaborated on the theory to include conditions that may increase the probability that a given adolescent will engage in risk-taking behaviors (see Figure 2). Biological factors thought to predispose adolescents to risk-taking behaviors include male gender, genetic predispositions, and hormonal influences. Psychological predisposing factors include sensation-seeking, risk perception, depression, and low self-esteem. Social environmental predisposing factors include maladaptive parenting styles, parental modeling of risk behaviors, peer behaviors, and socioeconomic status. Finally, adolescent vulnerability to risk-taking behaviors may be increased situationally by family disruption, school transitions, substance use, and peer initiation of risk-taking behaviors.

VIVIEN IGRA and CHARLES E. IRWIN, Jr.

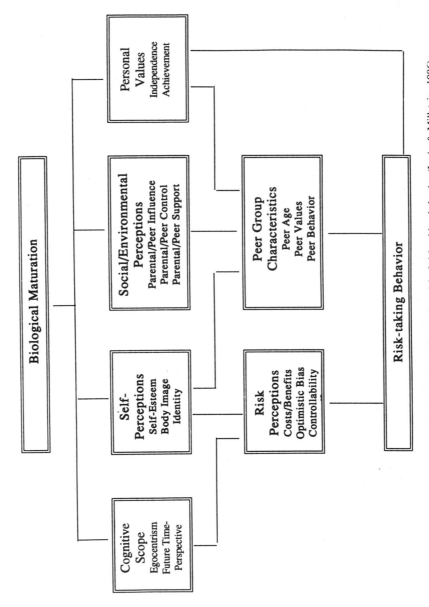

Figure 1. Model based on the biopsychosocial causal model of risk-taking behavior (Irwin & Millstein, 1986).

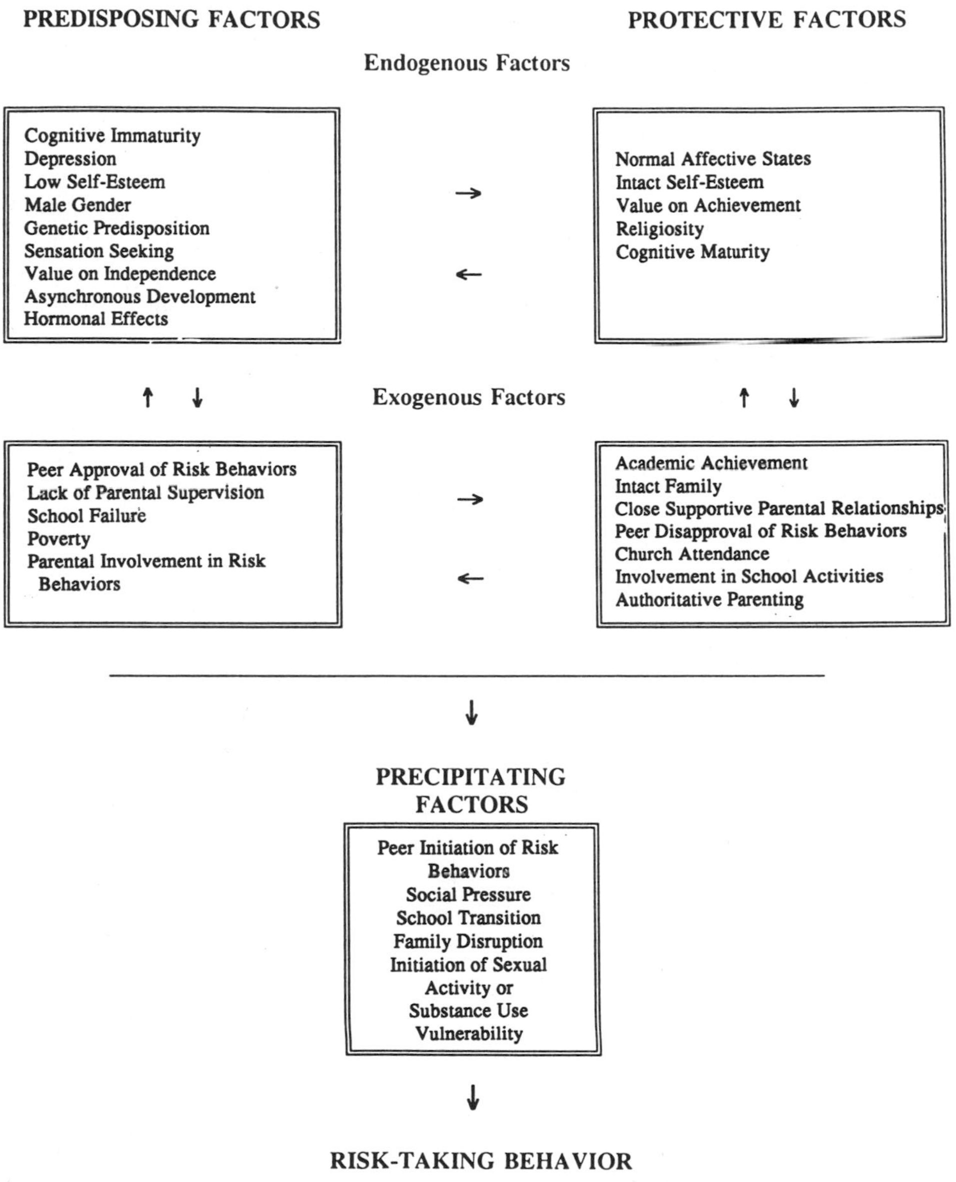

PREDISPOSING FACTORS   **PROTECTIVE FACTORS**

Endogenous Factors

| Cognitive Immaturity
Depression
Low Self-Esteem
Male Gender
Genetic Predisposition
Sensation Seeking
Value on Independence
Asynchronous Development
Hormonal Effects | →

 ← | Normal Affective States
Intact Self-Esteem
Value on Achievement
Religiosity
Cognitive Maturity |

↑ ↓   Exogenous Factors   ↑ ↓

| Peer Approval of Risk Behaviors
Lack of Parental Supervision
School Failure
Poverty
Parental Involvement in Risk
  Behaviors | →

 ← | Academic Achievement
Intact Family
Close Supportive Parental Relationships
Peer Disapproval of Risk Behaviors
Church Attendance
Involvement in School Activities
Authoritative Parenting |

↓

**PRECIPITATING
FACTORS**

Peer Initiation of Risk
Behaviors
Social Pressure
School Transition
Family Disruption
Initiation of Sexual
Activity or
Substance Use
Vulnerability

↓

RISK-TAKING BEHAVIOR

Figure 2. Factors contributing to the onset of risk-taking behaviors during adolescence (Irwin & Ryan, 1989; Irwin & Millstein, 1986).

CONCLUSION

Given a set of biological and psychological predispositions in a particular social environmental milieu, some adolescents will engage in risk-taking behaviors and some will not. Furthermore, some adolescents will experiment in a limited way and others will establish health-endangering life-styles that will jeopardize their futures. Clearly there are protective as well as predisposing biological, psychological, and social/environmental (or perhaps cultural) factors. Few theories of adolescent risk-taking have specifically incorporated these potentially mitigating factors. Further research is needed to understand the variable trajectories of risk-taking behaviors in adolescents and young adults.

Risk-taking behaviors can be viewed as alternate vehicles for achieving developmental tasks of adolescence such as individuation from the family, identification with a peer group, or achieving adult status. Given this perspective, motivations for engaging in the various behaviors will vary at different developmental stages during adolescence. Whereas alcohol use and sexual activity are "normative" by late adolescence, the onset of these behaviors in middle or early adolescence has a different significance for society, and has a different meaning for adolescents at different stages of their development. Similarly, the various factors found to be associated with the onset of risk behaviors may be more or less influential at different stages during adolescence.

The values and meanings adolescents assign to risk-taking behaviors at various stages in their development remain uncertain. Similarly, although rates of risk behaviors are known to vary in different cultural and ethnic groups, the cultural significance of, and the role that cultural factors play in risk-taking behaviors have not been addressed. Future research should focus on dynamic models that accommodate the changing biological, psychological, social, and cultural contexts in adolescents' development. Optimally this research will translate into more effective, developmentally based intervention strategies in the future.

ACKNOWLEDGMENT.   During the preparation of this manuscript, the authors were supported in part by a grant from the Maternal and Child Health Bureau (MCJ 000978).

REFERENCES

Adger, H. (1991). Problems of alcohol and other drug abuse in adolescents. *Journal of Adolescent Health, 12,* 606–613.
Andrucci, G. L., Archer, R. P., Pancoast, D. L., & Gordon, R. A. (1989). The relationship of MMPI and sensation seeking scales to adolescent drug use. *Journal of Personality Assessment, 53,* 253–266.
Bachman, J. G., Wallace, J. M., O'Malley, P. M., Johnston, L. D., Kurth, C. L. & Neighbors, H. W. (1991). Racial/ethnic differences in smoking, drinking, and illicit drug use among American high school seniors, 1976–89. *American Journal of Public Health, 81,* 372–377.
Baumrind, D. (1987). A developmental perspective on adolescent risk taking in contemporary America. In C. E. Irwin (Ed.), *Adolescent social behavior and health. New directions for child development* (pp. 93–125). Social and Behavioral Science Series, No. 37, Fall. San Francisco: Jossey Bass.
Baumrind, D. (1991). The influence of parenting style on adolescent competence and substance abuse. *Journal of Early Adolescence, 11,* 56–95.

Bijur, P. E., Kurzon, M., Hamelsky, V., & Power, C. (1991). Parent–adolescent conflict and adolescent injuries. *Journal of Developmental and Behavioral Pediatrics, 12,* 92–97.

Billy, J. O. G., & Udry, J. R. (1985). The influence of male and female best friends on adolescent sexual behavior. *Adolescence, 20,* 21–32.

Blum, R. W. (1991). Global trends in adolescent health. *Journal of the American Medical Association, 265,* 2711–2719.

Brooks-Gunn, J. (1988). Antecedents and consequences of variations in girls maturational timing. *Journal of Adolescent Health Care, 9,* 1–9.

Centers for Disease Control. (1991). Premarital sexual experience among adolescent women—United States, 1970–1988. *Morbidity and Mortality Weekly Report, 39*(Nos. 51 & 52), 929–932.

Centers for Disease Control and Prevention. (1993). Reduction in alcohol-related traffic fatalities—United States, 1990–1992. *Morbidity and Mortality Weekly Report, 42,* 905–909.

Cloninger, C. R. (1987). Neurogenetic adaptive mechanisms in alcoholism. *Science, 236,* 410–416.

Covey, L. S., & Tam, D. (1990). Depressive mood, the single-parent home and adolescent cigarette smoking. *American Journal of Public Health, 80*(11), 1330–1333.

Crockett, L. J., & Petersen, A. C. (1993). Adolescent development: Health risks and opportunities for health promotion. In S. G. Millstein, A. C. Petersen, & E. O. Nightingale (Eds.), *Promoting the health of adolescents: New directions for the twenty-first century* (pp. 13–37). London: Oxford University Press.

Dielman, T. E., Campanelli, P. C., Shope, J. T., & Butchart, A. T. (1987). Susceptibility to peer pressure, self-esteem, and health locus of control as correlates of adolescent substance abuse. *Health Education Quarterly, 14,* 207–221.

Donovan, J. E., Jessor, R., & Costa, F. M. (1988). Syndrome of problem behavior in adolescence: A replication. *Journal of Consulting and Clinical Psychology, 56,* 762–765.

Donovan, J. E., Jessor, R., & Costa, F. M. (1991). Adolescent health behavior and conventionality-unconventionality: An extension of problem-behavior theory. *Health Psychology, 10,* 52–61.

Dryfoos, J. G. (1990). *Adolescents at risk.* London: Oxford University Press.

Elkind, D. (1967). Egocentrism and adolescence. *Child Development, 38,* 1025–1034.

Elliott, D. S. (1993). Health-enhancing and health compromising lifestyles. In S. G. Millstein, A. C. Petersen, & E. O. Nightingale (Eds.), *Promoting the health of adolescents: New directions for the twenty-first century* (pp. 119–145). London: Oxford University Press.

Farrington, D. P., Loeber, R., & Van Kammen, W. (1990). Cited in U.S. Congress Office of Technology Assessment. (1991). *Adolescent health: Vol. II. Background and the effectiveness of selected prevention and treatment services* (OTA-H-466). Washington, DC: U.S. Government Printing Office.

Fischoff, B. (1992). Risk taking: A developmental perspective. In J. F. Yates (Ed.), *Risk-taking behavior* (pp. 132–162). New York: Wiley.

Flay, B. R. (1985). Psychosocial approaches to smoking prevention: A review of findings. *Health Psychology, 4*(5), 449–488.

Flewelling, R. L., & Bauman, K. E. (1990). Family structure as a predictor of initial substance use and sexual intercourse in early adolescence. *Journal of Marriage and Family, 52,* 171–181.

Forman, S., Irwin, C. E., Jr., & Turner, R. (1990). Family structure, emotional distancing and risk-taking behavior in adolescents. *Pediatric Research, 27,* 5A.

Friedman, I. M. (1985). Alcohol and unnatural deaths in San Francisco youths. *Pediatrics, 76,* 191–193.

Furby, L., & Beyth-Maron, R. (1990). *Risk taking in adolescence: A decision making perspective.* Washington, DC: Carnegie Council on Adolescent Development.

Greening, L., & Dollinger, S. J. (1991). Adolescent smoking and perceived vulnerability to smoking related causes of death. *Journal of Pediatric Psychology, 16*(6), 687–699.

Hawkins, J. D., & Fitzgibbon, J. J. (1993). Risk factors and risk behaviors in prevention of adolescent substance abuse. In M. Schydlower & P. D. Rogers (Eds.), *Adolescent medicine state of the art reviews: Adolescent substance abuse and addictions, 4*(2), 249–262.

Hayes, C. D. (1987). *Risking the future: Adolescent sexuality and child bearing.* Vol. I. Washington, DC: National Academy Press.

Irwin, C. E., Jr. (Ed.). (1987). Adolescent social behavior and health. *New Directions for Child Development, 37,* 1–12.

Irwin, C. E., Jr. (1990). The theoretical concept of at-risk adolescents. *Adolescent Medicine: State of the Art Reviews, 1,* 1–14.

Irwin, C. E., Jr., & Millstein, S. G. (1986). Biopsychosocial correlates of risk-taking behaviors during adolescence. *Journal of Adolescent Health Care, 7,* 82S–96S.

Irwin, C. E., Jr., & Ryan, S. A. (1989). Problem behaviors of adolescence. *Pediatrics in Review, 10,* 235–246.

Irwin, C. E., Jr., & Shafer, M. A (1992). Adolescent sexuality: The problem of negative outcomes of a normative behavior. In D. Rogers & E. Ginzberg (Eds.), *Adolescents at risk medical and social perspectives* (pp. 35–79). Boulder, CO: Westville Press.

Jessor, R. (1976). Predicting time of onset of marijuana use: A developmental study of high school youth. *Journal of Consulting and Clinical Psychology, 44,* 125–134.

Jessor, R. (1982). Problem behavior and developmental transition in adolescence. *Journal of School Health, May,* 295–300.

Jessor, R. (1991). Risk behavior in adolescence: A psychosocial framework for understanding and action. *Journal of Adolescent Health Care, 12,* 597–605.

Jessor, R., Chase, C. A., & Donovan, J. E. (1980). Psychosocial correlates of marijuana use and problem drinking in a national sample of adolescents. *American Journal of Public Health, 70,* 604–613.

Jessor, R., Costa, F., Jessor, S. L., & Donovan, J. E. (1983). Time of first intercourse: A prospective study. *Journal of Personality and Social Psychology, 44,* 608–626.

Jessor, R., & Jessor, S. L. (1977). *Problem behavior and psychological development: A longitudinal study of youth.* New York: Academic Press.

Johnston, L. D., O'Malley, P. M., & Bachman, J. G. (1993). *National survey results on drug use from the Monitoring the Future Study, 1975–1992* (NIH publication #93-3597). Rockville, MD: National Institute on Drug Abuse. U.S. Department of Health and Human Services, Public Health Service, National Institutes of Health.

Kandel, D. B. (1985). On processes of peer influences in adolescent drug use: A developmental perspective. *Advances in Alcohol and Substance Abuse, 4*(3–4), 139–163.

Kandel, D. B., & Logan, J. A. (1984). Patterns of drug use from adolescence to early adulthood: I. Periods of risk for initiation, continued use and discontinuation. *American Journal of Public Health, 74,* 660–665.

Kazdin, A. E. (1989). Developmental psychopathology: Current research, issues and directions. *American Psychologist, 44,* 180–187.

Keating, D. P. (1990). Adolescent thinking. In S. S. Feldman & G. R. Elliot (Eds.), *At the threshold: The developing adolescent* (pp. 54–89). Cambridge, MA: Harvard University Press.

Kegeles, S. M., Adler, N. E., & Irwin, C. E., Jr. (1988). Sexually active adolescents and condoms: Changes over one year in knowledge, attitudes and use. *American Journal of Public Health, 78,* 460–461.

McCord, J. (1990). Problem behaviors. In S. S. Feldman & G. R. Elliot (Eds.), *At the threshold: The developing adolescent* (pp. 414–429). Cambridge, MA: Harvard University Press.

Marlatt, G. A., Baer, J. S., Donovan, D. M., & Kivlahan, D. R. (1988). Addictive behaviors: Etiology and treatment. *Annual Review of Psychology, 39,* 223–252.

Millstein, S. G., Irwin, C. E., Jr., Adler, N. E., Cohn, L. D., Kegeles, S. M., & Dolcini, M. M. (1992). High-risk behaviors and health concerns among young adolescents. *Pediatrics, 89,* 422–428.

Moffitt, T. E. (1990). Cited in Earls, F., Cairns, R. B., & Mercy, J. A (1993). The control of violence and the promotion of nonviolence in adolescents. In S. G. Millstein, A. C. Petersen, & E. O. Nightingale (Eds.), *Promoting the health of adolescents: New directions for the twenty–first century* (pp. 285–304). London: Oxford University Press.

Mosher, W. D., & McNally, J. W. (1991). Contraceptive use at first premarital intercourse: United States, 1965–85. *Family Planning Perspectives, 23,* 108–128.

Mott, F. L., & Haurin, R. J. (1988). Linkages between sexual activity and alcohol and drug use among American adolescents. *Family Planning Perspectives, 20,* 128–136.

Muuss, R. E. (1988). *Theories of adolescence* (5th ed.). New York: McGraw–Hill.

Newcomb, M. D., & Bentler, P. M. (1989). Substance use and abuse among children and teenagers. *American Psychologist, 44,* 242–248.

Newcomb, M. D., & McGee, L. (1991). Influence of sensation seeking on general deviance and specific problem behaviors from adolescence to adulthood. *Journal of Personality and Social Psychology, 61,* 614–628.

Newcomer, S., & Udry, J. R. (1987). Parental marital status effects on adolescent sexual behavior. *Journal of Marriage and Family, 49,* 235–240.

Orr, D. P., Wilbrandt, M. L., Brack, C. J., Rauch, S. P., & Ingersoll, G. M. (1989). Reported sexual behaviors and self-esteem among young adolescents. *American Journal of Diseases of Children, 143,* 86–90.

Osgood, D. W., Johnston, L. D., O'Malley, P. M., & Bachman, J. G. (1988). The generality of deviance in late adolescence and early adulthood. *American Sociological Review, 53,* 81–93.

Perry, C. L., Kelder, S. H., & Komro, K. A. (1993). The social world of adolescents: Families, peers and school. In S. G. Millstein, A. C. Petersen, & E. O. Nightingale (Eds.), *Promoting the health of adolescents: New directions for the twenty-first century* (pp. 73–96). London: Oxford University Press.

Phinney, V. G., Jensen, L. C., Olsen, J. A., & Cundick, B. (1990). The relationship between early development and psychosexual behaviors in adolescent females. *Adolescence, 98,* 321–332.

Piaget, J. (1972). Intellectual evolution from adolescence to adulthood. *Human Development, 15,* 1–12.

Richardson, J. L., Dwyer, K., McGuigan, K., Hansen, W. B., Dent, C., Johnson, C. A., Sussman, S. Y., Brannon, B., & Flay, B. (1989). Substance use among eighth-grade students who take care of themselves after school. *Pediatrics, 84,* 556–566.

Rogers, P. D., & Adger, H., Jr. (1993). Alcohol and adolescents. In M. Schydlower & P. D. Rogers (Eds.), *Adolescent medicine state of the art reviews: Adolescent substance abuse and addictions, 4*(2), 295–304.

Schor, E. L. (1987). Unintentional injuries: Patterns within families. *American Journal of Diseases of Children, 141,* 1280–1284.

Sonenstein, F. L., Pleck, J. H., & Ku, L. C. (1991). Levels of sexual activity among adolescent males in the United States. *Family Planning Perspectives, 23,* 162–167.

Steinberg, L. (1990). Autonomy conflict and harmony in the family relationship. In S. S. Feldman & G. R. Elliot (Eds.), *At the threshold: The developing adolescent* (pp. 255–275). Cambridge, MA: Harvard University Press.

Tonkin, R. S. (1987). Adolescent risk-taking behavior. *Journal of Adolescent Health Care, 8,* 213–220.

Tschann, J. M., Adler, N. E., Irwin, C. E., Jr., Millstein, S. G., Turner, R. A., & Kegeles, S. M. (1994). Initiation of substance use in early adolescence: The roles of pubertal timing and emotional distress. *Health Psychology, 13,* 326–333.

Turner, R. A., Irwin, C. E., Jr., Tschann, J. M., & Millstein, S. G. (1993). Autonomy, relatedness, and early initiation of health risk behaviors in early adolescence. *Health Psychology, 12*(3), 200–208.

Udry, J. R. (1990). Biosocial models of adolescent problem behaviors. *Social Biology, 37*(1–2), 1–10.

Udry, J. R., Billy, J. O. G., Morris, N. M., Groff, T. R., & Raj, M. H. (1985). Serum androgenic hormones motivate sexual behavior in adolescent boys. *Fertility and Sterility, 43*(1), 90–94.

Udry, J. R., Talbert, L. M., & Morris, N. M. (1986). Biosocial foundations for adolescent female sexuality. *Demography, 23,* 217–227.

U.S. Preventive Services Task Force. (1989). *Guide to clinical preventive services.* Baltimore: Williams & Wilkins.

Werner, M. J. (1991). *Adolescent substance abuse.* Maternal and Child Health Technical Information Bulletin. Cincinnati: National Center for Education in Maternal and Child Health.

Wintemute, G. J. (1990). Childhood drowning and near-drowning in the United States. *American Journal of Diseases of Children, 144,* 663–669.

Yamaguchi, K., & Kandel, D. B. (1984a). Patterns of drug use from adolescence to young adulthood: II. Sequences of progression. *American Journal of Public Health, 74,* 668–671.

Yamaguchi, K., & Kandel, D. B. (1984b). Patterns of drug use from adolescence to young adulthood: III. Predictors of progression. *American Journal of Public Health, 74,* 673–681.

Zuckerman, M. (1979). *Sensation seeking: Beyond the optimal level of arousal.* Hillsdale, NJ: Erlbaum.

Zuckerman, M. (1990). The psychophysiology of sensation seeking. *Journal of Personality, 58,* 313–341.

Zuckerman, M. (1991). Sensation seeking: The balance between risk and reward. In L. P. Lipsett & L. L. Mitnick (Eds.), *Self-regulatory behavior and risk taking: Causes and consequences* (pp. 143–152). Norwood, NJ: Ablex Publishing.

4

Tobacco Use

CHERYL L. PERRY and MICHAEL J. STAUFACKER

INTRODUCTION

The purpose of this chapter is to review (1) the health consequences of adolescent tobacco use, (2) the epidemiology of tobacco use, (3) prevention strategies that have been successfully evaluated, and (4) tobacco cessation strategies applicable to adolescents. This chapter takes advantage of knowledge synthesized in the recent Surgeon General's report, *Preventing Tobacco Use among Young People* (USDHHS, 1994).

Consequences of Tobacco Use

The use of tobacco by children and adolescents deserves special attention. The adverse health consequences of tobacco use have recognized public health importance. The onset and development of cigarette smoking and smokeless tobacco use occurs primarily in adolescence. Tobacco use is highly addictive. Regular tobacco use in adolescence develops into nicotine dependency, and this behavior is likely to continue into adulthood, increasing the likelihood of long-term adverse health consequences. Recent research has provided sufficient information to support conclusions about the negative short-term effects of tobacco use during childhood and adolescence, as well as the adult health implications of smoking initiated earlier in life.

The adult health implications of smoking among young people are numerous. Smoking during childhood and adolescence appears to increase the risk for developing chronic obstructive pulmonary disease (COPD) in adulthood as well as at an earlier age (Tager *et al.,* 1985; Tager, Segal, Speizer, & Weiss, 1988). Epidemiologic and experimental studies also suggest that the risk of developing cancer, especially lung cancer, is most strongly associated with the duration of cigarette smoking, that is, the number of years

CHERYL L. PERRY and MICHAEL J. STAUFACKER • Division of Epidemiology, University of Minnesota School of Public Health, Minneapolis, Minnesota 55455. *Current address for M. J. S.:* StayWell Health Management Systems, Inc., St. Paul, Minnesota 55120.
Handbook of Adolescent Health Risk Behavior, edited by Ralph J. DiClemente, William B. Hansen, and Lynn E. Ponton. Plenum Press, New York, 1996.

that someone has smoked (Peto, 1977; Doll & Peto, 1978; USDHHS, 1982, 1989, 1990; International Agency for Research on Cancer, 1985). Therefore, the risk of smoking-related cancer is inversely proportional to the age of onset of smoking. Studies show that earlier onset of smoking is also related to heavier smoking in adulthood (Taioli & Wynder, 1991; Escobedo, Marcus, Holtzman, & Giovino, 1993). Heavier smokers are more likely to experience smoking-related morbidity and are the least likely to quit (Hall & Terzhalmy, 1984; USDHHS, 1989).

Effects of Smoking on the Respiratory System

The effects of cigarette smoking on the structure and function of the lung have been reported in both adults and young adults (USDHHS, 1984, 1990; Bates, 1989). Changes in lung structure resulting from smoking include the weakening of an individual's defenses against infectious organisms and inhaled particles and gases, changes in the numbers and types of cells in the lung, and the activation of potentially damaging proteolytic enzymes and the inactivation of the proteins that inhibit them. Manifestations of these effects are observable among adolescent smokers.

Symptoms of respiratory tract injury and disease related to smoking in adults are cough, increased sputum production, wheezing, and shortness of breath. Studies of children and adolescents who are regular smokers (those who have smoked in the past month) show that smoking is also a cause of respiratory symptoms in this age group. Studies over the past 20 years provide consistent evidence that smoking is associated with the occurrence of cough, increased phlegm production, wheezing, and shortness of breath (Holland & Elliott, 1968; Rush, 1974; Weiss, Tager, Speizer, & Rosner, 1980; Oechsli, Seltzer, & Van Den Berg, 1987).

Studies of adults have shown that smokers have a lower level of lung function, as measured by tests of lung mechanics and gas exchange, than persons who have never smoked (USDHHS, 1984; Bates, 1989). Long-term studies show that smoking increases or accelerates the age-related decline of lung function. Children and adolescents also experience the negative effects of smoking on lung function (Seely, Zuskin, & Bouhuys, 1971; Comstock & Rust, 1973; Spinaci et al., 1985) and on the rate of lung growth (Beck, Doyle, & Schachter, 1982; Woolcock, Peat, Leeder, & Blackburn, 1984).

Smoking is related to increased levels of illness in adults, as measured by indicators such as absenteeism from work, use of medical services, or by the frequency or severity of respiratory infections (USDHHS, 1990). Studies of young people also show that smoking increases respiratory illnesses in this age group (Finklea, Hasselblad, Sandifer, Hammer, & Lowrimore, 1971; Blake, Abell, & Stanley, 1988; Schwartz & Zeger, 1990). Comparisons were made in medical care use by smokers and nonsmokers in settings where all medical care was received at a single location (Haynes, Krstulovic, & Bell, 1966). All respiratory illnesses were more evident in the adolescent smokers. This was particularly the case for severe illnesses including COPD.

Cigarette Smoking and Heart Disease

The epidemiological evidence is clear that smoking is a cause of coronary heart disease and stroke in adults (USDHHS, 1989). Studies have shown that atherosclerosis starts in childhood and may become significant in young adulthood (McNamara, Molot, Stremple, & Cutting, 1971; Enos, Holmes, & Beyer, 1986; Strong, 1986). Autopsy studies have demonstrated that cigarette smoking is associated with increased atherosclerosis in young adults (Strong & Richards, 1976; Pathobiological Determinants of Atherosclerosis in Youth Research Group, 1990; Berenson *et al.*, 1992). Smoking among young people is also associated with serum lipids that are predictive of increased risk for cardiovascular diseases (Craig, Palomaki, Johnson, & Haddow, 1990).

More proximal to the cardiovascular health of young people are the effects of smoking on physical fitness. Cigarette smoking adversely affects physical fitness in the areas of both performance and endurance. Smoking reduces the oxygen-carrying ability of the blood and increases the heart rate and the basal metabolic rate. These changes counter the benefits of physical activity as a function of how long the young person has smoked and the total number of cigarettes smoked (Royal College of Physicians of London, 1992).

Nicotine Dependency

Nicotine dependency is one of the most common forms of drug addiction, causing more health problems than all other addictions combined (USDHHS, 1988). Nicotine is a psychoactive or mood-altering substance. In the short term, nicotine acts more like a stimulant than a depressant. Research on nicotine addiction has been done primarily with adults, but the basic biologic processes of this dependency appear to be similar in adolescents and adults. Each year, approximately 20 million people try to quit smoking in the United States (USDHHS, 1990), but only 3% have long-term success (Pierce, Fiore, Novotny, Hatziandreu, & Davis, 1989). The NIDA's 1985 National Household Survey on Drug Abuse (NHSDA) showed that 84% of 12- through 17-year-olds who smoke one pack or more of cigarettes per day felt that they "needed" or were "dependent" on cigarettes (Henningfield, Clayton, & Pollin, 1990). The survey showed that young smokers develop tolerance, increase the amount they smoke, and are unable to abstain from nicotine.

Nicotine dependence is inversely related to the age of initiation of smoking (Breslau, Fenn, & Peterson, 1993). The process of moving from first use to dependency during adolescence takes about 2 to 3 years (USDHHS, 1988; Leventhal, Fleming, & Glynn, 1988). First experiences with smoking are often negative and other social factors become important in keeping an adolescent experimenting until dependency develops (Haertzen, Kocher, & Miyasato, 1983). Data from recent research indicate that more than one out of three young people who try cigarettes increase to regular patterns of use (Hirschman, Leventhal, & Glynn, 1984; McNeill, 1991; Henningfield, Cohen, & Slade, 1991). The degree of addiction can be reliably measured with indicators including the degree of craving when denied, the number of cigarettes smoked daily, and the degree to which smoking persists despite inconvenience or its untoward side effects. For example, individuals who smoke first thing in the morning or who smoke when they are experiencing bad colds are usually considered severely addicted.

Regularity of smoking has been shown to be predictive of the ability of adolescent smokers to remain abstinent when they attempt to quit (Hansen, 1983). A special subgroup of smokers known as chippers, individuals who periodically smoke but never become addicted, have recently been identified. These individuals are very rare, constituting less than 5% of the total smoking population. It is not known what protects this group from addiction.

Smoking as a Risk Factor for Other Drug Use

The 1988 Surgeon General's Report (USDHHS, 1988) reviewed several decades' research on the gateway theory of drug use which has repeatedly demonstrated that cigarette smoking among young people is a risk factor in the development of alcohol use and illegal drug use. Tobacco is generally used by young people before they use marijuana and other illegal drugs (USDHHS, 1994). It is hypothesized that nicotine exposure may lead to a heightened sensitivity to the reinforcing effects of other drugs. This is supported by the finding that the development of tolerance to nicotine is accompanied by the development of tolerance ("cross-tolerance") to alcohol (Burch et al., 1988; Collins, Burch, Defiebre, & Marks, 1988). Research with animals shows that nicotine exposure may change the behavioral responses to alcohol and cocaine (Signs & Schechter, 1986; Horger, Giles, & Schenk, 1992). Therefore, there seems to be a biological basis for a causal role for tobacco use in the development of other substance abuse patterns.

Smokeless Tobacco Use

Various forms of advertising have promoted the benefits of smokeless tobacco with the implication that the use of these products is without danger. This is clearly not the case. The health consequences of smokeless tobacco use among young people are becoming better known. The primary adverse consequences among adults include bad breath, discoloration and abrasion of teeth, dental caries, gum recession, leukoplakia, nicotine dependence, and oral cancer (USDHHS, 1986, 1992; World Health Organization, 1988). Smokeless tobacco use may also be associated with cardiovascular disease and stroke by increasing blood pressure, vasoconstriction, and irregular heart beat (Hsu, Pollack, Hsu, & Going, 1980; Gritz, Baer-Weiss, Benowitz, Van Vunaikis, & Jarvik, 1981; Schroeder & Chen, 1985). Early indicators of all of these conditions are found among young people who use smokeless tobacco (USDHHS, 1994).

Smokeless tobacco users also develop nicotine dependency. The level of addiction is similar to that of smokers (Benowitz, Porchet, Sheiner, & Jacob, 1988), since smokeless tobacco users absorb at least as much nicotine as smokers do (Russell, Jarvis, & Feyerabend, 1980). The high pH of saliva allows efficient absorption of nicotine through the oral mucosa. Adolescents develop physical dependence from smokeless tobacco use as shown by documented withdrawal symptoms when they try to quit (Hatsukami, Gust, & Keenan, 1987).

Young people who use smokeless tobacco products are at greater risk to smoke cigarettes than are nonusers. Among smokeless tobacco users, 12 to 30% also smoke cigarettes (Eakin, Severson, & Glasgow, 1989; Williams, 1992; CDC, 1993). For young people who use both smokeless tobacco and cigarettes, cessation of one may lead to an increase in the other. Smokeless tobacco use is also predictive of other drug use. Smokeless tobacco users are significantly more likely to use cigarettes, marijuana, or alcohol than nonusers (Ary, Lichtenstein, & Severson, 1987).

EPIDEMIOLOGY

Despite at least three decades of efforts to prevent tobacco use among children and adolescents, large numbers of young people continue to smoke and use smokeless tobacco. Over 3 million adolescents currently smoke cigarettes, and over 1 million young males use smokeless tobacco products (USDHHS, 1994). Accurate data on levels of tobacco use and trends in use are essential for planning prevention programs.

The data for this section are derived from three national surveillance systems that document health behaviors among adolescents. These data were recently analyzed specifically around youth tobacco use (USDHHS, 1994). The first surveillance system, the National Teenage Tobacco Surveys (NTTS), was conducted by the U.S. Public Health Service and the U.S. Department of Education in 1968, 1970, 1972, 1974, and 1979. A similar version of this survey was done in 1989 as the Teenage Attitudes and Practices Survey (TAPS). The Monitoring the Future Project (MTFP) surveys have been conducted annually from 1976 for the National Institute on Drug Abuse by the University of Michigan's Institute for Social Research (Johnston, O'Malley, & Bachman, 1994).

Patterns of Cigarette Smoking

Based on data from TAPS and MTFP, approximately two-thirds of adolescents in the United States have ever tried smoking by age 18. The overall national prevalence of current smoking (i.e., having smoked within the last 30 days) for 12- to 18-year-olds was 16% in the 1989 TAPS. (This suggests that over 3 million young people in the United States are current smokers.)

All measures of smoking reveal that smoking consistently increases as a function of age and grade level. Among 12th grade students surveyed in 1991, 22% of TAPS and 40% of MTFP students reported that they had tried their first cigarette by age 14. About 60% of the young people in the MTFP and about 50% of those in the TAPS reported that they had smoked by their senior year, representing 80–90% of the potential adult smokers. Daily smoking began by age 16 for about 20% of the adolescents in the MTFP. By their senior year, 29% of these people had become daily smokers.

The TAPS surveys also show that the prevalence of ever smoking is greater among males than females. Current prevalence among males was equal to or slightly higher than current prevalence for females. This pattern is different from that reported in the late 1970s and mid-1980s, when the prevalence for young females was higher than that for males (USDHEW, 1979; USDHHS, 1989). Prior to the late 1970s, smoking among youth was primarily a male-dominated activity. The pattern of gender involvement in smoking generally reflects changes in sex stereotyping of society at large.

White students have the highest prevalence of ever smoking and black students the lowest prevalence. Both white males and white females show a considerably higher current smoking prevalence than black males and black females. In the 1989 TAPS, 8% of

12- to 18-year-olds were frequent smokers, that is, they had smoked on 20 or more of the 30 days prior to the survey. Ten percent of high school seniors in the 1992 MTFP were heavy smokers, smoking at least one-half pack per day. Young men were slightly more likely than females to be frequent or heavy smokers. White adolescents were more likely than black or Hispanic adolescents to be frequent or heavy smokers. Among whites, frequent and heavy smoking was 2.8 to 7.5 times more common than among blacks and 2.3 to 2.6 times more common than among Hispanic young people.

Sociodemographic factors such as age, socioeconomic status, gender, and ethnic group are important to the understanding of the onset and maintenance of adolescent tobacco use. These and other factors will be discussed in the section on etiology.

Trends in Cigarette Smoking

The prevalence of ever smoking among adolescents has declined since the 1970s as evidenced by data from the NTTS and the MTFP (USDHHS, 1994). Current smoking prevalence over the past 20 years shows that for both males and females, past month smoking declined considerably in the late 1970s or early 1980s (USDHHS, 1994). Since that time, the data show little or no change, with about 29% of seniors smoking in the past month. However, the most recent (1993) MTFP data suggest that tobacco use is even beginning to increase among adolescents (Figure 1).

For both black and white older adolescents (17–19 years), the prevalence of current smoking declined during the late 1970s or early 1980s (USDHHS, 1994). In the

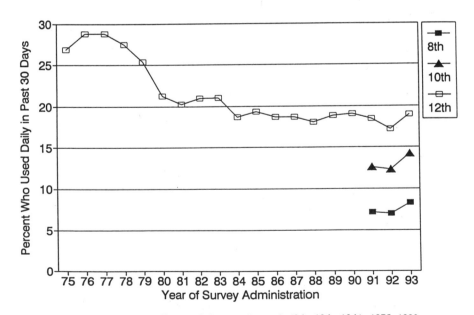

Figure 1. Trends in daily use of cigarettes by grade (8th, 10th, 12th), 1975–1993.

mid-1970s, current smoking prevalence was almost equal among blacks and whites. By the end of the decade, black adolescents were less likely to be current smokers than white adolescents; this trend continued into the 1980s.

Bachman, Johnston, and O'Malley (1991) used MTFP trend data to examine daily smoking among racial and ethnic groups. Generally, for Asian, black, white, Hispanic, and American Indian male and female high school seniors, the prevalence of daily smoking declined from 1976 through 1979 and from 1980 through 1984. The decline continued at a slower rate during the late 1980s for most groups and stopped altogether among white males.

Using national surveys conducted between 1955 and 1988 (NCHS, 1970; USDHEW, 1955; USDHHS, 1980, 1989, 1991; CDC, 1992b), the age at which people became regular smokers was measured. Data from these surveys generally show that people became regular smokers at progressively younger ages over the past four decades.

Stages of Smoking Initiation

Young people progress through a series of stages of smoking onset (Leventhal & Cleary, 1980; Flay, D'Avernas, Best, Kersell, & Ryan, 1983; Flay, 1993). During the *preparatory* or precontemplation stage, attitudes and beliefs about smoking are formed. The young person may begin to view smoking as serving some function, such as a way to appear mature, cope with stress, bond with a peer group, or show independence (Perry, Murray, & Klepp, 1987). The *trying* stage includes the first few times a young person smokes; encouragement of peers is usually involved in this stage (Conrad, Flay, & Hill, 1992). *Experimentation* includes repeated but irregular smoking and is generally in response to a particular situation (such as a party) or to a particular person (such as a date). The fourth stage, *regular use,* occurs when a young person smokes regularly (usually weekly) and smokes in a variety of settings and with a variety of people. Physiological need characterizes the last stage of *addiction.* This need includes tolerance of nicotine, withdrawal symptoms if the adolescent tries to quit, and a high likelihood of relapse if the person does quit (Flay, 1993).

Generally, it takes an average of 2 to 3 years from the time of the initial try of a cigarette to the stage of regular use (Leventhal *et al.,* 1988). This implies that it is important to study the risk factors related to first use as well as to regular use. If a young person can become a regular smoker in 2–3 years, then secondary school is the critical time in the life span for intervention programs (Evans *et al.,* 1978). A primary goal of these efforts should be to encourage, support, cajole, and expect nonsmoking until at least age 18.

Brand Preference

It is important to know which brands of cigarettes young people are using; this knowledge is useful for the development of smoking prevention and intervention programs. It also provides information about the influence of cigarette advertising and promotion on young people.

More than two-thirds (68.7%) of the 1989 TAPS respondents who usually purchased their own cigarettes bought Marlboro. There were no significant differences in this choice by gender, Hispanic origin, age, or region of the country. White adolescents were much more likely to smoke Marlboro than were black adolescents (71 versus 9%). During this period, Newport and Camel each accounted for only 8% (a relatively minor share of the overall market). Black smokers were more likely to smoke Newport than were white smokers (61 versus 6%). Smokers who lived in the Northeast and Midwest were more likely to smoke Newport cigarettes than were smokers in the South and West.

In a 1990 survey of 9th grade students in ten communities in the Community Intervention Trial for Smoking Cessation (COMMIT) evaluation, 43% of smokers who usually bought their own cigarettes bought Marlboro, 30% bought Camel, and 20% bought Newport (CDC, 1992a). This suggests that Camel cigarettes may be gaining in popularity among adolescent smokers. Studies by DiFranza et al. (1991) and Pierce, Naquin, Gilpin, Giovino, and Mills (1991) also show increased rates of Camel cigarette preference among young smokers similar to those found in the COMMIT survey. This increase in Camel's popularity coincides with the launch of the Joe Camel advertising campaign, which uses a cartoonlike character portrayed participating in high-pressure situations that has attracted national attention (DiFranza et al., 1991).

Smoking and Other Drug Use

In the MTFP data, cigarette smoking prevalence among alcohol, smokeless tobacco, marijuana, cocaine, and inhalant users was about 2 to 4 times greater than among non-users of these substances (USDHHS, 1994). The majority of marijuana (62%), cocaine (68%), and inhalant (56%) users were smokers. Although a majority of alcohol drinkers did not smoke, almost all smokers (88%) used alcohol. Forty-five percent of smokers were also marijuana users, 11% were cocaine users, 5% used inhalants, and 33% used smokeless tobacco. The prevalence of other drug use was from 1.6 to 5.2 times greater among cigarette smokers than nonsmokers.

The MTFP surveys from 1986 to 1989 show that among ever smokers, 61% first smoked and 53% had used smokeless tobacco by the 8th grade. Fewer users of alcohol, marijuana, and cocaine started use as early as users of cigarettes and smokeless tobacco. Thirty-four percent of alcohol users, 26% of marijuana users, and 6% of cocaine users first tried these drugs by the eighth grade. These data suggest that nicotine is a "gateway" drug and its use, either cigarettes or smokeless, is likely to precede use of other drugs (Kandel, 1975).

Patterns of Smokeless Tobacco Use

The national estimates for adolescents who had tried smokeless tobacco were 18% for 12- through 18-year-olds in the 1989 TAPS and 32% for high school seniors in the 1992 MTFP. Males were much more likely than females to have tried smokeless tobacco, and white males were more likely than any other subgroup. The prevalence of those who had used smokeless tobacco increased with increasing age. In the 1986 through 1989

MTFP surveys, high school seniors' past month use of smokeless tobacco declined slightly for all respondents (from 12 to 8%), for whites (from 13 to 10%), and for males (from 22 to 16%) (Bachman, Johnston, & O'Malley, 1987, 1991; Johnston, Bachman, & O'Malley, 1991, 1992).

PREVENTION

Tobacco prevention and cessation programs have been developed based on an understanding of the etiology of tobacco use. Interventions are designed to alter modifiable mediating processes, risk factors, and protective factors that influence the onset, development, and maintenance of tobacco use. Tobacco use among young people is explained by sociodemographic, environmental, behavioral, and personal factors that increase an adolescent's chances of initiating tobacco use and of experiencing the adverse health effects of continued use. These psychosocial factors can be conceptualized on a continuum of proximal and distal factors. Personal and behavioral factors that directly and immediately affect an adolescent's choice to use tobacco are considered proximal. Distal factors are those environmental and sociodemographic conditions and influences that are thought to act indirectly to affect tobacco use. However, distal factors, such as the effects of advertising, may influence proximal factors, such as the perceived benefits of smoking, and therefore strongly influence the ultimate use of tobacco.

The psychosocial factors related to smoking behavior are grounded in theories guided by the work of Levanthal (1968), Bandura (1977), Evans et al. (1978), McAlister, Perry, and Maccoby (1979), and McGuire (1984). Smoking is seen as a social behavior with social causes, functions, and reinforcements; previous theoretical and research efforts viewed cigarette smoking primarily as a health behavior.

Psychological Risk Factors of Cigarette Smoking

Smoking onset occurs in early adolescence. The peak age group for initiation and experimentation is ages 11 through 15 (sixth through ninth grades) (Alexander et al., 1983; Coombs, Fawzy, & Gerber, 1986). Socioeconomic status (SES) is an important risk factor (Conrad et al., 1992). Generally, lower-SES youth are at greater risk to begin smoking, possibly because they have fewer opportunities for healthy development and parental supervision. There is no longer a gender difference, another risk factor, but the functional meanings of cigarette use and the progress to regular use may be different by gender (Grunberg, Winders, & Wewers, 1991). Lastly, except for black adolescents, differences by ethnic group do not show a consistent pattern across communities, especially when income and cigarette availability are taken into account (Fiore et al., 1989; Bachman et al., 1991). Therefore, among sociodemographic factors, a young adolescent from a low-SES family is at highest risk to initiate smoking.

Conrad et al. (1992) conducted a review of 27 prospective studies of the onset of smoking. They found that the influence of peers, friends, and siblings is substantial in the initiation of adolescent smoking; these influences are considered proximal environmental factors. Smoking initiation seems to be a part of peer associations and peer bonding in this age group; smoking may be a shared behavior that certain groups use to differentiate themselves from other peers and from adults. Adolescents usually try their first cigarette with their peers; peers may then provide expectations, reinforcement, and opportunities for continuation. The influence of peers may be particularly strong during the preparatory, trying, and experimentation stages; during the regular use and addiction stages, personal and pharmacological factors may become more important.

Another proximal environmental factor, parental smoking, appears to have the strongest influence for white and female adolescents, especially in the early stages of smoking (Bauman, Foshee, Linzer, & Koch, 1990; Chassin, Presson, Montello, Sherman, & McGrew, 1990; Sussman, Dent, Flay, Hansen, & Johnson, 1987). A review of the literature suggests that this influence may also include other factors, such as parental approval or disapproval of smoking, parental involvement in adolescents' free-time supervision, the style and extent of parental communication on health-related matters, and whether or not parents promote academic achievement for their children.

The perceived social environment also has an influence on adolescent smoking behavior. Surveys consistently show that young people overestimate the number of their peers and adults who smoke and those with the highest estimates are more likely to become smokers (Gerber & Newman, 1989; Leventhal, Fleming, & Glynn, 1988; Collins et al., 1987). If young people feel that peers approve of smoking and adults do not disapprove, they are more likely to smoke. It is possible that the perceived environment accurately reflects the real environment; young people who start to smoke may be exposed to more smoking role models, more peer approval, and less adult disapproval than those adolescents who never start to smoke. However, it is equally likely that exaggerated norms promote experimentation independently of overt pressures to try smoking. The fact that beliefs held by young people about the prevalence and acceptability of smoking suggests that interventions might be successfully targeted at correcting these errors in perception (Hansen & Graham, 1991).

Proximal to cigarette smoking are a variety of behavioral factors. Several patterns of behavior are associated with smoking; these include alcohol and other drug use (Fleming, Leventhal, Glynn, & Ershler, 1989; Newcomb & Bentler, 1986), risk-taking and rebellious behavior (Conrad et al., 1992), and involvement in peer groups at a relatively early age (Brunswick & Messeri, 1984). Those behaviors that are associated with less risk of smoking include academic achievement (Gerber & Newman, 1989; Chassin, Presson, & Sherman, 1990), involvement in sports (for females) (Swan, Creeser, & Murray, 1990), healthy eating and physical activity patterns (Kelder, 1992), and the skills to resist offers of cigarettes (Conrad et al., 1992). By supporting and providing opportunities for healthy activities and academic achievement, prevention of some adolescent smoking may be achieved by fulfilling some "needs" that smoking might meet for young people.

A variety of personal factors are also thought to have proximal and direct influences on an individual's decision to smoke cigarettes. Although an adolescent's general knowledge of the adverse health consequences of smoking is a poor predictor of subsequent use, smoking risks that are personalized and individualized appear to be important. The perceived positive functions of smoking as well as an expected utility of cigarette use are significant predictors (Leventhal & Cleary, 1980; Perry et al., 1987; Bauman, Fisher,

Bryan, & Chenoweth, 1984). These factors are related to having a positive social image, bonding with peers, and being "mature"; all are socially relevant for teenagers. Those young people who start to smoke appear to have lower self-images and lower self-esteem than their nonsmoking peers (Conrad *et al.*, 1992). Self-efficacy in avoiding cigarettes seems closely linked with the ability to resist cigarette offers from peers (Stacy, Sussman, Dent, Burton, & Flay, 1992). There is limited evidence to support the predictive nature of some personality variables, including symptoms of depression, helplessness, aggression, pessimism, and an inability to consider future consequences. The most predictive personal factors are those related to the social environment, to peers, and to the functional meanings of cigarette smoking.

Other factors that strongly predict future smoking include intentions to smoke and prior experimentation (Conrad *et al.*, 1992). The initial adverse physiological reactions to initial smoking diminish with repeated tries, and tolerance to nicotine increases. Nicotine dependence is associated with a shift from social to more personal, individual reasons for smoking. The MTFP provides useful and interesting data on young people's expectations about smoking or not smoking in the future. Among high school seniors (1976–1986), about 1% said they "definitely" would be smoking in 5 years, 14% said they "probably" would, 27% said they probably would not, and 58% said they definitely would not. Five years after graduation, 32% of these former seniors were current smokers; 27% were daily smokers. Generally, seniors' expectations to smoke in the future were not predictive of future smoking behavior. The expectation of being a nonsmoker was associated with less subsequent smoking only among nonsmokers and very light smokers in high school, although few seniors in these groups reported an intention to smoke. Among daily smokers, the expectation to become a nonsmoker in 5 years was not as predictive of subsequent smoking as was their daily smoking behavior. These findings suggest the importance of prevention education and cessation efforts with young people that highlight the addictive nature of nicotine and its ability to overpower the notion that one can quit at any time.

Cultural and community-level research on the effects of taxation, restrictions of public smoking, vending machine regulations, and limiting access for underage buyers is necessary and under way (Chapman & Bloch, 1992; Sweanor *et al.*, 1992). Research is needed on which factors, such as rules, consistency of rule enforcement, grade structure, or discipline procedures, contribute to smoking onset (Best *et al.*, 1984; Semmer, Lippert, Fuchs, Cleary, & Schindler, 1987). These distal factors help determine the meaning and acceptability of cigarette use at the broader community level. They also determine the difficulty with which young people can obtain cigarettes or inhibit the continued use into adulthood.

Psychosocial Risk Factors of Smokeless Tobacco Use

The knowledge and research base on smokeless tobacco initiation is limited when compared with the literature on smoking. The factors associated with smokeless tobacco use are very similar to those associated with cigarette smoking. Most young people perceive that smokeless tobacco use can be harmful to health (USDHHS, 1986b); but most smokeless tobacco users do not perceive the risk to be great, especially compared with the risk of cigarette smoking (Ary *et al.*, 1987). Peer role modeling is strongly and consistently related to the onset and continued use of smokeless tobacco. Smokeless tobacco use also serves social functions within the peer group that may support experimentation and continued use (Ary *et al.*, 1987; Ary, 1989). Peer and parental acceptance of smokeless tobacco use is much higher than for cigarette smoking (USDHHS, 1986).

Risk-taking behavior and poor academic performance also appear to be related to the use of smokeless tobacco (Dent, Sussman, Johnson, Hansen, & Flay, 1987; Jones & Moberg, 1988). There is conflicting evidence that smokeless tobacco use is associated with participation in athletic activities. It is widely observed that members of particular male sports teams such as baseball players promote smokeless tobacco use as part of an informal ritual of group membership. It is clear, however, that membership on many other sports teams does not necessarily promote smokeless tobacco use. The perception that smokeless tobacco use is a healthier choice than cigarette smoking consistently arises from the research literature and indicates the need for prevention programs that emphasize the negative health consequences of smokeless tobacco use.

Smokeless tobacco use shares a common etiology with cigarette smoking among young adolescents. Smokeless tobacco use seems to be a function of the social world of adolescents who see this "adult" behavior as a way to improve their individual social image and thereby fit in. Therefore, peer use of smokeless tobacco is a strong motivator for initiation and continuation. The general misperceptions of both adolescents and adults about the health-compromising, addictive aspects of smokeless tobacco use are of great concern and should be a continued focus of intervention efforts.

Tobacco Advertising and Promotion

In 1990, cigarette companies spent almost 4 billion dollars on advertising and promotional activities (Federal Trade Commission, 1992). These expenditures made cigarettes the second most promoted consumer product (after automobiles) in the United States. Smokeless tobacco advertising and promotional expenditures have increased steadily from 80 million dollars in 1985 to over 104 million dollars in 1991 (Federal Trade Commission, 1992).

The tobacco industry claims that the purpose of advertising and promotional activities is to encourage brand-switching and to increase market shares of adult consumers. Yet, the evidence shows that some young people are recruited to smoking by brand advertising. This assertion is supported by data showing that adolescents consistently smoke the most heavily advertised brands of cigarettes (McCarthy & Gritz, 1984; Baker, Homel, Flaherty, & Trebilco, 1987; DiFranza *et al.*, 1991). In addition, after the introduction of advertisements that target young people, the prevalence of use of those brands increases. After the 1968 introduction of Virginia Slims, smoking prevalence among young females went from 8% in 1968 to 15% in 1974 (USDHHS, 1980). After an intensive advertising and promotion campaign in the 1970s that focused on "starters," smokeless tobacco use increased substantially among young men (Tye, Warner, & Glantz, 1987). In the past few years, Camel's Old Joe campaign has resulted in a greater percentage of young people who are now smoking Camel cigarettes (DiFranza *et al.*, 1991).

Cigarette advertising and promotional activities appear to influence psychosocial risk factors for adolescent tobacco use; these mechanisms are multiple and complementary (USDHHS, 1994). Most young people are aware of and recognize cigarette advertisements and brands. They develop preferences for particular advertisements. Some young people approve of tobacco advertising and are more likely to initiate smoking or already be smoking. Cigarette advertising uses images rather than information to portray the attractiveness and function of smoking. Advertisements provide images of smokers that are perceived by adolescents to have attributes they desire—independence, healthfulness, adventure-seeking, and youthful activities. These advertisements are particularly potent with adolescents whose lower self-images predispose them to initiate smoking. These images are found in abundance in the lives of young people through the print media such as youth-oriented magazines and billboards, in-store point-of-sale displays, distribution of specialty items, and at entertainment and sporting events.

Adolescents perceive cigarette advertising as promoting benefits of smoking; these perceptions are not solely related to young people's exposure to adult smokers (Pierce *et al.*, 1993). Advertising promotes an ideal self-image by portraying attributes or benefits of smoking that young people would like to possess. For those adolescents with a lower self-image, smoking is a way to close the gap between their actual and ideal self-image; the ideal self-image may closely resemble the images of smokers in advertisements (McCarthy & Gritz, 1984). Adolescents with the greatest distance between their actual self-image and their ideal self-image are most likely to have intentions to smoke (Burton, Moinuddin, & Grenier, 1992). Advertising also seems to affect the accuracy of young people's perceptions of smoking prevalence among their peers and among adults; young people with the greatest overestimations appear to be those most exposed to cigarette advertising and those most likely to begin to smoke (Botvin, Goldberg, Botvin, & Dusenbury, 1993). Many young people in the United States may consider smoking a normative experience and a desirable adult behavior because of the pervasiveness of cigarette advertising (Burton *et al.*, 1992).

Tobacco advertising and promotional activities appear to have an effect of influencing factors that increase the risk of smoking initiation among young people. These psychosocial risk factors—having a low-self image, attributing positive meanings or benefits to smoking, and perceiving smoking as prevalent and normative—strongly predict adolescent smoking intentions and smoking onset.

School-Based Approaches to Smoking Education and Prevention

Prevention strategies in the 1960s and early 1970s were often based on the assumption that young people who smoked did not understand the health-compromising effects of cigarette smoking (Thompson, 1978). It was thought that there was a deficit of information that could be addressed by presenting young people with health information that caught their attention and provided them with sufficient reason not to smoke. Improvement in knowledge would lead directly to changes in behavior. Fear-arousal techniques were often used to try to convince young people that smoking was associated with the risk of serious long-term physical consequences, including premature death in adulthood from cardiovascular disease and cancer.

Although expanded efforts in schools throughout the 1970s provided young people with various kinds of smoking-prevention messages, this information did not deter them from beginning to smoke. Comprehensive reviews concluded that smoking-prevention programs based on the information deficit model were not effective (Thompson, 1978; Goodstadt, 1978). Providing an accurate knowledge base regarding the negative health consequences of smoking is still important, but this single strategy is not sufficient to change most young people's behavior.

The 1970s marked a period of initial program development regarding smoking prevention during which alternative smoking-prevention approaches were considered in an attempt to correct the shortcomings of the information deficit model. One such group of programs were known as *affective education* models and were based on the premise that young people smoke cigarettes because their self-perceptions were compatible with health-compromising behaviors such as smoking (Durell & Bukoski, 1984). Interventions based on this model tried to increase adolescents' perceptions of self-worth and clarify a health-related value system that would support a young person's decision not to smoke. Reviews of research have concluded that affective educational interventions were no more effective in reducing adolescent smoking than the information deficit approach (Hansen, Collins, Johnson, & Graham, 1985).

A second line of prevention research, initiated during the 1970s (Evans *et al.*, 1978) and brought to fruition in the 1980s (Botvin & Dusenbury, 1989; Flay, 1985; Hansen, 1988; McAlister *et al.*, 1979), were programs that utilized social influence strategies. These programs utilized social, psychological, and behavioral theories as a basis for considering approaches that might work to modify patterns of smoking onset among adolescents. Researchers began to design intervention components based directly on findings from theory-based research on adolescent smoking. This led to an improved targeting of the most potent psychosocial risk factors for smoking behavior among adolescents. Much of what was learned focused on social influences, norms, competencies, and intentions that are associated with the maintenance of a nonsmoking life-style. Associated with this shift in orientation, the research methodology used to evaluate prevention programs became increasingly rigorous (Flay, 1985).

This social influences model recognizes the social environment as the most important determinant of smoking onset and focuses on the development of norms and skills to identify and resist social influences to smoke. An underlying assumption of this approach is that young people who smoke may lack skills to identify and deal with various social influences that support smoking. These influences include the misperception that most young people smoke, the perceived desirable social image of smoking, the notion that cigarette smoking is functional, the appeal of cigarette advertising and promotional activities, and the persuasive effects of sibling and peer smoking. Although there is considerable variation across school curricula, programs that instill skills needed to resist social influences have included a fairly consistent set of components that include training in resisting social pressures (e.g., advertising and promotional activities) and peer pressures to smoke and, training that enhances general assertiveness, decision-making, and communication skills (Botvin & Wills, 1985). These programs also promote healthful normative expectations and specifically correct the misperception that most adolescents smoke (Hansen & Graham, 1991). Multiple metaanalyses of smoking prevention programs also support the effectiveness of the social influences curriculum model (Hansen, 1992; Tobler, 1986, 1992; Rooney, 1992; Bruvold, 1993).

The positive effects of even the most successful prevention programs tend to diminish over time (Murray, Pirie, Luepker, & Pallonen, 1989; Pentz *et al.*, 1989; Flay *et al.*, 1989; Ellickson, Bell, & McGuigan, 1993). This has been particularly noted among school-based intervention studies that included little emphasis on booster sessions, few communitywide activities, or few mass media components (Botvin, Renick, & Baker, 1983; Perry, Klepp, & Shultz, 1988; Botvin & Botvin, 1992).

The National Cancer Institute convened a panel of experts in 1987 to reach consensus on the essential elements of school-based smoking-prevention programs (USDHHS, 1991). These elements are shown in Table 1. The emphasis is on the early adolescent grades in school, social influences to smoke, student and parental involvement in the program, adequate teacher training, and cultural sensitivity (Glynn, 1989).

In summary, multiple individual research reports (Botvin & Dusenbury, 1989; Flay *et al.*, 1989), several comprehensive literature reviews (Fay, 1985; Best, Thomson; Santi, Smith, & Brown, 1988), and the metaanalyses mentioned above, have all reported lower smoking rates among students in social influence programs compared with reference students in experimental and quasiexperimental studies. As Best *et al.* (1988) have noted, given the large number of research studies that have evaluated smoking-prevention programs, the variations in program implementation and style, the various communities and cultures in which these studies were undertaken, and the potential threats to validity in school-based research, the consistency of overall reductions in smoking prevalence across studies testing the social influences approach is noteworthy. Promising programs have been developed and are available for distribution, including *The Minnesota Smoking Prevention Program* developed by researchers at the University of Minnesota School of Public Health, *Project SMART* developed by researchers at the University of South California Institute for Prevention Research, *Life Skills Training* developed by Dr. Gil Botvin at the Institute for Prevention Research at Cornell University Medical College, and most recently, *All Stars* developed by Dr. William Hansen at Tanglewood Research (Clemmons, North Carolina).

Table 1. Essential Elements of School-Based Smoking Prevention Programs[a]

1. Classroom sessions should be delivered at least five times per year in each of two years in the sixth through eighth grades.
2. The program should emphasize the social factors that influence smoking onset, short-term consequences, and refusal skills.
3. The program should be incorporated into the existing school curricula.
4. The program should be introduced during the transition from elementary school to junior high or middle school (sixth or seventh grades).
5. Students should be involved in the presentation and delivery of the program.
6. Parental involvement should be encouraged.
7. Teachers should be adequately trained.
8. The program should be socially and culturally acceptable to each community.

[a]From Glynn (1989).

School-Based Approaches to Preventing Smokeless Tobacco Use

Because the increased use of smokeless tobacco among young people is a relatively recent issue, few programs for preventing adolescent use of these products have been evaluated. Those that have been evaluated are often one component of a broad tobacco use prevention program.

The prevention programs that have been evaluated have targeted both smoking and smokeless tobacco use among middle and high school students. The primary focus has been on middle school, grades 6–8. Smokeless tobacco prevention has also been included as part of more comprehensive curricula to prevent drug abuse, such as Here's Looking at You, 2000 (Roberts, Fitzmahan & Associates, Inc., 1986), or as part of community-based interventions to reduce drug use. Seldom have programs to prevent smokeless tobacco use been implemented independent of other substance-use prevention or of a more general tobacco-use prevention program.

In several studies, young people have received a preventive curriculum that targeted both smoking and smokeless tobacco use. Severson et al. (1991) reported on a social influences program that was delivered by regular classroom teachers and by same-age peer leaders in randomly assigned schools. The seven-session program significantly reduced smokeless tobacco use among males in both seventh and (to a lesser extent) ninth grades.

A study by Sussman, Burton, Dent, Stacy, and Flay (1993) reports positive results in their Toward No Tobacco Use (TNT) project for reducing smokeless tobacco use. The study compared four different prevention curricula developed to counteract three types of factors related to the onset of tobacco use: peer approval for using tobacco, incorrect social information about tobacco use, and lack of knowledge about physical consequences of tobacco use. Smokeless tobacco use was significantly less prevalent among students who had received the TNT intervention than among those who had not (Sussman et al., 1993). The results of the evaluation of this ten-lesson curriculum intervention suggest that learning about the physical consequences of smokeless tobacco use can be as successful as a social influences program and that a combination of both is probably best for preventing smokeless tobacco use.

Elder et al. (1993) developed Project SHOUT, a social influences program that has been evaluated in 22 junior high schools in San Diego County, California. Based on an operant conditioning model of tobacco use (Elder & Stern, 1986), the intervention was delivered in randomly assigned schools to seventh-grade students. Intervention and assessment continued for 3 years. Because of multiple school changes at the end of the eighth grade, Project SHOUT used telephone calls and program newsletters for the ninth-grade intervention.

At the 3-year follow-up, the intervention had a significant effect on cigarette use, smokeless tobacco use, and combined cigarette and smokeless tobacco use. The intervention effect was particularly strong during the ninth grade. The investigators concluded that the comprehensive 3-year tobacco-use prevention program has a modest but significant effect on the smokeless tobacco component for junior high school students at the end of ninth grade (Elder et al., 1993).

TREATMENT

The relatively few studies that have examined adolescent smoking cessation vary considerably in scientific quality; many are anecdotal or descriptive accounts of interventions. Various programs and materials for adolescent smoking cessation have been developed and implemented. Cessation programs are sometimes led by peers, teachers, or volunteers. Young smokers are recruited by school newsletters, classes, public address announcements, and posters and bulletin boards. Evidence from descriptive reports and formal research programs indicates that recruitment is difficult, and young smokers are hesitant to become involved in formal cessation programs. In some schools, young smokers are referred to cessation programs for breaking school smoking policies and therefore are not coming to these programs voluntarily.

Smoking Cessation among Young People

Perry, Killen, Telch, Slinkard, and Danaher (1980) conducted a school-based cessation intervention in California schools. Tenth-grade classes in three high schools ($N = 477$) received a program that focused on immediate physiological effects of smoking and on social cues that influence the adoption of smoking. At posttest, the experimental group, compared with the control group, had a significantly greater percentage of students who reported abstinence in the previous week (22 versus 16%) and month (30 versus 24%). Similar significant differences were also found for carbon monoxide measures.

The most comprehensive school-based adolescent smoking cessation study with rural and suburban high schools in Illinois and California was conducted by Burton *et al.* (1993). In each of the 16 treatment schools, students volunteering for a cessation clinic were randomly assigned to a clinic or to a wait-list control group. Clinic students were further randomly assigned to a clinic that addressed addiction or to one that addressed psychosocial issues. Clinics consisted of five sessions over a 1-month period. A follow-up session was held 3 months after the last session. At the 3-month follow-up, when corrected for biochemical verification, 6.8% of clinic participants and 7.9% of control students were abstinent. These negative results are more alarming because the investigators had conducted 31 focus groups to help form the intervention's recruitment strategies and program content (Sussman *et al.*, 1991). This study underscores both the difficulties in conducting adolescent smoking cessation programs and the urgent need for more research in this area.

There is only a small body of research on self-initiated smoking cessation among adolescents. Given the challenges of running organized clinics for adolescents, it is possible that the programs that augment attempted self-initiated cessation may be of increased importance in the future. One reason for placing increased emphasis on such approaches is that, even among adults, most people who quit do so on their own, meaning without the specific assistance of a formal organized group. One study of adolescent smokers (Hansen, Collins, Johnson, & Graham, 1985) found that three variables—holding attitudes that smoking was not moral, the presence of nonsmoking peers, and a lack of beliefs that smoking would result in positive outcomes—predicted smoking cessation. The different variables—a lack of belief that smoking would result in negative consequences, having parents who smoked, and being rebellious and risk-taking—were risk factors for relapsing among those who had made an attempt to quit. These findings and similar findings suggest that youths who smoke can quit on their own if they have appropriate attitudes and social support.

Smokeless Tobacco Cessation

The first published study of smokeless tobacco cessation was reported by Glover (1986), who adapted an American Cancer Society smoking cessation program for use with adults who used smokeless tobacco. Eakin *et al.* (1989) reported an intervention with adolescent male daily users, aged 14 through 18, who were recruited from high schools in Oregon. Of the 21 subjects who completed treatment, 2 subjects had quit using smokeless tobacco by the end of treatment, and 3 subjects were abstinent at the 6-month follow-up.

Burton *et al.* (1993) report results from their school-based cessation clinic model tested in 16 high schools in Illinois and California. When all students who volunteered to participate in the clinic were included in the denominator and the results corrected for biochemical verification, the quit rate for students in the smokeless tobacco clinic was 15%; none of the control students had quit at the 3-month follow-up.

Community Programs

Community-based interventions to prevent smoking are important adjuncts to school-based programs. The limited outcomes of the school-only programs suggest the need to involve parents and the community outside the schools to produce longer-term behavior change.

As part of the Minnesota Heart Health Program, cohorts of students in two communities were surveyed from their 6th grade year in school (1983) until high school graduation (1989). Class of 1989 students in one of the communities took part in 5 years of behavioral health education in schools, and were exposed to a communitywide program on cardiovascular health. The intervention students also had a peer-led, social influences smoking prevention program in the 7th through 9th grades. At each of the annual follow-up surveys from 1984 through 1989, youth from the intervention community had significantly lower smoking prevalence and intensities than youth from the reference community (see Figure 2). At the end of 12th grade, the intervention group had reduced its smoking prevalence by 40% (Perry, Kelder, Murray, & Klepp, 1992).

The Midwestern Prevention Project (MPP) reported by Pentz *et al.* (1989) tested the use of the communitywide implementation of programs designed to prevent the onset of tobacco use. The primary focus of the MPP program remained in the school and the school intervention was the only component experimentally manipulated. Nonetheless, the mobilization of the entire community as a support for the program has been interpreted to be important for the ultimate success of the project. Analyses from students in 42 schools ($N = 5008$) indicated a lower prevalence of past-month smoking at 1-year follow-up for those exposed to the school intervention than for the control group (17 versus 24%). These results demonstrate the feasibility of a large-scale, communitywide effort focused

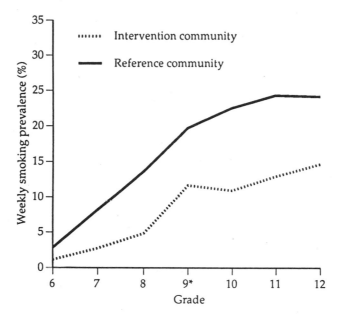

Figure 2. Smoking prevalence of the cohort sample, Class of 1989 Study. *Smoking prevalence adjusted for false negatives in ninth grade. From Perry *et al.* (1992).

exclusively on youth. The program has also demonstrated impact on those young people considered at high risk to initiate smoking.

At the University of Vermont, Worden and colleagues (1988) examined the added efficacy of youth-oriented antitobacco mass media in conjunction with a school-based social influences program. Communities in Montana and Vermont were assigned to a school program only, or to a school program plus a 4-year mass media campaign. At the end of 5 years, students who received both the mass media and school program were smoking at 34–41% lower rates than those with the school program alone (Flynn *et al.*, 1992).

These promising studies of communitywide approaches suggest that communitywide strategies are feasible and can be effective. They may also sustain the effects of the social influences programs in schools by actually changing the social environment of communities. Because of the limited number of such large-scale research studies, more research is needed that is devoted to communitywide strategies.

Policies to Reduce Tobacco Use among Adolescents

Nearly all adolescent smokers report buying their own cigarettes (Gallup Organization, 1993). Reducing the availability of tobacco to young people is critical to the success of prevention efforts. Making tobacco more difficult to obtain provides a significant barrier for young persons who are experimenting with smoking but not yet regular users. Laws that restrict availability to young people also add to the perceived social unacceptability of tobacco use among youth. This normative change could potentially result in lower tobacco use, as is suggested by evidence from two cross-sectional studies (Jason, Ji, Anes, & Birkhead, 1991; DiFranza, Carlson, & Caisse, 1992). Controlling the sale of tobacco to minors emphasizes the dangerous nature of tobacco and places it in the category of regulated products. These laws are consistent with the messages about tobacco that young people receive in school and other settings.

A Model Sale of Tobacco Products to Minors Control Act was proposed by former Secretary of Health and Human Services Louis Sullivan. It contains the following provisions (PHS, 1990): (1) institute 19 years as the minimum age for legal tobacco sales; (2) create a tobacco-sales licensing system similar to that used for alcohol; (3) establish a graduated schedule of penalties for illegal sales; (4) place primary responsibility for enforcement with a designated state agency; local law enforcement and public health officials should participate and have input; (5) use civil penalties and local courts to assess fines; and (6) ban cigarette vending machines. These provisions are currently being proposed as legislation within communities (such as vending machine bans), states (licensing systems), and the federal government. Together, the potential to dissuade underage teens from tobacco use could be greatly enhanced.

A second area of policy with the potential for prevention is in raising the price of tobacco through increased local, state, and federal taxes. Econometric studies consistently show that increasing the price of cigarettes reduces the prevalence of smoking. Adolescents appear to be at least as responsive to price increases as are adults (USDHHS, 1994). In this area, the United States can benefit from the Canadian experience where teenage smoking rates have dropped by 62% nationwide since 1980 (Sweanor, 1992).

SUMMARY

A large number of young people continue to initiate tobacco use in adolescence. The social environment of young people plays a critical role in the initiation process, affecting both distal and proximal factors. Efforts to prevent tobacco use onset need multiple, complementary strategies implemented at the national, state, and community levels. School-based smoking-prevention programs that identify social influences to smoke and teach skills to resist those influences have demonstrated consistent and significant reductions in adolescent smoking prevalence. Programs to prevent smokeless tobacco use that are based on the same model have also demonstrated modest reductions in the initiation of smokeless tobacco use. The effectiveness of school-based programs appears to be enhanced and sustained by communitywide programs that involve mass media, community organizations, or other elements of a young person's social environment. In an environment where tobacco is difficult to obtain and expensive to use, smoking and smokeless tobacco use by young people could substantially decline.

CONCLUSIONS

Since the 1964 Surgeon General's Report on smoking and health, the relationships between cigarette smoking, disease, and death, have become increasingly supported by

research data. Ensuing reports of the Surgeon General and others on the health consequences of smoking have shown that smoking is the most important modifiable risk factor
for coronary heart disease and lung cancer, is a major risk factor for stroke, and is a cause
of disease resulting from passive inhalation in healthy nonsmokers. Nicotine dependency
in the form of cigarette smoking is the most common form of drug addiction and causes
more disease and death than all other addictions combined. Smokeless tobacco users
develop nicotine dependency similar to that of smokers.

The tobacco use by young people is still unacceptably high in the United States. Based
on national surveys, approximately two-thirds of adolescents in the United States have
tried smoking by age 18. The national prevalence of current smoking for 12- to 18-year-
olds was approximately 16% in 1989; nearly 30% graduate from high school as current
smokers. The national estimate for adolescents who had tried smokeless tobacco was 32%
for high school senors in 1992. Current use estimates of smokeless tobacco show that 20%
of male high school seniors use smokeless tobacco in the United States.

The etiology of tobacco use can be explained by sociodemographic, environmental,
behavioral, and personal factors that increase a young person's chances of initiating and
continuing tobacco use. The effects of advertising on adolescents' normative expectations,
images, and functions of smoking need confirming research support. The higher use by low-
SES adolescents and those with lower academic achievement suggests higher risk groups to
target. The increasing influence of peers and their strong role in the onset process needs to be
underscored. Those adolescents with lower self-images, fewer social skills, and involvement in other risk-taking activities are particularly vulnerable to onset and these factors
suggest methods of intervention. This is particularly salient since these same adolescents are
at higher risk for use of alcohol, other drugs, and other problem behaviors.

The social influences model for tobacco use prevention recognizes the social environment as the most important determinant of smoking onset and focuses on the development of norms and skills to identify and resist social influences to smoke and use smokeless tobacco. This approach has been repeatedly demonstrated to reduce or delay
adolescent smoking. Programs that use this model have not achieved sustained positive
effects without additional education interventions, community components, or significant
policy changes.

Future research might focus on the following. First, efficacy studies are needed to
evaluate communitywide efforts that test the social influences program in schools in
combination with programs to reduce access to tobacco products, to increase prices, or to
restrict advertising and promotional activities. This combination of activities could thereby affect both supply of and demand for tobacco among young people. Second, the need
for strategies to encourage adolescent cessation is critical, particularly while young people
are underage and have fewer life-years of tobacco use. Third, studies to investigate the
lower rates of smoking among black adolescents are important and could illuminate
methods that might be applicable to other cultural or high-risk groups. Finally, the study
of nationwide strategies, such as differences in tax rates, the introduction of youth-
oriented counteradvertising, restrictive access legislation, penalties for underage use or
provision to those under age, or pack-size warning labels, might provide evidence of the
influence of distal factors that affect onset with adolescents, and potentially ways to lower
the prevalence of tobacco use at a national level.

REFERENCES

Alexander, H. M., Callcott, R., Dobson, A. J., Hardes, G. R., Lloyd, D. M., O'Connell, D. L., & Leeder, S. R. (1983). Cigarette smoking and drug use in schoolchildren: IV—Factors associated with changes in smoking behaviour. *International Journal of Epidemiology, 12*(1), 59–66.

Ary, D. V. (1989). Use of smokeless tobacco among male adolescents: Concurrent and prospective relationships. In National Cancer Institute, *Smokeless tobacco use in the United States*. Monograph No. 8. U.S. Department of Health and Human Services, Public Health Service, National Institutes of Health, National Cancer Institute. NIH Publication No. 89-3055, pp. 49–55.

Ary, D. V., Lichtenstein, E., & Severson, H. H. (1987). Smokeless tobacco use among male adolescents: Patterns, correlates, predictors, and the use of other drugs. *Preventive Medicine, 16,* 385–401.

Bachman, J. G., Johnston, L. D., & O'Malley, P. M. (1987). Monitoring the future: Questionnaire responses from the nation's high school seniors, 1986. Ann Arbor: Institute for Social Research, University of Michigan.

Bachman, J. G., Johnston, L. D., & O'Malley, P. M. (1991). Monitoring the future: Questionnaire responses from the nation's high school seniors, 1988. Ann Arbor: Institute for Social Research, University of Michigan.

Baker, W., Homel, P., Flaherty, B., & Trebilco, P. (1987). *The 1986 survey of drug use by secondary school students in New South Wales*. Sydney: New South Wales Drug and Alcohol Authority.

Bandura, A. (1977). *Social learning theory*. Englewood Cliffs, NJ: Prentice–Hall.

Bates, D. V. (1989). *Respiratory function in disease* (3rd ed.). Philadelphia: Saunders.

Bauman, K. E., Fisher, L. A., Bryan, E. S., & Chenoweth, R. L. (1984). Antecedents, subjective expected utility, and behavior: A panel study of adolescent cigarette smoking. *Addictive Behaviors, 9*(2), 121–136.

Bauman, K. E., Foshee, V. A., Linzer, M. A., & Koch, G. G. (1990). Effect of parental smoking classification on the association between parental and adolescent smoking. *Addictive Behaviors, 15,* 413–422.

Beck, G. J., Doyle, C. A., & Schachter, E. N. (1982). A longitudinal study of respiratory health in a rural community. *American Review of Respiratory Disease, 125,* 75–81.

Benowitz, N. L., Porchet, H., Sheiner, L., & Jacob, P. (1988). Nicotine absorption and cardiovascular effects with smokeless tobacco use: Comparison with cigarettes and nicotine gum. *Clinical Pharmacology and Therapeutics, 44*(1), 23–28.

Berenson, G. S., Wattigney, W. A., Tracy, R. E., Newman, W. P., III, Srinivasan, S. R., Webber, L. S., Dalferes, E. R., Jr., & Strong, J. P. (1992). Atherosclerosis of the aorta and coronary arteries and cardiovascular risk factors in persons aged 6 to 30 years and studied at necropsy (the Bogalusa Heart Study). *American Journal of Cardiology, 70*(9), 851–858.

Best, J. A., Flay, B. R., Towson, S. M. J., Ryan, K. B., Perry, C. L., Brown, K. S., Kersell, M. W., & D'Avernas, J. R. (1984). Smoking prevention and the concept of risk. *Journal of Applied Social Psychology, 14*(3), 257–273.

Best, J. A., Thomson, S. J., Santi, S. M., Smith, E. A., & Brown, K. (1988). Preventing cigarette smoking among school children. In L. Breslow, J. E. Fielding, & L. B. Lave (Eds.), *Annual review of public health*, Vol. 9. Palo Alto: Annual Reviews Inc.

Blake, G. H., Abell, T. D., & Stanley, W. G. (1988). Cigarette smoking and upper respiratory infection among recruits in basic combat training. *Annals of Internal Medicine, 109*(3), 198–202.

Botvin, G. J., & Botvin, E. M. (1992). Adolescent tobacco, alcohol, and drug abuse: Prevention strategies, empirical findings, and assessment issues. *Journal of Development and Behavioral Pediatrics, 13*(4), 290–301.

Botvin, G. J., & Dusenbury, L. (1989). Substance abuse prevention and the promotion of competence. In L. A. Bond & B. E. Compas (Eds.), *Primary prevention and promotion in the schools*. Newbury Park: Sage.

Botvin, G. J., Goldberg, C. J., Botvin, E. M., & Dusenbury, L. (1993). Smoking behavior of adolescent exposed to cigarette advertising. *Public Health Reports, 108*(2), 217–223.

Botvin, G. J., Renick, N. L., & Baker, E. (1983). The effects of scheduling format and booster sessions on a broad-spectrum psychosocial smoking prevention. *Journal of Behavioral Medicine, 6*(4), 359–379.

Botvin, G. J., & Wills, T. A. (1985). Personal and social skills training: Cognitive-behavioral approaches to substance abuse prevention. In C. S. Bell & R. Battjes (Eds.), *Prevention research: Deterring drug abuse among children and adolescents.* Monograph No. 63. U.S. Department of Health and Human Services, Public Health Service, Alcohol, Drug Abuse, and Mental Health Administration, National Institute on Drug Abuse. DHHS Publication No. (ADM) 85-1334.

Breslau, N., Fenn, N., & Peterson, E. (1993). Early smoking initiation and nicotine dependence in a cohort of young adults. *Drug and Alcohol Dependence, 33*(2), 129–137.

Brunswick, A. F., & Messeri, P. A. (1984). Origins of cigarette smoking in academic achievement, stress and social expectations: Does gender make a difference? *Journal of Early Adolescence, 4*(4), 353–370.

Bruvold, W. H. (1993). A meta-analysis of adolescent smoking prevention programs. *American Journal of Public Health, 83*(6), 872–880.

Burch, J. B., Fiebre, C. M., Marks, M. J., & Collins, A. C. (1988). Chronic ethanol or nicotine treatment results in partial cross-tolerance between these agents. *Psychopharmacology 95*(4), 452–458.

Burton, D., Chakravorty, B., Flay, B. R., Dent, C., Stacy, A., & Sussman, S. (1993). *The TNT tobacco-cessation program for high-school students: Main outcomes.* University of Illinois at Chicago Prevention Research Center. Unpublished data, University of Illinois, Chicago.

Burton, D., Moinuddin, M., & Grenier, B. (1992). *Advertising images and product symbolism as contributors to product desirability among black and white adolescents.* Unpublished data, University of Illinois, Chicago.

Centers for Disease Control. (1992). Comparison of the cigarette brand preferences of adult and teenaged smokers—United States, 1989, and 10 U.S. communities, 1988 and 1990. *Morbidity and Mortality Weekly Report, 41*(10), 169–81.

Centers for Disease Control. (1992b). Tobacco, alcohol, and other drug use among high school students—United States, 1991. *Morbidity and Mortality Weekly Report 41*(37), 698–703.

Centers for Disease Control and Prevention. (1993). Use of smokeless tobacco among adults—United States, 1990 and 1991. *Morbidity and Mortality Weekly Report, 42*(26), 504–507.

Chapman, S., & Bloch, M. (Eds.). (1992). *Tobacco Control,* (1 Suppl.), September S2–S3.

Chassin, L., Presson, C. C., Montello, D., Sherman, S. J., & McGrew, J. (1986). Changes in peer and parent influence during adolescence: Longitudinal versus cross-sectional perspectives on smoking initiation. *Developmental Psychology, 22*(3), 327–334.

Chassin, L., Presson, C. C., & Sherman, S. J. (1990). Social psychological contributions to the understanding and prevention of adolescent cigarette smoking. *Personality and Social Psychology Bulletin, 16*(1), 133–151.

Collins, A. C., Burch, J. B., Defiebre, C. M., & Marks, M. J. (1988). Tolerance to and cross tolerance between ethanol and nicotine. *Pharmacology, Biochemistry and Behavior, 29,* 365–373.

Collins, L. M., Sussman, S., Rauch, J. M., Dent, C. W., Johnson, C. A., Hansen, W. B., & Flay, B. R. (1987). Psychosocial predictors of young adolescent cigarette smoking: A sixteen-month, three-wave longitudinal study. *Journal of Applied Social Psychology, 17*(6), 554–573.

Comstock, G. W., & Rust, P. F. (1973). Residence and peak expiratory flow rates among Navy recruits. *American Journal of Epidemiology, 98*(5), 348–354.

Conrad, K. M., Flay, B. R., & Hill, D. (1992). Why children start smoking cigarettes: Predictors of onset. *British Journal of Addiction, 87*(12), 1711–1724.

Coombs, R. H., Fawzy, F. I., & Gerber, B. E. (1986). Patterns of cigarette, alcohol, and other drug use among children and adolescents: A longitudinal study. *The International Journal of the Addictions, 21*(8), 897–913.

Craig, W. Y., Palomaki, G. E., Johnson, A. M., & Haddow, J. E. (1990). Cigarette smoking-associated changes in blood lipid and lipoprotein levels in the 8- to 19-year-old age group: A meta-analysis. *Pediatrics, 85*(2), 155–158.

Dent, C. W., Sussman, S., Johnson, C. A., Hansen, W. B., & Flay, B. R. (1987). Adolescent smokeless tobacco incidence: Relations with other drugs and psychosocial variables. *Preventive Medicine, 16*(3), 422–431.

DiFranza, J. R., Carlson, R. R., & Caisse, R. E., Jr. (1992). Reducing youth access to tobacco. *Tobacco Control, 1*(1), 58.

DiFranza, J. R., Richards, J. W., Paulman, P. M., Wolf-Gillespie, N., Fletcher, C., Jaffe, R. D., & Murray, D. (1991). RJR Nabisco's cartoon camel promotes Camel cigarettes to children. *Journal of the American Medical Association, 266,* 3149–3153.

Doll, R., & Peto, R. (1978). Cigarette smoking and bronchial carcinoma: Dose and time relationships among regular smokers and lifelong non-smokers. *Journal of Epidemiology and Community Health, 32,* 303–313.

Durell, J., & Bukoski, W. (1984). Preventing substance abuse: The state of the art. *Public Health Reports, 99*(1), 23–31.

Eakin, E., Severson, H.,& Glasgow, R. E. (1989). Development and evaluation of a smokeless tobacco cessation program: A pilot study. In National Cancer Institute, *Smokeless tobacco use in the United States.* Monograph No. 8. U.S. Department of Health and Human Services, Public Health Service, National Institutes of Health, National Cancer Institute. NIH Publication No. 89-3055, pp. 95–100.

Elder, J. P., & Stern, R. A. (1986). The ABCs of adolescent smoking prevention: An environment and skills model. *Health Education Quarterly, 13*(2), 181–191.

Elder, J. P., Wildey, M., De Moor, C., Sallis, J. F., Eckhardt, L., Edwards, C., Erickson, A., Golbeck, A., & Hovell, M. (1993). Long-term prevention of tobacco use among junior high school students through classroom and telephone interventions. *American Journal of Public Health, 83*(9), 1239–1244.

Ellickson, P. L., Bell, R. M., & McGuigan, K. (1993). Preventing adolescent drug use: Long-term results of a junior high program. *American Journal of Public Health, 83*(6), 856–862.

Enos, W. F., Holmes, R. H., & Beyer, J. (1953). Coronary disease among United States soldiers killed in action in Korea. *Journal of the American Medical Association, 152,* 1090–1093.

Escobedo, L. G., Marcus, S. E., Holtzman, D., & Giovino, G. A. (1986). Sports participation, age at smoking initiation, and the risk of smoking among U.S. high school students. *Journal of the American Medical Association, 256*(20), 2859–2862.

Evans, R., Rozelle, R., Mittlemark, M., Rozelle, R. M., Hansen, W. B., Bane, A. L., & Hairs, J. (1978). Deterring the onset of smoking in children: Knowledge of immediate physiological effects and coping with peer pressure, media pressure, and parent modeling. *Journal of Applied Social Psychology, 8*(2), 126–135.

Federal Trade Commission. (1992). Report to Congress for 1990: Pursuant to the Federal Cigarette Labeling and Advertising Act. Washington, DC: Author.

Finklea, J. F., Hasselblad, V., Sandifer, S. H., Hammer, D. I., & Lowrimore, G. R. (1971). Cigarette smoking and acute non-influenza respiratory disease in military cadets. *American Journal of Epidemiology, 93*(6), 457–462.

Fiore, M. C., Novotny, T. E., Pierce, J. P., Hatziandreu, E. J., Patel, K. M., & Davis, R. M. (1989). Trends in cigarette smoking in the United States. The changing influence of gender and race. *Journal of the American Medical Association, 261*(1), 49–55.

Flay, B. R. (1985). Psychosocial approaches to smoking prevention: A review of findings. *Health Psychology, 4*(5), 449–488.

Flay, B. R. (1993). Youth tobacco use: Risks, patterns and control. In J. Slade & C. T. Orleans (Eds.), *Nicotine addiction: Principles and management.* London: Oxford University Press.

Flay, B. R., D'Avernas, J. R., Best, J. A., Kersell, M. W., & Ryan, K. B. (1983). Cigarette smoking: Why young people do it and ways of preventing it. In P. McGrath & P. Firestone (Eds.), *Pediatric and adolescent behavioral medicine.* Berlin: Springer-Verlag.

Flay, B. R., Koepke, D., Thomson, S. J., Santi, S., Best, J. A., & Brown, K. S. (1989). Six-year follow-up of the first Waterloo school smoking prevention trial. *American Journal of Public Health, 79*(10), 1371–1376.

Fleming, R., Leventhal, H., Glynn, K., & Ershler, J. (1989). The role of cigarettes in the initiation and progression of early substance use. *Addictive Behaviors, 14*(3), 162–272.

Flynn, B. S., Worden, J. K., Secker-Walker, R. H., Badger, G. J., Geller, B. M., & Costanza, M. C. (1992). Prevention of cigarette smoking through mass media intervention and school programs. *American Journal of Public Health, 82*(6), 827–834.

Gallup Organization. (1993, April). The public's attitudes toward cigarette advertising and cigarette tax increase. Poll conducted for the Coalition for Smoking OR Health. Princeton, NJ: Author.

Gerber, R. W., & Newman, I. M. (1989). Predicting future smoking of adolescent experimental smokers. *Journal of Youth and Adolescence, 18*(2), 191–201.

Glover, E. D. (1986). Conducting smokeless tobacco cessation clinics [letter]. *American Journal of Public Health, 76*(2), 207.

Glynn, T. J. (1989). Essential elements of school-based smoking prevention programs. *Journals of School Health, 59*(5), 181–188.

Goodstadt, M. S. (1978). Alcohol and drug education: Models and outcomes. *Health Education Monographs*, *6*(3), 263–279.

Gritz, E. R., Baer-Weiss, V., Benowitz, N. L., Van Vunaikis, H., & Jarvik, M. E. (1981). Plasma nicotine and cotinine concentrations in habitual smokeless tobacco users. *Clinical Pharmacology and Therapeutics, 30*, 201–209.

Grunberg, N. E., Winders, S. E., & Wewers, M. E. (1991). Gender differences in tobacco use. *Health Psychology, 10*(2), 143–153.

Haertzen, C. A., Kocher, T. R., & Miyasato, K. (1983). Reinforcements from the first drug experience can predict later drug habits and/or addiction: Results with coffee, cigarettes, alcohol, barbiturates, minor and major tranquilizers, stimulants, marijuana, hallucinogens, heroin, opiates and cocaine. *Drug and Alcohol Dependence 11*, 147–165.

Hall, E. H., & Terzhalmy, G. T. (1984). Oral manifestations of the smokeless tobacco habit. *U.S. Navy Medicine, 75*(3), 4–6.

Hansen, W. B. (1983). Behavioral predictors of abstinence: Early indicators of a dependence on tobacco among adolescents. *The International Journal of the Addiction, 3*, 913–920.

Hansen, W. B. (1988). Theory and implementation of the social influence model of primary prevention. In K. H. Rey, C. L. Gaegre, & P. Lowery (Eds.), *Prevention research findings: 1988*. Rockville, MD: DHHS, PHS, ADAMHA.

Hansen, W. B. (1992). School-based substance abuse prevention: A review of the state-of-the-art in curriculum, 1980–1990. *Health Education Research Theory & Practice, 7*(3), 403–430.

Hansen, W. B., Collins, L. M., Johnson, C. A., & Graham, J. W. (1985). Self-initiated smoking cessation among high school students. *Addictive Behaviors, 10*, 265–271.

Hansen, W. B., & Graham, J. W. (1991). Preventing alcohol, marijuana, and cigarette use among adolescents: Peer pressure resistance training versus establishing conservative norms. *Preventive Medicine, 20*, 414–430.

Hatsukami, D. K., Gust, S. W., & Keenan, R. M. (1987). Physiological and subjective changes from smokeless tobacco withdrawal. *Clinical Pharmacology and Therapeutics, 41*, 103–107.

Haynes, W. G., Krstnlovic, V. J., & Bell, A. L. (1966). Smoking habit and incidence of respiratory track infections in a group of adolescent males. *American Review of Respiratory Disease, 93*(5), 730–734.

Henningfield, J. E., Clayton, R., & Pollin, W. (1990). Involvement of tobacco in alcoholism and illicit drug use. *British Journal of Addiction, 85*, 279–292.

Henningfield, J. E., Cohen, C., & Stade, J. D. (1991). Is nicotine more addictive than cocaine? *British Journal of Addiction, 86*(5), 565–569.

Hirschman, R. S., Leventhal, H., & Glynn, K. (1984). The development of smoking behavior: Conceptualization and supportive cross-sectional survey data. *Journal of Applied Social Psychology, 14*, 184–206.

Holland, W. W., & Elliott, A. (1968). Cigarette smoking, respiratory symptoms, and anti-smoking propaganda. An experiment. *Lancet, 1*, 41–43.

Horger, B. A., Giles, M. K., & Schenk, S. (1992). Preexposure to amphetamine and nicotine predisposes rats to self-administer a low dose of cocaine. *Psychopharmacology, 107*, 271–276.

Hsu, S. C., Pollack, R. L., Hsu, A. F., & Going, R. E. (1980). Sugars present in tobacco extracts. *Journal of the American Dental Association, 101*, 915–918.

International Agency for Research on Cancer. (1985). Tobacco habits other than smoking: Betel quid and areca nut chewing; and some related nitrosamines. *IARC Monograph, 37*, 291.

Jason, L. A., Ji, P. Y., Anes, M. D., & Birkhead, S. H. (1991). Active enforcement of cigarette control laws in the prevention of cigarette sales to minors. *Journal of the American Medical Association, 266*(22), 3159–3161.

Johnston, L. D., Bachman, J. G., & O'Malley, P. M. (1991). Monitoring the future: Questionnaire responses from the nation's high school seniors, 1987. Ann Arbor: Institute for Social Research, University of Michigan.

Johnston, L. D., Bachman, J. G., & O'Malley, P. M. (1992). Monitoring the future: Questionnaire responses from the nation's high school seniors, 1989. Ann Arbor: Institute for Social Research, University of Michigan.

Johnston, L. D., O'Malley, P. M., & Bachman, J. G. (1993). *National Survey Results on Drug Use from*

Monitoring the Future Study, 1975–1992. NIH Publication No. 93-3597.

Jones, R. B., & Moberg, D. P. (1988). Correlates of smokeless tobacco use in a male adolescent population. *American Journal of Public Health, 78*(1), 660–666.

Kandel, D. (1975). Stages in adolescent involvement in drug use. *Science, 190*(4217), 912–914.

Kelder, S. H. (1992). Youth cardiovascular disease risk and prevention: The Minnesota Heart Health Program and the Class of 1989 Study [dissertation]. Minneapolis: University of Minnesota.

Leventhal, H. (1968). *Experimental studies of anti-smoking communications.* New York: Hawthorne.

Leventhal, H., & Cleary, P. D. (1980). The smoking problem: A review of the research and theory in behavioral risk modification. *Psychological Bulletin, 88*(2), 370–405.

Leventhal, H., Fleming, R., & Glynn, K. (1988). A cognitive-developmental approach to smoking intervention. In S. Maes, C. D. Spielberger, P. B. Defares, & I. G. Sarason (Eds.), *Topics in health psychology: Proceedings of the first annual expert conference in health psychology* (pp. 79–105). New York: Wiley.

McAlister, A. L., Perry, C. L., & Maccoby, N. (1979). Adolescent smoking: Onset and prevention. *Pediatrics, 63*(4), 650–658.

McCarthy, W. J., & Gritz, E. R. (1984). *Teenagers, cigarette smoking and reactions to selected cigarette ads.* Paper presented at the Western Psychological Association Meeting, Los Angeles, April 6.

McGuire, W. J. (1984). Public communication as a strategy to inducing health-promoting behavioral change. *Preventive Medicine, 13*(3), 299–319.

McNamara, J. J., Molot, M. A., Stremple, J. F., & Cutting, R. T. (1971). Coronary artery disease in combat casualties in Vietnam. *Journal of the American Medical Association, 216*(7), 1185–1187.

McNeill, A. D. (1991). The development of dependence on smoking in children. *British Journal of Addiction, 86*, 589–592.

Murray, D. M., Pirie, P., Luepker, R. V., & Pallonen, U. (1989). Five- and six-year follow-up results from four seventh-grade smoking prevention strategies. *Journal of Behavioral Medicine, 12*(2), 207–218.

National Center for Health Statistics. (1970). *Changes in cigarette smoking habits between 1955 and 1966.* Vital and Health Statistics, Series 10, No. 59. U.S. Department of Health, Education, and Welfare, Public Health Service, Health Services and Mental Health Administration. PHS Publication No. 1000, Series 10, No. 59.

Newcomb, M. D., & Bentler, P. M. (1986). Frequency and sequence of drug use: A longitudinal study from early adolescence to young adulthood. *Journal of Drug Education, 16*(2), 101–118.

Oechsli, F. W., Seltzer, C. C., & Van Den Berg, B. J. (1987). Adolescent smoking and early respiratory disease: A longitudinal study. *Annals of Allergy, 59*, 135–140.

Pathobiological Determinants of Atherosclerosis in Youth (PDAY) Research Group. (1990). Relationship of atherosclerosis in young men to serum lipoprotein cholesterol concentrations and smoking. *Journal of the American Medical Association, 264*(23), 3018–3024.

Pentz, M., MacKinnon, D. P., Dwyer, J. H., Wang, E. Y. I., Hansen, W. B., Flay, B. R., & Johnson, C. A. (1989). Longitudinal effects of the Midwestern Prevention Project on regular and experimental smoking in adolescents. *Preventive Medicine, 18*(2), 304–321.

Perry, C. L., Kelder, S. H., Murray, D. M., & Klepp, K.-I. (1992). Communitywide smoking prevention: Long-term outcomes of the Minnesota Heart Health Program and the Class of 1989 Study. *American Journal of Public Health, 82*(9), 1210–1216.

Perry, C. L., Killen, J., Telch, M., Slinkard, L. A., & Danaher, B. G. (1980). Modifying smoking behavior of teenagers: A school-based intervention. *American Journal of Public Health, 70*(7), 722–725.

Perry, C. L., Klepp, K. I., & Shultz, J. M. (1988). Primary prevention of cardiovascular disease: Communitywide strategies for youth. *Journal of Consulting and Clinical Psychology, 56*(3), 358–364.

Perry, C. L., Murray, D. M., & Klepp, K. I. (1987). Predictors of adolescent smoking and implications for prevention. *Morbidity and Mortality Weekly Report, 36*(4S), 41S–47S.

Peto, R., (1977). Epidemiology, multistage models, and short-term mutagenicity tests. In H. H. Hiatt, J. D. Watson, & J. A. Winsten. (Eds.), *Origins of human cancer. Book C. Human risk assessment, Vol. 4.* Cold Spring Harbor, NY: Cold Spring Harbor Laboratory.

Pierce, J. P., Farkas, A., Evans., N., Berry, C., Choi, W., Rosebrook, B., Johnson, M., & Bal, D. G. 1993. Tobacco use in California, 1992. A focus on preventing uptake in adolescents. Saramento: California Department of Health Services.

Pierce, J. P., Fiore, M. C., Novotny, T. E., Hatziandreu, E. J., & Davis, R. M. (1989). Trends in cigarette smoking in the United States. Projections to the year 2000. *Journal of the American Medical Association, 261*, 61–65.

Pierce, J. P., Naquin, M., Gilpin, E., Giovino, G., & Mills, M. S. (1991). Smoking initiation in the United States: A role for worksite and college smoking bans. *Journal of the National Cancer Institute, 83*(14): 1009–1013.

Public Health Service. (1990, May 24). Model Sale of Tobacco Products to Minors Control Act. A model law recommended for adoption by states and localities to prevent the sale of tobacco products to minors. U.S. Department of Health and Human Services.

Roberts, Fitzmahan & Associates, Inc. (1986). Comprehensive Health Education Foundation. *Here's looking at you, 2000*. Seattle, WA: Comprehensive Health Foundation.

Rooney, B. (1992). *A meta-analysis of smoking prevention programs after adjustment for study design* [dissertation]. Minneapolis: University of Minnesota.

Royal College of Physicians of London. (1992). *Smoking and the young.* London: Lavenham Press.

Rush, D. (1974). Respiratory symptoms in a group of American secondary school students: The overwhelming association with cigarette smoking. *International Journal of Epidemiology, 3*(2), 153–165.

Russell, M. A. H ., Jarvis, M. J., & Feyerabend, C. (1980). A new age of snuff. *Lancet, 1*, 474.

Schroeder, K. L., & Chen, M. S., Jr. (1985). Smokeless tobacco and blood pressure. *New England Journal of Medicine, 312*, 919.

Schwartz, J., & Zeger, S. (1990). Passive smoking, air pollution, and acute respiratory symptoms in a diary study of student nurses. *American Review of Respiratory Disease, 141*, 62–67.

Seely, J. E., Zuskin, E., & Bouhuys, A. (1971). Cigarette smoking: Objective evidence for lung damage in teenagers. *Science, 172*, 741–743.

Semmer, N. K., Lippert, P., Fuchs, R., Cleary, P. D., & Schindler, A. (1987). Adolescent smoking from a functional perspective: The Berlin–Bremen study. *European Journal of Psychology of Education, 2*(4), 387–401.

Severson, H. H., Glasgow, R., Wirt, R., Brozovsky, P., Zoref, L., Black, C., Biglau, A., Ary, O., & Weissman, W. (1991). Preventing the use of smokeless tobacco and cigarettes by teens: Results of a classroom intervention. *Health Education Research, 6*(1), 109–120.

Signs, S. A., Schechter, M. D. (1986). Nicotine-induced potentiation of ethanol discrimination. *Pharmacology, Biochemistry, and Behavior, 24*(3), 769–771.

Spinaci, S., Arossa, W., Bugiani, M., Natale, P., Bucca, C., & De Candussio, G. (1985). The effects of air pollution on the respiratory health of children: A cross-sectional study. *Pediatric Pulmonology, 1*, 262–266.

Stacy, A. W., Sussman, S., Dent, C. W., Burton, D., & Flay, B. R. (1992). Moderators of peer social influence in adolescent smoking. *Personality and Social Psychology Bulletin, 18*(2), 163–172.

Strong, J. P. (1986). Coronary atherosclerosis in soldiers. A clue to the natural history of atherosclerosis in the young. *Journal of the American Medical Association, 256*(20), 2863–2866.

Strong, J. P., & Richards, M. L. (1976). Cigarette smoking and atherosclerosis in autopsied men. *Atherosclerosis, 23*, 451–476.

Sussman, S., Burton, D., Dent, C. W., Stacy, A. W., & Flay, B. R. (1991). Use of focus groups in developing an adolescent tobacco use cessation program: Collective norm effects. *Journal of Applied Social Psychology, 21*(21), 1772–1782.

Sussman, S., Dent, C. W., Flay, B. R., Hansen, W. B., & Johnson, C. A. (1987). Psychosocial predictors of cigarette smoking onset by white, black, Hispanic, and Asian adolescents in Southern California. *Morbidity and Mortality Weekly Report, 36*(4S), 11S–7S.

Sussman, S., Dent, C. W., Stacy, A. W., Sun, P., Craig, S., Simon, T. R., Burton, D., & Flay, B. R. (1993). project "Towards No Tobacco Use:" 1-year behavior outcomes. *American Journal of Public Health, 83*(9), 1245–1250.

Swan, A. V., Creeser, R., & Murray, M. (1990). When and why children first start to smoke. *International Journal of Epidemiology, 19*(2), 323–330.

Sweanor, D. T. (1991). *The Canada tobacco tax project: 1985–1991. A review of a major public health success story.* Non-Smokers' Rights Association, Working Paper. Ontario, Canada: Non-Smokers' Rights Association.

Sweanor, D., Ballin, S., Corcoran, R. D., Davis, A., Deasy, K., Ferrence, R. G., Lahey, R., Lucido, S., Nethery, W. J., & Wasserman, J. (1992). Report of the tobacco policy research study group on tobacco pricing and taxation in the United States. *Tobacco Control*, (*1 Suppl.*), S31–S36.

Tager, I. B., Muñoz, A., Rosner, B., Weiss, S. T., Carey, V., & Speizer, F. E. (1985). Effect of cigarette smoking on the pulmonary function of children and adolescents. *American Review of Respiratory Disease*, *131*, 752–759.

Tager, I. B., Segal, M. R., Speizer, F. E., & Weiss, S. T. (1988). The natural history of forced expiratory volumes. Effect of cigarette smoking and respiratory symptoms. *American Review of Respiratory Disease*, *138*, 837–849.

Taioli, E., & Wynder, E. L. (1991). Effect of the age at which smoking begins on frequency of smoking in adulthood [letter]. *New England Journal of Medicine*, *325*(13), 968–969.

Thompson, E. L. (1978). Smoking education programs, 1960–1976. *American Journal of Public Health*, *68*(3), 250–257.

Tobler, N. S. (1986). Meta-analysis of 143 adolescent drug prevention programs: Quantitative outcome results of program participants compared to a control or comparison group. *Journal of Drug Issues*, *16*(4), 537–567.

Tobler, N. S. (1992). Drug prevention programs can work: Research findings. *Journal of Addictive Diseases*, *11*(3), 1–28.

Tye, J. B., Warner, K. E., & Glantz, S. A. (1987). Tobacco advertising and consumption: Evidence of a causal relationship. *Journal of Public Health Policy*, *8*(4), 492–508.

U.S. Department of Health, Education, and Welfare. (1955). *Tobacco smoking patterns in the United States: Public Health Monograph No. 45*. U.S. Department of Health, Education, and Welfare, Public Health Service, Office on Smoking and Health. DHEW Publication No. (PHS) 463.

U.S. Department of Health, Education, and Welfare. (1979). *Teenage smoking. Immediate and long-term patterns*. U.S. Department of Health, Education, and Welfare, National Institute of Education.

U.S. Department of Health and Human Services. (1980). *The health consequences of smoking for women*. A report of the Surgeon General. U.S. Department of Health and Human Services, Public Health Service, Office of the Assistant Secretary for Health, Office on Smoking and Health.

U.S. Department of Health and Human Services. (1982). *The health consequences of smoking: Cancer. A report of the Surgeon General*. U.S. Department of Health and Human Services, Public Health Service, Office on Smoking and Health. DHHS Publication No. (PHS) 82-50179.

U.S. Department of Health and Human Services. (1984). *The health consequences of smoking: Chronic obstructive lung disease. A report of the Surgeon General*. U.S. Department of Health and Human Services, Public Health Service, Office on Smoking and Health. DHHS Publication No. (PHS) 84-50205.

U.S. Department of Health and Human Services. (1986). *The health consequences of using smokeless tobacco. A report of the advisory committee to the Surgeon General*. U.S. Department of Health and Human Services, Public Health Service, National Institutes of Health. NIH Publication No. 886-2874.

U.S. Department of Health and Human Services. (1988). *The health consequences of smoking: Nicotine addiction. A report of the Surgeon General*. U.S. Department of Health and Human Services, Public Health Service, Centers for Disease Control, Center for Health Promotion and Education, Office on Smoking and Health. DHHS Publication No. (CDC) 88-8406.

U.S. Department of Health and Human Services. (1989). *Reducing the health consequences of smoking: 25 years of progress*. A report of the Surgeon General. U.S. Department of Health and Human Services, Public Health Service, Centers for Disease Control, Center for Chronic Disease Prevention and Health Promotion, Office on Smoking and Health. HHS Publication No. (CDC) 89-8411.

U.S. Department of Health and Human Services. (1990). *The health benefits of smoking cessation. A report of the Surgeon General*. U.S. Department of Health and Human Services, Public Health Service, Centers for Disease Control, Center for Chronic Disease Prevention and Health Promotion, Office on Smoking and Health. DHHS Publication No. (CDC) 90-8416.

U.S. Department of Health and Human Services. (1991). *Drug abuse and drug abuse research. The third triennial report to Congress from the Secretary, Department of Health and Human Services*. U.S. Department of Health and Human Services, Public Health Service, Alcohol, Drug Abuse, and Mental Health Administration. DHHS Publication No. (ADM) 91-1704.

U.S. Department of Health and Human Services. (1992). *Smokeless tobacco or health: An international perspective*. National Cancer Institute Monograph, NIH Monograph 2, NIH No. 92-3461.

U.S. Department of Health and Human Services. (1994). *Preventing tobacco use among young people: A report of the Surgeon General*. U.S. Department of Health and Human Services, Public Health Service, Centers for Disease Control and Prevention, National Center for Chronic Disease Prevention and Health Promotion, Office on Smoking and Health.

Weiss, S. T., Tager, I. B., Speizer, F. E., & Rosner, B. (1980). Persistent wheeze: Its relation to respiratory illness, cigarette smoking, and level of pulmonary function in a population sample of children. *American Review of Respiratory Disease, 122,* 697–707.

Williams, N. J. (1992). *A smokeless tobacco cessation program for postsecondary students* [dissertation]. Memphis, TN: Memphis State University.

Woolcock, A. J., Peat, J. K., Leeder, S. R., & Blackburn, C. R. B. (1984). The development of lung function in Sydney children: Effects of respiratory illness and smoking. A ten year study. *European Journal of Respiratory Diseases, 65(Suppl. 132),* 1–97.

Worden, J. K., Flynn, B. S., Geller, B. M., Chen, M., Shelton, L. G., & Secker-Walker, R. H. (1988). Development of a smoking prevention mass media program using diagnostic and formative research. *Preventive Medicine, 17*(5), 531–558.

World Health Organization. (1988). *Smokeless tobacco control. Report of a WHO study group*. WHO Technical Report Series 773, Geneva, Switzerland.

5

Disordered Eating

LYNN E. PONTON

INTRODUCTION

The continuum of adolescent behavior addressed by the term "disordered eating" is complex. For decades the term has been more commonly associated with the severe end of the spectrum of eating-disordered behavior represented in the psychiatric diagnoses of anorexia nervosa and bulimia nervosa. This is largely connected to the historical perspective that conceptualized the behavior in terms of "disease" and paid little or no attention to the milder symptoms of the full-range continuum of eating behavior (Lucas, 1981). It is important, however, to recognize that disordered eating is itself a risk-taking behavior with a wide spectrum, including various types of unhealthy restricted food intake such as dieting and many patterns of binging behavior.

Terms related to this behavior are often used in a generally cavalier fashion. It is particularly important that they be carefully understood and defined when applied to patients. Adolescents and their parents commonly use both "disordered eating" and "eating disorder" to describe any perceived fluctuation from what they view as normal eating. "Disordered eating" as a clinical term generally refers to any abnormal pattern from the most mild to the most severe. The term "eating disorder" represents an extreme of severity and is applied to diagnostic syndromes or a constellation of symptoms regularly found to occur together such as atypical binge disorder (Spitzer *et al.*, 1993). The term "eating disorder" is also used to refer to specific diseases such as anorexia nervosa (APA, 1994); these are relatively well-defined disorders that have been shown to have regularly recurring psychopathological correlates, clear genetic basis, a distinctive etiology, physical pathology, and shared prognosis. The term "eating disordered" is also used to refer to a condition of chronic disability when multiple relapses have occurred. While acknowledging the wide range of disordered eating behavior in adolescents, this chapter will primarily

LYNN E. PONTON • Langley Porter Psychiatric Institute, Division of Child and Adolescent Psychiatry, University of California, San Francisco, San Francisco, California 94117.

Handbook of Adolescent Health Risk Behavior, edited by Ralph J. DiClemente, William B. Hansen, and Lynn E. Ponton. Plenum Press, New York, 1996.

focus on the epidemiology, prevention, and treatment of anorexia nervosa and bulimia nervosa, the areas addressed by most studies. Obesity and atypical binge disorder will be covered briefly.

DEFINITIONS OF DISORDERED EATING

The diagnostic criteria for anorexia nervosa as defined by DSM-IV are: (1) refusal to maintain body weight over a minimal normal weight for age and height ($<85\%$ of what is expected) or failure to make expected weight gain during a period of growth (again $<85\%$ of what is expected); (2) intense fear of becoming fat even though underweight; (3) disturbance in the way in which one's body or shape is experienced, undue influence of body weight or shape on self-evaluation or denial of the seriousness of the current low body weight; and (4) amenorrhea in postmenarcheal females, i.e., the absence of at least three consecutive menstrual cycles. The DSM-IV specifies two types of anorexia nervosa: restricting, where the individual does not engage in binging or purging, and the subtype categorized as binge eating/purging type, where the individual regularly engages in binge eating or purging behavior during the current episode of anorexia nervosa.

The diagnostic criteria for bulimia nervosa as defined by the DSM-IV are: (1) recurrent episodes of binge eating characterized by eating an amount of food that is definitely larger than most people would eat during a similar period of time and a sense of lack of control over eating during the episode; (2) engaging in a method to prevent weight gain such as self-induced vomiting; misuse of laxatives, diuretics, enemas, and other medications; fasting; or excessive exercise; (3) behavior (both binging and compensatory behavior) occurs, on average, at least twice a week for 2 months; (4) self-evaluation is unduly influenced by body shape and weight; and (5) the disturbances do not occur exclusively during episodes of anorexia nervosa. There are two designated subcategories of bulimia nervosa; purging type and nonpurging (e.g., use of fasting or excessive exercise) type.

The DSM-IV lists a third diagnostic disorder, atypical binge eating, in a provisional category proposed for further study. The proposed criteria include: (1) recurrent episodes of binge eating characterized by eating an amount of food that is definitely larger than most people would eat during a similar period of time and a sense of lack of control over eating during the episode; (2) binge eating episodes include three of the five symptoms— eating more rapidly than normal; eating until feeling uncomfortably full; eating large amounts of food when not feeling physically hungry; eating alone because one is embarrassed by the amount; feeling self-disgust, depression, or guilt after the eating; (3) the individual feels markedly distressed about the binge eating; (4) the binge eating occurs at least 2 days a week for at least 6 months; and (5) the binge eating is not associated with regular use of inappropriate compensatory mechanisms (e.g., vomiting, laxative use). The validity of atypical binge eating disorder has been supported by its strong association with impairment in work and social functioning, overconcern with body shape and weight, general psychopathology, significant amount of time on diets, and an associated history of depression, drug and alcohol use, and periods of psychiatric treatment (Spitzer *et al.*, 1993). Individuals with anorexia nervosa, bulimia nervosa, and atypical binge eating disorder may all experience weight loss, but individuals with bulimia nervosa and atypical binge eating disorder are able to keep their weight at or above 85% of the expected weight.

Thinness is much admired in Western cultures, including among adolescents (Stunkard, d'Aquile, Fox, & Filion, 1972), and obese adolescents are frequently stigmatized (Canning & Meyer, 1966) as well as suffering increased risk for a variety of medical conditions (Tobias & Gordon, 1980). Obesity in adolescents is defined by a triceps fat fold thickness greater than the 95th percentile (Kleinman, 1987). Obesity is believed to be connected more strongly with environmental factors, particularly diet, lack of physical activity, and family patterns of feeding (Sevdula *et al.*, 1993).

The psychiatric diagnoses of anorexia nervosa and bulimia nervosa are now recognized as important but relatively uncommon syndromes or disease processes within a wide spectrum of disordered eating. Within this spectrum, dieting, and in particular unsupervised and unhealthy dieting patterns in adolescents, may be one of the most important pathways to eating disorders. Key influences may operate to initiate dieting rather than eating disorders specifically. As dieting appears to be a commonly reported behavior among adolescents and represents a risk factor that could be targeted in prevention programs (e.g., programs focused on healthy eating habits or life-style), understanding its role within the spectrum of disordered eating is particularly important.

Adolescent dieting is clearly not well understood. Studies indicate that dieting alone does not directly lead to the more severe findings of anorexia or bulimia nervosa. Schleimer's longitudinal follow up of 111 pathological dieters indicated that girls who diet in adolescence do not go on to develop an eating disorder without having been presented with some of the criteria for an eating disorder early in adolescence (Schleimer, 1984). Patton (1992) found that a rise in self-reported depressive symptoms correlated with the development of eating disorders in a group of adolescent dieters. Depressive symptoms have been found to predict progression in other risk behaviors in adolescence, including smoking, problem drinking or alcoholism, and substance abuse (Sharpe & Lowe, 1987).

EPIDEMIOLOGY OF DISORDERED EATING

Incidence and Prevalence

Studies report varying incidence (the number of new cases appearing during a given interval) and prevalence (total number of cases of the disease or behavior in a group at a specific time) of eating-disordered behavior among adolescents. Most of the studies in this area have focused on the most severe symptomatology, the psychiatric diagnoses of anorexia nervosa and bulimia nervosa. Reported prevalence rates vary for anorexia nervosa in adolescent females, from 1 in 100 females to 1 in 800 (APA, 1987). Halmi and her team of investigators (Halmi, Broadland, & Loney, 1973) reported the prevalence to be 1 in 100 adolescent girls and noted a bimodal pattern of onset with two risk periods, early adolescence (13–14 years of age) and late adolescence (17–19 years of age). Bulimia nervosa is more common and is reported to affect between 4 and 10% of adolescent college-age women (Pyle *et al.*, 1983). Varying prevalence rates for bulimia nervosa are reported for female adolescents (Yates, 1989). Obesity has been shown to have prevalence rates of 6–13% for all adolescents (Kleinman, 1967).

Many adolescents do not meet the diagnostic criteria for the psychiatric diagnoses or the medical criteria for obesity, but exhibit some form of disordered eating consisting of a preoccupation with food or weight that seriously interferes with their daily lives. Here again, reported prevalence varies based on the adolescent population sample, but 30–70% of adolescent females report that they are dieting (Felts, Tavasso, Chenier, & Dunn, 1992; King, 1989). Data from a self-report adolescent risk behavior survey given to 3437 high school students revealed that 25% of that population believed that they were "too fat" (Felts *et al.*, 1992). Adolescent girls constituted 75% of this group. Sixty-eight percent of the adolescents in the study reported currently being on a diet.

In a second study, which reported on the responses of over 6000 high school-age youth to a behavioral questionnaire focusing on eating behaviors, 33% of Caucasian and African-American youth reported that they binge at least twice a week (Ponton, Gruber, & DiClemente, 1994). Five percent of Caucasian youth, three percent of African-American youth, and nine percent of Native American youth reported that they have used diet pills. Four percent of Caucasian youth, three percent of African-American youth, and seven percent of Native American youth report that they have used vomiting for weight control. Thirty-two percent of Native American youth, twenty-five percent of Caucasian youth, and sixteen percent of African-American youth report that they skip meals (Ponton *et al.*, 1994).

Both of these studies describe a wide spectrum of eating-disordered behaviors, many of which do not fall into specific diagnostic categories. The equally high incidence of eating-disordered behavior among African-American and Native American youth indicates that the behavior is manifested across ethnic groups, and the higher rates of behavior among Native American youth indicate that certain cultural groups may be at higher risk at different points in time (Ponton *et al.*, 1994).

Within the past 10 years, there has been disagreement about the reported incidence of anorexia nervosa and bulimia nervosa. Several researchers have reported a doubling of the incidence of anorexia nervosa, and possibly bulimia nervosa, between 1960 and 1980 (Jones, Fox, Babigian, & Hutton, 1983; Willi & Grossmann, 1983). Williams and King (1987) questioned the increased incidence of eating disorders, and attributed the perceived increase to a large number of young women in the population. Lucas, Beard, O'Fallon, and Kurland (1991) explored the question of increased incidence in a population-based study in Minnesota. This study, focusing on the 50-year period from 1935 to 1984, found that while the overall incidence of anorexia nervosa had not increased, a significant temporal increase had occurred for 15- to 24-year-olds. The 10- to 19-year-old age group, which included premenarcheal girls, reported a high rate of anorexia nervosa in the 1930s, a lower rate in the 1950s, and a gradually increasing rate from 1964 until the end of the study in 1984. Lucas classified anorexia nervosa into two subtypes: Type I, a chronic, severe form of the illness with a largely biological etiology, and Type II, a less severe form with a more benign course. He believed that the increase in the incidence of anorexia nervosa among adolescent females is probably an increase in the more mild Type II (Lucas, 1992). This is consistent with Yates's hypothesis (Yates, 1989, 1990) that sociocultural pressures have played an important role in the increasing incidence among adolescent females.

Soundy, Lucas, Suman, and Melton (1994) have investigated the incidence of bulimia nervosa in a population-based study in Rochester, Minnesota, between 1980 and 1990. They found that the yearly incidence in females rose sharply from 7.4 per 100,000 in 1980 to 49.7 in 1983, and then remained relatively constant around 30 per 100,000 through 1990. The highest rates, 125 per 100,000 for girls ages 15–19, and 83 per 100,000 for women ages 20–24, were comparable to the reported incidence of a study conducted in Stockholm (Culberg & Engstrom-Lindberg, 1988), where an incidence of 65 per 100,000 was found for 16- to 24-year-old females. Soundy and colleagues proposed that case selection by selective contacts may have resulted in a lower incidence in the Stockholm study (Soundy et al., 1994).

Specific subgroups of individuals deserve special mention with respect to the topic of disordered eating: males because they are frequently ignored, prepubertal girls (approximately 8–13 years of age) because they are the group that precedes the group with the highest incidence (14- to 19-year-old adolescent females), and individuals who are diagnosed with an eating disorder and another psychiatric diagnosis concomitantly because of the severity of their combined disorders.

Although the presentation, history, and family dynamics of male and female patients with diagnosed eating disorders are reported to be remarkably similar (Lerner, Orlos, & Knapp, 1976), the epidemiology for males with eating disorders does not reflect the increases noted for young females during the past 20 years. For males in the Rochester, Minnesota, study (Soundy et al., 1994), the incidence of anorexia nervosa for the 50-year period from 1935 to 1984 was found to be 1.6 per 100,000 in contrast to the overall reported incidence for females of 13.5 per 100,000. Soundy and colleagues reported that the incidence of bulimia nervosa among males was rare: 0.8 per 100,000 compared with 26.5 per 100,000 for females. The suspected underlying pathology also appears to be different. Lerner et al. (1976) found that physical attractiveness predicts self-concept and self-esteem in adolescent girls, whereas physical effectiveness predicts self-concept in boys. Therefore, it is not surprising that male patients with eating disorders present with unconventional psychosexual development and gender identity issues. Male anorexia nervosa patients are reported to be more extroverted and score superfeminine on many of the personality scales. Yeager, Kurtman, Landsverk, and Wiesmeier (1988) found a high prevalence of binge eating problems, terror of being fat, and diuretic use in homosexual male college students, indicating another male group at higher risk for eating disorders.

Very little is known about the epidemiology of eating disorders or disordered eating in prepubertal children (Singer, Ambuel, Wade, & Jaffe, 1992). Certain characteristics have been found more commonly in this population when diagnosed with anorexia nervosa or bulimia nervosa (Irwin, 1984; Jemerin & Ponton, 1987). These include a more frequent association at the time of onset with a physical illness; the failure to make expected height and weight gain rather than a weight loss; a dramatic decrease in fluid intake; and a clinical picture that frequently shows a battery of other symptoms, including depression and anxiety. Jaffe and Singer (1989) propose that these children comprise a specific syndrome and do not fall into either diagnostic category.

Individuals who present with eating-disordered behavior and other psychiatric disturbances—most commonly affective, personality, substance abuse, or anxiety disorders—raise some interesting questions about the interaction between disordered eating and other types of psychiatric pathology. Do adolescents with disordered eating or eating disorders more commonly develop other psychopathology? Are adolescents who are struggling with other psychiatric problems more vulnerable to eating disturbance? The answers to these questions are not yet known, but we do recognize that there is significant overlap between individuals with eating disorders and other types of psychopathology. First-degree relatives of individuals with anorexia and bulimia nervosa are reported to have an increased frequency of affective disorders (APA, 1978). Vanderheyden and Boland (1987) emphasize, however, that neither anorexia nervosa nor bulimia nervosa should be considered as variants of affective illness. Although there is clearly an association between affective illness and eating disorders, the relationship between these diagnostic categories still is not well understood, and to identify eating disorders as subtypes or variants of affective disorder would be premature. Rather, the diagnoses can be made concomitantly. The co-morbidity of these two categories of illness is a growing area of study.

Pathogenesis

Any discussion of prevention and treatment of the linked conditions of eating disorders and disordered eating needs to be prefaced with a discussion of the complex biopsychosocial and cultural factors that have affected both the development of the problems themselves as well as our current understanding and treatment of them. The initial work on pathogenesis and theoretical perspective in this area focused on a specific illness, anorexia nervosa, so a historical review of theoretical perspective regarding this illness is useful. It mirrors changes in thinking which have also affected the broader field of disordered eating. The best historian is Alexander Lucas.

Lucas reviews the development of the field of eating disorders in his historical papers (Lucas, 1981; Ponton, 1994). He underscores the need for an integrative approach. He describes six eras wherein controversial data have led to polarized and dogmatic positions. The first, from 1868 to 1914, marks the discovery and acknowledgment of eating disorders in the literature and is titled "the descriptive era." The biological era followed in 1914 when Simmond, a pathologist, described "pituitary cachexia." The etiology developed from the autopsy of a young woman who died of cachexia with pituitary failure. Lucas describes the third era, from 1930 to 1961, as a period of rediscovery. It included the end of Simmond's disease when extensive pathological reports did not substantiate the diagnosis. This era also sparked the recognition of a certain psychopathological component in patients with eating disorders. The fourth era, that of the psychoanalytic perspective, followed the period of rediscovery. The lingering effect of Helene Deutsch's work (1944, 1981), characterized by descriptions of fears of impregnation and delayed adolescent sexuality, still hovers over the field. Lucas describes the fifth era of eating disorders from 1961 to 1980 and highlights the importance of the work of Hilde Bruch, a clinical theoretician who worked to define the diagnoses, develop clinical strategies, and educate patients and their families. He introduces the sixth era in the study of eating disorders crediting the biopsychosocial model and the importance of a developmental approach. He details the complex interactions and genetic determinants that lead to a variable degree of biologic vulnerability in persons who are at risk for experiencing the illness. He states:

> Anorexia nervosa is the ideal paradigm for the study of these interacting factors, and
> such a model is herein proposed. . . . Specific early experiences and family influences
> may create intrapsychic conflicts that determine a psychologic predisposition. Societal
> influences and expectations play their role in setting the social climate that is condu-
> cive to the development of the disease. The biologic factors may be mediated by
> pubertal endocrine changes that initiate the disorder. Psychologic conflicts lead to
> personality and behavioral changes that promote and support the dieting. Social fac-
> tors, such as the cultural obsession with thinness, tend to reinforce the psychologic
> motivation. Each of these factors has greater or less importance for the person in whom
> the disease may manifest itself in degrees of severity. [Lucas, 1981]

Although Lucas is one of the great theoretical and clinical integrationalists in the field of eating disorders, much has happened since he wrote his thoughtful and predictive descriptions, and his historical perspective can also be expanded upon. During the 1980s, there was a growing awareness of the importance of cultural factors in eating disorders and other illnesses. At the end of that decade the model could more aptly be described as a biopsychosocial and cultural model.

Research efforts in the late 1980s and early 1990s have focused on multivariate analyses of risk factors, often examining larger populations than previously studied; these populations are frequently nonclinical. These studies of risk factors have contributed significantly to knowledge of the field and are summarized below before addressing these specific trends.

A number of risk factors have been reported to be associated with disordered eating, among them dieting (Patton, 1992; Polivy & Herman, 1985), early pubertal development in adolescent girls (Irwin & Shafer, 1991), athletics (Taub & Blinde, 1992), sexual abuse (Miller, McClusky-Fawcett, & Irving, 1993), specific patterns of psychological defense (Smith, Thienemann, & Steiner, 1992), family patterns (Kenny & Hart, 1992), female socialization (Striegel-Moore, Silberstein, & Rodin, 1986), and acculturation to Western society (Bulik, 1987b). Although the relationships between these factors and disordered eating are not well understood, the existing knowledge suggests that there is a complex but as yet unknown interaction among many factors.

The knowledge that we have regarding the interaction between dieting and disor-dered eating supports the idea of complex interaction among multiple factors in the etiology of disordered eating. Although we know that dieting may increase the risk of developing binging (Polivy & Herman, 1985), overall, dieting does not appear to be associated with the development of the psychiatric diagnoses of anorexia nervosa and bulimia nervosa without the presence of cofactors such as depression (Patton, 1992). Patton's study of London school girls (1988, 1992) supports a view that dieting in adolescence, although for the most part unproblematic, is in some instances a precursor to the more extreme methods of weight control and concerns about weight.

Similarly, female pubertal development has been found to be associated with the presence of eating disorders (Killen et al., 1992), yet it is probable that disordered eating is only one of a spectrum of risks that affects girls going through puberty. Factors such as early puberty and pubertal discomfort interact with other factors to increase the risk of psychopathology (Irwin & Shafer, 1991), but it is questionable as to whether early puberty by itself is a risk factor without interaction with other factors.

Originally it was believed that certain sports activities (such as ballet dancing, gymnastics, horseback riding, wrestling, and running) were associated with a much higher risk of disordered eating. Sundgot-Borgen (1993) demonstrated that even so-called "protected" sports activities such as swimming were associated with a higher rate of disordered eating. McDonald and Thompson (1992), however, again demonstrated the importance of interactive effects in determining risk when they investigated underlying motivations for engaging in athletic activities. They found that exercising "for health" was associated with low rates of eating disturbance and positive self-esteem for both sexes, whereas exercising "for fitness" in men was correlated with high self-esteem and lower rates of eating disturbance, but in women the findings were significantly different, demonstrating high rates of disordered eating and disturbed body image. Recognition of gender-specific problems for women related to fitness can increase educative and prevention efforts for this population.

Although investigators (Miller et al., 1993) have reported increased rates of sexual abuse associated with women who binge versus controls, one should be skeptical of the interpretation of the results until the interaction between risk factors is better understood. It is possible that the higher rates of sexual abuse are related to underlying psychopathology rather than to disturbed eating behavior. Single-factor studies in this complex area may confuse rather than elucidate the etiology. Pope and Hudson (1992) believe that methodologic factors in specific studies have been responsible for the misperception that childhood sexual abuse is a risk factor for bulimia nervosa.

Defensive styles have been examined as a potential risk factor in a population of adolescent girls diagnosed with eating disorders and affective disorders (Smith et al., 1992). Maturity of defensive style was correlated with overall level of adaptation and was found to be independent of either diagnosis within this population. This result is interesting because it counters early work that suggested that individuals diagnosed with eating disorders had specific defensive styles (Bruch, 1982). This finding is also consistent with the conceptualization of disordered eating as a spectrum affecting individuals very differently and with wide variations in adaptation.

The examination of risk factors related to families has also evolved. Initially, research in this area focused on descriptive studies of families who presented with an adolescent with an eating disorder (Minuchin, Rosman, & Baker, 1980). More recent examinations of family factors have utilized independent rating scales and have focused on rating scales that evaluate parental bonding. Kenny and Hart (1992) found that for college-age adolescent females with eating disorders and a control group of college-age adolescent females without an eating disorder, the presence of an affectively positive and emotionally supportive parental relationship, in conjunction with parental fostering of autonomy, was inversely associated with weight preoccupation, bulimic behavior, and feelings of ineffectiveness. Studies such as those that utilize standardized measures and controls are increasing the knowledge base regarding specificity of risk factors.

In terms of sociocultural influences, it is ironic in this era when women are beginning to feel more empowered in the work arena that they appear to have a heightened sense that their efforts should attain greater success in the domain of beauty and "thinness" as a desired characteristic of beauty as well (Striegel-Moore et al., 1986). The contribution to this pressure from many aspects of the media world (e.g., magazines, television, movies) has increased dramatically during the past 20 years (Yates, 1989), transmitting the value that thinness for women and girls is equated with higher beauty and vocational status.

When considering adolescents, it is important to remember that this trend of cultural valuation begins in childhood, and is pervasive in early adolescence. Tobias and Gordon (1980) found that children devalue obese children and that obesity connotes social isolation for girls. This trend develops even further in adolescence: studies (Eisele, Hertsgaard, & Light, 1986) indicate that 78% of adolescent girls wish to weigh less and only 14% are satisfied with their weight. The thin ideal for girls and women not only appears to be unattainable, but leads to widespread dissatisfaction with their bodies. Cross-cultural studies suggest comparing heavily Westernized cultures with those that are not, but these studies are becoming increasingly difficult to conduct as Western cultural values and the Western media extend through the world (Pate, Pumareiga, Hester, & Garner, 1992). It is clear, however, that these values play some role in the development of eating disorders.

Finally, patients with co-morbidity demand a carefully conducted assessment phase of treatment. Major depression is the most commonly diagnosed co-morbid disorder (Herzog, Keller, Sacks, Yeh, & Lavore, 1992; Hoffman & Halmi, 1993). Patients diagnosed with both anorexia nervosa and bulimia nervosa exhibited the most chronicity and psychiatric co-morbidity (Herzog et al., 1992). Although the patients in this study would be regrouped into anorexia nervosa with binge–purge subtype, this pattern suggests a group at high risk that should be treated with attention to its high rate of severity. Early detection and appropriate treatment of co-morbid disorders increase the likelihood of a good prognosis (Herzog et al., 1992).

Bulimia nervosa has also been linked to alcohol use (Bulik, 1987a) and substance abuse (Lipscomb, 1987). Pope, Frankenburg, Hudson, Jonas, and Yurgelun (1987) failed to find a correlation between bulimia nervosa and borderline personality disorder using the Diagnostic Interview for Borderlines, but other investigators have found co-morbidity (Herzog et al., 1992).

These findings have clear implications for treatment but also suggest areas for future epidemiological studies. Better clarifications of the interactive role of disordered eating and psychiatric diagnoses would, importantly, better outline high-risk groups with whom prevention and treatment efforts could be conducted.

Temporal Trends and Age, Gender, and Ethnic Issues

The carefully constructed epidemiological studies by Lucas (1991), Soundy et al. (1994), and their colleagues in Minnesota suggest several temporal patterns for the diagnostic grouping of anorexia nervosa and bulimia nervosa. As mentioned, Lucas and his colleagues found a gradually increasing incidence of anorexia nervosa in the adolescent population between 1964 and 1984, the last year of their study. Soundy and his colleagues, also in Minnesota, found a parallel pattern regarding the incidence of bulimia nervosa with a peak year in 1983, the highest rates of bulimia nervosa among adolescent females and a moderately increased incidence across the female age spectrum from 1983 to 1990 when the study ended. This suggests that certain factors are affecting the incidence of these two illnesses in the adolescent age group and increasing the incidence of "disordered eating" among the younger adolescent girls.

These studies suggest that we should look at how adolescents, particularly adolescent females, feel about their bodies and their adolescent development, as well as focusing on which unhealthy behaviors related to body image and eating they are engaging in.

In keeping with Lucas's biopsychosocial, and now cultural, model for eating disorders, the etiology of the problem is not simple. The confluence of many factors appears to increase the incidence of this problem in adolescent females. Progressively early puberty in adolescent females gives them mature bodies before they are psychologically ready to cope with the attention that female bodies receive in the current cultural milieu. On the other hand, adolescence is a time when girls develop almost twice as much body fat as boys (in childhood, the difference is only 10–15% greater in girls; Marino & King, 1980). Physical maturation in adolescent boys, with its associated increase in muscle and lean tissue, brings them closer to the masculine ideal. For many girls, however, adolescent development, with its coincident fat deposits, is a move away from the current feminine ideal (Striegel-Moore *et al.,* 1986).

Biological changes are also compounded by psychological issues for adolescent girls. The psychological tasks of adolescence include separation and individuation from parents and important adult figures, identity formation, exploration of intimate relationships, and acquisition of control and mastery over drives and impulses (Lamb, 1986). Adolescent girls and boys pursue these tasks differently. Most notably, adolescent girls seem to be more interpersonally oriented than are boys (Gilligan, 1982). This orientation has several advantages in terms of achieving intimacy, but girls may also worry more about what people think of them, and may be more willing to please others and work hard to avoid perceived negative reactions (Simmons & Rosenberg, 1975). Losing weight may allow them to defy their pubertal development and fulfill society's current feminine ideal through pleasing others, a psychological process with which they are quite familiar.

Societal factors also affect this problem. The 1980s were associated with increased incidence of eating disorders in adolescent females. Snow and Harris (1985) noted an increasing trend in slim models between 1950 and 1983. Contemporary television and film portray the successful woman as being thin (Garner & Garfinkel, 1980). Increased emphasis on slender-as-successful combines with the very real lack of opportunities to achieve power that are presented to young women to encourage pursuit of thinness as one pathway. Young women with eating disorders comment repeatedly that they are engaging in the eating-disordered behavior to gain "power" or "control" over their lives (Bruch, 1982). Becoming a slender object is an opportunity for a certain kind of female power in this society, that of achieving or exemplifying the popular physical feminine ideal. Adolescent girls with psychological vulnerabilities—low self-esteem, coincident depression, histories of sexual abuse, or other psychological disturbance—are more likely to develop eating disorders (Ponton, 1993).

Notions about eating disorders affecting specific cultural or socioeconomic groups have existed for over a century. In 1880, Fenwick observed that anorexia nervosa was more common in the "wealthier classes of society than those who have to procure their bread by daily labor" (p. 107). Bruch (1966) was one of the first investigators to connect the onset of eating disorders in families with the values of strong achievement and upward mobility. As early as 1970, investigators (Rowland, 1970) were reporting a growing percentage of eating-disordered patients from lower- and middle-class backgrounds. Theander (1970) suggested that disordered eating may develop in a specific ethnic group or social class as attitudes about achievement, appearance, weight changes, and female role. Theander's additional prediction about shifts in populations affected by disordered eating has taken place. There are now reports of eating disorders in African-Americans (Pumareiga, Edwards, & Mitchell, 1984), in Asians (Kope & Sack, 1987), Latinos/Hispanics (Silber, 1986), and Native Americans (Yates, 1989). Similar patterns have been noted in various cultures worldwide as adherence to Western culture and values grows. Our current understanding is that this shift represents an increase in incidence in nonwhite populations, not simply increased reporting (Pate *et al.*, 1992).

Studies of a population in transition to Western values reveal that the diagnosable eating disorders are just a part of the picture. In a study of risk behaviors in a large population of American youth, Ponton *et al.* (1994) found that large numbers of Native American youth were reporting high rates of disordered eating behavior and normal to low body weight most commonly associated with anorexia nervosa and bulimia nervosa. These results differ from the high incidence of obesity formerly found in Native American youth during this century (Ponton *et al.*, 1994a). Adolescent girls are the most likely to manifest this pattern consisting of restricting and/or binging for weight control. Why these symptoms are occurring with this group at this particular time is interesting and important for targeted prevention efforts.

In summary, certain groups seem to be at high risk for developing both eating disorders and disordered eating. At highest risk are adolescent females in a cultural group that is adopting Western values. Epidemiological patterns observed have also been altered by the rapidly changing knowledge base in this field. A decade ago, Native American adolescents may not have been studied, but recent studies suggest that they might be a population at risk. Future studies will continue to alter how we see both the spectrum of disordered eating in adolescents and the specific diagnoses of anorexia nervosa and bulimia nervosa.

PREVENTION

Literature Review

In contrast to other risk behaviors discussed in this volume, the development of the field of prevention with respect to the continuum of disordered eating is very limited. In some respects it makes for a simple discussion of the topic because the existing prevention programs can be presented and discussed expeditiously. However, the lack of prevention programs makes identification of important aspects for future prevention efforts quite difficult. Even though there is not a large number of papers on prevention, a broad spectrum of ideas on the topic of prevention can be found scattered throughout articles on epidemiology, pathogenesis, or treatment.

Prevention programs are often aided by preliminary investigative literature which identifies the antecedents of a behavior. Even investigating the antecedents of the spectrum of eating-disordered behaviors is complex. There is a body of literature concerning investigations or descriptions of the antecedents of full-fledged eating disorders focused on the diagnoses of anorexia and bulimia nervosa (Garner & Garfinkel, 1980). There are few studies, however, that address the largest category: the antecedents of the symptoms of disordered eating (Patton, 1992).

Part of the reason for this is because most of the research in the field of disordered eating has been conducted on clinical populations which already carry the diagnosis of an eating disorder or an eating disorder coexisting with other psychiatric diagnoses. Prevalence studies have examined nonclinical populations, but have often been quite restrictive, focusing on populations at risk—schoolgirls, patients in a general practice clinic, university students, and athletes. During the past decade, the limitations of studies in identified patient or high-risk groups have been recognized and have led to research on the continuum of disordered eating in nonclinical populations. Recent epidemiological studies have concentrated their efforts in this area and a small number of prevention studies have followed.

A second category of study contributing to the area of prevention has focused on factors contributing to some aspect of the continuum of eating-disordered behavior such as exercise, dieting, or parental attachment. Many of these studies comment on widespread but vague prevention efforts aimed at educating the general population about the behavior and associated risks. A third category of prevention studies, that of piloted interventions, including pre- and postassessment, has grown during the past decade but is still limited.

Populations that have already been mentioned as having high rates of eating-disordered behavior include schoolgirls (Johnson-Sabine, Wood, Patton, Mann, & Wakeling, 1988), patients in a general practice clinic (King, 1989; Whitehouse, Cooper, Vize, Hill, & Vogel, 1992), university students (Herzog & Copeland, 1985; Schotte & Stunkard, 1987), and athletes (Benson, Alleman, Thintz, & Howard, 1990; McDonald & Thompson, 1992; Taub & Blinde, 1992). The studies examining clinical populations suggested a variety of early detection techniques. Whitehouse *et al.* (1992) studied a population of 540 women attending a general practice clinic and found that half of the cases of bulimia nervosa (8 cases total) and partial bulimia nervosa (29 cases total) had not been identified by the general practitioner even though some of the patients had been referred to medical specialists for treatment of secondary complications of the eating disorder. They suggest developing and distributing a rudimentary assessment tool that general practitioners could use for detection of eating disorders as well as for educating general practitioners about disordered eating. Studies that identify athletes as a high-risk group also suggest prevention strategies. Benson *et al.* (1990) found that certain groups of adolescent athletes such as swimmers, heretofore believed to be at low risk for eating-disordered behavior, may have rates as high as "high-risk" athletes—dancers, wrestlers, runners, and gymnasts. They suggest the development of tailored intervention programs highlighting the risk of eating-disordered athletes for all adolescent athletes.

Studies that focus on risk factors such as dieting, exercise, early puberty, and the link between substance abuse and eating disorders as contributing to some aspect of disordered eating behavior also provide information about prevention. In this category studies focusing on dieting are the most well known. Dieting is commonly and falsely believed to be a successful strategy for weight reduction. Hueneman, Shapiro, Hampton, and Mitchell (1966) studied a group of adolescents over 4 years and found that adolescent dieters retained the same proportion of body fat. Studies examining weight loss indicate that effective weight loss must include an integrated weight reduction approach utilizing behavior techniques, skill-building, nutritional counseling, and exercise aimed at changing adolescents' patterns or life-style (Mellin, 1993). The Centers for Disease Control (1991) recognizes that both unhealthy weight gain and reduction are serious problems for adolescents and represent one of the most important health concerns in the United States today (Public Health Service, 1988; Shisslak, Crago, & Neal, 1987). To develop appropriate weight management practices among adolescents, the CDC recommends the development and implementation of programs about assessment and maintenance of healthy body weight involving families, teachers, school administrators, nurses, counselors, public health officials, pediatricians, and family practitioners. They recommend that this goal be implemented through the development of family-based adolescent obesity programs. Although their conceptualization of the magnitude of the problems regarding weight and adolescents is good, their recommended prevention program for obesity would probably be frightening to young girls who fear that they are becoming obese. However, the CDC recognizes the full extent of disordered eating among adolescents and suggests that a range of individuals, including both care-givers and adolescents, need to be targeted in prevention efforts. Family practitioners and specialists in adolescent medicine are often very conscious of the wide range of risk behaviors that today's adolescents face. They are beginning to recommend integrating concerns about disordered eating into general programs addressing risk reduction in the adolescent population. They underscore the lack of exercise among the adolescents of today and believe that effective prevention programs should include exercise as one of their main components (Gilchrist, 1991).

Onset of puberty may be an important risk factor for eating-disordered behavior among adolescent females, the high-risk group. Killen *et al.* (1992) found an association between sexual maturation (using self-reported Tanner staging) and disordered eating, suggest targeting prevention efforts toward pre- and peripubertal girls. Their study and general knowledge about overall increased risk behavior among early developing females (Irwin & Shafer, 1991) suggest that we should examine how pubertal development is introduced to girls. It is possible that initial education efforts on puberty which occur in the fourth or fifth grade could be modified and appended with a section on normal female body development and associated risks. This type of program might also be an opportunity to educate teachers and parents about the risks for early developing girls.

Watts and Ellis (1992) believe that we cannot separate prevention efforts regarding disordered eating from those addressing substance abuse. Like many others, they believe that the same impulsivity and need to control that is thought to underlie substance abuse also underlies eating disorders. They believe that substance abuse and eating disorders can be best explained by the concept of addiction (i.e., the anorexic addicted to food restriction, the bulimic to food binges, and the substance abuser to the intake of substances). Whether or not you agree with their underlying assumption, they make some interesting recommendations regarding prevention, suggesting that peer-based prevention groups which have been used effectively with substance and alcohol use could be part of a more complex strategy. They also recommend coordination of the peer-based program with a program for families which addresses the role that families play in addictive behaviors.

Effective Prevention Programs

Although there are many ideas and even recommendations concerning prevention of disordered eating, there are few piloted prevention programs. The programs that have been tested are presented here with special attention paid to whether they can be modified and more widely implemented. Three of the four existing programs (Killen *et al.*, 1993; Moreno & Thelan, 1993; Paxton, 1993) target disordered eating in junior high school girls using the school setting. The intervention developed by Moreno and Thelan was conducted among junior-high school girls (135 control group subjects and 82 experimental group subjects) in a home economics class, and consisted of viewing a 6-minute videotape on bulimia and participating in a group discussion for the remainder of the hour. All subjects were pretested, then tested again at 4 days and 1 month. Knowledge, attitudes, and behavioral intentions regarding disordered eating were assessed utilizing a 23-item questionnaire. Based on comparisons of the experimental and control groups, they found that even this brief intervention was successful in changing girls' knowledge, attitudes, and behavioral intentions regarding some aspect of their eating behavior. The factors that were most affected by the intervention were the attitudes and knowledge about weight and diet. The intervention group reported a significantly reduced likelihood that they would diet in order to lose weight. The intervention group also acquired a significantly greater knowledge base regarding purging. There was only minimal difference reported between the two groups on attitudes about purging because the baseline attitude about purging for both groups was already very negative prior to the intervention. Attitudes about exercise and weight loss were also not greatly affected by the intervention as measured by differences between the control and experimental groups.

There are several limitations to this study. First, it is a very brief intervention. Populations of junior high school girls would have to be followed over time to find out if the intervention continued to make a significant difference. It would also be important to find out if the intervention alters more than behavioral intention, i.e., behavior. Only a longitudinal study could demonstrate this. (Moreno and Thelan did raise the idea of adding on "booster sessions" at a later point to maintain and build on the positive effects of their original effort.) Another serious limitation is the sole measure of the 23-item questionnaire. Moreno and Thelan's results are more positive than the other two studies implemented by Paxton and by Killen and colleagues, but part of the difference may be related to their more limited questionnaire. A larger battery of measures which could have included the Eating Disorder Index, for example, would have provided us with more information about this intervention.

The intervention of junior high school girls developed and piloted by Killen and colleagues was much more extensive. In their study, 963 sixth- and seventh-graders were randomized to intervention and control groups. The intervention group participated in an 18-hour curriculum developed around three components: instruction on the harmful effects of unhealthful weight regulation, promotion of healthful weight regulation through the practice of sound nutrition and dietary principles and regular physical activity, and the development of coping skills for resisting sociocultural influences related to weight. They utilized a number of measures including a scale to measure knowledge developed by the authors, the 64-item Eating Disorder Index Scale, the revised Dietary Restraint Scale developed by Herman, Polivy, Pliner, and Threlkeld (1978), a self-report measure of eating disorder symptoms, and the Body Mass Index measure.

Although they did observe a significant increase in knowledge among girls receiving the intervention, there was only a small, albeit statistically significant, effect on body mass index. The girls participating in the intervention were divided into high- and low-risk groups for disordered eating based on their responses to the self-report measure examining weight concerns. The high-risk group manifested greater benefit from the intervention than did the low-risk intervention group or the high- and low-risk controls. They exhibited a significant gain in knowledge and showed a significantly smaller gain in body mass index than did the control group, indicating that they were gaining weight in a developmentally appropriate way, with lower levels of fat gain. Body mass index is considered to be the preferred index of relative body weight as a reflection of adiposity.

Based on this study, Killen and colleagues believe that interventions similar to theirs need to be targeted to identified high-risk junior high school girls. A simple measure of self-report questioning girls about dieting patterns and weight concerns could be used to locate girls at risk who would then be targeted with a healthy weight curriculum designed to modify typical eating attitudes and unhealthy weight reduction practices. They recommend that these future interventions be even more intensive than the one they piloted because even after the intervention, the weight concerns of the high-risk students were still twice those of the lower-risk students. They also raise the idea of attaching prevention programs to treatment sites. How the prevention and treatment components fit together is clearly important. When Shisslak et al. (1987) moved in the opposite direction and incorporated a treatment component into a pilot eating disorder prevention intervention for high school students, even extensive advertising services did not yield more than minimal use of the treatment option. Killen et al. (1993) suggest an alternative strategy to embed a more intensive curriculum within a general curriculum that provides health information to all students. The interface between prevention and treatment is important and will be discussed more extensively at the end of this section.

A third intervention again piloted junior high school girls, this time 107 ninth-grade girls in Australia, and presented them with five specialized classes addressing media images of women, determinants of body size, healthy and unhealthy weight control, and eating and emotions (Paxton, 1993). The girls completed self-report questionnaires assessing eating behavior and body image prior to the intervention and at 1- and 12-month follow-up. They were unable to detect any measurable effect of the intervention using their measures. What is remarkable about this intervention is that there was a very small control group of 29 students from a different school. The different school environment and extremely small number are serious problems in the study. It also made no attempt to define or target high-risk girls, who may have received significantly greater benefit, a factor that would be lost when their results are included in the larger population.

A fourth disordered eating prevention program—the only one not conducted with middle school girls—was developed in Germany by Gerlinghoff, Backmund, Angenendt, and Linington (1991) and combined prevention and treatment components. They developed a three-stage program targeted to eating-disordered patients and consisting of 1–2 months of outpatient motivation, an 8-week day hospital program, and a 1- to 2-year outpatient group therapy phase. A prevention component was part of the outpatient program. Their preliminary results indicated that this prevention/treatment model was effective and they are awaiting follow-up data. I mention this program because it underscores the importance of linking prevention components to treatment efforts; this is appropriate for eating disorders such as bulimia and anorexia nervosa which have a high rate of chronicity, and individuals coming for treatment by definition are high risk for recurrent episodes. In this context, prevention is targeted toward chronicity.

What Works: Development of Future Programs

Although there are only a limited number of existing prevention programs, several conclusions can be made from both general and specific studies. First, developing targeted programs for adolescents at risk (i.e., school girls, university students, athletes, and girls visiting general practice clinics) is an important idea. Nonspecific studies of high-risk populations (Benson et al., 1990; Herzog & Copeland, 1985; King, 1989; McDonald & Thompson, 1992; Schotte & Stunkard, 1987; Taub & Blinde, 1992; Whitehouse et al. 1992) suggest this, and the intervention developed by Killen et al. (1993) found the greatest benefit with the girls at higher risk. Second, the interface between dieting and disordered eating also bears further investigation and development. Adolescent dieters may be a high-risk population that would benefit from targeted intervention. We also need to develop methods for imparting to adolescents the important prevention message that dieting is not a strategy for weight control that is likely to prove successful. As puberty itself appears to be a risk factor for disordered eating, girls who are pre- and peripubertal should be assessed and monitored for manifestations of disordered eating. A second important prevention message to deliver is that pubertal development in girls is normally accompanied by changes in body composition including body fat composition. The need for this fact to become an accepted and acceptable reality clearly underscores the negative effects of the current sociocultural media message which is its opposite.

Specific intervention studies suggest other important strategies for future prevention efforts. Interventions need to be reproducible and effected with sufficiently large intervention and control groups. Paxton's study which utilized a control population of 29 subjects from a different school illustrates potential problems in this arena. One session or cluster of sessions may not be adequate and the idea of "booster sessions" at a later point to build on the positive effects as proposed by Moreno and Thelan should be considered. Measures utilized in the interventions have to be very carefully considered. Including measures that assess more than change in knowledge or attitudes such as measures of behavioral intention (Moreno & Thelan, 1993) or monitoring the body mass index (Killen et al., 1993) is valuable. Refining and utilizing existing measures would offer uniformity and help standardize prevention efforts. Attaching and integrating prevention programs with treatment is also important. Shisslak and colleagues' failure to have treatment offers accepted in the high school population indicates that the marketing of treatment and prevention efforts for adolescent girls must be carefully considered. Prevention components targeted at behavior patterns and future episodes should also be attached to all treatment services to decrease chronicity. Detecting middle school girls—the population most at risk for disordered eating—and tracking them into well-marketed, specialized interventions in the school setting appears to be valuable. Full-fledged disorders have not yet developed or are in the early stages at this point, and the school site allows greater accessibility to the intervention rather than requiring that the girls attend a treatment setting.

One also has to be aware of the overall cultural and media context in which the interventions occur. Paxton (1993) raised a significant concern when he stated that he believes that their intervention was ineffective because it was conducted in a cultural and media milieu that promoted unhealthy eating habits. He suggests the important strategy of combining on-site school interventions with a larger media-focused prevention effort.

Ethnic and Gender Issues in Prevention Programs

Taking into account the limited number of prevention programs, it is not surprising that there has been only minimal discussion of how ethnic and gender issues affect prevention programs. Although ethnic and gender issues do not yet play a large role in prevention, they seriously impact on the overall topic of disordered eating.

A common misconception is that these disorders affect only white females. There are dramatically increasing numbers among Hispanic (Silber, 1986), African-American (Pumareiga et al., 1984), and Asian (Kope & Sack, 1987) females. Currently, Native American adolescent females are reporting some of the highest rates of disordered eating (with normal or lower than normal body weights) (Ponton et al., 1994), indicating that specialized interventions need to be developed for nonwhite adolescent females who appear to be at high or higher risk for disordered eating as they assimilate the thin-body ideals of Western culture. Further research may demonstrate culturally specific risk factors that would be important to target in interventions. For example, Native American adolescent females appear to exhibit an increase in risk behaviors overall as the rate of disordered eating increases.

The diagnoses of anorexia nervosa, bulimia nervosa, and atypical binge-eating disorder affect females ten times more commonly than males. To date, the limited number of interventions have ignored males. Certain groups of males—models, actors, gymnasts, wrestlers, jockeys, and runners—are at significantly higher risk for eating disorders and would benefit from targeted interventions. In developing programs to target men, an initial strategy should include an educational component which educates the public about the presence of these disorders in men and simultaneously works to decrease the stigma for men having these disorders. Prevention programs in this subgroup would need to target an array of risk behaviors, including steroid use and high-risk careers and exercise patterns for men who develop eating disorders.

Because the disorders primarily affect adolescent females, there is also a lack of recognition of the disorders in younger girls and older women. Recognition of how the disorders are manifested in these other age groups is important, and interventions would have to be modified appropriately for these populations. For example, younger girls with this disorder often have a very concrete but age-appropriate approach to nutrition and dieting. Interventions would have to understand their perspective and be able to address the girls' misconceptions about eating.

Summary: Highlighting Limitations of Current Programs

Most of the limitations of prevention programs have been mentioned in earlier sections, but I will highlight them here. There have been only a few prevention programs piloted to date. Several of these (Killen *et al.*, 1993; Paxton, 1993) have not shown significant changes. Many of the researchers make the point that the interventions are conducted in an overall cultural milieu that encourages unhealthy eating and overly thin body types. Investigators suggest that time-limited interventions need to be combined with media and cultural interventions.

Several other areas have been noted in this section and deserve efforts in the near future. First, adding prevention components to treatment efforts is promising and merits further research. Second, screening high-risk populations such as middle school girls, and channeling them into school-based interventions developed and targeted specifically for them, is crucial. Designing tailored interventions for high-risk groups that target cultural, gender, and age-related factors is also necessary. All prevention efforts should include assessment measures so that our knowledge of this limited area can be expanded further. They should also include the two important prevention messages to date: that dieting is not a successful method for weight control, and that female pubertal development is normally accompanied by body changes that include increased body fat composition. As a final consideration, interventions that target disordered eating behavior and utilize the media should be developed and evaluated.

TREATMENT

Although there is a whole spectrum of severity, from mild to severe, in patients presenting with disordered eating, many of those with anorexia nervosa and bulimia nervosa are extremely difficult to treat and respond best to combined modalities. And although many papers are written about treating adults with eating disorders, Wachsmuth and Garfinkel (1983) underscore the point that there are only a limited number of articles available on the treatment of adolescents. They emphasize the importance of the treating physician or therapist being able to set and prioritize clear treatment goals for this age group. The goals they outline include establishing and maintaining a treatment alliance based on trust; weight restoration or a cessation of binging, vomiting, or other unhealthy weight reduction methods; improvement in eating behavior; and improvement in social behavior.

Assessment

The treatment of these difficult patients responds best to an approach that integrates several modalities, including physical assessment and laboratory testing, nutritional assessment, and evaluation of individual psychopathology and family functioning. Ideally the treatment team should have considerable experience working together and should be able to address each of these important areas. A possible combination for members of the treatment team would include a pediatrician or primary care physician, a nutritionist, and a psychiatrist or other trained mental health professional, all with expertise in this area. The basic history and physical examination gathered and conducted by the physician should include a weigh-in, vital signs, and evaluation of daily activities including exercise, eating, and sports and school activities (Kreipe & Uphoff, 1992). Baseline collaborating data would include a complete blood count, a serum electrolyte determination, urinalysis, an electrocardiogram, T_4 and TSH, LH and FSH (Fisher, 1992). Additional tests such as an MRI brain scan may be prescribed when the diagnosis is unclear to rule out other clinical entities. All members of the team should question the patient about weight loss examining methods and signs and symptoms. The nutritionist should begin an educational program explaining methods of weight reduction or weight maintenance and, emphasizing the keeping of a daily food journal, should help the patient initiate a healthy dietary plan. A nutritional assessment includes an assessment of daily nutritional intake combined with eating attitudes, behaviors, and habits, and an anthropoietic assessment, which might include skinfold caliper measurements of subcutaneous body fat (Schebendach & Nussbaum, 1992). A nutritional assessment might also include laboratory and metabolic assessment, areas that may overlap with the basic physical examination. Evaluation by the mental health professional should include an individual assessment and evaluation of the family, which covers developmental issues and makes psychiatric diagnoses such as anorexia or bulimia nervosa as well as other co-morbid diagnoses. The mental health professional should also evaluate and oversee the utility of psychopharmacologic agents. Once the initial assessment has been conducted, the treatment team should meet, share recommendations, and establish or refer to an ongoing treatment program.

Inpatient treatment is determined by the presence of specific criteria that Herzog and Copeland (1985) define as: weight loss greater than 30% over a 3-month period; metabolic disturbances manifested by vital sign changes, or changes in the potassium or bound urea nitrogen; suicidal risk; severe purging with a risk of aspiration; or the presence of psychosis and the existence of a family crisis that puts the adolescent's physical health or safety in jeopardy. A combined methodologic approach to inpatient treatment should be adopted, including the implementation of an eating disorder protocol to restore eating, and a combined approach utilizing individual family, group, nutritional, and biological therapy. The inpatient hospitalization might begin with a behavioral modification plan that reinforces weight gain by offering a levels system with increasing responsibility and privilege. Nasogastric feeding is also frequently employed if the severity of weight loss mandates it (Larocca & Goodner, 1986). The inpatient unit also offers an opportunity for intensive education about faulty eating behaviors and can utilize group, milieu, family, and individual therapy; diet and exercise counseling; and psychoeducational material to promote changes in eating and social behavior.

Outpatient treatment is also aided by a team approach where team members (physician, nutritionist, and psychiatrist or psychologist) continue to collaborate at regular intervals (Kreipe & Uphoff, 1992).

Before any effective treatment program can be developed, it is important that the treatment team understand the biological, psychological, social, and cultural components of these illnesses.

Biological Treatment Modalities

In addition to understanding the diverse etiology of these illnesses, it is important to have a clear grasp of physical changes commonly associated with them. Physiological changes with eating disorders are well summarized in the review articles by Herzog and Copeland (1985), Halmi (1983), and Yates (1990). I will highlight some of the areas important to focus on clinically.

Biological theories are most frequently based on studies that have been conducted on individuals maintained on semistarvation diets. They report that starving individuals undergo sleep disturbance, impaired concentration, indecisiveness, withdrawal, mood lability, anxiety, and depression (Garfinkel & Kaplan, 1985). There are a host of abnormal neuroendocrine axes in anorexic patients who are self-starved, and, in fact, the whole endocrine axis is very much affected by the starvation process. In starvation, the hypothalamus secretes a larger amount of corticotropin-releasing factor that stimulates the adrenal cortex. The degree of elevation of corticotropin-releasing hormone in the CSF of anorexic patients correlates with the degree of their depression (Gold & Rubinow, 1987).

Kaye, Picker, Naber, and Ebert (1982) demonstrate that endogenous opiates are elevated in the CSF of anorexics although certain β-endorphins are reported to be within the normal limits. Through the disruption of the endocrine axis, β-endorphins could possibly be implicated in these disorders, creating the inhibition of CNS catecholamine that is characteristic of anorexia. Underweight anorexic women also have low levels of another neurotransmitter, serotonin. Serotonin is important in the regulation of sleep, pain, appetite, and mood. All of these factors indicate the important role that the biological aspects play in the maintenance of this illness.

Anorexia nervosa in many ways parallels other "starvation states." There are many changes consistent with this including differences in total sodium, potassium loss, and decreased T_3 and T_4. Decreased production of blood cells of all types is a frequent phenomenon. Anemia, leukopenia, and thrombocytopenia are associated with changes in the bone marrow. The anemia may contribute to fatigue. In patients with bulimia nervosa, hypokalemic alkalosis is one of the most serious physical problems. Careful monitoring of serum creatinine and BUN is important. Also quite serious are EKG changes increased by electrolyte abnormalities. Most remarkable are flattening of the T wave, ST segment depression, and lengthening of the QT interval. Long-term presence of anorexia nervosa may lead to cardiac changes, including thinning of the wall of the left ventricle. EEG changes are also notable revealing moderate to marked slowing. Vomiting is more significant in patients with EEG changes, indicating that it might reflect CSF changes. For bulimics, many gastrointestinal abnormalities—tears from vomiting, erosion of dental enamel, and gastric dilation with the risk of rupture—present significant risk. Renal changes that reflect dehydration and a reduced glomerular filtration rate may also be present. The incidence of renal calculi is increased.

Hormonal abnormalities are also found with these disorders. If amenorrhea, one of the diagnostic criteria for anorexia nervosa, is present, it may appear associated with hypothalamic abnormalities even before weight loss. Amenorrhea in anorexia nervosa is associated with a revision of gonadotropin secretion to the prepubertal pattern (Boyer, Katz, & Finkelstein, 1974). Specifically, there is a decrease in the pattern of gonadotropin pulsations, and the development of what is quite similar to a prepubertal pattern. Gonadotropin secretion is decreased in both male and female adolescents. Other hormonal changes include a change in growth hormone, which is elevated in response to the decreased levels of somatomedin C.V., and abnormal temperature regulations that occur regularly secondary to the loss of body fat and/or a hypothalamic defect. The complexity of physiological changes in adolescent patients with eating disorders necessitates that the treating therapist be informed about the condition and either be fully trained or work with someone who is fully trained in the medical aspects of these illnesses.

Psychological Treatment Modalities

Recent studies (Agras *et al.*, 1992; Fairburn, Jones, Peveler, Hope, & O'Connor, 1993; Garner *et al.*, 1993) indicate that a structured psychotherapy specifically designed for the treatment of bulimia nervosa is most beneficial in comparative studies. Fairburn and colleagues compared cognitive behavioral therapy (CBT), interpersonal therapy (ITP), and behavioral therapy (a modified program separate from CBT) and found that patients in the groups receiving CBT and ITP respectively made the most substantial and long-lasting changes across all symptom areas at a 12-month follow-up point. Although CBT and ITP achieved roughly equivalent results, it is believed that they work through different mediating mechanisms with clear temporal differences in areas of response. A further comparison of CBT and IPT would be beneficial.

Garner and colleagues compared the effectiveness of 4 months of CBT and supportive expressive therapy for bulimia. They found that both were effective in leading to significant improvement in specific eating disorder symptoms and psychosocial disturbances. CBT was found to be more effective, however, in promoting long-term abstention from vomiting. They recommend further refinement of the psychotherapy treatment modalities for eating disorders, repeat studies that clearly differentiate diagnostic groupings (anorexia nervosa versus bulimia nervosa versus subclinical but symptomatic and normals), and longer-term follow-up.

Another study, conducted by Agras *et al.* (1992), compared pharmacologic treatment (specifically desipramine), CBT, and a group that received both desipramine and CBT. After 4 months of treatment the patients in the CBT group and the combined group were doing better than the controls and the group given medication alone. However, at the 8-month point, only the combined treatment program was superior to the other single treatment modality groups and the controls. It is important to understand that all of the controlled medication or psychotherapy studies have been conducted with adult females. Although we believe the information is applicable to the adolescent population, it is important to repeat the studies with adolescents.

Family therapy may be an important component of both inpatient and outpatient treatment. It is particularly important in the treatment of adolescents. In a randomized study of discharged inpatients with eating disorders (Russell, Szmukler, & Dare, 1987), family therapy was found to be most effective in patients whose illness was not chronic and where the onset of the illness occurred at 19 years of age or younger. Family therapy also appears to be particularly helpful if the patient needs to attain autonomy from the family.

The cornerstone of treatment for individuals with anorexia nervosa and bulimia nervosa continues to be individual psychotherapy focusing on both the individual's symptoms and underlying psychological problems associated with the illness. Bruch (1982) introduced the importance of this type of work which focuses on building individual autonomy in contrast to analytically uncovering psychological issues. The therapist working with these patients actually performs several roles. One role is clearly that of providing education about the impact of societal expectations regarding body image, but equally important, and often more difficult, is to help the young patient understand how societal expectations and the patient's own issues result in a pattern of disordered eating. An additional role for the individual therapist is to help the patient see the disordered eating behavior as risk-taking, and then to help him or her develop an internal process of risk assessment (Ponton, 1993). These are complex functions which require individual therapists with medical knowledge, societal awareness, psychological understanding, and an ability to address risk-taking behavior in the adolescent population.

Medications Commonly Used in Treatment

Psychotropic therapy may be an important component but should be carefully integrated with the use of other therapies. Anorexic patients who are depressed have lowered urinary excretion of *3-methoxy-4 hydroxy phenylglycol,* which suggests a greater responsiveness to norepinephrine-reuptake blockers such as imipramine or desipramine (Herzog & Copeland, 1985). However, there are to date no published controlled trials of the use of tricyclic antidepressants in adolescents with eating disorders (Wachsmuth & Garfinkel, 1983). Imipramine and phenelzine have been found to be superior to placebo in reducing depressive and bulimia symptoms in the treatment of bulimia (Bond, Crabbes, & Sanders, 1986), but more controlled studies are needed in the pharmacotherapy of eating disorders. In general, restrictor anorexics experience more side effects than bulimics with medications. Therefore, careful attention to the side effect profile must occur when treating that population. Medications that have some utility in treating patients with eating disorders include: antidepressants, phenothiazines, anxiolytics, cyproheptadine marketed as periactin, clonidine, naloxone, and lithium. Tricyclics and other newer antidepressant agents are frequently used in the treatment of bulimia nervosa and are recommended in the treatment of anorexia nervosa when a concomitant affective disorder has been diagnosed. Treating adolescents diagnosed with anorexia nervosa with tricylic medication necessitates a careful monitoring of cardiac function with serial EKGs. Adolescents' greater proclivity for cardiac changes makes the consideration of alternatives to tricyclic antidepressants such as fluoxetine important.

The use of fluoxetine and other serotonergic agents is also important in patients with bulimia nervosa, where they have been shown to decrease binging and associated cravings. It is believed that fluoxetine accomplishes this by increasing serotonin levels in the brain. Patients who respond successfully claim that they get full faster and crave binge foods less. It is important to note that antidepressant medication may decrease either depressive symptoms or binging patterns. Current understanding indicates that there is an independent relationship between the two factors so one, both, or neither may improve.

A major impediment to fluoxetine use has been the reported side effect of increased suicidality. Wheadon *et al.* (1992) conducted a controlled study where they looked at suicidality associated with fluoxetine use in individuals being treated for bulimia. They found no increased incidence of suicidality in the population treated with fluoxetine compared with the control group. New serotonergic agents continue to be piloted and tested in patients with bulimia nervosa. Pilot studies have been conducted with fluoxamine (Faverin) in patients diagnosed with atypical binge eating disorder and bulimia nervosa with favorable results, including decreased binging and reported improved affect (Gardiner, Freeman, Jesinger, & Collins, 1993). It is important to underscore that these studies have not been conducted with adolescents, and that the Food and Drug Administration has only recently indicated that serotonergic agents could be used specifically for treating binging rather than the more common usage for depression.

Phenothiazines are occasionally used in the treatment of low-weight patients with anorexia nervosa who also present with symptoms of severe anxiety or delusional material. Attention to side effect profile and lowered dosage should be utilized because the patients are quite sensitive to medications. Pimazide (Vandereycken & Pierloot, 1982) has been shown to be slightly better than placebo at increasing weight gain. Occasionally patients with anorexia nervosa who are in the hospital on bedrest may benefit from mild anxiolytics to decrease anxiety prior to meals. Xanax has been used for that purpose. Cyproheptadine (Periactin) is an antihistamine and antiserotonergic agent which competes with histamine and serotonin for receptor sites. This blockage of serotonin supposedly leads to an increased appetite, helping the patients to eat. The medication is manufactured in 4-mg capsules and given 4–20 mg/day (Mitchell, 1987; Yates, 1990). Other agents that have demonstrated some utility include clonidine (Catapres), which is an adrenergic potentiator that may act centrally to assist individuals with strong binge cravings during the withdrawal period. The common dosage is 0.1 mg given twice a day, but the dose range may be as high as 0.2 to 0.8 mg. Naloxone hydrochloride is a narcotic antagonist, a synthetic congener of oxymorphone. It is also supposed to decrease cravings in doses of 0.4 to 2 mg daily possibly acting through stimulation of β-endorphins (Yates, 1990).

Lithium carbonate is the treatment of choice for patients co-diagnosed with an eating disorder and bipolar affective disorder. Caution must be exercised in using this medication with either bulimic or anorexic patients because of the risk associated with neurological and cardiac toxicity in the population (Bond *et al.*, 1986).

Treatment Programs for Obesity

Obesity is believed to be connected most strongly with environmental factors, particularly diet, lack of physical activity, and family patterns of feeding. Psychological explanations have been formulated by Hilde Bruch, who states that feeding becomes a substitute for other sources of satisfaction (Bruch, 1974). Most notably, obese children who are heavily stigmatized exhibit a greater sensitivity and lower self-esteem (Kalucy, 1976).

A recent paper (Epstein, Valoski, Wing, & McCurley, 1994) summarizing 10-year treatment outcomes for children in four randomized behavior studies has yielded some important results. Ten years after treatment, 34% of the obese children had a decreased percentage over normal weight, and 30% were no longer obese. These results sharply contrast with treatment outcome studies of obese adults. Treatment efforts that involved a parent and/or the addition of exercise were the most successful. Given that these studies involved 10-year follow-up and were initiated in 1977, the interventions were quite old and did not represent state-of-the-art treatment. What the study does underscore is that treatment efforts initiated early are invaluable.

Outcomes

The outcome in patients with anorexia nervosa remains guarded. Hsu (1980) found that 50% of hospital-treated patients relapsed within a 12-month period. Studies (Bryant-Waugh, Knibbs, & Fosson, 1988; Hawley, 1985) conducted in Great Britain examining early to mid-adolescent onset of eating disorder in girls found that 65 to 76% of the girls were within 15% of ideal body weight at greater than 5-year follow-up; however, regular menses were found in only 50%. There appears to be the continued presence of psychosocial difficulties and eating disturbance. The outcome research in bulimia nervosa focuses on different factors examining changed eating behavior. Norman and Herzog (1986) note a reduction in core symptoms, somatic complaints, and depressive symptoms in their study examining treatment versus nontreatment groups. Two studies (Brotman, Herzog, & Hamburg, 1988; Wozniak & Herzog, 1993) document both high rates of relapse and recovery.

Better understanding of the chronicity of the illness and promoting the use of terms such as "relapse" and "remission" instead of "cure" serve to enhance clinical understanding and to further prevention. Understanding the wide range of severity included within the spectrum of eating-disordered patients is crucial.

The earliest outcome studies focusing on anorexia nervosa described a chronic condition with a poor prognosis. Several of these earlier studies reported that over a third of the patients were incapacitated at 5 years (Kreipe & Uphoff, 1992). Recent outcome studies (Nussbaum *et al.*, 1985; Steiner, Mazer, & Litt, 1990) of adolescents with anorexia nervosa who were treated in inpatient settings reveal that 71% of these adolescents had a satisfactory outcome. Both programs utilized a multidisciplinary approach combining psychotherapies, nutritional education, and medical management, and both utilized the same assessment tool, the Global Assessment Score (Garfinkel, Moldofsky, & Garner, 1977), allowing for comparability of data. There are a number of predictors of poor outcome in adolescents with anorexia nervosa—long duration of illness, disturbed parent–child relationship, coexisting personality disorders, and the presence of vomiting (Wozniak & Herzog, 1993). Even with early treatment the clinician should expect treatment to last 6 months to 2 years or more (Kreipe & Uphoff, 1992).

Age, Gender, and Ethnic Differences in Treatment Outcome

Treatment efforts are just beginning to address the needs of adolescents with psychiatrically diagnosable eating disorders, obesity, or unhealthy eating behavior (Wachsmuth & Garfinkel, 1983; Yates, 1990). To expect specific treatment efforts aimed at age, gender, and ethnic subgroups at present is even more unlikely. An important first step would be to develop both treatment and prevention programs aimed at adolescent girls, the group currently at highest risk for both abnormal eating behavior and associated psychopathology. Prevention efforts could identify adolescents at risk (e.g., through programs in the schools) and channel them toward treatment programs. To date, there have been some rudimentary efforts in this direction (Shisslak *et al.*, 1987), but this opportunity should be much more extensively investigated.

Programs should also be tailored to be sensitive to detection of male adolescents at risk—adolescent males involved in high-risk athletic activities such as wrestling and adolescent males with gender identity issues (Lerner *et al.*, 1976; Yeager *et al.*, 1988).

Treatment programs for prepubertal girls (ages 8–13) who are either pre- or early adolescent are also important. There is some evidence to indicate that the earlier the age at which an individual with an eating disorder begins treatment, the better is the long-term prognosis (Halmi *et al.*, 1973). As treatment programs are developed for the adolescent and preadolescent age group, ethnic components should be integrated. And because it now seems clear that adolescents are at risk as they assimilate to Western culture, this too should be recognized and programs should be developed as needed (Ponton *et al.*, 1994).

SUMMARY AND CONCLUSIONS

There are many review articles that address the diverse and rapidly developing field of disordered eating but there are far fewer articles addressing the specific at-risk population of adolescents. The social contributors (desire for thinness amplified by the media) to this behavior and associated illnesses are considerable and affect all adolescent and latency-age girls to some degree. Understanding the full range of behavior and those at high risk to develop pathology is important. Developing prevention programs that target adolescent girls and their families, schools, and the relevant media is also important. Prevention has been a much neglected area within the field of eating disorders.

The chronic nature of eating disorders characterized by remission and relapse bears further study. Attention to the factors that provoke a symptomatic period is crucial. Along with relapse and remission are shifts between diagnostic categories within the field of disordered eating and co-morbid illnesses. A better understanding of the factors that cause these shifts to occur would be quite valuable.

Outcome and prospective studies would provide valuable information about the course of the illnesses and further identify the individuals at high risk. Certain groups of adolescents are known to be at high risk, such as girls involved in specific athletics (e.g., gymnastics) or career activities, but recent investigations have indicated that girls involved in what was previously believed to be a low-risk activity such as swimming may also be at risk (Benson *et al.*, 1990). Further investigation of these factors is crucial.

Cultural factors play a role in these illnesses and cross-cultural studies provide crucial information. Understanding when cultural groups such as Native American adolescents are at high risk is crucial in order to develop prevention programs. We must also continue to explore the biological and psychological correlates of these illnesses, and further define their complex and heterogeneous etiology. Their study promises to yield exciting challenges.

Increased public awareness regarding the spectrum of risk behavior associated with disordered eating, the high incidence in adolescent females, and the need for treatment of these illnesses all ought to be high priorities. If untreated, chronicity appears inevitable. Examination and study of the most cost-effective methods of treatment is very important.

REFERENCES

Agras, W. S., Rassiter, E. M., Arnow, B., Schneider, J. A., Telch, C. F., Raeburn, S. D., et al. (1992). Pharmacologic and cognitive-behavioral treatment for bulimia nervosa: A controlled comparison. *American Journal of Psychiatry, 149*(1), 82–87.

American Psychiatric Association. (1987). *Diagnostic and statistical manual of mental disorders* (3rd ed., revised). Washington, DC: American Psychiatric Association Press.

American Psychiatric Association. (1994). *Diagnostic and statistical manual of mental disorders* (4th ed.). Washington, DC: American Psychiatric Association Press.

Benson, J. E., Alleman, Y., Thintz, G. E., & Howard, H. (1990). Eating problems and caloric intake levels in Swiss adolescent athletes. *International Journal of Sports, 11*(4), 249–252.

Bond, W. C., Crabbes, E. C., & Sanders, M. C. (1986). Pharmacotherapy of eating disorders: A critical review. *Drug Intelligence & Clinical Pharmacy, 20,* 659–662.

Boyer, R. M., Katz, J., & Finkelstein, J. W. (1974). Anorexia nervosa: Immaturity of the 24-hour luteinizing hormone secretory pattern. *New England Journal of Medicine, 291,* 861–865.

Brotman, A. W., Herzog, D. B., & Hamburg, P. (1988). Long-term course in fourteen bulimic patients treated with psychotherapy. *Journal of Clinical Psychiatry, 49,* 157.

Bruch, H. (1966). Anorexia nervosa and its differential diagnosis. *Journal of Nervous and Mental Disorders, 141*(5), 555–566.

Bruch, H. (1974). *Eating disorders: Obesity, anorexia and the person within.* London: Routledge & Kegan Paul.

Bruch, H. (1982). Anorexia nervosa: Therapy and theory. *American Journal of Psychiatry, 139*(12), 1531–1538.

Bryant-Waugh, R., Knibbs, J., & Fosson, A. (1988). Long-term follow-up of patients with early onset anorexia nervosa. *Archives of Diseases of Children, 63*(5), 5–9.

Bulik, C. M. (1987a). Alcohol use and depression in women with bulimia. *American Journal of Drug and Alcohol Abuse, 13*(3), 343–355.

Bulik, C. M. (1987b). Eating disorders in immigrants: Two case reports. *International Journal of Eating Disorders, 6*(1), 133–147.

Canning, H., & Meyer, J. (1966). Obesity: Its possible effect on college acceptance. *New England Journal of Medicine, 285,* 1407.

Canning, H., & Meyer, J. (1967). Obesity: An influence on high school performance. *American Journal of Clinical Nutrition, 20,* 352–354.

Casper, R. C., Hedeker, R. C., & McClough, J. F. (1992). Personality dimensions in eating disorders and their relevance for sub-typing. *Journal of Child and Adolescent Psychiatry, 31*(5), 830–840.

Centers for Disease Control. (1991). Body-weight perceptions and selected weight management goals and practices of high school students: United States. *Journal of the American Medical Association, 266*(20), 2812–2813.

Chatour, I. (1989). Infantile anorexia nervosa: A developmental disorder of separation and individuation. *American Academy of Child and Adolescent Psychiatry, 17*(1), 43–64.

Chisholm, D. (1978). Obesity in adolescence. *Journal of Adolescence, 1,* 177–194.

Culberg, J., & Engstrom-Lindberg, M. (1988). Prevalence and incidence of eating disorders in a suburban area. *Acta Psychiatrica Scandinavica, 78,* 314–319.

Deutsch, H. (1944). *The psychology of women: A psychoanalytic interpretation* (Vol. 1). New York: Grune & Stratton.

Deutsch, H. (1981). Anorexia nervosa. *Bulletin of the Menninger Clinic, 45,* 499–511.

Eisele, J., Hertsgaard, D., & Light, H. K. (1986). Factors related to eating disorders in young adolescent girls. *Adolescence, 28,* 283–290.

Epstein, L. H., Valoski, A., Wing, R. R., & McCurley, J. (1994). Ten-year outcomes of behavioral family-based treatment for childhood obesity. *Health Psychology, 13,* 373–383.

Fairburn, C. G., Jones, R., Peveler, R. C., Hope, R. A., & O'Connor, M. (1993). Psychotherapy and bulimia nervosa: Longer term effects of interpersonal psychotherapy, behavior therapy, and cognitive behavior therapy. *Archives of General Psychiatry, 50*(6), 419–428.

Felts, M., Tavasso, D., Chenier, T., & Dunn, P. (1992). Adolescents' perceptions of relative weight and self-reported weight loss activities. *Journal of School Health, 62*(8), 372–376.

Fenwick, S. (1880). *On atrophy of the stomach and on the nervous affections of the digestive organs.* London: Churchill Foster.

Fisher, M. (1992). Medical complications of anorexia and bulimia nervosa. *Adolescent Medicine: State of the Art Reviews, 3*(3), 487–502.

Gardiner, H. M., Freeman, C. P., Jesinger, D. K., & Collins, S. A. (1993). Fluoxamine: An open pilot study in moderately obese female patients suffering from atypical eating disorders and episodes of binging. *International Journal of Obesity, 17*(5), 301–305.

Garfinkel, P. E., & Kaplan, A. S. (1985). Starvation based perpetuating mechanism in anorexia nervosa and bulimia. *International Journal of Eating Disorders, 4,* 661–665.

Garfinkel, P. E., Moldofsky, H., & Garner, D. M. (1977). The outcome of anorexia nervosa: Significance of clinical features, body image, and behavior modification. In R. A. Vigersky (Ed.), *Anorexia nervosa* (pp. 315–330). New York: Raven Press.

Garner, D. M., & Garfinkel, P. E. (1980). Socio-cultural factors in the development of anorexia nervosa. *Psychological Medicine, 10,* 647–656.

Garner, D. M., Rickert, W., Davis, R., Garner, M. V., Olmstead, M. P., & Eagle, M. V. (1993). Comparison of cognitive-behavioral supportive-expressive therapy for bulimia nervosa. *American Journal of Psychiatry, 150*(1), 27–46.

Gerlinghoff, M. E., Backmund, H., Angenendt, J., & Linington, A. (1991). Tagklinisches Therapie modell fur psychosomatische EssStorungew (A day hospital model for treating psychosomatic eating disorders). *Verhattens Therapie, 1*(1), 61–65.

Gilchrist, G. (1991). Prevention health care for the adolescent. *American Family Physician, 43*(3), 869–878.

Gilligan, C. (1982). *In a different voice: Psychological theory and women's development.* Cambridge, MA: Harvard University Press.

Gold, D. W., & Rubinow, D. R. (1987). Neuropeptide function in affective illness. In H. W. Meltzer (Ed.), *Psychopharmacology: The third generation of progress.* New York: Raven Press.

Halmi, K. (1983). Anorexia nervosa and bulimia. *Psychosomatics, 24*(2), 111–129.

Halmi, K., Broadland, G., & Loncy, J. (1973). Prognosis in anorexia nervosa. *Annals of Internal Medicine, 78,* 907–909.

Hawley, R. M. (1985). The outcome of anorexia nervosa in younger subjects. *British Journal of Psychiatry, 146,* 657.

Herman, C. P., Polivy, J., Pliner, P., & Threlkeld, J. (1978). Distractibility in dieters and nondieters: An alternative view of "externality." *Journal of Personality and Social Psychology, 5,* 536–548.

Herzog, D. B., & Copeland, P. M. (1985). Eating disorders (a review). *New England Journal of Medicine, 313*(5), 295–303.

Herzog, D. B., Keller, M. B., Sacks, M. R., Yeh, C. J., & Lavore, P. W. (1992). Psychiatric co-morbidity in treatment-seeking anorexics and bulimics. *Journal of the American Academy of Child and Adolescent Psychiatry, 31*(5), 810–818.

Hoffman, L., & Halmi, K. (1993). Co-morbidity and course of anorexia nervosa. In M. Lewis & J. L. Woolsten (Eds.), *Child and adolescent clinics of North America, January,* 129–145.

Hsu, K. L. (1980). Outcome of anorexia nervosa: A review of the literature (1954–1978). *Archives of General Psychiatry, 37,* 1041–1046.

Hueneman, R. L., Shapiro, L. R., Hampton, M. C., & Mitchell, B. W. (1966). A longitudinal study of gross body composition and body conformation and their association with food and activity in a teen-age population. *American Journal of Clinical Nutrition, 18,* 335–338.

Irwin, C. E., & Shafer, M. (1991). Somatic growth and development during adolescence. In A. Rudolph (Ed.), *Pediatrics* (19th ed.). Norwalk, CT: Appleton & Lange.

Irwin, M. (1984). Early onset anorexia nervosa. *Southern Medical Journal, 77*(5), 611–614.

Jaffe, A., & Singer, L. (1989). Atypical eating disorders in young children. *International Journal of Eating Disorders, 8,* 575–582.

Jemerin, J., & Ponton, L. E. (1987). *Eating disorders in children.* Presentation at Child Psychiatry Grand Rounds, Langley Porter Psychiatric Institute, University of California, San Francisco.

Johnson, C., Lewis, C., & Hagman, J. (1984). The syndrome of bulimia: Review and synthesis. *Psychiatric Clinics of North America, 7,* 247–273.

Johnson-Sabine, E., Wood, K., Patton, G., Mann, A., & Wakeling, A. (1988). Abnormal eating attitudes in London school girls. *Psychological Medicine, 18,* 615–622.

Jones, D. J., Fox, M. M., Babigian, H. M., & Hutton, H. E. (1983). Epidemiology of anorexia nervosa in Monroe County, New York, 1960–1976. *Psychosomatic Medicine, 42,* 551–558.

Kalucy, R. (1976). Obesity: An attempt to find a common ground among some of the biological, psychological and sociological phenomena of the obesity/overeating syndrome. In O. Hill (Ed.), *Modern trends in psychosomatic medicine* (Vol. 3, pp. 404–429). London: Butterworths.

Kaye, W. H., Picker, D. M., Naber, D., & Ebert, M. H. (1982). Cerebrospinal fluid opioid activity in anorexia nervosa. *American Journal of Psychiatry, 139,* 643–645.

Kenny, M. E., & Hart, K. (1992). Relationship between parental attachment and eating disorders in an inpatient and a college sample. *Journal of Counseling Psychology, 39*(4), 521–526.

Killen, J. D., Barr Taylor, C., Hammer, L. D., & Litt, J. (1993). An attempt to modify unhealthful eating attitudes and weight reduction practices of young adolescent girls. *International Journal of Eating Disorders, 13*(4), 369–384.

Killen, J. D., Hayward, C., Litt, J., Hammer, L., Wilson, D. M., & Miner, B. (1992). Is puberty a risk factor for eating disorders? *American Journal of Diseases of Children, 146*(3), 323–325.

King, M. B. (1989). Eating disorders in a general practice population: Prevalence, characteristics, and follow-up at 12–18 months. *Psychological Medicine Supplement, 14,* 463–469.

Kleinman, R. E. (1987). Obesity. In A. Rudolph (Ed.), *Pediatrics.* Norwalk, CT: Appleton & Lange.

Kope, T. M., & Sack, W. H. (1987). Anorexia nervosa in southeast Asian refugees: A report on three cases. *Journal of the American Academy of Child and Adolescent Psychiatry, 26*(5), 795–797.

Kreipe, R. E., & Uphoff, M. (1992). Treatment and outcome of adolescents with anorexia nervosa. *Adolescent Medicine: State of the Art Reviews, 3*(3), 519–540.

Lamb, D. (1986). *Psychotherapy with adolescent girls.* New York: Plenum Press.

Larocca, F. E., & Goodner, S. A. (1986). Tube feeding: Is it ever necessary? *New Directions for Mental Health Services, 31,* 87.

Lerner, R. M. Orlos, J. B., & Knapp, J. R. (1976). Physical attractiveness, physical effectiveness, and self-concept in late adolescents. *Adolescence, 11,* 313–316.

Lipscomb, P. A. (1987). Bulimia: Diagnosis and management in the primary care setting. *Journal of Family Practice, 24*(2), 187–194.

Lucas, A. R. (1981). Toward the understanding of anorexia nervosa as a disease entity. *Mayo Clinic Proceedings, 56,* 254–264.

Lucas, A. R. (1992). The eating disorder "epidemic": More apparent than real. *Pediatric Annals, 21*(11), 746–751.

Lucas, A. R., Beard, M., O'Fallon, W. M., & Kurland, L. T. (1991). 50-year trends in the incidence of anorexia nervosa in Rochester, Minnesota: A population-based study. *American Journal of Psychiatry, 148*(7), 917–922.

McDonald, K., & Thompson, J. K. (1992). Eating disturbance, body image dissatisfaction, and reasons for exercising: Gender differences and correlational findings. *International Journal of Eating Disorders, 11*(3), 289–292.

Marino, D. P., & King, J. C. (1980). Nutritional concerns during adolescence. *Pediatric Clinics of North America, 27,* 125–139.

Mellin, L. M. (1993). To: President Clinton Re: Combating childhood obesity. *Journal of the American Dietetic Association, 93*(3), 265–266.

Miller, D. A., McClusky-Fawcett, K., & Irving, L. M. (1993). The relationship between childhood sexual abuse and subsequent onset of bulimia nervosa. *Child Abuse and Neglect, 17*(2), 305–314.

Minuchin, S., Rosman, B., & Baker, L. (1980). *Psychosomatic families: Anorexia nervosa in context.* Cambridge, MA: Harvard University Press.

Mitchell, J. E. (1987). Pharmacology of anorexia nervosa. In H. Y. Meltzer (Ed.), *Psychopharmacology: The third generation of progress.* New York: Raven Press.

Moreno, A. M., & Thelan, M. H. (1993). A preliminary prevention program for eating disorders in a junior high school population. *Journal of Youth and Adolescence, 22*(2), 109–124.

Norman, D. K., & Herzog, D. B. (1986). A three-year outcome study of normal weight bulimics: Assessment of psycho-social functioning and eating attitudes. *Psychiatric Research, 19,* 199.

Nussbaum, M., Shenker, R., Baird, D. (1985). Follow-up investigation in patients with anorexia nervosa. *Journal of Pediatrics, 106,* 835.

Pate, J. D., Pumareiga, A. J., Hester, C., & Garner, D. M. (1992). Cross cultural patterns in eating disorders: A review. *Journal of the American Academy of Child and Adolescent Psychiatry, 31*(5), 802–809.

Patton, G. W., Johnson-Sabine, E., Wood, K., Mann, A. H., & Wakeling, A. (1988). Abnormal eating attitudes in London schoolgirls: A prospective epidemiological study, outcome at 12 months. *Psychological Medicine, 20,* 383–394.

Patton, G. W. (1992). Eating disorders: Antecedents, evolution, and course. *Annals of Medicine, 24,* 281–285.

Paxton, S. J. (1993). A prevention program for disturbed eating and body dissatisfaction in adolescent girls: A one-year follow-up. *Health Education Research, 8,* 43–51.

Polivy, J., & Herman, C. P. (1985). Dieting and binging: A causal analysis. *American Psychologist, 40,* 193–201.

Ponton, L. E. (1993). Issues unique to psychotherapy with adolescent girls. *American Journal of Psychotherapy, 47*(3), 353–372.

Ponton, L. E. (1994). A review of eating disorders in adolescents. *Adolescent Psychiatry, 20,* 267–285.

Ponton, L. E., Gruber, E., & DiClemente, R. (1994). Reported symptoms of eating disorders among Native American adolescents contrasted with white and black youth. *Proceedings of the Society for Adolescent Medicine,* 25–26 (Abstract).

Pope, H. G., Frankenburg, F. R., Hudson, J. I., Jonas, J. M., & Yurgelun, T. D. (1987). Is bulimia associated with borderline personality disorder? *Journal of Clinical Psychiatry, 8*(5), 181–184.

Pope, H. G., & Hudson, J. I. (1992). Is childhood sexual abuse a risk factor for bulimia nervosa? *American Journal of Psychiatry, 149*(4), 455–463.

Public Health Service. (1988). *The Surgeon General's Report of Nutrition and Health.* Department of Health and Human Services, Public Health Service. PHS 88-50210. Washington, DC.

Pumareiga, A. J., Edwards, P., & Mitchell, C. B. (1984). Anorexia nervosa in black adolescents. *Journal of the American Medical Association, 258,* 1213–1215.

Pyle, R. L., Mitchell, J. E., Eckert, E. D., Halvorson, P. A., Newman, P. A., & Goff, G. M. (1983). The incidence of bulimia in freshman college students. *International Journal of Eating Disorders, 2*(3), 75–85.

Rowland, C. (1970). Anorexia and obesity. *International Psychiatry Clinics, 7,* 37–137.

Russell, G. F. F., Szmukler, G. L., & Dare, C. (1987). An evaluation of family therapy in anorexia and bulimia nervosa. *Archives of General Psychiatry, 44,* 1047–1053.

Schebendach, J., & Nussbaum, M. P. (1992). Nutrition management in adolescents with eating disorders. *Adolescent Medicine State of the Art Reviews, 3*(3), 541–558.

Schleimer, K. (1984). Dieting in teenage girls. *Acta Pediatrica,* Suppl. 312.

Schotte, D. E., & Stunkard, A. J. (1987). Bulimia vs. bulimic behaviors on a college campus. *Journal of the American Medical Association, 258,* 1213–1215.

Serdula, M. K., Ivery, D., Coates, R. J., Friedman, D. S., Williamson, D. F., & Byers, T. (1993). Do obese children become obese adults? A review of the literature. *Preventive Medicine, 22*(2), 167–177.

Sharpe, D. J., & Lowe, G. (1987). Adolescents and alcohol: A review of British research. *Journal of Adolescence, 12,* 295–307.

Shisslak, C. M., Crago, M., & Neal, M. E. (1987). Prevention of eating disorders among adolescents. *Journal of Consulting and Clinical Psychology, 55,* 660–667.

Silber, T. J. (1986). Anorexia nervosa in blacks and Hispanics. *International Journal of Eating Disorders, 5*(1), 121–128.

Simmons, R., & Rosenberg, F. (1975). Sex, sex-roles, and self-image. *Journal of Youth and Adolescence, 4,* 229–258.

Singer, L. T., Ambuel, B., Wade, S., & Jaffe, A. C. (1992). Cognitive behavioral treatment of health-impairing food phobias in children. *Journal of the American Academy of Child and Adolescent Psychiatry, 31*(5), 847–852.

Smith, C., Thienemann, M., & Steiner, H. (1992). Defense style and adaptation in adolescents with depressions and eating disorders. *Acta Paedopsychiatrica, 55*(3), 185–186.

Snow, J. T., & Harris, M. B. (1985). *An analysis of weight and diet content in five women's interest magazines.* Unpublished manuscript. University of New Mexico, Albuquerque.

Soundy, T. J., Lucas, A. R., Suman, V. J., & Melton, L. J., III. (1994). Bulimia nervosa in Rochester, Minnesota, 1980–1990. Personal communication.

Spitzer, R., Yanovski, S., Wadden, T., Wing, R., Marcus, M. D., Stunkard, A. (1993). Eating disorder: Its further validation in a multisite study. *International Journal of Eating Disorders, 13*(2), 137–153.

Steiner, H., Mazer, C., & Litt, I. (1990). Compliance and outcome in anorexia nervosa. *Western Journal of Medicine, 153,* 133–138.

Striegel-Moore, R. H., Silberstein, L. R., & Rodin, J. (1986). Toward an understanding of risk factors of bulimia. *American Psychologist, 4*(3), 246–263.

Stunkard, A., d'Aquile, E., Fox, S., & Filion, R. (1972). Influence of social class on obesity and thinness in children. *Journal of the American Medical Association, 221,* 579–584.

Sundgot-Borgen, J. (1993). Prevalence of eating disorders in elite female athletes. *International Journal of Sport Nutrition, 3*(1), 29–40.

Taub, D. E., & Blinde, E. M. (1992). Eating disorders among adolescent female athletes. *Adolescence, 27*(108), 833–848.

Theander, S. (1970). Anorexia nervosa: A psychiatric investigation of 94 female patients. *Acta Psychiatrica Scandinavica, 214,* 1–194.

Tobias, A., & Gordon, J. (1980). Social consequences of obesity. *Journal of the American Dietetic Association, 76,* 338–342.

Vandereycken, W., & Pierloot, R. (1982). Pimazide combined with behavior therapy in the short-term treatment of anorexia nervosa. *Acta Psychiatrica Scandinavica, 66,* 445–450.

Vanderheyden, D. A., & Boland, F. J. (1987). A comparison of normals, mild, moderate, and severe binge eaters and binge vomiters using discriminant functional analysis. *International Journal of Eating Disorders, 6,* 331–337.

Wachsmuth, J. R., & Garfinkel, P. E. (1983). The treatment of anorexia nervosa in young adolescents. In M. Lewis & J. L. Woolston (Eds.), *Child and adolescent psychiatric clinics of North America.* Philadelphia: Sanders.

Watts, D. W., & Ellis, A. M. (1992). Drug abuse and eating disorders: Prevention implications. *Journal of Drug Education 22*(3), 223–240.

Wheadon, D. E., Rampey, A. H., Thompson, V. L., Potvin, J. H., Masica, D. N., & Beasley, C. M. (1992). Lack of association between fluoxatine and suicidality in bulimia nervosa. *Journal of Clinical Psychiatry, 53*(7), 235–241.

Whitehouse, A. M., Cooper, P. J., Vize, C. V., Hill, C., & Vogel, L. (1992). Prevalence of eating disorders in three Cambridge general practices: Hidden and conspicuous morbidity. *British Journal of General Practice, 42,* 355; 57–60.

Willi, J., & Grossmann, S. (1983). Epidemiology of anorexia nervosa in a defined region of Switzerland. *American Journal of Psychiatry, 140,* 564–567.

Williams, P., & King, M. (1987). The "epidemic" of anorexia nervosa: Another medical myth? *Lancet, 1,* 205–207.

Wozniak, J., & Herzog, D. B. (1993). The course and outcome of bulimia nervosa. In M. Lewis & J. L. Woolston (Eds.), *Child and adolescent psychiatric clinics of North America* (pp. 109–127). Philadelphia: Saunders.

Yates, A. (1989). Current perspectives on the eating disorders: I. History, psychological and biological aspects. *Journal of the American Academy of Child and Adolescent Psychiatry, 28*(6), 813–828.

Yates, A. (1990). Current perspectives on the eating disorders: II. Treatment, outcome, and research directions. *Journal of the American Academy of Child and Adolescent Psychiatry, 29*(1), 1–9.

Yeager, J., Kurtman, F., Landsverk, J., & Wiesmeier, E. (1988). Behaviors and attitudes related to eating disorders in homosexual male college studies. *American Journal of Psychiatry, 145,* 495–497.

6

Alcohol Use

MICHAEL WINDLE, JEAN THATCHER SHOPE, and OSCAR BUKSTEIN

INTRODUCTION

The majority of adolescents have used alcohol on at least some occasions (e.g., at parties) by their senior year of high school, with more than a few teens abusing alcohol on a regular basis. It has been estimated that 4.6 million adolescents (i.e., 3 out of 10) annually have problems related to alcohol use (Bowen, 1988). Higher levels of adolescent alcohol use have been associated with the three most frequent forms of mortality among adolescents, namely, accidental deaths (e.g., fatal automobile or boating crashes), homicides, and suicides. Nearly 9 out of 10 teenage automobile accidents involve the use of alcohol. Higher levels of adolescent alcohol use are also associated with higher rates of a number of other pressing problems on the public health agenda, including an increased risk of contracting human immunodeficiency virus (HIV) infection and other sexually transmitted diseases, teenage pregnancy, and poor school performance or school dropout. Alcohol use has been characterized as a "gateway" substance, preceding the use of marijuana and then other illegal substances such as cocaine or heroin (e.g., Kandel, 1985). Given the widespread use of alcohol among adolescents, and its significant relations to a host of other health-related problems, it must be considered pivotal in preventive intervention approaches seeking to reduce health-compromising behaviors among adolescents.

MICHAEL WINDLE • Research Institute on Addictions, Buffalo, New York 14203.   **JEAN THATCHER SHOPE** • University of Michigan Transportation Research Institute, Ann Arbor, Michigan 48109.   **OSCAR BUKSTEIN** • University of Pittsburgh Medical Center, Western Psychiatric Institute and Clinic, Pittsburgh, Pennsylvania 15213.
Handbook of Adolescent Health Risk Behavior, edited by Ralph J. DiClemente, William B. Hansen, and Lynn E. Ponton. Plenum Press, New York, 1996.

EPIDEMIOLOGY OF ALCOHOL USE

This section discusses the prevalence of alcohol use among adolescents. In order to provide epidemiologic information on a broad range of adolescents, several different datasets were used to refer to recent trends for subgroups based on grade level. The age (grade level) trends were deemed to be of importance because age of onset of drinking is a risk factor for the subsequent development of more serious problems with alcohol use, delinquent activity, and other substance use. Furthermore, age of onset is of importance in the consideration of age-targeted preventive interventions. In addition to age (grade level) trends, subgroup comparisons of alcohol use were provided for gender and racial/ethnic groups. Prevalence data were provided not only for the use of (versus abstention from) alcohol, but also for "binge drinking," defined as consuming five or more drinks consecutively on at least one occasion. Binge drinking among adolescents has been associated with more severe and pervasive problems in key social contexts (e.g., at school, in the home, with legal authorities) and poses heightened risk for serious alcohol problems. Finally, data are presented on the prevalence of alcohol problems (e.g., missing school because of drinking, passing out) among adolescents. Much research has focused on patterns of adolescent alcohol use, but recent research suggests the value of also examining levels and patterns of alcohol problems (e.g., Bailey & Rachal, 1993; White, 1987; Windle, 1994).

The majority of the information used for estimating adolescent prevalence rates were derived from four large survey datasets that are identified in Table 1. Two of the datasets referred to in Table 1—Monitoring the Future surveys (Bachman *et al.*, 1991) and the National Adolescent Student Health Survey (American School Health Association, 1989)—are nationally representative sample surveys. The third dataset referred to in Table 1—the New York State Survey (Barnes & Welte, 1986a)—is a state representative sample of over 27,000 seventh- to twelfth-graders in New York State. The final survey consists of two representative samples of fourth-graders from the Washington, D.C. area. Whereas there are differences across these four datasets with regard to the frame for the representative sampling (i.e., local, state, or national), each dataset involves careful sampling procedures to increase representativeness, and each provide unique characteristics to facilitate a more comprehensive evaluation of the prevalence of alcohol use spanning the grades 4 through 12, and have sufficient sample sizes for meaningful gender and racial/ethnic group comparisons. In addition to the four datasets referenced in Table 1, other datasets are referenced to illustrate findings of relevance to specific issues, such as the prevalence of alcohol problems.

Prevalence of Alcohol Use

The data in Figure 1 illustrate the lifetime prevalence of alcohol use (i.e., the proportion who have ever used alcohol) for four different grade levels. It should be noted that the data were not collected in exactly the same years for each of these samples and thus the prevalence rates are not adjusted for cohort effects (see Bachman *et al.*, 1991, for a discussion of this issue). Nevertheless, the trends are generally consistent with "same" cohort studies for alcohol use in the literature (e.g., Barnes & Welte, 1986a); trend data

Table 1. Adolescent Surveys Used for Prevalence Data Estimates

Dataset	N	Gender		Ethnicity		Grade levels
Washington DC Study (Bush & Iannotti, 1993)						
Sample 1 (1988/89)	4,675	Girls	50.0%	Black	84.1%	4th
		Boys	50.0%			
Sample 2 (1990/91)	4,678	Girls	50.0%	Black	85.7%	4th
		Boys	50.0%			
National Adolescent Student Health Survey (American School Health Association, 1989)	11,400	Girls	50.4%	White	72.7%	8th and 10th
		Boys	49.6%	Black	12.6%	
				Hispanic	8.6%	
				Asian	2.5%	
				Native American	1.1%	
				Other	2.4%	
New York State Survey (Barnes & Welte, 1986a)	27,335	Girls	50.3%	White	74.4%	7th through 12th
		Boys	49.7%	Black	11.5%	
				Hispanic	8.9%	
				West Indian	2.7%	
				Asian	2.0%	
				Native American	0.5%	
Monitoring the Future survey (Bachman et al., 1991)	17,000 (annual)	Gender is approximately equal		White	82.0%	12th
				Black	11.1%	
				Hispanic	4.2%	
				Asian	1.6%	
				Native American	1.2%	

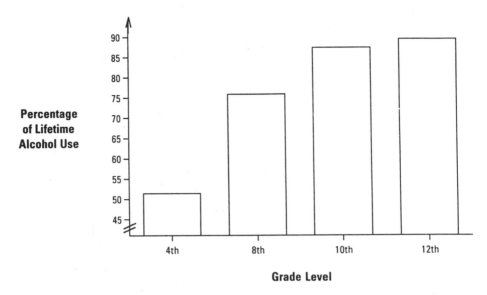

Figure 1. Lifetime adolescent alcohol use by grade level. Fourth-grade data from Bush and Iannotti (1993); 8th and 10th from ASHA (1989); 12th from Johnston *et al.* (1991).

for adolescents have indicated cohort effects and changes, less so with regard to alcohol and more so with regard to substances other than alcohol use (see Johnston, O'Malley, & Bachman, 1991). The data in Figure 1 indicate that by 4th grade, approximately one-half of the students have already used alcohol at least once. By 8th grade, the prevalence increases to almost 76%, and by 10th and 12th grade the prevalence is 87 and 89%, respectively. These findings suggest that the early onset (at least initiation) of alcohol use is typical among a large number of youngsters, and statistically normative use can be observed by 10th grade.

Prevalence of Use by Subgroup

It has been suggested that the gender gap in adolescent drinking practices is diminishing. This statement is reasonably accurate if reference is made simply to the percentage of adolescents who have used alcohol at least once in their lifetime (e.g., Johnston *et al.*, 1991). However, gender differences emerge when heavy alcohol use or alcohol-related problems are considered. When thus considered, males manifest a more severe pattern of alcohol misuse. Data on gender differences in ever used alcohol in one's lifetime are reported in Figure 2 for different racial/ethnic groups of high school seniors. Whereas male use is equivalent to or exceeds female use for all racial/ethnic groups, the size of this difference is relatively small. Therefore, there are minimal gender differences with regard to having ever used alcohol in one's lifetime, with both boys and girls endorsing a positive response to this probe at high levels. However, gender differences do emerge when high-

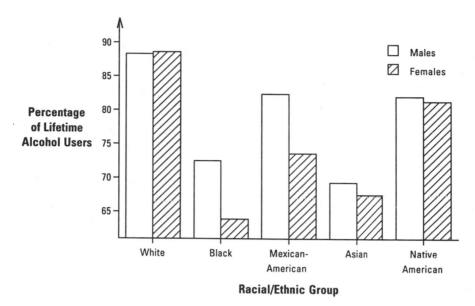

Figure 2. Lifetime adolescent alcohol use by gender and racial/ethnic group for seniors. Data from Monitoring the Future surveys (Bachman *et al.*, 1991).

volume drinking or alcohol-related problems are considered (e.g., Robbins, 1989; Windle, 1994).

The racial/ethnic group differences reported in Figure 2 indicate some subgroup differences. White adolescents reported the highest prevalence of alcohol use, followed by Mexican-American and Native American youth. Consistent with prior studies (e.g., Barnes & Welte, 1986b), black and Asian adolescents have the lowest prevalence of having ever used alcohol. The data reported in Figure 2 are from seniors in the Monitoring the Future surveys (Bachman *et al.*, 1991); by contrast, the data reported in Figure 3 are from 7th- to 12th-graders in New York State (Barnes & Welte, 1986a). These data are generally in agreement with the senior data for racial/ethnic differences in the prevalence of ever used alcohol. However, the data in Figure 3 represent the pooled scores for 7th-through 12th-graders and yet the prevalence rates are almost as high for some subgroups (e.g., Native Americans, blacks) as they are for the 12th-graders.

One may have anticipated lower prevalence rates for the data in Figure 3 relative to Figure 2 given the pooled sample of 7th- to 12th-graders that included younger adolescents in the population sample of New York State. Two factors may contribute to the absence of stronger sample differences. First, there are regional differences in drinking practices that reveal higher drinking levels among adolescents in the Northeast and on the West Coast. In addition, there may be differences in subcultural practices for specific subgroups (e.g., the use of alcohol among Native American tribes in New York may differ from those in other regions of the country). Second, the senior data in Figure 2 may exclude a number of adolescents who have dropped out of school, for example because of pregnancy, and yet are included in a majority of grade levels for the sample in New York

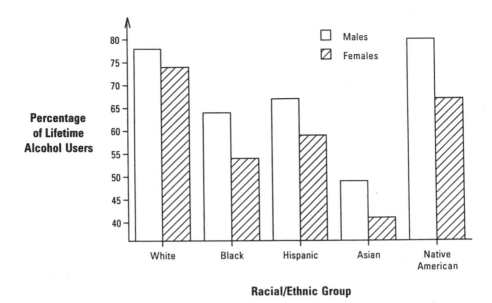

Figure 3. Lifetime adolescent alcohol use by gender and racial/ethnic group for 7th- to 12th-graders in New York State. Data from Barnes and Welte (1986a).

State. By focusing exclusively on any one survey, it is difficult to draw inferences about adolescent drinking practices in general. In some locales where the school dropout rates exceed 40%, a focus on seniors only may underestimate the extent of alcohol use and alcohol problems among adolescents. Furthermore, there is a strong need to consider alcohol use and misuse in special populations (e.g., adolescent unwed mothers, school dropouts) and to devise preventive interventions to facilitate health-enhancing behaviors for these adolescents, as well as their offspring, in the instance of unwed mothers.

Heavy or Binge Drinking

There has been increasing concern not only with the number of adolescents who are consuming alcohol, but also with the number engaging in heavy drinking episodes, referred to as binge drinking. Binge drinking is often defined for adolescents as consuming five or more drinks on a single occasion. Such binge drinking is associated with higher levels of problems in other domains (e.g., poor school performance, problems with family) and with increased risk for prolonged alcohol misuse. The most obvious effect of binge drinking is clearly defined intoxication. (For many adolescents, intoxication, which implies a loss of motor control, judgment ability, and reduced inhibition, can easily occur with much less than five drinks in a row.) Figure 4 summarizes the percentage of binge drinkers for samples of 8th- and 10th-graders. Subgroup breakdowns are provided for gender and three racial/ethnic groups. The data indicate high rates of binge drinking within the last 2 weeks for a number of subgroups. Hispanic and white males manifested the highest levels (in excess of 40% for 10th-graders), and Hispanic females were nearby

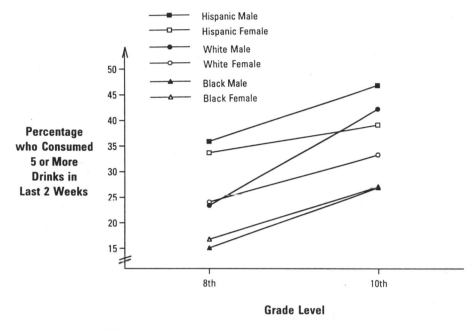

Figure 4. Prevalence of binge drinking by gender and racial/ethnic group for 8th- and 10th-graders. Data from ASHA (1989).

(approximately 38% for 10th-graders). Black males and females had the lowest rates of binge drinking and 8th-graders had a lower rate of binge drinking than 10th-graders (see also Windle, 1991).

These findings indicate serious levels of alcohol misuse for a significant percentage of adolescents, especially white males and Hispanic males and females. A focus on the reduction of binge drinking would be a beneficial objective of preventive intervention programs.

Epidemiology of Alcohol Problems

The preceding section identified high rates of alcohol use among adolescents and the tendency for a significant subset of youths to engage in "binge" or heavy drinking episodes. In this section the emphasis is on the prevalence of alcohol-related problems among adolescents, including negative or adverse social consequences, and dependency symptoms. These alcohol-related problems generally have not been a major focus of large-scale, national surveys of adolescent substance use, in part because such clinical assessments are difficult to make. Survey items assessing these problems have either been omitted completely or limited to a few items, thus precluding a comprehensive evaluation of the prevalence of adolescent alcohol-related problems with a nationally representative sample. Nevertheless, several large (though not nationally representative) adolescent sample surveys have been concluded that included a large number of alcohol problems and are cited in this section.

The consideration of alcohol-related problems is of importance to prevention planning for two reasons. First, the overall level of association (i.e., the Pearson correlation) between alcohol use and alcohol problems is approximately 0.50 (Sadava, 1985), thus suggesting that alcohol use is not a useful proxy for alcohol problems. Findings by Barnes and Welte (1986b) further substantiate this point. They reported that one moderator of the relationship between adolescent alcohol use and alcohol problems was ethnicity; at the same levels of alcohol consumption, black adolescents reported more alcohol problems than white adolescents. Therefore, even though proportionally fewer black than white adolescents may consume alcohol, the rate of alcohol problems was heightened for those black adolescents consuming the same amount of alcohol as white adolescents. Second, alcohol problems are important because they may signify more severe and pervasive current difficulties, as well as pose increased risk for the subsequent development of an alcohol disorder. Adolescents experiencing alcohol-related problems may require supplemental individual or group level interventions in addition to global intervention efforts targeted at larger social or institutional units (e.g., school-based curriculum).

White (1987) suggested that four distinct dimensions have been identified to classify problem drinking in adolescence. These include: (1) heavy and frequent use of alcohol, (2) frequent intoxication, (3) escapist coping by drinking, and (4) specific negative consequences (e.g., blackouts and morning drinking; adverse social, interpersonal, and legal consequences). The findings of Bailey and Rachal (1993) also indicate multiple problem dimensions for adolescent alcohol use behaviors, including level or frequency of alcohol use, adverse social consequences, and dependency symptoms. Boyle *et al.* (1992) used two dimensions of alcohol use behaviors to identify *regular users* of alcohol with a representative sample of community adolescents in Ontario. Regular use was defined by the consumption of alcoholic beverages at least once a week for a continuous 4-week period or longer, and reported intoxication or the consumption of at least two drinks on at least one of those occasions. Using these criteria, Boyle *et al.* reported regular alcohol use among 7% of the boys and 5% of the girls in 1983 (when subjects were between 12 and 16 years old), and 39.3% for boys and 35.6% for girls in 1987 (when subjects were between 16 and 20 years old). Hansen (1993) recently reported in a survey of North Carolina youths that the relative proportion of drinkers who reported drunkenness increased with age; about 70% of high school seniors who drank reported intoxication in the previous month compared to 50% of eighth-grade student drinkers.

Windle (1994) also used multiple criteria to identify subgroups of adolescent drinkers with a sample of over 1100 high school juniors and seniors. *Heavy drinkers* met the criteria by having consumed 45 or more alcoholic beverages in the last 30 days or by consuming six or more drinks on at least three occasions in the last 30 days. *Problem drinkers* met the criteria by reaching or exceeding the same alcohol misuse criteria as the heavy drinkers, but also by reporting five or more alcohol problems (e.g., passing out, missed school because of drinking) in the last 6 months. Data summarized in Table 2 provide the percentage of male and female adolescents endorsing an affirmative response

Table 2. Alcohol Problems Index: Frequency of Item Endorsement among Those Who Drink[a]

	Percentage endorsing affirmative response[a]			
	Total N	Boys	Girls	χ^2 (1 df)
1. Drank before or during school	12.1	16.6	8.5	12.61[c]
2. Missed school because of drinking	8.9	11.2	7.1	4.05[b]
3. Had a fight with parents about your drinking	16.1	19.3	13.4	5.36[b]
4. Did things while you were drinking that you regretted the next day	47.4	49.9	45.4	1.59
5. Thought about cutting down on your drinking	24.0	30.2	18.9	14.16[c]
6. Got drunk or high from alcohol several days in a row	28.3	36.8	21.4	23.42[c]
7. Passed out from drinking	29.1	33.1	25.8	5.10[b]
8. Had a fight with your girlfriend or boyfriend about your drinking	15.9	16.1	15.8	0.01
9. Got into a fight or heated argument with someone you didn't know while drinking	16.1	25.1	8.7	40.21[c]
10. Got into trouble with the law (other than driving related) while drinking	6.4	11.2	2.4	25.75[c]
11. Drank alone	21.6	25.3	18.5	5.61[b]
12. Drank alcohol to get rid of a hangover	7.2	8.7	6.0	2.20
13. Drank to forget your troubles	36.9	34.9	38.5	1.16

[a]Abstainers were excluded from these analyses. Time referent for alcohol problems was the last 6 months. Total number of subjects was 695 (321 boys, 374 girls).
[b]$p < 0.05$.
[c]$p < 0.01$.

to each of 13 alcohol-related problems. Consistent with other data (e.g., Bailey & Rachal, 1993; White, 1987), alcohol-related problems occurred with a relatively high frequency among adolescents. Furthermore, the prevalence rates for some of the problems (e.g., did things you regretted the next day, passed out) indicate fairly severe difficulties for a subset of adolescents. With regard to the prevalence of drinker status categories, 13.3% of boys and 7.1% of girls were identified as heavy drinkers, and 17.3% of boys and 8.4% of girls were identified as problem drinkers. In the study by Windle, problem drinkers not only had high rates of alcohol problems, but also had high rates of delinquent activity and depressed affect.

These findings regarding high rates of adolescent alcohol problems echo earlier comments that a substantial minority of adolescents have serious alcohol-related problems *during* adolescence. The delay of early onset alcohol use via prevention programs may be influential in reducing the number of adolescents experiencing alcohol-related problems, or the occurrence of the number of alcohol problems among those who drink. Clearly increased attention by mental health professionals needs to be directed toward the reduction of such health-compromising alcohol-related behaviors among a significant subset of adolescents. Booster sessions or supplemental intensive and extensive preventive interventions may facilitate health promotion objectives for these adolescents.

Risk Factors for Adolescent Alcohol Use

The prevalence data presented in previous sections of this chapter indicate high rates of alcohol use among adolescents, as well as the manifestation of serious and sometimes persistent alcohol-related problems among a substantial minority of adolescents. In this section, we briefly describe some of the major risk factors that have been associated with features of adolescent drinking such as the onset of drinking, or the escalation to alcohol misuse. The consideration of these risk factors is important for two reasons. First, they provide some conceptual framework for considering the multiple factors that may contribute to adolescent alcohol use and abuse. Second, they provide a context for evaluating the focus (or foci) of adolescent alcohol preventive intervention programs so as to facilitate what specific behaviors are being targeted that may reduce risk. Parenthetically, no single prevention program is likely to target all of these risk factors simultaneously; nevertheless, because many of these risk factors are often highly correlated with one another, the reduction of one risk behavior may attenuate the risk of other risk factors (e.g., a higher commitment to school achievement may result in the peer selection of lower-alcohol-using friends).

A large number of risk factors for adolescent substance use have been identified in the research literature and were recently summarized in a review article by Hawkins, Catalano, and Miller (1992). Much of the data provided in Table 3 was extracted from the Hawkins *et al.* article. For this chapter, risk factors were separated into five domains contingent on their social locus and included the levels of societal–community, school, family, peers, and individual. This social-ecological orientation was used because it provides a useful organizational structure and corresponds to alternative targets of prevention research. For instance, social resistance prevention programs are directed more toward the modification of refusal skills within the peer context, whereas laws focused on minimum drinking age are targeted more toward the societal and community contexts.

The information provided in Table 3 identifies a number of different risk factors within each of the five social-ecological domains. Further, the examples provided in Table 3 refer to the processes and mechanisms involved in the expression of these risk factors. The processes and mechanisms associated with the expression of risk factors are diverse and the examples are not comprehensive—these are just a "sampling" of some prominent modes of risk factor expression.

There are three major points to highlight with regard to the risk factors for adolescent alcohol use provided in Table 3. First, it is evident that there are a variety of determinants from different spheres (domains) within the biopsychosocial matrix of risk factors for teen drinking. These factors span from genetic and biochemical vulnerability to societal norms and laws. Second, a number of these risk factors do not occur independently, but rather often cluster together to undermine adolescent functioning and increase risk for alcohol use and abuse. Thus, there is often a cascading effect of risk factors that may contribute to both the onset of alcohol use, as well as the escalation and maintenance of heavy and problematic alcohol use. Third, while not explicitly noted in Table 3, it is important to consider age differences in the potential risk that these factors may have, for example, for early versus late adolescents. Adolescence is a period in the life span characterized by multiple changes in biological, cognitive, and social spheres; changes in these develop-

Table 3.   Risk Factors for Adolescent Alcohol Use[a]

Risk factors	Examples
Societal–Community	
1. Laws and normative behavior	Encouragement of youthful drinking via media sources; absence of legal enforcement of underage drinking
2. Availability	Easy access via the home or adults (e.g., siblings) purchasing liquor for minors
3. Extreme economic deprivation	Escapist drinking to cope with harsh realities of everyday life
4. Neighborhood disorganization	Undermine sense of security and purpose in life
School	
5. Low commitment to school	School expectations and career expectations very low
6. Academic failure	Poor attendance, poor grades, underachievement
7. Early persistent behavior problems	High aggression, attentional problems
Family	
8. Family members alcohol users (abusers)	Role modeling influences
9. Family management practices	Failure to monitor children; inconsistent parenting practices and/or harsh discipline
10. Family conflict	Marital dysfunction or partner violence
11. Low bonding to family	Lack of reciprocal nurturing and open communication
Peers	
12. Peer rejection in elementary grades	Rejected or neglected by peers undermines positive self-concept
13. Associating with alcohol-using peers	Peer selection fosters cycles of negative behaviors
14. Friends with attitudes favorable to alcohol use	Peer selection fosters cycles of negative attitudes and beliefs
Individual	
15. Physiological	Genetic susceptibility to alcohol via enhanced tension reduction or misjudgment about level of intoxication
16. Alienation and rebelliousness	Removed from normative attitudes and values of society, and commitments toward societal goals
17. Early onset deviant behavior	Early onset deviant behaviors consolidate earlier and perpetuate negative spiraling cycles
18. Problem-solving coping skills	Absence of strong problem-solving skills may contribute to adaptation of less desirable negotiating strategies (e.g., an aggressive coercive interpersonal style).

[a]See Hawkins, Catalano, and Miller (1992) for expanded discussion of these risk factors.

mental spheres may yield a differential potency for various risk factors. For example, associating with alcohol-using peers may pose a more heightened risk for alcohol use onset among 12-year-olds relative to 19-year-olds. The consideration of the differential potency of risk factors for different age groups (or preferably for different developmental levels) may facilitate the optimal selection of targets for prevention programs.

Epidemiology Summary

It is evident that a large portion of adolescents have used alcohol prior to the completion of their senior year of high school. There are minimal gender differences among adolescents with regard to the prevalence of ever used in lifetime. Racial/ethnic group comparisons indicated elevated rates among whites, Hispanics, and Native Americans, and lower rates among blacks and Asians. The occurrence of binge drinking (i.e., five or more drinks on a single occasion) was high, with over 40% of Hispanic and white tenth-grade males reporting instances of binge drinking in the last 2 weeks preceding the survey assessment. Data that included the identification of regular, heavy, and problem drinkers suggested that a substantial minority of adolescents (approximately 30–35%) have serious problems associated with their alcohol use. A number of risk factors were identified at five different interrelated social-ecological levels—societal–community, school, family, peers, and individual. A consideration of these risk factors suggests the multiple potential influences on adolescent alcohol use. They further delineate the multi-faceted tasks confronting preventive interventionists in attempting to prevent the onset of, or mitigate the problems associated with, adolescent alcohol use. In the next section, attention is directed toward prevention programs that have attempted to modify adolescent alcohol use practices.

PREVENTION

Because of the extent of adolescent alcohol use and misuse, and the severity of alcohol-related problems mentioned at the beginning of this chapter, much effort has been expended to deter adolescents from use of this particular drug. To help clarify the goals of prevention efforts, Figure 5 emphasizes the stages along a continuum through which too many, but by no means all, adolescents may proceed. This process starts with no alcohol use, then may be accelerated by the presence of the risk factors mentioned above, which can then lead to early first use of alcohol. Regular alcohol use follows, with misuse and binge drinking (five or more drinks in a row) the next stage. The occurrence of alcohol-related problems (i.e., injuries, fatalities) as well as problems that disrupt the social development of young people (i.e., school performance, early pregnancy), and alcohol-ism constitute the final stages of the continuum. Prevention efforts may be targeted at several stages along the continuum, with the goal being to prevent adolescents' progress to subsequent stages. Preventing the risk factors or enhancing the protective factors for adolescents' future alcohol problems would be targeting the first stage of the continuum. Other stages are and have been targeted by various prevention approaches. It is important to realize that the particular target of any prevention effort is only one stage of a continuum of alcohol use.

Primary prevention is the term used for prevention directed at stopping a problem from occurring, while *secondary prevention* is the term used for prevention directed at identifying problems and reducing the severity of their consequences. The goal of primary prevention in the adolescent alcohol field is to prevent adolescents from moving along the continuum toward alcohol-related problems (Figure 5). Primary prevention efforts can therefore be directed at reducing risk factors or enhancing protective factors, preventing

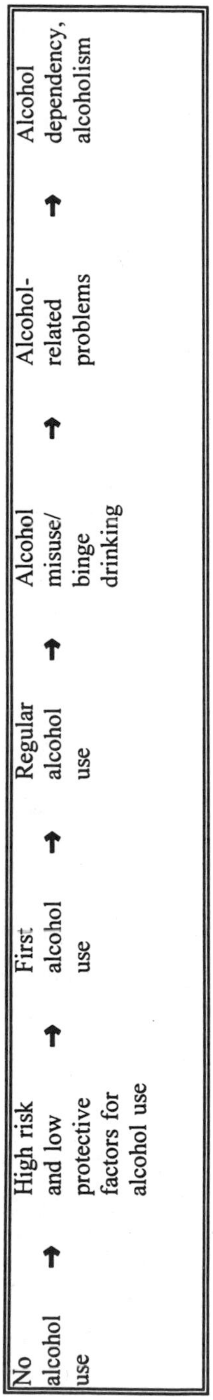

| No alcohol use | → | High risk and low protective factors for alcohol use | → | First alcohol use | → | Regular alcohol use | → | Alcohol misuse/ binge drinking | → | Alcohol-related problems | → | Alcohol dependency, alcoholism |

Figure 5. The continuum of adolescent alcohol use.

first or regular use of alcohol, and preventing alcohol misuse. An example of primary prevention is school-based alcohol prevention programming, an approach directed at all students, with the goal of preventing them from drinking alcohol. Secondary prevention efforts (identifying problems and reducing consequences) can be directed at preventing adolescents who use alcohol from misusing it, or preventing those who misuse alcohol from experiencing alcohol-related problems or becoming dependent. An example of secondary prevention is a program that identifies adolescents who misuse alcohol, and provides them with a program to prevent them from having motor vehicle accidents.

For prevention efforts to be most effective, they must be theoretically grounded; that is, a mechanism through which the problem occurs has been found, and the process by which the prevention approach will prevent the problem has been explicated. The risk and protective factors (often found as correlates or precursors) for adolescent substance use noted earlier and described by Hawkins *et al.* (1992) are most valuable in that the factors have been collected from the contributions of many fields and organized into a useful framework that can guide prevention efforts in the modification of factors that are amenable to change. Similarly, Petraitis, Flay, and Miller (1995) have reviewed, described, and integrated the various theories of adolescent experimental substance use. Three types of influence (social/interpersonal, cultural/attitudinal, and intrapersonal) were outlined, each with ultimate, distal, and proximal levels of influence. Such categorizations are useful for program developers and implementers to understand the mechanisms through which prevention is expected to take place. Both Hawkins and Petraitis with their colleagues have grouped alcohol with tobacco and other drugs in their discussions of adolescent substance use. While for many purposes this approach is justified because the behaviors are highly correlated, that is not always the case. Some studies have developed combined measures and do not report results for alcohol use. One should carefully weigh the applicability of drug use findings to alcohol use and vice versa because of key differences among the substances studied.

Several factors about alcohol itself should be acknowledged before discussing prevention efforts with adolescents, let alone developing or conducting prevention programs. Alcohol is a drug, but a unique one. It is widely used in our society, its use far more prevalent than the use of tobacco or illicit drugs. Unlike the use of tobacco, the moderate, responsible use of alcohol has not been shown to lead to serious health problems. The messages delivered to young people about alcohol are therefore not at all as clear-cut as are those about tobacco. Unlike illicit drugs which are illegal for all to use, alcohol use is legal for adults, but not for people under 21. While there is more than adequate justification for that age restriction, it is challenging to convince underage youth of its rationale, and enforcing a standard of nonuse has proven difficult at best. Unfortunately for program developers, alcohol is not a substance the use of which can be thoroughly discouraged at all times. Instead, there are more complex teaching points to make regarding who, when, and where, and how much of its use is inappropriate. Used by adults in moderation and responsibly, alcohol produces what many people regard as pleasant effects. Denying this fact makes prevention programs less credible. These complex factors about alcohol cannot be glossed over or ignored. They must be appreciated and dealt with, whether in a separate alcohol program or an alcohol section of programs on several substances. Young people already have learned much about alcohol and deserve a thoughtful approach that respects their ability to understand the complexities they have already observed.

Prevention Programs

Prevention efforts in the area of adolescent alcohol use can use as program goals any of the stages of the continuum in Figure 5. The continuum has been abbreviated somewhat, however, for use in Table 4, a summary of prevention programs, with alcohol risk factors, alcohol use/misuse, and alcohol problems being the main prevention goals of most programs and listed across the top row. (Alcoholism or alcohol dependence has not been included for two reasons. First, the prevalence among young people is quite low. Second, efforts directed solely at the goal of preventing alcoholism are more appropriately considered treatment, and would target those heavy drinkers with alcohol-related problems.) Prevention efforts that address the whole range of the continuum are needed because there are adolescents all along the continuum. Those programs that address risk factors or alcohol use can be considered primary prevention. Those that address alcohol misuse or alcohol problems can be considered secondary prevention.

The settings, or social systems in which most prevention efforts take place are listed down the first column: families (parents, siblings), school (peers, teachers), clinics/hospitals (physical and mental health care providers), community (local neighborhoods, organizations, towns), society (norms and practices), and the legal/policy system (laws, policies). While the individual adolescent and his or her welfare is the target of all of the programs in Table 4, few are directed solely to an individual. Most programs work toward positively affecting individuals through one of the social systems or structures listed. Prevention programs are needed in all settings, targeting all stages of the continuum. Individually, programs can have an impact on behavior (Hansen, 1992). However, it is clear that programs work best when multiple individual programs are allied into a larger

Table 4. Adolescent Alcohol Prevention Programs by Prevention Goals and Prevention Setting

Prevention setting	Prevention goal		
	Risk factor modification	Alcohol use/misuse prevention	Alcohol problem prevention
Families	Parent communication training[a] Parenting skills, family therapy, family conflict reduction, strengthen family bonding, referral[a] Parent involvement and support in school achievement, commitment[a] Training in role model effects[c]	Parent training: family policy, resistance skills, self control, active involvement[b] Parent prevention groups: foster antialcohol attitudes and norms[b] Parent components of school programs: homework, after-school meetings[b]	Safe-ride contracts[c] Family norms against riding/driving after drinking[c]

(continued)

Table 4.   (*continued*)

Prevention setting	Prevention goal		
	Risk factor modification	Alcohol use/misuse prevention	Alcohol problem prevention
School	Observe and refer students with behavior problems[a] Student Assistance Programs[d] Social competence training, anger management[a] Promote academic achievement and school commitment[a]	Curricula: social influence, refusal skill training, norm setting, life-skill training (multiple other components which include these)[a] Policies: foster antialcohol norms, attitudes[c]	Identification and referral of high-risk students[b] Student Assistance Programs[c] Students Against Drunk Driving[b]
Clinics and hospitals	Anticipatory guidance by nurses and physicians[c] Problem identification and referral[c]	Anticipatory guidance by nurses and physicians[c] *Guidelines for Adolescent Preventive Services* (GAPS)[c]	Screen and refer for high-risk behaviors[b] *Guidelines for Adolescent Preventive Services* (GAPS)[c] Hospital-based trauma program[b]
Community	Programs for youth[c] Latchkey programs: homework, self-esteem, supervised free play, dramatics[b]	Strengthen community norms[c] Reduce alcohol billboards[c] Observe and enforce laws against sales to minors, reduce outlet density[a] Server training[b] Youth groups, supervised recreation[b] Community coalitions[b]	Reduce outlet density[a] Server training[d] Alternative transportation[d] Change norms and enforcement about drunk driving and riding[c] Community-based high-risk youth alternative programs[c]
Society		Reduce alcohol advertising and positive alcohol portrayals on TV and in movies[c] Anti-alcohol advertising[c]	Public service announcements about avoiding drinking and driving[c]
Legislation and policy		Minimum legal drinking age, enforcement of laws[a] Increase taxation[a] Alcohol warning labels[b]	Minimum legal drinking age, older minimum legal driving age, curfews, graduated licensing, administrative license revocation, increase enforcement[a] Reduced or zero-tolerance BAC for young drivers[a] Increased taxation[a] Juvenile court diversion programs[a] *Per se* laws[c]

[a]Effectiveness demonstrated.
[b]Effectiveness not demonstrated, but some positive results.
[c]Effectiveness not evaluated.
[d]Little potential for effectiveness.

strategic plan in which these approaches work together to solve the problems of alcohol abuse and alcoholism. Adolescents need consistent messages about drinking from the several settings in which they live their lives.

The prevention approaches highlighted in Table 4 focus on factors that are amenable to change through prevention, rather than listing all alcohol-related factors, some of which are individual characteristics (such as genetics and sociodemographic status) and not amenable to change. Such individual characteristics are useful in identifying subpopulations at special risk, and for whom targeted, appropriate prevention programs should be selected.

A wide range of adolescent alcohol prevention programs will be briefly described below by prevention goal (what the program tries to prevent) and prevention setting (where the program takes place). An overview of each approach will be given, as well as its implementation status and effectiveness. Program effectiveness has also been included in Table 4 in a very abbreviated fashion. It is presumed that prevention targeted toward risk factors will also prevent the alcohol use and alcohol problems that could follow along the continuum. Similarly, prevention of alcohol use will also prevent the alcohol problems that could follow.

Programs' Impact on Changing Risk and Protective Factors

This section describes effects of programmatic efforts on changing risk and protective factors associated with developing alcohol use, misuse, and abuse.

Families

Several risk factors for subsequent adolescent alcohol problems involve early patterns of socialization and communication within families (Kumpfer & DeMarsh, 1986). It is therefore appealing that prevention programs be developed that seek to reduce such early risk factors. These programs will be discussed in this section; others that seek to directly focus on preventing alcohol use will be discussed below.

Parent training in the Parent Communication Project (Shain, Suurvali, & Kilty, 1980) provided parents with skills in active listening, constructive confrontation, and problem solving, the goal being to develop familial conditions that would encourage more informed decisions about alcohol use by children. Positive changes in parents' skills and children's perceptions of family life were found in the short term, but had deteriorated by the 2-year follow-up.

Several prevention efforts summarized by Hawkins et al. (1992) were also found to be effective in their goals of reducing family-related risk factors: parent skills training (including improving family interaction and promoting monitoring, contingent discipline, rewards of prosocial behavior), functional family therapy, reduction of family conflict, and strengthening of family bonding. If family conflict cannot be reduced through programs such as these, families should be referred for services to address the problem.

School achievement and commitment to school, protective factors against alcohol use, were also improved with parent involvement and family support approaches (Hawkins et al., 1992).

Another risk factor that should be addressed in prevention approaches that involve families is that of alcohol behavior modeled by parents and siblings of adolescents. Some parents are unaware of the impact of such role models on their adolescents' subsequent drinking behavior, and might consider their child's future welfare in decisions about their own current behavior. Including this component in parent training merits study.

School

School-based student assistance programs have rapidly increased recently in response to several psychosocial problems noted among students. Families, school staff, or students themselves may identify students in need of assistance because of their status as "at risk" for subsequent school or social problems. Frequently the "at risk" status is based on the same risk factors that predispose to subsequent alcohol use and related problems, and teachers can be trained to improve their early identification of such students (McLaughlin, Holcomb, Jibaja-Rusth, & Webb, 1993). Students with family backgrounds that include alcohol problems should also be considered "at risk." The students may participate in individual counseling or group prevention (Emshoff, 1989) or may be referred to community agencies for specific needs. Klitzner, Fisher, Stewart, and Gilbert (1992) concluded after a review of studies, that despite their wide popularity and active promotion, there is little evidence that student assistance programs effectively reduce rates of underage drinking. The studies reviewed, however, were methodologically flawed, so their effectiveness may yet be demonstrated.

The risk factors of early social, peer, and behavioral problems can be addressed by schools through effective approaches (Hawkins *et al.*, 1992), including social competence training and anger management. The risk factor of poor school achievement has also been addressed successfully in studies supporting the merit of several approaches (Hawkins *et al.*, 1992): early childhood education; active teachers' instruction and direct supervision of learning; interactive teaching, proactive classroom management, cooperative learning, and tutoring of socially rejected low achievers; school governance and management teams; and interventions to help students manage school transitions. A final risk factor, that of low commitment to school, has also been positively affected in studies that suggest the following effective approaches (Hawkins *et al.*, 1992): interactive teaching, cooperative learning, and proactive classroom management; curricular restructuring; transition programs; and a multicomponent program that included shared decision-making, student services, and academic innovations.

Clinics/Hospitals

Children and young people are seen somewhat regularly by health professionals for illness episodes, required immunizations, and physical exams, if not for routine well-child visits. Nurses and physicians have opportunities at these visits to screen for risk factors or problems as described above. They can then provide anticipatory guidance (enabling families to adapt and cope) themselves, or refer young people to other health professionals if indicated (O'Neal, 1993).

Community

The multitude of activities and programs for young people that many communities offer may provide those children who participate with certain factors protective against subsequent alcohol use. For other children perhaps at greater risk, such opportunities should also be offered and evaluated. Early prevention of precursors of substance use was tried with latchkey youth in sessions held at schools and including supervised homework, self-esteem-building exercises, free play, and creative dramatics (Ross, Saavedra, Shur, & Winters, 1992). No measurable positive effects were found on any personality variables (self-esteem, depression, risk-taking), in-classroom behavior, or standardized achievement tests. There was, however, a significant interaction effect between participation in self-esteem-building exercises and improvement on standardized achievement tests. Further work in this area is needed.

Society and Legal/Policy

Both of these settings are lacking in established programs directed toward the prevention of alcohol risk factors for children and adolescents. Some public television programming includes efforts toward building self-esteem among young children, and toward early childhood education, but these efforts are not explicit in their prevention goals. Most of the legal/policy approaches are aimed directly at alcohol itself—controlling access to it by young people—and do not lend themselves to controlling early risk factors.

Preventing Alcohol Use and Misuse

This section summarizes findings from evaluations of programs that have specifically targeted reductions in alcohol consumption, including the promotion of abstinence, reduced quantity and frequency of use, and reduced misuse of alcohol.

Families

Preparing for the Drug (Free) Years is a parent training program that includes alcohol prevention in its goals (Hawkins, Catalano, & Kent, 1991). After exposure to the four-session program, parents are expected to (1) establish a family position or policy on alcohol and other drug use, (2) teach children social influence resistance skills, (3) use self-control skills to reduce family conflict, and (4) create opportunities for children entering adolescence to contribute and learn through active involvement in the family. Positive changes in parents' attitudes, motivations, intentions to use the program's strategies, and reported behavior were found immediately after each session, but no comparison group or long-term follow-up was reported.

Concerned parents have formed groups to try to prevent youth alcohol and drug use (Klitzner, Bamberger, & Gruenewald, 1990a). Typically, these groups try to restore parental control, reduce peer influence, manipulate peer group and community norms, and influence the policies of schools and other community agencies (Klitzner, Bamberger, & Gruenewald, 1990b). Evaluation showed positive changes in families' communication and discipline, but only weak evidence of an impact on adolescent alcohol use. Many groups were, however, effective in altering the alcohol-related practices of schools, police, courts, and other agencies, which may have had an important impact.

Parent components of school- and community-based prevention programs have been considered important, but difficult to implement successfully. One report describes the parent component of the Midwestern Prevention Program in which 73% of the parents participated. Importantly, at follow-up parental participation was negatively associated with adolescent use of alcohol and friends' and siblings' substance use (Rohrbach, Hodgson, Broder, & Montgomery, 1994).

School

One of the most active areas of prevention for adolescents has been school-based alcohol prevention. The very earliest curricular programs were primarily information only, and although they increased students' knowledge, evaluations showed that they did not produce the desired behavioral outcomes. In the last decade or so, programs have been developed with more attention to sound theoretical bases, as well as improved evaluation methodology. The results are somewhat promising as several reviewers have recently summarized (Botvin & Botvin, 1992; Hansen, 1992, 1993; Tobler, 1986), although usually the reviews combined other drug education as well, which might make for less clear interpretations when the prevention focus is solely on alcohol. The various curriculum approaches used were categorized differently; however, types of programs effective against adolescent alcohol use emerged from each review. Tobler (1986) concluded that peer programs (those promoting positive peer influence, teaching, and counseling; refusal skills, and social/life skills) were the most effective for the average school-based population, whereas the alternatives programs (those emphasizing activities, personal competence, and perceived control) were effective for "at risk" adolescents. Botvin and Botvin's review (1992) found that approaches that teach adolescents skills for resisting the social influences promoting substance use and for enhancing general individual competence demonstrated effectiveness.

Hansen (1992, 1993) found that 14 of the 35 programs reviewed were effective in reducing students' alcohol use. The prevention programs were classified by their "building block theoretical concepts," the program content means by which behavior would be affected. Each of these content areas could also be considered a risk factor that influences substance use and that the program aimed to moderate. A successful program should target factors that statistically account for adolescent alcohol use and are modifiable (Hansen, 1993; Kline & Canter, 1994). Hansen found that two types of programs were most successful: those that were comprehensive (including a broad spectrum of prevention strategies) and those that included the social influence content area (peer and other social pressures, resistance skills). Hansen's later analysis of the school-based prevention programs (1993) further suggested that strategies were most successful when several program components were included, and when at least one component was aimed at changing normative beliefs about alcohol consumption—the incorrect belief that alcohol use and abuse is prevalent and acceptable among young people (Hansen & Graham, 1991; MacKinnon *et al.,* 1991; Shope, Kloska, Dielman, & Maharg, 1994). Donaldson, Graham, and Hansen (1994) suggest that successful social influence-based prevention programs may be driven primarily by their ability to foster social norms that reduce adolescents' social motivations to use alcohol.

Although fairly widely implemented, school-based programs to prevent adolescent alcohol use are not always carefully selected by schools based on theoretically grounded approaches and methodologically sound evaluation results. The DARE program, for example, has been widely supported and implemented, yet recent studies show no effects on students' alcohol use (Ennett, Tobler, Ringwalt, & Flewelling, 1994; Rosenbaum, Flewelling, Bailey, & Ringwalt, 1994).

Schools have opportunities other than curricula to prevent students' alcohol use/misuse. School policies that clearly prohibit alcohol use and spell out the consequences for violation have been strongly recommended and widely implemented. The school community can also do much to influence the norms and attitudes regarding young people's drinking of its students, faculty, staff, and parents.

Clinics/Hospitals

Anticipatory guidance that can prevent future alcohol use has become part of the *Guidelines for Adolescent Preventive Services* (GAPS) developed by the American Medical Association (1992). A preventive services health visit should take place once a year between the ages of 11 and 21 years, and include health guidance for the parents which, among other things, provides information about methods for helping adolescents avoid potentially harmful behaviors, such as monitoring social and recreational activities for the use of alcohol (Recommendation 4, p. 5). The American Medical Association is offering workshops on the Guidelines for practitioners.

Community

Community activism has been directed toward the prevention of adolescent alcohol use in several ways. Community norms against providing alcohol to adolescents or allowing unsupervised parties where drinking can take place can be strengthened through parent groups and concerned citizens, but such efforts have not been evaluated. Local efforts have been strong, but also not evaluated, in reducing the number of billboards advertising alcoholic beverages. In addition, local community members often pressure retail sellers and servers of alcohol to obey the minimum legal drinking age laws, as well as pressuring local law enforcement officials to enforce those laws. While essential to a community's comprehensive approach to responsible alcohol service, these efforts have also not been evaluated (McKnight, 1993). Local communities control planning and zoning ordinances and conditional use permits that relate to the sale of alcohol. Reductions in the consumption of alcohol can be achieved by restrictions on the growth of the number or density of sales outlets (Gruenewald, Madden, & Janes, 1991; Gruenewald, Ponicke, & Holder, 1991). Server training (McKnight, 1993), mandated in some localities, is a prevention program for those who work in bars and restaurants that sell alcohol. Servers are trained in age identification and how to handle underage purchase attempts. Server training has not affected the incidence of service to underage patrons (Saltz & Hennessy, 1991).

Prevention programs could be implemented within existing youth groups. One study reports some success in 13-year-olds' alcohol-related behavior and attitudes after the Stay SMART program in Boys and Girls Clubs (St. Pierre, Kaltreider, Mark, & Aikin, 1992). Recreational activities such as parties, rock concerts, and wilderness challenges have been promoted for adolescents under the theory that such experiences could offer safer alternatives to alcohol use for achieving excitement, challenge, and relief from boredom (Cohen, 1980). Others (Schaps & Slimmon, 1975) suggested alternatives that created opportunities for youth to become involved in meaningful service and community activities. Evaluations have not yet supported the effectiveness of this intuitively appealing approach.

Community-based coalitions are developing rapidly as it becomes clear that isolated prevention programs rarely solve the adolescent alcohol problem. What is sought is a comprehensive, coordinated, consistent prevention approach by all of the relevant community groups (schools, law enforcement agencies, social services, judicial system, regulatory agencies, and citizen groups). This model is being promoted nationally by both federal and private sponsors. Community-based prevention approaches have great potential while at the same time presenting considerable challenges to evaluation (Giesbrecht & Ferris, 1993; Giesbrecht, Krempulec, & West, 1993). Few evaluations of community coalitions have been done to date. The Midwest Prevention Project (Star) in Kansas City, Missouri, and Indianapolis, Indiana, is a current, ambitious example, in which mass media, school-based education, parent education and organization, community organization, and health policy components are integrated. Pentz *et al.* (1989) found the community context to strengthen a school-based project's ability to prevent adolescent alcohol use. The community-based approach to youth drinking and two large-scale randomized community trials in progress are discussed further by Wagenaar and Perry (1994).

While it is tempting to conclude that community-based approaches may help solve the alcohol problem, it should be noted that these efforts have their own special problems. Community coalitions tend to represent diverse political forces within communities that have diverse views about the importance and nature of alcohol problems. When unified, coalitions have the potential to bring tremendous massed resources to the problem. However, if diverse goals compete, coalitions may block or stop efforts that could, if left alone, have potential impact. Significant work for understanding how coalitions operate and for distinguishing effective from ineffective coalitions remains to be completed.

Society

The numerous portrayals of alcohol use and alcohol advertising or promotion on television have been regarded, but not conclusively demonstrated, to influence the alcohol-related beliefs and behavior of young people (Grube, 1993). Over 2 years of televised sports programming, more commercials appeared for alcoholic products than for any other beverage (Madden & Grube, 1994). In a study of 5th and 6th graders, awareness of televised beer advertising was related to more favorable beliefs about drinking, to greater knowledge of beer brands and slogans, and to increased intentions to drink as an adult, suggesting that alcohol advertising may predispose young people to drinking (Grube & Wallack, 1994). Much of the alcohol-related material on television makes drinking seem appealing by subtly using highly valued personal attributes (attractiveness, elegance, fame) linked with positive outcomes (success, romance, or adventure). In order to lessen these influences on young people's drinking, several strategies can be tried, although adequate evaluation would be challenging. Efforts to reduce the amount of both the portrayal of drinking, as well as the advertising of beer and wine during prime viewing hours for children could be considered. Reducing advertising's appeal to youngsters would require cooperation of the alcohol advertisers, a condition that is likely to go against the economic self-interest of the alcohol industry in the current economic climate.

Efforts could also be expended to produce appealing counteradvertising (Bochner, 1994) or to add health warnings directly to the alcohol advertising. A final prevention strategy is to help children develop and improve their critical skills regarding alcohol advertisements. This approach, including developing countermessages, has been included in several school-based alcohol prevention curricula with modest success.

Legal/Policy

The minimum legal drinking age in all states is now 21. Improved enforcement of the minimum age would enhance the prevention of alcohol use by young people (Klitzner, Stewart, & Fisher, 1993). Several enforcement strategies directed at alcohol retailers, bars, and restaurants are used, although their effects on adolescent alcohol use directly have not been evaluated. Operations using "decoys" or "stings" send underage young people into establishments to attempt to purchase alcohol. Penalties are inflicted on those establishments that sell to the underage purchaser. Stings that are well publicized may prevent alcohol sales to young people (Insurance Institute for Highway Safety, 1992).

State laws regarding the sale to and purchase by underage youth should be freed of loopholes, which too often make enforcement complex (Hingson, 1993; Klitzner et al., 1993). Some police departments expend effort to prevent or break up parties where young people drink alcohol (Preusser, Preusser, & Ulmer, 1992). Although no formal outcome data are available, some police departments believe these techniques to be successful.

Studies have shown that the price of alcoholic beverages influences levels of consumption (Chaloupka, 1993; Klitzner et al., 1993). Because federal excise taxes have been raised only modestly and infrequently, the real prices of alcoholic beverages have decreased, increasing consumption. As demonstrated in simulation studies, increasing price with inflation-equalization taxation would be an efficient means of deterring youthful drinking at all levels and is estimated to be even more effective than the minimum legal drinking age (Coate & Grossman, 1988; Grossman, Chaloupka, Saffer, & Laixuthai, 1994).

Since November, 1989, four rotating warning labels have been required on alcoholic beverage containers sold in the United States (Greenfield, Graves, & Kaskutas, 1993). Evaluations of this prevention policy have been carried out primarily with people 18 and older. Young adults (18–29 years) reported fairly high rates of having seen the labels. In general, the evaluation results are only mildly promising that behavioral outcomes are being achieved. MacKinnon, Pentz, and Stacy (1993) evaluated the effectiveness of the warning labels on a sample of adolescents up to 1 year after the labels were required. They found increases in awareness, exposure, and recognition memory, but there were no substantial changes in alcohol use or beliefs about the risks identified on the warning labels. The warning label prevention approach is, however, inexpensive and could be effective in synergy with other approaches.

Preventing Alcohol-Related Problems

This section reviews findings from prevention programs that have specifically targeted harm reduction. The primary concern addressed by many of these programs is drinking and driving.

Families

The problem of young people riding with drivers who have been drinking deserves prevention efforts that are evaluated. Within families, contracts can be made with parents whereby a ride will be provided no questions asked, rather than have an adolescent ride with someone who has been drinking. The establishment of family norms against riding with a drinking driver or driving after drinking is a prevention area deserving development and evaluation. Beck and Lockhart (1992) have presented a model of parental involvement in the prevention of teenage drinking and driving. They suggest that parents' effectiveness at preventing alcohol use and alcohol-impaired driving among their teenagers depends on their stage of involvement (awareness, acceptance, action, and consequences). Parents may be unaware of the true extent of teen drinking and thus less prone to intervention. This prevention approach has been underutilized and deserves development and evaluation.

School

Student assistance and other school-based programs can be helpful in preventing alcohol-related problems for students who are already using alcohol (Newman, Henry, DiRenzo, & Stecher, 1988–89). Trained teachers showed greater confidence in their ability to identify student substance abuse problems, greater willingness to intervene in student substance abuse problems and to make more referrals of students with suspected problems (Kantor, Caudill, & Ungerleider, 1992).

Some programs to prevent riding with a drinking driver are based in schools, an alternative ride program sometimes included. The national, school-based Students Against Driving Drunk organization aims to prevent students who have been drinking from driving. The goal of this program is to impact school and community norms with regard to drinking. While a strong relationship is known to exist between norms and both underage drinking and impaired driving, evidence that the program is effective in changing those norms or behaviors is lacking. Program effectiveness on outcome (behavior) or on mediating variables (beliefs) was not demonstrated in one evaluation, although the programs studied in the quasiexperimental design were not fully implemented (Klitzner, Gruenewald, Bamberger, & Rossiter, 1994). In another school-based program to prevent driving while intoxicated, significant improvements in target behaviors were found among high-risk subjects (Farrow, 1989).

Although not targeted at problem alcohol use, a program that focused on preventing use through the establishment of conservative normative beliefs (Hansen & Graham,

1991) demonstrated an effect on self-reported alcohol-related problems among seventh-graders. The rate of reported problem use among students who received an information only program and a program that focused on teaching students how to resist peer pressure doubled between seventh and eighth grade. In contrast, a program that included strategies for establishing and reinforcing intolerant attitudes about alcohol use and misuse resulted in no increase in reported alcohol problems between seventh and eighth grade. Such findings suggest that even problem use, which might be considered to reflect underlying psychological problems, is also subject to the influence of group norms and is amenable to preventive intervention.

Clinics/Hospitals

Because adolescents may avoid raising sensitive issues themselves with physicians, routine screening for high-risk behavior such as alcohol use/misuse has promise for identifying those adolescents who could benefit from prevention counseling or even a brief intervention. One screening program (Paperny, Aono, Lehman, Hammar, & Risser, 1990) is completed by the adolescent on a computer, which produces a printout and specific health advice and referral information. The program was well received, but not yet evaluated in terms of alcohol outcomes.

The *Guidelines for Adolescent Preventive Services* (GAPS) has a guideline in place to prevent adolescent alcohol problems. Recommendation 15 states that "all adolescents should be asked annually about their use of alcohol. . ." (AMA, 1992, p. 7). It is further recommended that adolescents who report any use of alcohol should be assessed further regarding family history, circumstances surrounding use, amount and frequency of use, attitudes and motivation about use, other drug and tobacco use, sexual behavior, and the adequacy of physical, psychosocial, and school functioning. Adolescents should receive counseling and mental health treatment as appropriate.

In an effort to prevent high-risk-taking adolescents from experiencing alcohol-related trauma, a hospital-based program sponsors a tour of a shock trauma unit (Dearing, Caston, & Babin, 1991). Evaluation results showed marked changes from pretest to posttest up to 1 year later on attitudes toward driving after drinking, riding with someone who has been drinking, and preventing a friend from driving after drinking. Behavior should be assessed as well.

Community

Restricted outlet density, under local community control, has been related to reductions in various alcohol problems, including alcohol-related traffic crashes (Gliksman & Rush, 1986). Alcohol beverage server training attempts to prevent intoxication among those patrons of bars and restaurants purchasing alcohol (McKnight, 1993). Although adolescents should not have been served if properly identified, preventing their becoming intoxicated if served would help prevent motor vehicle crashes, injuries, and fatalities. It remains to be demonstrated that server training can reduce the incidence of intoxication or service to already intoxicated patrons. The alternative transportation arrangements often offered as part of responsible alcohol beverage service introduce complexities as well, and have not demonstrated positive results, although the approach fits with preventing harm as a result of alcohol use. Communities as a whole can do much to influence citizens' norms and attitudes regarding young people's drinking-related problems and injuries. But awareness of the problems, and organization to address those problems, is a necessary first step.

Community-based programs to prevent and treat alcohol and other drug abuse and to rehabilitate alcohol and other drug abusers have been funded under the high-risk youth initiative by the Office for Substance Abuse Prevention within the Alcohol, Drug Abuse and Mental Health Administration of the U.S. Department of Health and Human Services. Several lessons learned from these programs are reported by Lorion and Ross (1992). First, preventive interventions appear to maximize their potential for lowering rates of alcohol use when targeted toward youth with several risk factors. Second, the authors point out the extraordinarily complicated tasks that development and implementation of a community-based prevention intervention involve. And third, the evaluation involves far more than solely outcome measures of alcohol and other drug use. Much is to be learned from these ambitious programs, as they strive to maintain community support to achieve their goals.

Society

Public service announcements regarding avoiding drinking and driving are occasionally broadcast on television. While not a strong prevention approach alone, they could serve to enhance other prevention approaches and should be evaluated as a component of a more comprehensive program.

Prevention Legislation

Increasing the minimum legal drinking age to 21 reduced alcohol-related crashes among young people (U.S. General Accounting Office, 1987), positively affected drinking behavior and other alcohol-related health problems (Jones, Pieper, & Robertson, 1992), and promoted lower rates of drinking by age 25 (O'Malley & Wagenaar, 1991). Many young lives have been saved since the onset of the nationwide effort to raise the minimum drinking age (National Highway Traffic Safety Administration, 1991).

Increases in taxes on beer have reduced motor vehicle fatality rates for 15- to 24-year-olds (Saffer & Grossman, 1987). This research has also estimated that there would have been a 15% decrease in the number of 18- to 20-year-olds killed in alcohol-related traffic crashes if the federal excise tax on beer had been indexed to inflation since 1951. Further, there would have been a 21% decrease if the alcohol content in beer had been taxed at the same rate as the alcohol content in distilled spirits. And finally, if both of these strategies had been implemented, a 54% decrease in fatalities would have been seen. Simulation studies show that increased taxation would reduce the heavy drinking among young people that predisposes them to injuries and fatalities (Coate & Grossman, 1988; Grossman *et al.*, 1994).

Another legal approach to preventing alcohol-related traffic problems is the establishment of lower legal blood alcohol concentration levels for drivers under age 21 (Hingson, 1993). Several states have recently established new, lower levels based on the fact that young people are impaired by smaller amounts of alcohol (Hingson & Howland, 1986). In states with the lower limits, traffic fatalities among young drivers decreased 42%, while decreasing only 29% in comparison states without the lower limits (Hingson, 1992). Public awareness campaigns enhanced the effectiveness of the new laws. Another deterrent to driving while alcohol-impaired is new laws adopted by most states which make it a criminal offense *per se* to drive with blood alcohol concentrations above the legal limit (Hingson, 1993).

The effectiveness of these new laws can be further enhanced by administrative license suspension and revocation, whereby the arresting officer can confiscate the license of drivers who test over the legal blood alcohol limit, or who refuse to take the test. This administrative, rather than legal (court system) approach to license revocation is effective (Nichols & Ross, 1990; Zador, Lund, Fields, & Weinberg, 1989), and a stronger deterrent to impaired driving than the judicial process where penalties are imposed slowly or not at all (Stewart & Sweedler, 1992). Jail sentences, vehicle impoundment and confiscation, and withdrawal of vehicle registration, although not found to be effective in one study (Popkin & Parker, 1992), could be further deterrents for adolescent driving after drinking—if young people are aware of the laws and believe that they will be enforced. The combined effects of these and other laws and programs are at least in part responsible for decreases in alcohol-related traffic fatalities among young people (Hingson, 1993).

Because of the serious consequences resulting from alcohol consumption by young drivers, another approach to preventing these problems is to limit youthful driving, rather than, or as well as, addressing the alcohol directly as the approaches above have. Minimum driving ages that are higher, provisional licensing and curfews (Williams, Karps, & Zador, 1983), and graduated licensing are approaches to reducing the driving exposure of young people that can reduce their traffic fatalities (Insurance Bureau of Canada and Traffic Injury Research Foundation of Canada, 1991). A 23% reduction in motor vehicle injuries among young people during curfew hours documents the merit of this approach to injury prevention (Preusser, Williams, Lund, & Zador, 1990).

A good example of secondary prevention of alcohol-related problems is the juvenile court diversion program offered by some communities as a way of avoiding prosecution of an adolescent for alcohol possession or other minor alcohol charges (Klitzner *et al.*, 1992). Instead, the offender can participate in an educational program, presumably designed to prevent further alcohol-related problems. Evaluation of these approaches is needed, although one educational intervention for juveniles found guilty of driving under the influence has demonstrated improved attitudes and less risky behaviors regarding alcohol and driving (Kooler & Bruvold, 1992). Another program that compared talk-based and behavioral alcohol education courses found positive results among court-referred young offenders, but the low percentage of subjects who completed the program suggests that self-selection was a factor (Baldwin, Heather, Lawson, & Robertson, 1991).

Gender, Cultural, and Ethnic Issues

There is a dearth of published information on adolescent alcohol prevention programs that address gender, cultural, or ethnic issues. Schinke, Orlandi, Botvin, and Gilchrist (1988) have described a bicultural competence skills approach for preventing substance abuse among Native American adolescents. Data from an evaluation of that approach suggest its efficacy, showing increased knowledge, improved attitudes and interactive skills, and reduced rates of self-reported alcohol use among those who received the prevention compared to those adolescents who served as controls.

Other authors have discussed differences among adolescents in alcohol use that may have implications for prevention approaches. In one study, high school students who were Mexican-Americans born in Mexico, born in the United States, and Caucasians were compared (Boles, Casas, Furlong, & Gonzalez, 1994). Female Mexican-born students abstained the most from alcohol use. Male Mexican-born students reported lower alcohol use than their U.S.-born Mexican-American and Caucasian counterparts, whose rates of use were similar. Caucasian students were more likely to report having had a substance abuse prevention program. In another study, drug use was compared among Cuban-American, African-American, and white non-Hispanic boys (Vega, Gil, & Zimmerman, 1993). First use of alcohol was at fifth grade for all groups. White non-Hispanics had the highest lifetime levels of alcohol use and African-Americans the lowest. Foreign-born Cuban-Americans had a lower lifetime prevalence of alcohol use than U.S.-born Cuban-Americans. Higher acculturation level was related to first use of alcohol. The relationship between neighborhood setting and drug use was examined among minority junior high students (Blount & Dembo, 1984). Knowledge of peer use was predictive of alcohol use regardless of how tough or drug-involved the neighborhood was thought to be.

Influences on alcohol use that vary between genders and among ethnic groups would have important implications for prevention programs. Newcomb, Chou, Bentler, and Huba (1988) studied cognitive motivations for alcohol use, finding them significantly correlated with alcohol use, but showing no gender differences. Scheier, Newcomb, and Skager (1994) also searched for gender differences in risk, protection, and vulnerability to adolescent drug use, which was represented by a construct of eight measures of alcohol and drug use. Vulnerability was strongly related to drug use for both genders. Both gender and cultural values regarding alcohol use were examined in focus group studies of Chicana/Latina high school and university students (Flores-Ortiz, 1994). The roles of cultural values and family communication in the ability to prevent high-risk behaviors were examined in the groups. Cultural values that highly prize modesty and virginity decreased the probability that these young women would (or could) discuss issues of sexuality and alcohol use with their parents. Furthermore, traditional double-standard gender values decreased the probability of assertive behavior (e.g., suggesting condom use) by these women because such behavior may be misconstrued as a general distrust of the male involved, or of an unsavory past on the part of the woman. Thus, cultural values inadvertently prevented the women from negotiating safe sex or alcohol abstinence.

In a study of family influences on black and white adolescents' drinking patterns (Barnes, Farrell, & Banerjee, 1994), black adolescents were found to have higher abstention rates and lower rates of alcohol abuse and other deviance than white adolescents in spite of black families having more single-parent households and lower family incomes. The same parenting factors (i.e., support, monitoring, and parent–adolescent communication) were important predictors for both black and white adolescents. There is evidence that blacks are protected from alcohol abuse by religion, and whites are susceptible to peer drinking influences. Another study of family influences (Peterson, Hawkins, Abbott, &

Catalano, 1994) found that for both black and white youth, parental drinking when the subjects were 12–13 years old was a predictor of alcohol use at 14–15 years old. Good family management practices decreased the likelihood of adolescent alcohol use. The parents of black youth drank less frequently, held stronger norms against alcohol use, perceived alcohol use as more harmful, and involved their children less frequently in family alcohol use than did parents of white youth.

Still other researchers have discussed the implications of ethnic and cultural minority group membership for the treatment of adolescent alcohol dependence (Delgado, 1988; Sweet, 1988–89; Thompson & Simmons-Cooper, 1988). The added stresses of poverty and discrimination (Sweet, 1988–89), the need for culture-specific approaches (Delgado, 1988), and increasing use but later problem-identification among black youth (Thompson & Simmons-Cooper, 1988) all highlight the need for enhanced prevention efforts including culturally appropriate approaches. While implications of these treatment reports may be drawn for prevention programs, more research is badly needed to ensure that prevention programming is culturally relevant for the several diverse backgrounds represented in our contemporary society.

Status of Prevention and Prevention Research

An overview of programs to prevent adolescent alcohol risk factors, use/misuse, and problems has been presented. While the summary was comprehensive, it was not necessarily exhaustive, so some programs may have been missed. In addition, programs are constantly being developed, implemented, and evaluated, and there is considerable lag time before their reports are readily available. The necessary abbreviated assessment of program evaluations and demonstrated effectiveness has omitted much of interest that should be explored further before pursuing or not pursuing specific prevention goals in particular prevention settings. Some programs have not been evaluated. When evaluations are done that have weak methodologies, invalid conclusions may be drawn. The purpose of this summary was not to thoroughly critique all of the evaluation methodology, but to present a useful overview of many types of prevention activities directed toward adolescent experiences with alcohol.

It is apparent that the most prevention programming has been done in school settings and in the legal/policy system. In schools, programs have been targeted toward the prevention both of risk factors and of alcohol use. Many of those programs were evaluated and shown to be effective at least to some degree in reducing risk factors and alcohol use. In the legal/policy system, programs have been targeted toward both the prevention of alcohol use and alcohol problems among adolescents. Most evaluated programs have been shown to be quite effective in reducing alcohol use and alcohol problems. It is worth considering whether the programs with demonstrated effectiveness are indeed being actively implemented in these areas. Lack of support or funding, or the choice of less effective programs may be limiting the potential impact on the adolescent alcohol problem.

Relatively little risk factor-focused prevention programming has been done on a societal scale and within the legal/policy system. While it is probably inappropriate to involve the legal system in the prevention of risk factors, society as a whole should definitely be more involved through awareness, media attention, programming through television, and a higher sense of commitment to doing something to prevent children from experiencing risk factors that may lead to subsequent alcohol use and alcohol problems. Another setting that is important for further prevention programming is the community, which is able to target all stages of the adolescent alcohol continuum. Communities are also ideal settings in which to coordinate the prevention efforts made in the other settings, and in fact encouraging efforts in this direction are being made. The most effective prevention strategies are probably those that are comprehensive. Such approaches are best able to consider all of the ecological and cultural forces that impact on local adolescents' risk factors, alcohol use, and alcohol problems, and promote appropriate comprehensive prevention approaches that do not rely on one small program for an impact on the problem being addressed (Gruenewald, Millar, & Treno, 1993).

Prevention research includes preintervention work as well as program development, implementation, and evaluation (Howard, 1993). Each new effort should clarify and state which stage along the adolescent alcohol continuum the prevention is targeting and which setting is most appropriate. Because the focus is on adolescents, their development and the need for developmentally appropriate approaches must be constantly considered. Research should focus on factors with the most predictive power, developing and testing prevention that prevents those factors from leading to adolescent alcohol problems. Because programs targeting alcohol use for prevention have had but limited success, more work is needed regarding prevention of the risk factors that precede alcohol use. Unfortunately, longitudinal studies would have to be very long indeed (and require much support) to track young people from early childhood throughout adolescence in order to measure the ultimate outcomes of alcohol use and alcohol problems. It would be more practical to accept reduction of the risk factors as good enough evidence that ultimately alcohol use and problems could also be reduced. The quality of prevention evaluation has improved greatly. Nonetheless, there is still a need for all prevention efforts to use the best methodology possible and to make sure their results are available for others.

Prevention Summary

The prevention of adolescent alcohol problems was addressed in terms of the need for a strong theoretical base, approaches that target factors that account for a large portion of the targeted behavior, and excellent evaluation methodology. A broad review of adolescent alcohol prevention was undertaken, categorizing the many prevention approaches by prevention goal along an adolescent alcohol continuum (risk factors, alcohol use, and alcohol problems) and by prevention setting (families, school, clinics/hospitals, community, society, and legal/policy). Programs were briefly described, and effectiveness noted if evaluations had been conducted. Gender, cultural, and ethnic issues were examined, although lacking in the literature. Prevention has been most active and effective in school and legal settings. In schools, programs have been targeted toward the prevention both of risk factors and of alcohol use. In the legal/policy system, programs have been targeted toward both the prevention of alcohol use and alcohol problems among adolescents. Prevention program adopters should consider evaluation results more before selecting, supporting, and implementing programs. Because comprehensive approaches will probably be more effective, community-based prevention programs deserve attention from both researchers and practitioners. Although very challenging to develop, implement, and evaluate, these approaches show promise and are worth the effort to evaluate.

TREATMENT FOR ADOLESCENT ALCOHOL ABUSE AND DEPENDENCE

The Unique Needs of Adolescents in Alcohol Treatment

Despite past efforts to provide youth with treatments for alcohol abuse or dependence that were originally designed for adults, there is an increasing understanding that adolescents have special needs and therefore require specific, developmentally appropriate treatment modalities. Perhaps the most salient aspect of adolescent life is their position as a dependent member of a family system. Adolescents look to their families to model appropriate behavior (including appropriate drinking behaviors), provide consistent behavioral limits, and provide support, especially in stressful times. Deficits in family functioning including parental alcoholism or other substance abuse, the absence of firm behavioral limits, and the lack of support need to be addressed in adolescent-oriented treatment.

Another critical treatment-relevant difference is the importance of considering the psychosocial and developmental contexts of the adolescent. Treatment programs for adolescents should consider promoting interventions that facilitate the successful and adaptive attainment of adolescent developmental tasks. Important considerations include achieving a separate identity and independence from their parents and preparing themselves for appropriate societal and developing individual relations to achieve the adult developmental tasks of job, marriage, and family. Education or vocational training is another unique characteristic of youth. In order to become a successful adult in today's economy, adolescents must learn at least a basic level of academic or vocational skills. To have a chance for success, treatment programs for adolescents must deal with risk factors promoting alcohol abuse or dependence as well as developmental issues concerning family, peer social development, and education or vocational training.

Adolescent or early onset alcohol abuse appears to be predicted or accompanied by the presence of other behavioral and emotional problems such as antisocial, aggressive behavior, depression, and some anxiety disorders (Bukstein, Brent, & Kaminer, 1989). Attention to comorbid psychopathology is crucial in treatment programs for youth. The high probability of coerced treatment by either parents, school, or the juvenile justice system is always an important consideration in adolescent treatment. In such cases, questionable motivation and insight may adversely affect participation in treatment and ultimate positive outcomes.

The unique needs of adolescents who enter treatment for alcohol abuse or dependence can create formidable obstacles for treatment. The ability of their family or other support systems to promote entry into treatment, participate in treatment, and provide adequate structure and limit-setting following treatment is often difficult because of the frequent high levels of family dysfunction and alcoholism. Compared with adults, adolescents are more likely to use and abuse multiple substances in addition to alcohol and are less likely to suffer from the medical consequences of alcohol dependence including chronic medical problems and psychological withdrawal symptoms (Bukstein & Van

Hasselt, 1993). The existence of additional behavioral and emotional problems requires concurrent attention to these problems. Unfortunately, not all treatment programs have the resources or ability to assess and treat multiproblem youth.

As with alcohol and drug treatment in older populations, treatment for adolescents is currently undergoing rapid change and transition. In 1990, 52,457 youth under 18 years of age were admitted to treatment units or programs with at least some state funding (NIDA, NIAAA, 1992). Such units represent a majority of, but usually not all, treatment programs in most states. Another 72,923 youth were admitted to *drug* treatment units in 1990. Presumably many of these adolescents also had significant problems with alcohol.

A previous emphasis on inpatient and residential treatment is currently being replaced by outpatient and briefer treatments. Many traditional 28- or 35-day inpatient or residential programs are decreasing their lengths of stay and are establishing expanded outpatient services such as partial hospitalization. Many programs that are unable to achieve this transition are closing or downsizing.

The Goals of Treatment and Treatment Modalities

While the primary goal of treatment for adolescents with substance abuse problems is achieving and maintaining abstinence from substance use, clinicians should consider targeting problems and deficits in other areas of the adolescent's life such as coexisting psychopathology, social skills, family functioning, academic and school functioning, and the ability to find and participate in prosocial activities. Goals for alcohol abuse treatment are becoming more comprehensive, commonly including the broad goal of a total change in the adolescent's life-style.

There exists a broad range of different treatment settings for adolescent alcohol abuse (Table 5). Inpatient or residential treatment represent the most restrictive settings and serve those youth with the most severe problems. Reasons for choosing inpatient or residential treatment include: (1) control of the environment by preventing the adolescent from running away, preventing exposure to substance-promoting influences such as music, radio or television, and deviant peers or bringing in contraband such as alcohol or other drugs, (2) separation from often problematic family circumstances, and (3) increasing the intensity of treatment by having each daily activity assume a therapeutic role in which the adolescent must participate.

Indications for inpatient treatment include adolescents who present with ideation or behavior indicating an actual or potential danger to self or others (e.g., suicidal ideation or

Table 5. Treatment Settings for Adolescents with Alcohol Abuse/Dependence

Inpatient

Residential, including therapeutic community

Partial or day hospitalization

Outpatient

Intensive case management/wraparound services (may include in-home therapy) and, for behavioral and emotional problems, parent management training, and social services such as academic assistance, vocational training behavior, more extreme forms of aggressive behavior), adolescents requiring acute medical attention (e.g., withdrawal or significant medical complications of substance use), and adolescents with significant coexisting psychopathology, especially psychotic symptoms.

A history of treatment failure should also be strongly considered, within the context of other severity factors, as an indication for inpatient treatment. While inpatient settings are usually acute, hospital-based programs, free-standing rehabilitation programs remain popular. These programs were based on a set time period, ranging from 28 days to as much as 60 days. Reimbursement limits and managed care have shifted the basis of lengths of stay to meet individual adolescent needs. Not only are programs required to justify admission to programs based on medical, psychiatric, or substance abuse severity, they also need to justify continued stay based on response to treatment and the continued documentation of severity factors. Such a variability in the lengths of stay between patients makes it difficult to develop and maintain specific programming or treatment curriculum. As a result, treatment has become increasingly individualized and flexible in many settings.

The difficulty in achieving success in short-term substance abuse treatment for adolescents has prompted the development of intermediate- and long-term treatment options. Residential care or intermediate care settings include therapeutic communities and offer lengths of stay that may range from 1 to 9 months, while long-term treatment can last as long as 2 years. They are less structured and usually less staff-intensive than inpatient programs.

Outpatient treatment settings and modalities for adolescent substance abusers range from very intensive day-care and partial hospitalization to regular or occasional follow-up (weekly or less often) by an individual therapist. While some outpatient settings may be every bit as intensive as some inpatient or residential treatment programs, the essential difference is that the adolescents reside either at home or in a less restrictive residential placement such as foster care or a group home. In outpatient settings, a significant amount of control may be sacrificed. However, the primary advantage (and in some ways disadvantage) of outpatient settings is that the adolescents participate in treatment while remaining in the community with exposure to the circumstances, stressors, and problems that may have contributed to the development and maintenance of alcohol problems. Given the concern about generalization of treatment progress from a protected, controlled inpatient setting to the exposed community or home environment, one might expect appropriate outpatient treatment to be preferable in being able to actively address problems in the adolescent's environment rather than in the artificial confines of an inpatient unit or residential setting.

School-based programs dealing with alcohol use are usually concerned with prevention. However, Student Assistance Programs (SAPs) often provide aftercare counseling and/or groups for high-risk youth. Several school-based programs offer support groups and more intensive intervention experiences than prevention programs (Fleisch, 1991).

Treatment should ideally provide the individual adolescent with the right modalities at the appropriate intensity in the best environment and would produce the optimal outcome in terms of targeting and improving specific treatment targets. The idea of treatment–patient matching has received much attention for the treatment of adult substance abusers (McLellan & Alterman, 1991). The concept of treatment–patient matching suggests that different groups of adolescents may have different treatment needs and that the philosophy of "one size fits all" treatment for adolescents may not be appropriate, efficacious, or cost-effective. Without treatment research to guide us in the selection of appropriate settings for individual adolescents, clinicians will need to rely on the experience and guidance of others. The American Society for Addiction Medicine has developed placement criteria based on explicit decision-making rules (Mee-Lee & Hoffman, 1992). While not strictly based on research involving substance-abusing adolescents, the criteria do provide a reasonable departure point for considering treatment–patient matching.

Age, Gender, and Ethnic Factors

Adolescent alcohol abuse is not a unitary or homogeneous phenomenon. Factors such as comorbid psychopathology, history of parental substance abuse, and other environmental factors can greatly influence the presentation, development, response to typical treatments, and, ultimately, the prognosis of an individual adolescent's psychoactive substance abuse disorder. Specific populations of adolescents, as defined by age, gender, or ethnic status, have differing types and levels of risk factors for the development of substance use and abuse. Because these differences can affect the screening, assessment, and treatment of adolescent substance use or abuse, the clinician should become familiar with the special population characteristics.

Age is a very important patient characteristic for adolescent substance abusers. The young adolescent, age 12 or 13, is very different from the 18-year-old on a variety of characteristics including cognitive development and level of independence from parents and other adult authority figures. Unfortunately, treatment programs need to aim their curriculum at some developmental level which may not be optimal for a given age group. Similarly, gender status or roles can play an important part in treatment. Sexual attraction and the importance of social standing with peers can distract the adolescents from treatment concerns.

In dealing with or providing any type of intervention for any specific racial, ethnic, or cultural group, the clinician must understand the cultural realities and context for that specific group. Both the process and the content of interventions and treatment must be culturally relevant and must target the specific needs and cultural experiences of the particular racial or ethnic group of adolescents (Table 6). Approaches to the screening, assessment, treatment, and aftercare of substance-abusing adolescents from different racial and ethnic backgrounds need to consider several basic factors in order to provide effective services. These factors include: (1) developing cultural sensitivity in terms of knowledge of the racial/ethnic population characteristics, values, and behaviors, (2) having minority staff from the specific racial/ethnic group to serve as role models, (3) maintaining sufficient numbers of similar minority youth within the treatment population served, (4) developing modified intervention approaches to serve the needs of the racial/ethnic population served, and (5) increasing emphasis on comprehensive services to address the significant environmental and social needs of many racial/ethnic youth and their families.

Alcohol abuse, like other deviant behavior, is not found in equal proportions among all groups of adolescents as defined by racial or ethnic status, sexual orientation, or adequacy of living arrangements. The level of risk is often defined in terms of such characteristics as race, environment, and sexual activity.

Interventions, whether they are to prevent or treat, must be relevant to the individual adolescent, his or her family and social/economic environment. In the spirit of "treatment matching," interventions should be individualized to address these characteristics. Treatment for the adolescent is most relevant to the adolescent when it involves those to whom he or she relates best, i.e., his or her peers. Treatment settings should develop appropriate programming for groups of similar adolescents. Adolescents should not feel isolated from peers with similar characteristics. This need speaks to the development of specialized treatment not only for specific adolescent populations but also in the specific communities where the adolescents live and where sensitive and relevant treatments can be best delivered.

Treatment Modalities

The types of modalities available for the treatment of adolescent alcohol abuse or dependence are many and varied (Table 7). The predominant inpatient and residential treatment approach remains the so-called Minnesota Model based on the tenets of Alcoholics Anonymous (AA) and a 12-step program of recovery (Wheeler & Malmquist, 1987). Such programs are largely group-oriented. In these groups, participants discuss issues relating to the disease of alcoholism and the participants' progress in their ongoing plan for recovery. Other functions of the treatment groups are confrontation of the adolescents' denial and motivation in treatment and to the life-style changes necessary for recovery. Attendance at AA meetings, psychoeducation which includes information about alcoholism and related problems, family therapy both with individual families and in multifamily groups, and the use of 12-step workbooks are usually components of these types of programs. Aftercare or follow-up treatment is variable in content and often merely centered around expected attendance at community AA meetings.

Therapeutic communities usually have a similar orientation as other inpatient and residential programs; however, therapeutic communities are usually longer-term and serve more multiproblem youth with more severe substance abuse and other psychosocial problems.

Table 6. Racial and Ethnic Factors and Intervention for Adolescents

Group	Factors	Intervention
African-American youth	Eye contact, touching, time perspective, social distance, alienation	Directional Confrontational Action-oriented
Hispanic youth	Group centered, ties to extended family, acculturation, bilingual	Family, social concrete, structured short-term goals
Native American youth	Bicultural isolation	Community-tribal orientation concrete, structured

Table 7. Current Treatment Approaches/Modalities

Modality	Content
12-step model	AA meetings
	Groups
	STEP workbooks
	Family sessions or groups
Behavioral	Relapse prevention
	Refusal skills
	Social skills
	Problem-solving skills
	Anger control
	Leisure-time management
Family therapy	
Behavioral	Parent management training
	Contingency contracting
Strategic-structural	Restructure maladaptive patterns
Systemic	Address boundary and generational issues
Contextual	Integration of emotional, behavioral, cognitive, and spiritual aspects of family
Mixed	A combination of various family modalities
Educational and vocational assistance/rehabilitation	
Medication[a]	
Depression or mood disorder	Antidepressants, lithium
Attention-deficit hyperactivity disorder	Stimulants
Severe aggression	Antidepressants, lithium

[a]This is not a complete list of indications or useful medications.

Despite a previous tendency of many 12-step, AA model programs to eschew other treatment modalities, there appears to be an increased acceptance of cognitive-behavioral modalities and medication for youth with coexisting psychiatric disorders (Bukstein & Van Hasselt, 1993). Many behavioral interventions have an origin in the prevention literature and have been adapted to serve treatment populations. Examples of behavioral interventions include social skills training, problem-solving, anger control training, and behavioral family therapy, including contingency contracting (Bukstein & Van Hasselt, 1993). Social skills training may include communication skills, and assertiveness skills. Contingency contracting involves an explicit agreement between parent(s) and adolescent as to the rules and expectations of the household. Contracts specify the consequences if the rules are violated and rewards if the rules are obeyed.

The increasing recognition of the frequent presence of coexisting psychiatric disorders in adolescent alcohol abusers has prompted more aggressive efforts to use psychotropic medications with this population. The use of antidepressants, lithium, and other agents appears to be more accepted by many treatment programs. The use of stimulants such as methylphenidate for adolescent alcohol abusers with attention-deficit hyperactivity disorder (ADHD) remains controversial because of the potential for abuse of the stimulant agent (Bukstein & Van Hasselt, 1993).

There is currently an increased emphasis on alternative treatment settings such as partial or day hospitalization and outpatient clinics. Many of these treatment programs incorporate 12-step model principles as well as a variety of family, behavioral treatments, vocational and educational services, recreational activities, and health services. There are initiatives to serve alcohol-abusing youth as part of an intensive system of services for difficult-to-serve, multiproblem adolescents and their families. In these programs, case managers and multidisciplinary teams representing local social service agencies and treatment programs attempt to coordinate services and care.

Evidence of Treatment Efficacy

The research into the effectiveness of treatment for adolescents with alcohol abuse or dependence is remarkable for its paucity and lack of evidence to support the superiority of any general or specific approach. Several other treatment studies point to the benefits of treatment in general while failing to identify the superiority of one approach over others (Catalano, Hawkins, Wells, Miller, & Brewer, 1991). Many attempts at establishing treatment effectiveness have been severely hampered by a variety of methodological problems including poor preassessment measures, the lack of clear, valid definitions or measures of treatment success or relapse, and poor follow-up procedures including very low rates of follow-up.

As part of the Drug Abuse Reporting Program (DARP) study in which youth were followed up 4 to 6 years after admission to 52 different treatment programs across the United States, Sells and Simpson (1979) reported that adolescents using alcohol were generally unaffected by treatment although a reduction in heavy alcohol use was reported for drug-free outpatient programs. In a treatment outcome study for the Pennsylvania Substance Abuse System, individuals with better psychosocial functioning did better during outpatient treatment and had lower rates of relapse on follow-up than those requiring inpatient or residential treatment (Rush, 1985). Finally, in the Treatment Outcome Prospective Study (TOPS), significant improvements in drug-related problems, depression, and education were noted (Hubbard, Cavanaugh, Craddock, & Rachel, 1985). Drug-free outpatient clients reported reductions in heavy alcohol use although these reductions were less than those in residential treatment settings.

In the one available study examining the efficacy of treatment in an AA/NA model inpatient treatment program, Alford, Koehler, and Leonard (1991) found that both completers of the program and noncompleters demonstrated less substance use after treatment than before. Completers showed lower rates of relapse at 6 and 12 months and 2 years postdischarge than noncompleters although relapse rates had exceeded 60% for males in both groups by the 1-year follow-up. Interestingly, 17% of relapsed adolescents reported functioning successfully in their social-civil behavior at the 2-year follow-up. However, most of this group were using alcohol in the follow-up period.

In a review of the adolescent treatment research, Catalano *et al.* (1991) identified factors associated with relapse or lack of relapse back to alcohol use. Studies report that younger age of onset, more serious alcohol use, the abuse of multiple drugs, deviant behavior, and criminal involvement are associated with noncompletion of treatment. Among treatment factors, time in treatment is related to reduced alcohol and other drug use in residential programs. Staff characteristics (including staff attitudes and level of training), the availability of special services, and family participation are also associated with improved outcomes. Posttreatment predictors of relapse include thoughts, feelings, and cravings about alcohol, less involvement in school or work, and less satisfactory leisure time activities.

Based on existing studies, a number of basic recommendations can be made as to the general content of adolescent treatment programs. Treatment for adolescents should have achieving and maintaining abstinence from alcohol and all illicit substances as the primary goal for treatment. Treatment should also seek to improve the overall psychosocial functioning of the adolescent. Although improved functioning is obviously a worthwhile goal in itself, improvements in specific areas of functioning may directly or indirectly improve the adolescent's prospects for maintaining abstinence and preventing relapse.

There are treatment program characteristics associated with improved abstinence rates and lower relapse rates (Fleisch, 1991; Friedman & Beschner, 1985). These characteristics provide guidelines for the treatment of adolescents with substance use problems and include the following.

1. Treatment programs should be intensive and of sufficient duration to achieve changes in attitude and behavior.

2. Aftercare or follow-up treatment after a more intensive level of treatment are essential. Adequate transition and continuity between treatment components involves reinforcing changes that are achieved earlier in treatment.

3. Treatment approaches should be as comprehensive as possible and potentially target psychosocial dysfunction within multiple areas or domains of the adolescent's life. These areas include coexisting psychiatric disorders, vocational or educational needs, recreational or leisure-time activities, birth control services, and education/information about alcohol and other substance abuse and medical issues, particularly HIV/AIDS education.

4. Treatment programs should be sensitive to and address the cultural issues and the socioeconomic realities of the adolescent, his or her family, and environment. Examples of relevant interventions include having treatment program staff representative of the racial and/or ethnic groups of the adolescents, assisting families obtain additional social services or financial resources such as welfare assistance. The adolescent, the family, and staff should perceive the program as practical to real-life circumstances.

5. Treatment programs should encourage family involvement and work with families to improve interpersonal communication between family members, to improve the ability of parents to consistently provide structure and limit-setting for their children, and to address addiction patterns in the parents through both referral of the parents for treatment and acknowledgment of the role of parents in the adolescent's problems.

6. Treatment programs should attempt to obtain and use a wide range of social services such as juvenile justice, child welfare, and recreational programs to assist the adolescent and his or her family in planning and preparing for an alcohol- and drug-free life-style. Programs should require or strongly encourage adolescent attendance and participation in self-support groups such as AA and/or NA to develop a drug-free peer group and models for abstinence.

Future Directions for Adolescent Alcohol Treatment and Treatment Research

The available research indicates that adolescents can benefit from treatment and that treatment, at least in general, is effective for many adolescents. Many types of treatment are effective in producing some level of change in youth. However, there are significant portions of the adolescent alcohol-abusing population who do not appear to benefit from treatment with desired outcomes such as abstinence from alcohol, reduced drinking, or improvements in adaptive functioning in other life areas.

As with adults, it appears likely that certain types and levels of treatment may be more suitable for certain types of adolescents. Research into treatment-matching will be a critical element of treatment research. However, we are at a very early stage in the development of research into adolescent alcohol treatment services. We need a greater willingness to support and conduct treatment studies utilizing more rigorous research methodology and experimental designs which include standardized assessments (prior, during, and after treatment), manual specific control of intervention content and consistency, the use of randomized assignment to specific treatment conditions or modalities, and the use of "control" interventions. Treatment research needs to compare outcomes between types of treatments including a variety of modalities such as cognitive-behavioral therapy and intensity of treatment.

Whether actively involved in research or not, adolescent treatment programs should improve data collection procedures with a more standardized and comprehensive evaluation before treatment, thorough inventories of treatment content during treatment (that is, what kind of modalities are used and in what intensity), comprehensive outcome or aftertreatment evaluation and careful follow-up for at least several years. Outcome needs to be broadened to include not only abstinence or relapse status but also other changes in drinking patterns as well as changes in adaptive functioning within multiple life areas such as mental health and behavior, school functioning, family functioning, and use of nondeviant forms of recreation.

Treatment research needs to include specific populations of adolescents with regard to age, sex, race, ethnicity, socioeconomic status, and comorbid psychiatric status. More nontraditional treatments such as behavioral interventions (e.g., social and problem-solving training, cognitive therapy, and parent management training) and medication treatments should receive careful evaluation, especially in populations showing resistance to more traditional approaches.

Treatment Summary

In summary, a wide variety of modalities and settings are available for the treatment of adolescent alcohol problems. Unfortunately, treatment of adolescent alcohol abuse and dependence has not been proven by research to change overall levels of alcohol use. Parents, clinicians, school personnel, and others who deal with adolescents should consider other, more comprehensive targets for treatment, especially general psychosocial functioning. Treatment should be targeted to the adolescent's needs and should consider differences such as age, gender, racial and ethnic status, and coexisting psychopathology. Finally, treatment should consider the adolescent's place in the community, the status of the community itself, and other macroenvironmental factors in developing and delivering effective treatment interventions.

Most adolescents use alcohol, many of them on a regular basis. Many of these adolescents develop problematic alcohol use behaviors that require some level of intervention or treatment. Many adolescents are helped by the many treatment programs that are currently available. Nevertheless, further research is needed to establish what kind of treatment, at what level of intensity and duration, is necessary to improve both alcohol use behavior and the adolescent's adaptive functioning.

ACKNOWLEDGMENT. This work was supported in part by Research Grant Nos. AA07861 and AA09026 from the National Institute on Alcoholism and Alcohol Abuse.

REFERENCES

Alford, G. S., Koehler, R. A., & Leonard, J. (1991). Alcoholic Anonymous–Narcotics Anonymous model inpatient treatment of chemically dependent adolescents: A 2-year outcome study. *Journal of Studies on Alcohol, 52,* 118–126.

American Medical Association. (1992). *Guidelines for adolescent preventive services* (NLO18292). Chicago: Author.

American School Health Association, Association for the Advancement of Health Education, and Society for Public Health Education, Inc. (1989). *The National Adolescent Student Health Survey: A report on the health of America's youth.* Oakland, CA: Third Party Publishing Co.

Bachman, J. G., Wallace, J. M., O'Malley, P. O., Johnston, L. D., Kurth, C. L., & Neighbors, H. W. (1991). Racial/ethnic differences in smoking, drinking, and illicit drug use among American high school seniors, 1976–89. *American Journal of Public Health, 81,* 372–377.

Bailey, S. L., & Rachal, J. V. (1993). Dimensions of adolescent problem drinking. *Journal of Studies on Alcohol, 54,* 555–565.

Baldwin, S., Heather, N., Lawson, A., & Robertson, I. (1991). Comparison of effectiveness: Behavioural and talk-based alcohol education courses for court-referred young offenders. *Behavioural Psychotherapy, 19*(2), 157–172.

Barnes, G. M., Farrell, M. P., & Banerjee, S. (1994). Family influences on alcohol abuse and other problem behaviors among black and white adolescents in a general population sample. *Journal of Research on Adolescence, 4*(2), 183–201.

Barnes, G. M., & Welte, J. W. (1986a). Patterns and predictors of alcohol use among 7–12th grade students in New York State. *Journal of Studies on Alcohol, 47,* 53–62.

Barnes, G. M., & Welte, J. W. (1986b). Adolescent alcohol abuse: Subgroup differences and relationships to other problem behaviors. *Journal of Adolescent Research, 1,* 79–94.

Beck, K. H., & Lockhart, S. J. (1992). A model of parental involvement in adolescent drinking and driving. *Journal of Youth and Adolescence, 21*(1), 35–51.

Blount, W. R., & Dembo, R. (1984). The effect of perceived neighborhood setting on self-reported tobacco, alcohol, and marijuana use among inner-city minority junior high school youth. *International Journal of the Addictions, 19*(2), 175–198.

Bochner, S. (1994). The effectiveness of same-sex versus opposite-sex role models in advertisements to reduce alcohol consumption in teenagers. *Addictive Behavior, 19*(1), 69–82.

Boles, S., Casas, J. M., Furlong, M., & Gonzalez, G. (1994). Alcohol and other drug use patterns among Mexican-American, Mexican, and Caucasian adolescents: New directions for assessment and research. *Journal of Clinical Child Psychology, 23*(1), 39–46.

Botvin, G. J., & Botvin, S. M. (1992). Adolescent tobacco, alcohol, and drug abuse: Prevention strategies, empirical findings, and assessment issues. *Journal of Developmental and Behavioral Pediatrics, 13*(4), 290–301.

Bowen, O. R. (1988). *Opening remarks. Surgeon General's Workshop on Drunk Driving Proceedings* (pp. 9–11). Washington, DC: U.S. Department of Health and Human Services.

Boyle, M. H., Offort, D. R., Racine, Y. A., Szatmari, P., Fleming, J. E., & Links, P. S. (1992). Predicting substance use in late adolescence: Results from the Ontario child health study follow-up. *American Journal of Psychiatry, 149*, 761–767.

Bukstein, O. G., Brent, D. A., & Kaminer, Y. (1989). Comorbidity of substance abuse and other psychiatric disorders in adolescents. *American Journal of Psychiatry, 146*, 1131–1141.

Bukstein, O. G., & Van Hasselt, V. B. (1993). Alcohol and drug abuse in A. S. Bellack & M. Hersen (Eds.), *Handbook of behavior therapy in the psychiatric setting* (pp. 453–475). New York: Plenum Press.

Bush, P. J., & Iannotti, R. J. (1993). Alcohol, cigarette, and marijuana use among fourth-grade urban school children in 1988/89 and 1990/91. *American Journal of Public Health, 83*, 111–114.

Catalano, R. F., Hawkins, J. D., Wells, E. A., Miller, J., & Brewer, D. (1991). Evaluation of the effectiveness of adolescent drug abuse treatment, assessment of risks for relapse, and promising approaches for relapse prevention. *International Journal of the Addictions, 25*, 1085–1140

Chaloupka, F. J. (1993). Effects of price on alcohol-related problems. *Alcohol Health and Research World, 17*(1), 46–53.

Coate, D., & Grossman, M. (1988). The effects of alcoholic beverage prices and legal drinking ages on youth alcohol use. *Journal of Law and Economics, 31*(1), 145–171.

Cohen, A. Y. (1980). Alternatives to drugs: New visions for society. In S. Einstein (Ed.), *The community's response to drug use.* New York: Pergamon Press.

Dearing, B., Caston, R. J., & Babin, J. (1991). The impact of a hospital based educational program on adolescent attitudes toward drinking and driving. *Journal of Drug Education, 21*(4), 349–359.

Delgado, M. (1988). Alcoholism treatment and Hispanic youth. *Journal of Drug Issues, 18*(1), 59–68.

Donaldson, S. I., Graham, J. W., & Hansen, W. B. (1994). Testing the generalizability of intervening mechanism theories: Understanding the effects of adolescent drug use prevention interventions. *Journal of Behavioral Medicine, 17*(2), 195–216.

Emshoff, J. G. (1989). A preventive intervention with children of alcoholics. *Prevention in Human Services, 7*(1), 225–253.

Ennett, S. T., Tobler, N. S., Ringwalt, C. L., & Flewelling, R. L. (1994). How effective is Drug Abuse Resistance Education? A meta-analysis of Project DARE outcome evaluations. *American Journal of Public Health, 84*(9), 1394–1401.

Farrow, J. A. (1989). Evaluation of a behavioral intervention to reduce DWI among adolescent drivers. *Alcohol, Drugs and Driving, 5*(1), 61–72.

Fleisch, B. (1991). *Approaches in the treatment of adolescents with emotional and substance abuse problems.* Rockville, MD: U.S. Department of Health and Human Services.

Flores-Ortiz, Y. G. (1994). The role of cultural and gender values in alcohol use patterns among Chicana/Latina high school and university students: Implications for AIDS prevention. *International Journal of the Addictions, 29*(9), 1149–1171.

Friedman, A. S., & Beschner, G. M. (1985). *Treatment services for adolescence substance abusers.* Rockville, MD: National Institute on Drug Abuse, U.S. Department of Health and Human Services.

Giesbrecht, N., & Ferris, J. (1993). Community-based research initiatives in prevention. *Addiction, 88* (Suppl.), 83S–93S.

Giesbrecht, N., Krempulec, B. A., & West, P. (1993). Community-based prevention research to reduce alcohol-related problems. *Alcohol Health and Research World, 17*(1), 84–88.

Gliksman, L, & Rush, B. R. (1986). Alcohol availability, alcohol consumption and alcohol-related damage. II. The role of sociodemographic factors. *Journal of Studies of Alcohol, 47*(1), 11–18.

Greenfield, T. K., Graves, K. L., & Kaskutas, L. A. (1993). Alcohol warning labels for prevention: National survey findings. *Alcohol Health and Research World, 17*(1), 67–75.

Grossman, M., Chaloupka, F. J., Saffer, H., & Laixuthai, A. (1994). Effects of alcohol price policy on youth: A summary of economic research. *Journal of Research on Adolescence, 4*(2), 347–364.

Grube, J. W. (1993). Alcohol portrayals and alcohol advertising on television. *Alcohol Health and Research World, 17*(1), 61–66.

Grube, J. W., & Wallack, L. (1994). Television beer advertising and drinking knowledge, beliefs, and intentions among schoolchildren. *American Journal of Public Health, 84*(2), 254–259.

Gruenewald, P., Madden, P., & Janes, K. (1991). *Alcohol availability and the formal power and resources of state Alcohol Beverage Control Agencies.* Berkeley, CA: Prevention Research Center, Pacific Institute for Research and Evaluation.

Gruenewald, P. J., Millar, A. B., & Treno, J. J. (1993). Alcohol availability and the ecology of drinking behavior. *Alcohol Health and Research World, 17*(1), 39–45.

Gruenewald, P. J., Ponicke, W., & Holder, H. D. (1991). *The dynamic relationship of outlet density to alcohol consumption: A time series cross-sectional analysis.* Berkeley, CA: Prevention Research Center, Pacific Institute for Research and Evaluation.

Hansen, W. B. (1992). School-based substance abuse prevention: A review of the state of the art in curriculum, 1980–1990. *Health Education Research, 7,* 403–430.

Hansen, W. B. (1993). School-based alcohol prevention programs. *Alcohol Health and Research World, 17*(1), 54–60.

Hansen, W. B., & Graham, J. W. (1991). Preventing alcohol, marijuana, and cigarette use among adolescents: Peer pressure resistance training versus establishing conservative norms. *Preventive Medicine, 20*(3), 414–430.

Hawkins, J. D., Catalano, R. F., & Kent, L. A. (1991). Combining broadcast media and parent education to prevent teenage drug abuse. In L. Donohew, H. E. Sypher, & W. J. Bukoski (Eds.), *Persuasive communication and drug abuse prevention.* Hillsdale, NJ: Lawrence Erlbaum Associates.

Hawkins, J. D., Catalano, R. F., & Miller, J. Y. (1992). Risk and protective factors for alcohol and other drug problems in adolescence and early adulthood: Implications for substance abuse prevention. *Psychological Bulletin, 112*(1), 64–105.

Hingson, R. (1992). *Effects of lower BAC levels on teenage crash involvement.* Paper presented at the 71st Annual Meeting of the Transportation Research Board, Washington, DC.

Hingson, R. (1993). Prevention of alcohol-impaired driving. *Alcohol Health and Research World, 17*(1), 28–34.

Hingson, R., & Howland, J. (1986). Prevention of drunk driving crashes involving youth drivers: An overview of legislative countermeasures. In T. Benjamin (Ed.), *Proceedings of International Symposium on Youth Drivers Impaired by Alcohol or Other Drugs* (pp 337–348). London: Royal Society of Medicine Services.

Howard, J. (1993). Alcohol prevention research: Concepts, phases, and tasks at hand. *Alcohol Health and Research World, 17*(1), 5–9.

Hubbard, R. L., Cavanaugh, E. R., Craddock, S. G., & Rachel, J. V. (1985). Characteristics, behaviors and outcomes for youth in TOPS. In A. S. Friedman & G. M. Beschner (Eds.), *Treatment services for adolescent substance abusers* (pp. 49–65). Washington, DC: U.S. Department of Health and Human Services.

Insurance Bureau of Canada and Traffic Injury Research Foundation of Canada. (1991). *New to the road: Prevention measures for young or novice drivers.* Toronto: Author.

Insurance Institute for Highway Safety. (1992). Sting curbs alcohol sales to minors. *Denver Status Report, 29*(14), 1–3.

Johnston, L. D., O'Malley, P. M., & Bachman, J. G. (1991). *Drug use among American high school seniors, college students and young adults, 1975–1990.* Rockville, MD: National Institute on Drug Abuse.

Jones, N., Pieper, C. F., & Robertson, L. J. (1992). The effect of legal drinking age on fatal injuries of adolescents and young adults. *American Journal of Public Health, 82,* 112–115.

Kandel, D. B. (1985). Stages in adolescent involvement in drug use. *Science, 190,* 912–914.

Kantor, G. K., Caudill, B. D., & Ungerleider, S. (1992). Project Impact: Teaching the teachers to intervene in student substance abuse problems. *Journal of Alcohol and Drug Education, 38*(1), 11–29.

Kline, R. B., & Canter, W. A. (1994). Can educational programs affect teenage drinking? A multivariate perspective. *Journal of Drug Education, 24*(2), 139–149.

Klitzner, M., Bamberger, E., & Gruenewald, P. (1990a). The assessment of parent-led prevention programs: A national descriptive survey. *Journal of Drug Education, 20*(2), 111–125.

Klitzner, M., Bamberger, E., & Gruenewald, P. (1990b). The assessment of parent-led prevention programs: A preliminary assessment of impact. *Journal of Drug Education, 20*(1), 77–94.

Klitzner, M., Fisher, D., Stewart, K., & Gilbert, S. (1992). *Substance abuse early intervention for adolescents: Research, theory, and practice.* Princeton, NJ: The Robert Wood Johnson Foundation.

Klitzner, M., Gruenewald, P. J., Bamberger, E., & Rossiter, C. (1994). A quasi-experimental evaluation of Students Against Driving Drunk. *American Journal on Drug Alcohol Abuse, 20*(1), 57–74.

Klitzner, M., Stewart, K., & Fisher, D. (1993). Reducing underage drinking and its consequences. *Alcohol Health and Research World, 17*(1), 12–18.

Kooler, J. M., & Bruvold, W. H. (1992). Evaluation of an educational intervention upon knowledge, attitudes, and behavior concerning drinking/drugged driving. *Journal of Drug Education, 22*(1), 87–100.

Kumpfer, K. L., & DeMarsh, J. (1986). Family environmental and genetic influences on children's future chemical dependency. *Journal of Children in Contemporary Society (Childhood and Chemical Abuse: Prevention and Intervention), 18*(1 & 2), 49–91.

Lorion, R. P., & Ross, J. G. (1992). Programs for change: A realistic look at the nation's potential for preventing substance involvement among high-risk youth. *Journal of Community Psychology, OSAP Special Issue,* 3–9.

MacKinnon, D. P., Johnson, C. A., Pentz, M. A., Hansen, W. B., Flay, B. R., & Yang, Y. F. I. (1991). Mechanisms in a school-based drug prevention program: First year effects of the Midwestern Prevention Project. *Health Psychology, 10,* 164–172.

MacKinnon, D. P., Pentz, M. A., & Stacy, A. W. (1993). The alcohol warning label and adolescents: The first year. *American Journal of Public Health, 83*(4), 585–587.

McKnight, A. J., (1993). Server intervention: Accomplishments and needs. *Alcohol Health and Research World, 17*(1), 76–82.

McLaughlin, R. J., Holcomb, J. D., Jibaja-Rusth, M. L., & Webb, J. (1993). Teacher ratings of student risk for substance use as a function of specialized training. *Journal of Drug Education, 23*(1), 83–95.

McLellan, A. T., & Alterman, A. I. (1991). *Patient Treatment Matching: A conceptual and methodological view with suggestions for future research in National Institute on Drug Abuse, improving drug abuse treatment* (pp. 114–135). Washington, DC: U.S. Department of Health and Human Services.

Madden, P. A., & Grube, J. W. (1994). The frequency and nature of alcohol and tobacco advertising in televised sports, 1990 through 1992. *American Journal of Public Health, 84*(2), 297–299.

Mee-Lee, D., & Hoffmann, N. G. (1992). *American Society of Addiction Medicine Adolescent Admission and Continued Stay Criteria.* St. Paul, Minnesota: CATOR/New Standards.

National Highway Traffic Safety Administration. (1991). *Tools for community action: Youth traffic safety program* (DOT HS 807 769). Washington, DC: Author.

National Institute on Drug and Alcohol Abuse; National Institute on Alcohol Abuse and Alcoholism State Resources and Services Related to Alcohol and Other Drug Abuse Problems, Fiscal Year 1990. (1992). Rockville, MD: U.S. Department of Health and Human Services.

Newcomb, M. D., Chou, C., Bentler, P. M., & Huba, G. J. (1988). Cognitive motivations for drug use among adolescents: Longitudinal tests of gender differences and predictors of change in drug use. *Journal of Counseling Psychology, 35*(4), 426–438.

Newman, L., Henry, P. B., DiRenzo, P., & Stecher, T. (1988–89). Intervention and student assistance: The Pennsylvania model. *Journal of Chemical Dependency Treatment, 2*(1), 145–162.

Nichols, J., & Ross, H. L. (1990). The effectiveness of legal sanctions in dealing with drinking drivers. *Alcohol, Drugs, and Driving, 6*(2), 33–61.

O'Malley, P. M., & Wagenaar, A. C. (1991). Effects of minimum drinking age laws on alcohol use, related behaviors, and traffic crash involvement among American youth: 1976–1987. *Journal of Studies on Alcohol, 52*(5), 478–491.

O'Neal, K. J. (1993). Anticipatory guidance: Alcohol, adolescents, and recognizing abuse and dependence. *Issues in Comprehensive Pediatric Nursing, 16*(4), 207–218.

Paperny, D. M., Aono, J. Y., Lehman, R. M., Hammar, S. L., & Risser, J. (1990). Computer-assisted detection and intervention in adolescent high-risk health behaviors. *Journal of Pediatrics, 116*(3), 456–462.

Pentz, M., Dwyer, J., MacKinnon, D., Flay, B., Hansen, W., Wang, E., & Johnson, C. A (1989). A multicommunity trial for primary prevention of adolescent drug abuse. *Journal of the American Medical Association, 26*(22), 3259–3266.

Peterson, P. L., Hawkins, J. D., Abbott, R. D., & Catalano, R. F. (1994). Disentangling the effects of parental drinking, family management, and parental alcohol norms on current drinking by black and white adolescents. *Journal of Research on Adolescents, 4*(2), 203–227.

Petraitis, J., Flay, B. R., & Miller, T. Q. (1995). Reviewing theories of adolescent substance use: Organizing pieces in the puzzle. *Psychological Bulletin, 117*(1), 67–86.

Popkin, C. L, & Parker, E. W. (1992). *Deterrence and rehabilitation: Research needs for the next decade.* Paper presented at the National Research Council on Transportation, Research Board Workshop on Transportation, Irvine, CA, July 27–29.

Preusser, D., Preusser, C., & Ulmer, R. (1992). *Obstacles to enforcement of youthful impaired driving.* Prepared for the National Highway Traffic Safety Administration, U.S. Department of Transportation.

Preusser, D. F., Williams, A. F., Lund, A., & Zador, P. (1990). City curfew ordinances and teenage motor vehicle injury. *Accident Analysis and Prevention, 22*(4), 391–397.

Robbins, C. (1989). Sex differences in psychosocial consequences of alcohol and drug abuse. *Journal of Health and Social Behavior, 30,* 117–130.

Rohrbach, L. A., Hodgson, C. S., Broder, B. I., & Montgomery, S. B. (1994). Parental participation in drug abuse prevention. Results from the Midwestern Prevention Project. *Journal of Research on Adolescence, 4*(92), 295–317.

Rosenbaum, D. P., Flewelling, R. L., Bailey, S. L., & Ringwalt, C. L. (1994). Cops in the classroom: A longitudinal evaluation of drug abuse resistance education (DARE). *Journal of Research in Crime and Delinquency, 31*(10), 3–31.

Ross, J. G., Saavedra, P. J., Shur, G. H., & Winters, F. (1992). The effectiveness of an after-school program for primary grade latchkey students on precursors of substance abuse. *Journal of Community Psychology,* Special Issue: Programs for change: Office for Substance Abuse Prevention demonstration models, 22–38.

Rush, T. V. (1985). Predicting treatment outcomes for juvenile and young-adult clients in the Pennsylvania substance abuse system. In G. M. Beschner & A. S. Friedman (Eds.), *Youth drug abuse: Problems, issues and treatment* (pp. 629–656). Lexington, MA: Lexington Books.

Sadava, S. W. (1985). Problem behavior theory and consumption and consequences of alcohol use. *Journal of Studies on Alcohol, 46,* 392–397.

Saffer, H., & Grossman, M. (1987). Beer taxes, the legal drinking age, and youth motor vehicle fatalities. *Journal of Legal Studies, 16,* 351–374.

Saltz, R. F., & Hennessy, M. (1991). *Reducing intoxication in commercial establishments: An evaluation of responsible beverage service practices.* Berkeley, CA. Prevention Research Center.

Schaps, E., & Slimmon, L. (1975). Balancing head and heart: *Sensible ideas for the prevention of drug and alcohol abuse, Book 2.* Lafayette, CA: Prevention Materials Institute Press.

Scheier, L. M., Newcomb, M. D., & Skager, R. (1994). Risk, protection, and vulnerability to adolescent drug use: Latent-variable models of three age groups. *Journal of Drug Education, 24*(1), 49–82.

Schinke, S. P., Orlandi, M. A., Botvin, G. J., & Gilchrist, L. D. (1988). Preventing substance abuse among American-Indian adolescents: A bicultural competence skills approach. *Journal of Counseling Psychology, 35*(1), 87–90.

Sells, S. B., & Simpson, D. D. (1979). Evaluation of treatment outcome for youths in the drug abuse reporting program (DARP): A follow-up study. In G. M. Beschner & A. S. Friedman (Eds.), *Youth drug abuse: Problems, issues and treatment* (pp. 571–628). Lexington, MA: Lexington Books.

Shain, M., Suurvali, H., & Kilty, H. (1980). *The Parent Communication Project: A longitudinal study of the effects of parenting skills on children's use of alcohol.* Toronto: Addiction Research Foundation of Ontario.

Shope, J. T., Kloska, D. D., Dielman, T. E., & Maharg, R. (1994). Longitudinal evaluation of an enhanced Alcohol Misuse Prevention Study (AMPS) curriculum for grades six–eight. *Journal of School Health, 64*(4), 160–166.

St. Pierre, T. L., Kaltreider, D. L., Mark, M. M., & Aikin, K. J. (1992). Drug prevention in a community setting: A longitudinal study of the relative effectiveness of a three-year primary prevention program in Boys and Girls Clubs across the nation. *American Journal of Community Psychology, 20*(6), 673–706.

Stewart, K., & Sweedler, B. (1992). *Reducing drinking and driving through administrative license revocation.* Paper presented at the 12th International Conference on Alcohol, Drugs and Traffic Safety, Cologne, Germany.

Sweet, E. S. (1988–89). The chemically dependent adolescent: Issues with ethnic and cultural minorities. *Journal of Chemical Dependency Treatment 2*(1), 239–264.

Thompson, T., & Simmons-Cooper, C. (1988). Chemical dependency treatment and black adolescents. *Journal of Drug Issues, 18*(91), 21–31.

Tobler, N. S. (1986). Meta-analysis of 143 adolescent drug prevention programs: Quantitative outcome results of program participants compared to a control or comparison group. *Journal of Drug Issues, 16*(4), 537–567.

U.S. General Accounting Office. (1987). *Drinking-age laws: An evaluation synthesis of their impact on highway safety.* Washington, DC: Supt. of Documents, U.S. Government Printing Office.

Vega, W. A., Gil, A. G., & Zimmerman, R. S. (1993). Patterns of drug use among Cuban-American, African-American, and white non-Hispanic boys. *American Journal of Public Health, 83*(2), 257–259.

Wagenaar, A. C., & Perry, C. L. (1994). Community strategies for the reduction of youth drinking: Theory and application. *Journal of Research on Adolescence, 4*(2), 319–345.

Wheeler, K., & Malmquist, J. (1987). Treatment approaches in adolescent chemical dependency. *Pediatric Clinics of North America, 34,* 437–447.

White, H. R. (1987). Longitudinal stability and dimensional structure of problem drinking in adolescence. *Journal of Studies on Alcohol, 48,* 541–550.

Williams, A., Karps, R., & Zador, P. (1983). Variations in minimum licensing age and fatal motor vehicle crashes. *American Journal of Public Health, 73*(12), 1401–1403.

Windle, M. (1991). Alcohol use and abuse: Some findings from the National Adolescent Student Health Survey. *Alcohol Health and Research World, 15,* 5–10.

Windle, M. (1994). Coexisting problems and alcoholic family risk among adolescents. In T. F. Babor, V. Hesselbrock, R. E. Meyer, & W. Shoemaker (Eds.), *Types of alcoholics: Evidence from clinical, experimental, and genetic research* (pp. 157–164). New York: New York Academy of Sciences.

Zador, P. L., Lund, A. K., Fields, M., & Weinberg, K. (1989). Fatal crash involvement and laws against alcohol impaired driving. *Journal of Public Policy, 10,* 467–485.

7

Drug Use

WILLIAM B. HANSEN and PATRICK M. O'MALLEY

INTRODUCTION

Illicit drug use and abuse are serious problems for society. The use of these substances—marijuana, inhalants, amphetamines, hallucinogens such as LSD, tranquilizers, cocaine, opiates such as heroin, and steroids—have health, social, emotional, legal, and behavioral consequences that are serious and far-reaching for adolescents. In this chapter, we summarize prior research on epidemiology, prevention, and treatment research to provide an accurate albeit brief picture of the state-of-the-art.

EPIDEMIOLOGY

This section discusses the epidemiology of adolescent use of illicit drugs. The focus is on nationally representative samples of 8th, 10th, and 12th grade students, from both public and private schools. Prevalence rates and recent trends are discussed for subgroups based on gender and racial/ethnic groups. The term "illicit drugs" includes controlled substances, both those that are essentially proscribed for everyone (e.g., marijuana, LSD, heroin) and those that are available by prescription (e.g., tranquilizers). In this section, the drugs of interest are marijuana, LSD, cocaine, heroin, amphetamines, and tranquilizers. In addition, inhalants will be discussed; although the substances themselves may not be illegal, they are used for the purpose of getting intoxicated (and are a serious problem among adolescents). Finally, anabolic steroids will also be discussed. Alcohol and tobacco are dealt with in other chapters.

The data to be discussed come primarily from the Monitoring the Future surveys (Johnston, O'Malley, & Bachman, 1994). That series of surveys, which began in 1975,

WILLIAM B. HANSEN • Department of Public Health Sciences, Bowman Gray School of Medicine, Winston-Salem, North Carolina 27157.   **PATRICK M. O'MALLEY** • Survey Research Center, Institute for Social Research, The University of Michigan, Ann Arbor, Michigan 48106.

Handbook of Adolescent Health Risk Behavior, edited by Ralph J. DiClemente, William B. Hansen, and Lynn E. Ponton. Plenum Press, New York, 1996.

provides the most complete consistent reporting of trends in use of drugs among America's young people. Until 1991, the youngest students included were in grade 12; beginning in 1991, students in grades 8 and 10 were added, and this section will concentrate on the results of the survey in 1993. The core of the study consists of annual surveys of nationally representative samples of 8th, 10th, and 12th grade students; in-school questionnaires are administered by professional interviewers to over 45,000 students in approximately 420 public and private schools per year.

Prevalence and Incidence

Figure 1 shows 1993 lifetime prevalence (proportion who have ever used a drug) for eight classes of drugs, by grade level; the drugs are ordered by 12th grade prevalence. Figure 2 provides a similar demonstration for current use, i.e., the proportion who used in the past 30 days. These figures demonstrate a prevalence of substance use that has defined the scope of the national problem, especially for marijuana and inhalant use.

Marijuana

Among the various illicit drugs, the most prevalent is marijuana. As shown in Figure 1, in 1993 about one in three American high school seniors had used marijuana (35.3%) in their lifetime, one in four 10th-graders (24.4%), and one in eight 8th-graders (12.6%). Current use (prevalence of use in the past 30 days) stood at one in six seniors (15.5%), one in nine 10th-graders (10.9%), and one in twenty 8th-graders (5.1%) (Figure 2). It is clear from these data that there is substantial use of marijuana by American secondary school students.

Inhalants

Inhalants, though not necessarily illicit drugs, are sometimes used illicitly to get high.* Unlike almost all other substances used to get high, use of inhalants is generally seen more often among younger students than among high school seniors. As Figure 1 shows, lifetime use of inhalants is higher among 8th-graders (19.4%) than among 10th- (17.5%) or 12th-graders (17.4%). Current use of inhalants is proportionately even more disparate, with 5.4% of 8th-graders having used in the past month, compared to 3.3% of 10th-graders and 2.5% of seniors. It is important to note that whenever there are differences observed between the grades in reported drug use, there are always several alternative possible explanations. One is that there is an age effect, another is a cohort effect, and another is that there is a sample composition effect. Particularly with respect to reported lifetime use, there are several other possibilities as well, including simple forgetting of events that may have happened a long time previously. In the case of inhalants, we believe that there is an age effect, in that this is a behavior that seems especially likely to occur among younger students, and to become less common as students get older. However, the

*The question asks, "On how many occasions, if any, have you sniffed glue, or breathed the contents of aerosol spray cans, or inhaled any other gases or sprays in order to get high . . . ."

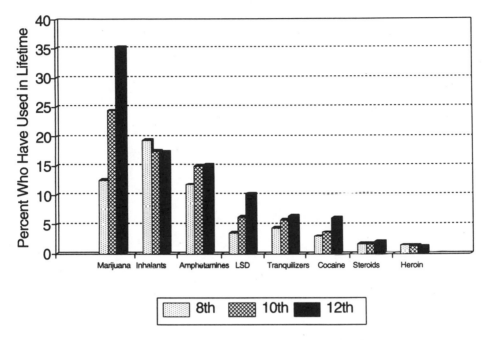

Figure 1. Lifetime prevalence in 1993 by grade for marijuana, LSD, cocaine, heroin, amphetamines, tranquilizers, inhalants, and steroids.

difference observed in Figure 1 in lifetime prevalence could also be related in part to a cohort effect and in part to differential sample composition. The latter is possible if those students who tend to use inhalants are more likely to drop out of school prior to late in their senior year; thus, they may be captured in the 8th grade samples, but not in the 12th grade samples. A cohort effect can occur when, for whatever reasons, a particular 8th grade cohort, for example, has a particularly high (or low) rate of substance use compared to earlier birth cohorts. Data from smaller samples of 6th through 12th grade students collected in Winston-Salem, North Carolina, show just such an effect (Hansen & Rose, 1995). Therefore, such an effect cannot be ruled out. The past history of substance use has found relatively few cohort effects (cigarette smoking being the major exception), as compared to secular trends or age effects (O'Malley, Bachman, & Johnston, 1988). In the end, all of these explanations combined may contribute to the recently observed differences. Whatever the explanation, the increases that have been observed make inhalant use worthy of attention.

Amphetamines

The next highest lifetime prevalence is that for amphetamines (Figure 1). About the same proportions of seniors and 10th-graders have tried amphetamines (15.1 and 14.9%, respectively); 11.8% of 8th-graders have tried them. There is not much difference among

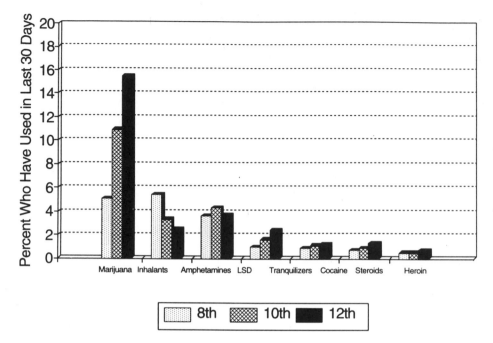

Figure 2. Current prevalence in 1993 by grade for marijuana, LSD, cocaine, heroin, amphetamines, tranquilizers, inhalants, and steroids.

the grades in current use figures: 3.7, 4.3, and 3.6% for 12th, 10th, and 8th grade, respectively.

LSD

The use of LSD continues to be relatively common among American secondary school students. Lifetime use of LSD in 1993 was 10.3% among seniors, 6.2% among 10th-graders, and 3.5% among 8th graders (Figure 1). Considering the potential problems of LSD use, it must be considered troublesome that one in ten students graduating from secondary school in 1993 had tried this substance. Current use levels are much lower, reflecting the episodic rather than chronic use pattern for this drug.

Tranquilizers

Tranquilizers are not unknown among secondary school students, with a little more than 5% of seniors (6.4%) and 10th-graders (5.7%) having tried a tranquilizer, compared to a little less than 5% of 8th-graders (4.4%). Nonetheless, tranquilizers are not a class of drugs that are widely used.

Cocaine

Cocaine is one substance that has shown a strong positive association with age (up to young adulthood), and Figure 1 demonstrates that the association holds for students. Seniors have a lifetime prevalence of 6.1%, compared to 3.6% for 10th-graders and 2.9% for 8th-graders. Cocaine has been the focus of much law enforcement activity and is associated with considerable economic gains by dealers. Nonetheless, compared to marijuana and inhalants, cocaine is less prevalent.

Heroin

Heroin is like inhalants in that its use shows a negative association with age (Figure 1). In 1993, 8th-graders reported a higher lifetime prevalence (1.4%) than 10th-graders (1.3%), who reported a higher level than 12th-graders (1.1%). The differences are not necessarily all statistically significant, but they are quite consistent over the last 3 years in showing a lower rate among seniors than among the younger students. The explanation probably lies in the fact that the younger grades include some individuals who will become dropouts (and who therefore will not be represented in the senior class populations); some of these individuals tend to be more deviant than average, and more likely to be and to become drug abusers.

Anabolic Steroids

Anabolic steroids represent another class of substances that are potentially abused by adolescents and should be mentioned. Anabolic steroids are not used to get high, but instead to get "big," although continued use can lead to some psychoactive symptoms such as tolerance and dependency (Brower, Blow, Young, & Hill, 1991). Use of these substances has received quite a bit of publicity in recent years, with some estimates suggesting a very serious level of use; however, the first nationally representative sample of high school seniors did not occur until 1989. That survey showed about 3% of seniors (mostly male seniors) in 1989 having used an anabolic steroid in their lifetime; the figure had declined to 2.0% by 1993. Thus, although use of this class of substances clearly bears watching, it does not appear to present an increasing problem at this time. The recent trends are similar for younger students, as well, at slightly lower levels of use. In 1993, 1.6% of 8th-graders and 1.7% of 10th-graders reported ever having used an anabolic steroid (Figure 1).

Prevalence of Drug Use by Sociodemographic Variables

Table 1 provides 1993 annual prevalence levels for eight classes of drugs by grade for the total samples and for subgroups defined by gender and racial/ethnic identification.

Gender

In general, males use substances of all kinds more than females. However, the differences are much smaller, and the direction sometimes reversed, for younger adoles-

Table 1. Annual Prevalence of Illicit Drugs by Grade, Gender,
and Racial/Ethnic Group, 1993

		Gender		Race/ethnic category[a]		
	Total	Male	Female	White	African-American	Hispanic
Marijuana						
Grade 8	9.2	10.5	8.0	7.8	5.7	13.9
Grade 10	19.2	21.2	16.9	18.0	8.7	21.3
Grade 12	26.0	29.0	22.4	25.9	14.2	23.5
LSD						
Grade 8	2.3	2.5	2.1	2.3	0.4	3.7
Grade 10	4.2	5.1	3.2	4.6	0.5	4.1
Grade 12	6.8	8.4	5.1	7.4	0.6	5.1
Cocaine						
Grade 8	1.7	1.9	1.5	1.3	0.7	4.0
Grade 10	2.1	2.5	1.6	2.0	0.6	3.7
Grade 12	3.3	4.0	2.3	3.1	0.8	5.8
Heroin						
Grade 8	0.7	0.8	0.5	0.6	0.3	1.4
Grade 10	0.7	0.9	0.4	0.7	0.4	0.7
Grade 12	0.5	0.7	0.3	0.5	0.4	0.7
Amphetamines						
Grade 8	7.2	5.6	8.8	7.4	3.4	7.7
Grade 10	9.6	8.2	10.9	10.1	3.0	7.0
Grade 12	8.4	8.2	8.5	9.0	2.3	6.2
Tranquilizers						
Grade 8	2.1	1.8	2.4	2.0	1.1	3.1
Grade 10	3.3	3.2	3.2	3.8	0.9	3.3
Grade 12	3.5	3.5	3.3	3.7	1.0	2.0
Inhalants						
Grade 8	11.0	10.4	11.9	11.3	4.6	11.5
Grade 10	8.4	9.1	7.7	8.8	3.7	8.3
Grade 12	7.0	9.2	4.8	7.6	2.2	5.7
Steroids						
Grade 8	0.9	1.4	0.3	1.0	0.6	1.1
Grade 10	1.0	1.7	0.3	1.0	0.8	1.4
Grade 12	1.2	2.5	0.1	1.2	1.0	1.6

[a]The data for the racial/ethnic groups are averages of 1992 and 1993, except for steroids, which are averages of 1991 through 1993.

cents. This tendency for younger females to be closer to males in rates of substance use may have to do with their slightly earlier maturing, and to their tendency to associate with slightly older males.*

Marijuana use is distinctly higher among males than females at all three grade levels.

---

*These data are based on cross-sectional comparisons. Thus, grade differences could be related to cohort effects rather than age effects, or to differential sample composition. Cohort effects are unlikely, because that would require a gender by birth year interaction, which seems improbable. The major source of composition differences would be differential dropout rates. Census estimates suggest very small differences between genders in dropout rates in recent years.

But the differences are slight in 8th grade (10.5 versus 8.0% annual prevalence) and larger by 12th grade (29.0 versus 22.4%).

The patterns of gender differences for LSD and cocaine use are similar to marijuana: higher rates among males, with the differences getting larger in the later grades.

Heroin use is low in general (annual rates less than 1%), with higher rates among males than females at all three grade levels.

Amphetamine use is an exception to the general pattern: more females report using amphetamines at all three grade levels. Annual use is 8.5% for senior females, compared to 8.2% for males. In eighth grade, the corresponding figures are 8.8 and 5.6%.

The 1993 pattern for tranquilizers shows rates of use for males equal to or higher than those for females in 10th and 12th grades. In 1991 and 1992, tranquilizers followed the pattern of amphetamines, with slightly higher rates among females than males at all three grade levels.

Inhalant use, as indicated previously, is actually higher among 8th-graders than 12th-graders; annual use in 1993 was 11.0 versus 7.0%. Much of the decline between 8th and 12th grade is due to females, whose use in 8th grade is slightly higher than males (annual prevalence 11.9 versus 10.4%), but then declines more sharply (to 4.8%, versus 9.2%). Anabolic steroid use is very low among females, 0.3% or less. Annual use rises from 1.4% in 8th grade to 2.5% in 12th grade among male students.

To summarize the data on gender differences, use of illicit drugs (marijuana, LSD, cocaine, heroin, inhalants) is generally higher among males than females, with the differences greater at 12th grade than at 8th grade. Use of psychotherapeutic drugs (amphetamines and tranquilizers) tends to be about equal or very slightly higher among female students. Use of anabolic steroids is distinctly higher among males at all grade levels; very few female students report using anabolic steroids.

Race/Ethnicity

One of the more interesting findings from population-based epidemiological studies is that African-American students tend to report lower rates of illicit drug use than other racial/ethnic groups. This finding is not consistent with the impressions that many Americans have about drug use rates. But a number of investigations have supported these findings: in general, the evidence supports the conclusion that drug use rates are indeed lower among young African-Americans than among European-Americans (Bachman *et al.*, 1991; USDHHS, 1993; Wallace & Bachman, 1994). The data for other ethnic groups are more variable. In part, this is because the other ethnic groups do not comprise sufficiently large enough proportions of the U.S. population to be represented accurately in most national surveys. In the Monitoring the Future surveys, it has been deemed necessary to combine 2 years of data in order to provide sufficient numbers of cases to allow reasonable inferences regarding the population of Hispanics, as a whole.* (For ease of discussion, the following sections discuss the findings for 8th and 12th grades only.

---

*We recognize that Hispanics, like other broad ethnic categorizations, are a diverse group, and that treating them as a single category may not provide an accurate representation of important subcategories. Unfortunately, the small numbers in smaller categories (e.g., Mexican-Americans, Cuban-Americans, and so forth) preclude accurate descriptions of these groups.

The findings for 10th grade tend to be as one would expect, intermediate between the two extremes.)

Among 12th-graders, annual prevalence of marijuana use is distinctly lower among African-American students than among white students (14.2 versus 25.9%, 1992 and 1993 combined, as shown in Table 1). Hispanic students report a slightly lower rate than white students (23.5%). Among 8th-graders, however, Hispanic students report a substantially higher rate of use (13.9%) than white students (7.8%); African-American students report the lowest rate (5.7%). LSD follows the same pattern of lowest use rates among African-American students for both grades, with the highest rates for 8th-grade Hispanic students and highest rates for white seniors.

Cocaine is similar for 8th-grade rank ordering: African-Americans lowest (0.7%), Hispanic students highest (4.0%), and white students intermediate (1.3%). However, the 12th-grade ordering for this substance is the same as for 8th grade: Hispanic, white, and African-American students report annual prevalence of 5.8, 3.1, and 0.8%, respectively. The rank ordering for heroin use (Table 1) parallels that for cocaine. Hispanic students are highest and African-American students lowest at both grade levels (but only the 8th-grade Hispanic students exceed an annual prevalence of 1%). The rank ordering for amphetamines and tranquilizers parallels that for marijuana: Hispanic students highest at 8th grade, intermediate at 12th; white students intermediate at 8th grade, highest at 12th; African-American students lowest at both grades. A similar pattern obtains for inhalants: Among 12th-graders, white students are highest (7.6%), African-American students lowest (2.2%), and Hispanic students are slightly lower than white students (5.7%). Among 8th-graders, Hispanic students are highest (11.5%), African-American students lowest (4.6%), and white students intermediate (11.3%).

Anabolic steroids are asked about on only one form (of six forms used in 12th grade; of two forms in 8th and 10th), making the racial/ethnic data more variable than the data for other substances. Consequently, the data and discussion are based on 1991 through 1993 data combined. As with the other illicit substances, anabolic steroid use is lowest among African-American students. Hispanics are highest in all three grades, with white students intermediate.

To summarize, the pattern of findings for racial/ethnic groups is quite consistent. African-American students are lowest at both grades for all drugs. Hispanic students are highest at 8th grade for all illicit drug classes. At 12th grade, Hispanics are highest only for cocaine, heroin, and steroids. An extensive series of analyses has led us to the conclusion that some of the differences among racial/ethnic groups in findings between 8th and 12th grades have to do with differential dropout rates (Wallace, Bachman, O'Malley, & Johnston, 1995). In particular, Hispanic students have higher dropout rates than either white or African-American students (U.S. Department of Education, 1992). Therefore, the smaller differences (and for some drug classes, a reversal of differences) between white seniors and Hispanic seniors, compared to differences observed in 8th grade, are very likely related to the fact that Hispanic seniors represent a distinctly smaller proportion of their age cohort. African-American students do not have rates of dropping out that are very different than white students; hence, the lower rates reported by African-American students in both 8th and 12th grade are not likely related to differential dropout rates.

Age of Initiation

Eighth-grade students are the youngest surveyed in the Monitoring the Future study. However, we can use retrospective reports of grade of first use to determine when substance use behavior begins. (These data have all of the problems of retrospective data, but we believe that they provide information that is approximately correct in most instances.) Among eighth-graders who reported having used any of the eight illicit drug classes by 1993, only one was initiated by more than 50% of users in sixth grade or earlier. This class is the inhalants; of all eighth-graders (not just users), 11.0% had used an inhalant by the end of sixth grade.

Just about one-third of marijuana smokers had initiated by sixth grade (32.5% of the 12.6% who used, or 4.1% of all eighth-graders). Of the other illicit substances, only amphetamines exceeded 3% of the cohort having used by sixth grade. One implication of these data is that the inhalants are clearly the earliest drug used (other than alcohol and tobacco). And marijuana and amphetamines are by no means unknown at this early age.

Temporal Trends in Use among 8th-, 10th-, and 12th-Graders

An epidemic of illicit drug use emerged among American young people in the 1960s and continued to expand through the 1970s. Marijuana was the most popular illegal drug, with use among high school seniors gaining majority status; in the high school class of 1979, 60.4% reported having used marijuana (Johnston et al., 1994). Use of marijuana peaked around 1979 or 1980, and the decade of the 1980s saw a long consistent general decline to a point where annual prevalence was cut in half, going from one in two seniors in the class of 1979 to one in four seniors in the class of 1991. A particularly striking trend in marijuana use occurred between 1975 and 1978, when the proportion of seniors reporting use of marijuana on a daily or near-daily basis in the past 30 days rose from 6.0% to an unprecedented 10.7%. Fortunately, that figure subsequently declined by more than 80%, reaching 2.0% in 1991. More recently, there has been a substantial turnaround. Between 1991 and 1993, *all three grade levels showed significant increases in use of marijuana.* Whether these trends portend a continuing increase of marijuana use is, of course, not clear at this writing.

Although the 1980s witnessed a long-term decline in marijuana use, not all of the signs were so encouraging. Cocaine in particular did not decline until after 1986, having increased dramatically in the late 1970s and staying fairly level among adolescents in the early 1980s. The advent of crack cocaine in the mid-1980s changed the epidemiology of cocaine in certain areas in a dramatic way; however, crack had relatively little effect on the data discussed in this report. A more detailed analysis is presented elsewhere (Johnston et al., 1994). The early 1990s have seen no new increases in cocaine use, though there has not been much in the way of declines, either.

One substance that generally increased throughout the 1980s is inhalants. Among high school seniors, the annual use rate observed in 1993 was 7.0%, the highest since observations began in 1975. As indicated earlier, this class of drug has become the most used substance (other than tobacco and alcohol) among younger students. Another substance that has shown recent signs of a reemergence is LSD, which had an annual prevalence among high school seniors in 1993 of 6.8%; this was the highest level recorded since 1975 (when it was 7.2%). Use rates increased for all three grades between 1991 and 1993. Amphetamines are yet another class of drugs that showed increases in use for all three grades between 1991 and 1993.

In sum, there are many disturbing aspects of the recent trends in use of illicit drugs among American students. Only a short time ago, it appeared that illicit drug use may have been on a trajectory that was very comforting for parents, teachers, and others who have an interest in the health and well-being of adolescents. The recent trajectories for a number of drugs—drugs that are important because of their considerable potential for serious damage, including marijuana, inhalants, LSD, amphetamines—are clearly not so comforting in 1994.

Patterns of Substance Use Onset

The relationship among multiple substances, including sequencing of use, is well documented (Ellickson, Hays, & Bell, 1992; Graham *et al.*, 1991; Kandel, 1978; Kandel, Yamaguchi, & Chen, 1992; Weber *et al.*, 1989). There is significant evidence that alcohol is the first drug of use. More commonly used substances, tobacco, marijuana, and perhaps inhalants, follow in sequence and precede experimentation with cocaine, heroin, hallucinogens, amphetamines, and other "hard" drugs. This order of progression is known as the Gateway Theory of substance use onset.

The result of these findings is that prevention programs target tobacco and alcohol in addition to illicit substances. Indeed, most prevention programs have focused on "gateway" substances, tobacco, alcohol, and marijuana. Particularly at risk are youth who are problem-prone to begin with (Weber *et al.*, 1989). These young people consume more alcohol, experience more drunkenness, and use more other drugs than their nonproblem counterparts.

Inhalant use during early adolescence has not been extensively researched. However, because of the recent evidence about when experimentation begins, inhalants may prove to play a significant "gateway" role in the development of use of cocaine, heroin, and other illicit psychoactive drugs (Edwards, 1993; Hansen & Rose, 1995; Johnston *et al.*, in press).

PREVENTION

This section focuses on the prevention of illicit substances, including marijuana, inhalants, amphetamines, cocaine, heroin, LSD, tranquilizers, and steroids. The goal of prevention has been to deter or at least delay the occurrence of use of these substances and reduce the prevalence of use in the population generally. While the focus will be on these illicit substances, it is widely recognized that few efforts to prevent the initiation or development of these substance will stand alone. In nearly all cases, substance use prevention will of necessity include the prevention of alcohol and tobacco as well.

With the exception of marijuana, there has been little or no research emphasis placed on the prevention of any of these drugs separately. Cocaine has received extensive media coverage and is the target of interdiction by law enforcement. However, little emphasis is found that examines cocaine as the sole substance targeted in adolescent research programs. In most cases, prevention of illicit substance co-occurs with the prevention of alcohol and tobacco. The reason for this has been twofold. First, there is a recognition that the prevention of rare phenomena is more difficult to implement and evaluate logistically. Second, there is an awareness that there is a statistical relationship between the use of illegal drugs and alcohol and tobacco, which are legally sold, but not to minors.

Research on the Etiology of Drug Use

The goal of prevention is to deter the onset and development of societal and individual ingestion of substances. The common logic for all prevention program development is to create an intervention that is designed to alter personal, social, and environmental characteristics that cause, influence, or account for substance use. To accomplish this goal, program developers have relied extensively on psychosocial theories and data from etiologic studies.

Theories Used to Explain Substance Use

Theory not only defines the language used to describe, predict, and explain substance abuse, but is also the source of intervention development. It is important to understand the extent to which theory is used, and particularly, which theories have predominated in order to gain a full perspective of the state of the field's practice.

To gain an understanding of the breadth of theory in research, two sets of literature were examined. Studies included those from the research on correlates and those reporting findings of programmatic interventions. Overall, eight theories predominate in the literature. These include the following.

- *Social Learning Theory.* Bandura's (1977) Social Learning Theory postulates that behaviors are learned through symbolic verbal and vicarious reinforcement. Behaviors are executed when the person believes that the action will be reinforced, places value on that reinforcement, and perceives the self as capable of performing the behavior.
- *Theory of Reasoned Action.* The Theory of Reasoned Action (Ajzen & Fishbein, 1980) postulates that behavior is determined by an individual's intentions which in turn are determined by the relative weight of his or her attitudes and normative beliefs. The theory further proposes that attitude results from the interaction between perceptions about perceived consequences of an event and the evaluation of those consequences; normative beliefs result from the interaction between beliefs about what relevant others believe and an individual's motivation to comply with external demands.
- *Social Control Theory.* Social Control Theory (Hirschi, 1969) focuses on the bonds that an individual establishes with society. Bonding is influenced by four elements: (1) attachment, the affective ties one has with those likely to express conventional norms; (2) commitment, the participation in and evaluation of activities considered

conventional; (3) involvement, the amount of time spent in conventional activities; and (4) beliefs, the acceptance of the central social value system of society.

- *Inoculation Theory.* McGuire's (1972) Inoculation Theory postulates that an individual's resistance to persuasive, threatening arguments may be enhanced with knowledge beforehand about the content and strategy of the argument.
- *Problem Behavior Theory.* Problem Behavior Theory (Jessor & Jessor, 1977) postulates that behavior results from the interaction within and between three dynamic systems, personality, perceived environment, and the behavior system. An individual's values, expectations, beliefs about self, and attitudes comprise the personality system. The perceived environment system incorporates support, control, influence, and approval by parents and peers. The behavior system includes problem as well as conventional behaviors.
- *Peer Cluster Theory.* Peer Cluster Theory (Oetting & Beauvais, 1987) postulates that the socialization process that accompanies adolescent development results in the formation of small, cohesive groups. It further postulates that other variables such as family sanctions, religious identification, and school adjustment affect substance use only indirectly through their effect on the peer clusters.
- *The Health Belief Model.* The Health Belief Model (Becker, 1974) postulates that health behaviors are primarily a function of several factors. These include an assessment of perceived risk or harm, an assessment of potential ability to avoid harm through the adoption of appropriate behaviors, and the perceived ability to access needed resources.
- *Social Influence Model.* The Social Influence Model (Flay, 1985; Flay & Petrakis, in press; Hansen, 1988) represents an emergent model that consists of a body of yet-to-be-codified explanations which generally guide the field. The model borrows heavily from many of the theories previously described, e.g., Social Learning Theory, the Theory of Reasoned Action, Social Control Theory, and Peer Cluster Theory. The primary focus of the theory is on the influence of social forces (peers, parents, and media) on individuals in their situational interactions and their perceptions about norms related to substance use and abuse.
- *Social Developmental Model.* A Social Developmental Model has recently been proposed by Hawkins, Catalano, and Miller (1992) that includes an assemblage of 16 risk factors which are classified according to their potential to influence behavior within relevant domains. Within the community domain, for instance, community laws and norms, the availability of substances, economic deprivation, neighborhood disorganization, and mobility are postulated to be important factors. Within the family domain, family history, family management, family conflict, and parental attitudes are important. Within the school domain, academic performance, school bonding, and early and persistent antisocial behavior are important. Finally, within the peer group and individual domain, rebelliousness, peer drug use, personal attitudes, and prior behavior are important predictors. This model clearly incorporates many elements that are derived from previously mentioned theories. It provides a framework for expanding from individual focus through community focus in prevention.

We examined 242 studies reviewed in a paper prepared for the Congressional Office of Technology Assessment (Hansen, Rose & Dryfoos, 1993). Problem Behavior Theory (Jessor & Jessor, 1977) was the most frequently represented theoretical approach, underlying the work in 45 studies. The Social Learning Theory was discussed in 18 studies as the underlying orientation. Other theories represented included Bandura's Social Learning Theory (1977) and Ajzen and Fishbein's Theory of Reasoned Action (1980), in 16 studies each, Hirschi's Social Control Theory (1969) in 8 studies, and Oetting and Beauvais's Peer Cluster Theory (1987) in 4 studies. The Health Belief Model was mentioned in 10 studies. At the time of this review, no studies mentioned either the Social Influence Model or the Social Development Model. Nonetheless, many concepts that are central to these models were discussed.

Programmatic studies referenced in a previous review (Hansen, 1992) were examined to determine the theoretical approach underlying the intervention. Of the 81 studies reviewed, 26 studies did not refer to a specific theory guiding the intervention. Bandura's Social Learning Theory was mentioned in 11 studies. Nine studies represented Jessor and Jessor's Problem Behavior Theory. McGuire's Inoculation Theory was specifically referred to in 8 studies and Ajzen and Fishbein's Theory of Reasoned Action was represented in 6 studies. The Health Belief Model was not mentioned, although a number of programs targeted health beliefs in particular and could be thought of as reflecting the underlying assumptions of this model.

Direct tests of the formal theory have been relatively rare in the field. More commonly, theories are used to suggest variables that should be measured for subsequent correlation with substance use outcome variables. Frequently, multiple theories were represented within the same study. The exceptions to this were several etiologic studies that made direct tests of Problem Behavior Theory and the Theory of Reasoned Action. In practice, theories are often used as a means of orienting readers to domains of variables rather than for the purpose of demonstrating how measures or interventions are derived. Critical tests of theories with specific regard to substance use have not been conducted. In practice, once a theory is presented, it serves the role of providing a guiding set of principles rather than as a focus of scientific scrutiny.

Grounded theories and eclectic aggregations of theory have been used by etiologic researchers and program developers. A key to understanding prevention programming is an understanding of any given program's theoretical roots. The most prominent theoretical orientations are those that are based in social psychology which address the potential for social influence and control.

Empirical Findings

Prevention programmers have used their assumptions about cause and effect to develop preventive interventions. Research on substance abuse etiology has examined numerous variables that serve as markers of these concepts, and empirical findings can be used to demonstrate the potential for prevention programs to have an impact on behavior. The essential logic of this approach is that a program must target a variable that statistically accounts for behavior. Variables that do not account for differences between users and nonusers, or users and abusers, hold little promise for being able to influence programmatic outcomes.

Researchers interested in understanding the causes of substance use and abuse have used a number of different terms for describing the relationships that they have observed. Because methods of study and inference have differed, five terms have evolved that are used to describe relationships between independent and dependent variables. Common terms that are in use include (1) *risk factors,* (2) *protective factors,* (3) *mediating processes,* (4) *correlates,* and (5) *predictors.* We have chosen the terms *correlates* and *predictors* to use in describing the relationships we will discuss because these terms predominate in the empirical literature. For the most part, *correlates* will refer to relationships in which both a theoretical construct and substance use or abuse were measured simultaneously. *Predictors* will be used exclusively to describe longitudinal relationships, particularly cases in which the independent variable was measured prior to the measurement of substance use.

Studies have tended to address marijuana as the primary outcome in etiologic research on use of drugs (other than alcohol or tobacco). We examined over 1800 statistical findings from 242 studies and found that 80% addressed marijuana or hashish. Only 5% addressed opiates and another 5% addressed amphetamines as dependent variables. Thus, findings reported directly address marijuana and only indirectly address other substances of abuse. Drugs such as cocaine and inhalants, which form the core of substances about which recent social attention has been given, have been relatively ignored.

The primary measures from etiologic research assess use as opposed to abuse. Even for drugs such as cocaine and heroin, abuse was not measured. In part, this may reflect the relative difficulty in recruiting truly abusive individuals into research. Adolescent youth who are truly abusive tend to drop out of conventional institutions, such as schools, through which researchers often work to recruit subjects. It may also reflect the precision with which use, as opposed to abuse, can be defined. It must also be remembered that extremely high levels of use provide one measure of abuse. As such, these analyses do address some issues relevant to understanding the causes of abuse. That is, differences between nonusers and low-level users compared to high-level users provide one means of comparison that can be used to understand the causes of substance abuse. The data reported here do not address abuse exclusively and directly, but must nonetheless be considered to address abuse to a large degree.

Eleven major types of variables have been examined in etiologic studies (Hansen *et al.,* 1993). These include (1) previous drug use, (2) intentions to use drugs, (3) cognitive factors, (4) competency factors, (5) personality factors, (6) institutional influences, (7) drug use by others, (8) pressures to use drugs, (9) peer group characteristics, (10) home factors, and (11) demographics such as age, gender, and ethnicity.

There were meaningful differences among the categories in the average correlations observed. Overall, the highest mean correlation coefficient was observed for prior or current other substance use (average correlation = 0.36). Drug use has long been known to be the single best correlate of the concurrent use of other substances and the best predictor of future drug use behavior. Substance use is habitual and addictive. These two factors in combination explain this finding. However, it is important to note that habit and addiction do not account for everything and, in fact, leave plenty of room for other things to matter.

Drug use by others had a relatively strong correlation (average correlation = 0.27). Drug use by peers was more strongly correlated with self-reported drug use (average correlation = 0.37) than was parental drug use (0.16) and drug use by siblings (0.28). Beliefs about psychological (0.30) and social consequences (0.29) and attitudes toward drug use (0.29) also had strong average correlations. Beliefs about health consequences were not as strongly correlated (0.20). Reported pressures to use substances which included offers from peers and parents (0.38) as well as perceived attitudes about drug use among others (0.38) had very large average correlations. Bonding and commitment to school (0.27) had a strong correlation with substance use. Deviance (0.32) also had a strong correlation with substance use.

Several categories of variables would be characterized as having a weak relationship with substance use. The weakest observed category of variables were home factors which had an average correlation of 0.13. This category included the psychological traits of parents, parent–child relationships, parental marital status, parental education, family composition, and socioeconomic status. Other variable groups had average correlation coefficients which were all less than 0.20. These included institutional influences such as church attendance and affiliation and participating in sports and other structured activities (0.14). Competence (0.16), personality variables including self-esteem (0.17), moodiness (0.19), and locus of control (0.17), and demographic variable such as race (0.20) and gender (0.07) all had average correlations less than or equal to 0.20. This suggests that overall, a weak relationship exists between each of these categories and substance use.

The accumulated research points to two general factors that influence substance use. First, it is clear that prior use of a substance is a major predictor of subsequent use. Many substances create addictions which are real in terms of creating withdrawal symptoms if discontinued as well as increased psychopharmacologic tolerance. Previous research also demonstrates that social processes are important as an etiologic mechanism for the onset *and* progressive development of substance use. Many of the strongest correlates of substance use reflected either the positive or negative influence of peers on behavior. It is quite likely that the use of substances is a key marker that defines group membership. Groups in which substance use is common may use substances as a social identifier and may use drugs as part of established social rituals. This is more likely to be the case in groups of established users than experimental users.

Preventive Interventions

The need for effective substance abuse prevention is great, partly because alcohol, tobacco, and drug abuse pose serious threats to the health and welfare of the nation, and partly because throughout the 1980s the call for public action, manifested by the commitment of public and private dollars, steadily increased. Schools, because of their guaranteed access to young people, are most routinely considered as the focus of programming. Recently a number of other formats for prevention have also emerged including a variety of approaches that focus on community-based prevention. These innovative approaches, which are needed and promising, have not been evaluated.

Much of what is known about effective school-based curricular approaches has been learned from researcher-initiated intervention trials. Information about commercially available prevention programs which have proliferated since the availability of Drug-free Schools and Communities funds, in contrast, is relatively limited. This review will focus on two aspects of curriculum. First, what is known from evaluation studies will be documented. Second, curricular approaches that are common but unresearched will be identified.

Numerous reviews have been completed about the effectiveness of curricular approaches to prevention. These reviews have spanned the review methodology spectrum and have made their own unique contribution to understanding the field of prevention. Tobacco prevention studies have been extensively reviewed (e.g., Best, Thomson, Santi, Smith, & Brown, 1988; Botvin & Wills, 1985; Evans & Raines, 1982; Flay, 1985; Leventhal & Cleary, 1980; Schinke, Gilchrist, & Snow, 1985; Thompson, 1978). Alcohol has been the focus of several reviews (Goodstadt, 1980, 1986; Gordon & McAlister, 1982; Moskowitz, 1989). Reviews that are specific and limited to examining the prevention of marijuana or cocaine use do not exist. However, several reviews have included an examination of the prevention of multiple substances (Bangert-Drowns, 1988; Bruvold & Rundall, 1988; Moskowitz, 1989; Schaps, DiBartolo, Moskowitz, Palley, & Churgin, 1981; Tobler, 1986). Even these reviews typically have a primary focus on tobacco and alcohol. Because marijuana, cocaine, and other illegal drugs share etiologic roots with tobacco and alcohol, the findings from studies that include these substances provide the best available evidence of prevention program effectiveness.

At the root of all curricular activities is the assumption that behavioral effects are the result of changing causal processes that underlie the onset of substance use. Most of these assumptions incorporate the correlates that have been described previously. It is interesting to note, however, that there is not a one-to-one correspondence between what people have tried to do programmatically and the variables that have emerged from etiologic research. Nonetheless, there has been significant borrowing and use of etiologic statistical facts and etiologic theory in the creation of prevention programs.

- *Information* programs target knowledge and beliefs about the consequences of using substances and personal beliefs that substance use puts one at risk. Included as targets of program intervention are the three cognitive factors that address (1) beliefs about health consequences, (2) beliefs about social consequences, and (3) beliefs about the psychological consequences of drug use.
- *Decision-making* programs teach a process for making rational decisions about substance use. In the typology of correlates, decision-making programs target competency factors related to self-management. Decision-making programs typically teach young people a strategy for identifying problems, creating solutions, and making choices among alternatives. Decision-making skills are taught as rational responses to specific situations. Making decisions about more general life issues may also be addressed. Decision-making frameworks may or may not be directly applied to an individual's drug use. Correlates that are expected to change as a result of decision-making programs are skills for making rational decisions and

the application of rational procedures for dealing with problem situations. Distinctly emphasized is the *process* of making the decision.

- *Commitment* programs encourage participants to adopt a personal commitment not to use substances. The correlate addressed by these programs is intentions to use or not use substances; students are expected to develop a strong personal commitment to stay drug- or alcohol-free.
- *Values clarification* programs examine the relationship between individuals' values and the consequences of their behavior and demonstrate that personal values are incompatible with substance use (Rokeach, 1968). In the independent variable typology presented above, values programs address correlates such as general values and religious values. Values clarification programs are postulated to operate by placing an individual's values in a central position to influence life choices and by developing beliefs that drug use is inconsistent with an individual's overall life objectives.
- *Goal setting* programs teach skills for setting and attaining goals and encourage the adoption of an achievement orientation. Goal setting may be placed within a realistic framework of resources, skills, time, and rewards. Goal setting programs are postulated to prevent drug and alcohol use through the development of achievement values. Also mediating the prevention effects are the application of skills for setting and achieving positive life goals. Values clarification approaches may appear similar to, but differ from, goal setting approaches in that goal setting is oriented toward building a specific set of skills whereas values clarification programs are oriented to setting priorities and ordering life choices accordingly.
- *Stress management* programs teach skills for coping with and managing stress. Stress management focuses on teaching students skills to cope with psychologically difficult situations. Stress management programs are postulated to operate by increasing an individual's perceived self-efficacy for coping with life difficulties and through the application of coping skills to dealing with problem situations. A reduction in perceived stress is also expected to deter the development of substance use.
- *Self-esteem* programs focus on developing an individual's feelings of self-worth and value. Program success is expected to be mediated by the degree to which self-esteem in individuals is improved.
- *Resistance skills training* teaches students to identify and assertively resist pressure and influences to use substances from peers, siblings, parents, adults, and the media. The focus of instruction may be to develop skills to deal with pressure from peers as well as pressure from advertising, parents, or siblings to use drugs. Assertiveness training is included in this category. Resistance skills training programs are postulated to be effective in altering the onset of substance use and abuse through the development of personal skills for refusing offers to use substances, through the development of general invulnerability to social pressure, and through the development of perceived self-efficacy for resisting peer pressure.
- *Life skills training* programs teach broad social skills including communication skills, human relations skills, and skills for solving interpersonal conflict. Correlates targeted by these programs include a diverse mixture of constructs, including

altering social personality traits and facilitating peer bonding. Life skills training programs are postulated to mediate substance use onset by improving communication and skills for gaining social acceptance, and developing skills for resolving interpersonal problems. The latter variables addressed by these program components have not been extensively measured in etiologic studies and did not emerge as a variable category or subcategory in the meta-analysis above.

- *Norm setting* programs establish conservative norms regarding use. Norm setting programs focus on correcting erroneous perceptions of the prevalence and acceptability of drug and alcohol use and establishing conservative group norms. Norm setting programs are postulated to operate through lowering perceptions of drug use by peers, reducing perceived social availability, and reducing perceptions about peer attitudes about drug use.

- *Assistance* programs provide students with skills for dealing with life problems. Curriculum-based assistance programs are differentiated from Student Assistance Programs described below (see the section on treatment, below). Curriculum-based assistance programs are postulated to affect drug use by providing social support to at-risk individuals. The meta-analysis found no variables that assessed these characteristics.

- *Alternatives* programs provide experience in activities that are incompatible with substance use. Alternatives programs are postulated to mediate the development of substance use through reducing time of exposure to at-risk situations and through providing skills to pursue activities that run counter to drug use (e.g., activities that require physical endurance and coordination). These programs also address participation in structured and nonstructured activities.

These 12 topics describe program components. However, even a cursory review of the literature reveals that programs rarely focus on only one component. Most prevention programs that have been developed have addressed at least 2, and often between 3 and 7 of these program components simultaneously. In order to understand what we know about the effectiveness of curriculum programs, a simplified conceptual framework for evaluating the content of substance abuse prevention curricula is critical. Previous reviewers, particularly those who have attempted meta-analyses, have also faced the problem of creating a meaningful classification scheme. For example, Tobler (1986) examined what appeared to be major themes by researchers reporting results and proposed five summary categories to describe functional content grouping: Knowledge Only programs, Affective Only programs, Peer programs, Knowledge Plus Affective programs, and Alternatives programs. Bangert-Drowns (1988) similarly classified programs based on functional content into three types: Information Only, Affective Education Only, or Mixed. On the other hand, Bruvold and Rundall (1988) based their classification on theory types rather than program types and came up with four types of program components: Rational components, Social Reinforcement components, Social Norm components, and Developmental components. Bruvold and Rundall (1988) demonstrated that there is some similarity between their conceptualization of the theoretical underpinnings of prevention programs and those suggested by other reviewers (Bernstein & McAlister, 1969; Leventhal & Cleary, 1980; Moskowitz *et al.*, 1983; Schaps *et al.*, 1981; Thompson, 1978). While there is some intersection among function-based and theory-based classification schemes, such categorizations are yet too broad to allow for a theoretically precise classification of programs.

In recent reviews, Hansen (1992) and Tobler (1995) have independently presented categorization schemes that are highly similar to those presented above. Four functional categories of programs were identified by each author. For Hansen (1992) classification schemes were based solely on program content. Resulting groups of curricula included (1) information and values clarification programs, (2) affective programs which also included information components, (3) social influence programs which also tended to include information, and (4) multiple-component programs, usually including some element of all three of the previous groups but emphasizing social influence in conjunction with additional affective strategies.

Tobler's classification scheme included (1) knowledge programs, (2) programs that included knowledge, decision-making, and affective education, (3) programs that focused exclusively on social influences, and (4) programs that added social life skills components. Differences in classification focused on the inclusion of teaching methodologies (didactic versus interactive), the use or nonuse of peer opinion leaders, and the relative weighting given to each component. Thus, several programs that may have included social influence components were reclassified as affective because of their relative minor emphasis on these topics and the primary reliance on didactic teaching approaches and failure to include peer opinion leaders. Given the current state of the art, these classification schemes are sufficiently similar and well recognized to allow most curricular programs to be adequately classified with little discrepancy.

Curriculum Effectiveness

Numerous curricula have been developed. Researcher-generated programs have been more likely to be evaluated than commercially developed programs. The effectiveness of school-based curricular approaches has been widely questioned (Moskowitz, 1989). It is clear that the primary difficulty in gaining an understanding of which strategies hold promise has to do with methodological difficulties in conducting field trials needed to evaluate the effectiveness of these projects. Nonetheless, two recent reviews (Hansen, 1992; Tobler, 1995) suggest that despite these difficulties, there are promising findings, particularly among the program types that include social influences approaches.

In a review by Hansen (1992), the effects of programming on outcome variables were reviewed from 45 published and unpublished studies. Programs outcomes were coded using a three-point system. Positive program effects, those that reduced substance use compared to control or comparison groups, that were statistically significant received a plus (+). Negative outcomes (the program increased substance use compared to controls) that were statistically significant received a minus (−). Programs that had no statistically determinable effect were coded as zeros (0). Each analysis that was reported for each program was included as one of these three outcomes. Therefore, because some programs had multiple analyses within a report and may have had multiple reports, more than 45 analyses were categorized.

The results of this analysis revealed that 31% of outcomes for information programs,

19% of outcomes for affective education programs, 51% of outcomes for social influence programs, and 50% of outcomes for multiple-component programs were positive. In contrast, 25% of the information program outcomes, 19% of the affective education programs, 11% of the social influence programs, and none of the multiple-component programs were negative. Outcomes that were neither positive nor negative were common among all program categories; information programs (44%), multiple-component programs (50%), and affective programs (62%) had more nonsignificant results than social influence programs (38%). Overall, social influence and multiple-component programs (which also typically featured social influence strategies as major components) had more positive results than did either information-based approaches or affective education approaches. This overall pattern was maintained when studies that were judged to have methodological weaknesses (probable selection bias or lack of statistical power) were deleted. Among these analyses, 30% of information, 42% of affective, 63% of social influence, and 72% of multiple-component strategies had significant positive findings.

Tobler (1995) used means and standard deviations to calculate effect size statistics for each of the studies reviewed above. In addition, slight modifications in the classification scheme were introduced. The studies included in Hansen's (1992) review were analyzed for effect sizes and then were reanalyzed using the Tobler classification scheme. Tobler's review increased the number of studies in the analysis and conducted analyses on two datasets. The first included all reported studies for which effect sizes could be determined. The second included only those studies from the larger group that met methodological standards for inclusion (e.g., adequate follow-up, control groups).

A summary of results is presented in Table 2. Values that are given are effect sizes, which provide a description of the magnitude of difference that was made due to the program. Larger positive values indicate larger positive effects. As can be seen, there is overall concurrence between both reviews and all analyses. Programs that were primarily informational or affective in nature had relatively small effect sizes. Programs that feature social influences approaches or include life skills approaches in addition to social influences approaches are, in comparison, relatively strong programs. Such programs as *Project SMART* and *Project STAR,* available from the University of Southern California (Hansen & Graham, 1991; Pentz, MacKinnon, *et al.,* 1989), *Life Skills Training,* available from Gilbert Botvin of Cornell University (Botvin, Baker, Dusenbury, Tortu, &

Table 2. Effect Size Meta-analysis Results from Two Prevention Intervention Outcome Reviews

Source of studies	Hansen		Hansen		Tobler large		Tobler restricted	
Categorization method	Hansen		Tobler		Tobler		Tobler	
	N	ES	N	ES	N	ES	N	ES
Information	8	0.07	5	0.17	14	0.09	3	0.05
Affect	5	0.01	11	−0.01	25	0.05	14	0.02
Social influence	12	0.14	12	0.19	37	0.18	16	0.27
Multicomponent	11	0.08	3	0.13	25	0.37	20	0.37

Botvin, 1990), and *ALL STARS,* available from William Hansen at Tanglewood Research, Clemmons, North Carolina (W. B. Hansen, V. S. Uebersax, & L. A. Rose, unpublished), are examples of interactive social influence prevention programs.

Only recently have commercially available programs been evaluated. Three circular programs in particular have captured a sizable segment of the prevention program market, *D.A.R.E.* (Drug Abuse Resistance Education), *Quest: Skills for Living,* and *Here's Looking at You, 2000.* Of these only evaluations of *D.A.R.E.* have been reported in sufficient numbers to draw conclusions.

The *D.A.R.E.* program consists of materials created by the Los Angeles Unified School district that consist largely of materials borrowed from research-based programs that were developed in the early 1980s. The program is delivered by uniformed police officers who have received extensive training at one of five regional training centers. *D.A.R.E.* is delivered annually to approximately 5,000,000 students in the United States. The program is delivered in all 50 states and has made international connections as well.

The magnitude of the program notwithstanding, there is little evidence to support *D.A.R.E.* as a viable or effective approach to substance abuse prevention. In a recent review by Ennett, Ringwalt, and Flewelling (1993), 17 published and unpublished manuscripts documenting evaluations of *D.A.R.E.* were examined. Of the 17, only 11 met minimal standards for methodological rigor and were used to form the basis of interpreting findings. None of these studies have demonstrated any outcome effectiveness of *D.A.R.E.* The average calculated effect-size reported was 0.06, indicating very small average effects. Overall, drug use among controls schools and *D.A.R.E.* schools was roughly equal. Several of these studies were longitudinal and found neither short-term nor long-term results.

D.A.R.E. has important strengths, not the least of these is widespread political support and funding. Community residents and community leaders almost uniformly find that *D.A.R.E.* promotes good school–police relations. The observed quality of program implementation is high. Finally, the program has been expertly marketed. However, the strengths of *D.A.R.E.* do not compensate for its lack of effectiveness as a prevention program. Plans currently exist for revising the *D.A.R.E.* curriculum. This must be considered a positive step. However, revision *per se* may not be sufficient to make the program effective. Given the expense and widespread distribution of the program, high priority should be given to conducting multiple scientifically rigorous outcome evaluations of future versions of the program.

The United States Department of Education currently funnels $500,000,000 annually to states and school districts through the Drug-free School and Communities program. Many districts use these funds to pay for curricula and curriculum training. The Government Accounting Office (1993) estimated that approximately one-fourth of the funds spent under the Drug-free School and Communities funding given to school districts went toward purchasing and delivering school curricula. It is alarming that this funding has paid for such widespread distribution of a number of curricular approaches that have no evaluative results whatsoever, most of which have doubtful potential to prevent substance use.

Packages that have been widely adopted such as *Quest: Skills for Living, Here's Looking at You, 2000, Project Adventure, Ombudsman, B.A.B.E.S., Project CHARLIE,* and *Children Are People* have no adequate evaluation results by which program effectiveness can be judged (Thorne, personal communication). Evaluations that have been conducted have primarily been short-term evaluations for dissertations and theses and lack interpretable behavioral endpoints (Swisher, personal communication). Given the breadth of dissemination of these curricula, the potential for quality evaluation studies is great. This lack of evaluation reflects a low priority by organizations that spend public funds for actually solving the substance use and abuse problem.

Curriculum-based prevention, if effective, offers a significant means for reducing the costs of drug abuse and for improving the quality of life throughout the nation. Nonetheless, like all human endeavors, developing a truly effective technology for prevention will require significant knowledge-based effort. The field to date can be characterized as showing promise (Hansen, 1992; Tobler, 1986, 1995). Nonetheless, there are those (Moskowitz, 1989) who suggest that significant difficulties remain. Many of these difficulties are methodological, difficulties that are inherent in all field trial research and evaluation. There are individual studies that provide encouragement that school-based prevention might ultimately be effective. However, there are no proven technologies that are sufficiently well refined and tested that can guarantee the success of school-based preventive efforts.

The standards for judging programmatic success are well developed. That is, to be successful, programs must demonstrate a reduction in the rates of substance use onset of students in schools receiving the program compared to students in schools where the program has not been delivered. The criteria for determining the validity of such evaluation trials are now well defined (Hansen, 1992). The same standards must be applied to evaluating all programmatic efforts.

In the end, success in school-based prevention requires the development of a significant knowledge base. The importance of this technical capability cannot be overemphasized. Without it, preventive approaches will fail more often than they succeed. The fact that failure characterizes nearly all non-research-based curricular approaches underscores this point. Currently, the school-based prevention field is characterized and dominated by individuals and groups who believe strongly in the value of prevention. More often than not, however, such activist approaches to prevention substitute adequate technical knowledge with a determination to succeed. Unfortunately, such approaches seldom, if ever, achieve prevention goals. No matter how widespread, politically viable, or popular a program may be, effectiveness in preventing the onset of substance use and abuse must remain the primary and sole criterion by which programs are judged.

Priorities should be directed away from programs that are based on marketing, persuasive philosophy, or testimonials-as-evidence and toward those that are based on solid empirical research and proven effectiveness. Approaches that have demonstrated promise should form the basis for refinements and experimentation until a technology of prevention can be fully developed. In the end, empirically grounded theory and extensive field testing will result in the development of effective programs. The promise of a quick fix must be understood to be an illusion. The demand for ready solutions should be met with the development of technically sound solutions.

Curriculum-based efforts have dominated the field. This is so for two reasons: (1) curricular approaches are simple to identify and understand, and (2) the methods available to evaluate curricula have become standardized. Nonetheless, there are several noncurricular approaches that have recently emerged that deserve some attention. Unfortunately, evaluation of these approaches is relatively lacking and only the most conjectural of conclusions can be drawn regarding the effectiveness of these approaches.

Schools may also play a role in prevention in conjunction with other normal institutions within society, notably the family and the community. The past decade has produced some, albeit limited research that has addressed the potential of these forums to work with schools to prevent substance use and abuse.

Since the earliest studies (Evans *et al.*, 1978), school-based curriculum prevention research has included parent issues. These studies primarily focused on instruction to students about pressures that family members may give to use substances through modeling of unwanted behaviors. More recently, parents have been included as participants in prevention programming through the use of homework assignments (Hansen & Graham, 1991) and parent-focused ancillary activities, such as parent nights (Rohrback, Hansen, & Pentz, 1992) and special parent programs (Brannon *et al.*, 1989). Sufficiently robust information to demonstrate effectiveness is not yet available. Typical of the problems experienced by these programs is low parent participation. From a methodological perspective, the "best" parents or the parents whose children have defined problems are expected to be overrepresented in parent gatherings. Such biases severely complicate any analyses of data to date.

A major federal program to involve communities in prevention is currently funded by CSAP (The Center for Substance Abuse Prevention, SAMHSA, PHS, DHHS). The focus of this approach is the development of community partnerships for prevention. To date, 251 partnership programs have been funded. Over 60% of these actively involve schools as coalition members, providing significant opportunity for school and community interventions to be developed. Each site is required to have a local evaluator. Further, a national evaluation has begun. The methodological sophistication of local evaluations varies markedly and the field of community program research has not developed sufficiently to have established widely accepted standards. The national evaluation of this endeavor will specifically monitor the effects of programs on substance use among school-age youth. Programmatic activities will be monitored both by national evaluators and by local evaluators. This program is too young to have provided any outcome findings.

A number of other model community programs exist. The Midwest Prevention Project (Pentz, Johnson, *et al.*, 1989) includes school-based interventions in the greater Kansas City metropolitan area and Marion County (Indianapolis), Indiana, that were based on *Project SMART* program materials (Hansen & Graham, 1991). The evaluation results to date speak directly only to the impact of the school-based curricular interventions (Pentz, MacKinnon, *et al.*, 1989). Because of constraints in the study design, community organization, parental, and media intervention components cannot be evaluated. Nonetheless, this approach directly addresses the potential for communities to support school-based prevention efforts.

Cities-in-Schools is a national nonprofit organization devoted to preventing dropout through partnerships between schools, local government, and businesses. Cities-in-Schools operates in 122 communities in 21 states with 384 schools participating in the program. The focus of this organization's activities is to bring health, social, and employment services into schools with the goal of helping high-risk youth find jobs, tutors, and counseling and to motivate high-risk youth to stay in school. Cities-in-Schools has a national staff that provides assistance to local boards. In each site, a prominent person in business presides over each program and directs fund-raising and organizes a team of professionals to assist potential dropouts. In most programs, a case manager is assigned to each high-risk child. Beyond these basics, programs vary greatly, focusing on a diversity of prevention and intervention strategies. Several Cities-in-Schools sites have achieved national attention. Although little concrete evaluation data are available about overall effects of this program or its effects on substance use, this appears to be a promising model that deserves the attention of research and evaluation.

In addition to those mentioned, there are numerous alternative educational environments and educational strategies that may, through changing the social or physical climate, have an impact on substance use. Research and theory have not yet considered the wide variety of structures that exist that can conceivably impact substance use. Possible areas of future research may include open versus closed campuses, alternative schools, and afterschool care programs. Each of these approaches is deserving of evaluation to determine the extent to which they may help contribute to solving the student drug and alcohol problem.

TREATMENT

The need for treatment to address adolescent substance use has become increasingly important during the past few decades. In response, numerous approaches for treating substance abuse have been developed and marketed. As is typical with all fields in which there is rapid development and a high demand for service, research has tended to lag behind practice. Indeed, there are numerous models for treatment that address a spectrum of needs for which crucial outcome data are just becoming available.

The variety of treatment programs span the spectrum from low-intensity school-based student assistance programs and school-based health clinics, to residential hospital and therapeutic community programs. The primary purpose of this section is to review the spectrum of services available and discuss research findings where available.

Student Assistance Programs

Student assistance programs are among the most common programs to be found in schools, accounting for approximately half of the expenditures of Drug-free Schools and Communities funds in six evaluated urban school districts (GAO, 1993). Overall, student assistance programs remain unevaluated despite their popularity and the diffusion of the approach across the United States.

The focus of student assistance programs is on providing early intervention to students who use substances through a variety of intervention strategies including referral to treatment, providing social support, and increasing skill and competence at dealing with a variety of life problems. A common feature of these programs is the involvement of peers who often play active roles in the program. Among the variety of roles that peers play are those of crisis managers, small group facilitators, and referral agents. Adults are also often involved as program facilitators and counselors. Typical programs include such activities as group counseling for children of alcoholics, counseling for students who use alcohol or drugs dysfunctionally, counseling for students who have poor school performance (identified as a risk factor for initiating substance abuse), and working with families to assist parents in addressing their children's needs.

In all, we were able to identify four (and obtain three) reports that dealt directly with the evaluation of student assistance programs. Two of these studies (Kim, McLeod, Rader, & Johnston, 1992; Pollard, Horowitz, & Houle, 1991) address only process issues. Only one report (Kleinman, Tobler, Morehouse, Eschbach, & Kleinman, 1992) addresses program outcomes. This outcome study differs markedly from the typical student assistance program; it addresses the effects of an intervention program on students in six residential facilities, one of which was a locked correctional facility. Nonetheless, the content and structure of this program reflect approaches often adopted by student assistance programs.

Results of this single-group, pretest–posttest design found that marijuana and tobacco use declined among program participants in five of the six facilities. Alcohol declined in half of the sites; two sites remained unchanged and one site saw a slight rise in alcohol consumption. The decline in use was observed at two posttests, one approximately 9 months and one approximately 15 months after receiving the program. These results suggest promise.

Given the popularity and level of funding allocated for these programs, evaluations should proliferate and yet are universally absent. High priority should be given to assessing the variety of structures and strategies employed by student assistance programs. The effectiveness of programs should be evaluated. Program elements that account for program effectiveness should be thoroughly researched.

School Health Clinics

There are concerns about group-based interventions, such as student assistance programs. These concerns focus on the possibility that low-problem users may actually experience a strengthening of the drug subculture by associating with high-problem users in therapy group. An alternative is to develop individualized service care strategies. Many different kinds of health and social services are being provided in schools that may directly or indirectly address the problem of substance abuse. Community agencies are bringing services into schools to help educators deal with social and health problems, such as sexually transmitted diseases, drug use, violence, and depression. This reflects an awareness that many social and health problems are interrelated (they co-occur) and share common causes and cures. School-based clinics and other types of youth service centers are being organized by service providers to provide comprehensive, integrated, one-stop health and social services. This new wave of programming has been supported by state governments, local school districts, and private foundations.

School-based clinics were developed in response to several specific issues. First, the proportion of youth who live in poverty or otherwise have limited access to health care facilities is large and increasing. Brindis et al. (1993) indicate that the percent of adolescents defined as living in poverty increased from 15% in 1979 to 19% in 1986. An additional five million youths have no health insurance. Second, the prevalence of violence, teen pregnancy, and substance use remain high. In many cases, the solutions to these problems require direct one-on-one medical or social intervention.

In response to these needs, a wide range of activities fall under the rubric of school-based health and social services. These services target a range of issues, including the promotion of healthy development, prevention of high-risk behaviors, screening, diagnosis, and treatment of illness, and early intervention in the entire spectrum of health and social problems. School-based health and social service models include those that are administered directly by school personnel, including school nurses and counselors, as well as those that supplement or provide the entire spectrum of services by nonschool agencies. Providers may include nurses, guidance counselors, psychologists, social workers, health educators, substance abuse counselors, clinical nurse practitioners, physicians, physician assistants, public health nurses, and volunteers.

There is as yet no single model for school-based clinics. In a recent review (Brindis et al., 1993), 306 school-based health centers were identified in operation in 33 states and Puerto Rico. Most of these were in high schools. Fewer were found in junior high or middle schools. This review also notes that medical reasons (injuries and acute illnesses) account for about half of the visits to school-based clinics, with approximately 40% of the visits for counseling purposes and 10% for obtaining birth control supplies or receiving counseling regarding reproductive issues. The extent to which school-based clinics deal directly with drug abuse prevention and treatment issues has not been documented.

The self-referral and other available data suggest that school-based clinics are a needed resource for health care and social support generally. To date, no evaluations exist about the potential efficacy of school-based clinics to assist with the treatment or prevention of substance abuse problems. Given the multiple roles that clinics serve, the diversity of treatment that might be provided, and the lack of substance use-specific programmatic details, significant efforts to define, refine, and test the effects of school-based clinic programs on substance use are needed. Substance use will not, and perhaps should not, be the primary focus of school-based clinics. Nonetheless, to the extent that these programs may become widespread during the coming years, research should document the potential for these services to address substance abuse problems and give insights about how services can be structured and rendered in order to maximize potential benefit.

Because program documentation, theories of program action, and research on program mechanisms and outcomes are entirely lacking, significant efforts to advance understanding of school-based clinic and student assistance programs are needed. Evaluations of service programs, which may have a heavy self-selection bias built in, are inherently difficult to evaluate. This is so because finding an appropriate and equivalent control or comparison group is a serious challenge which evaluators must be prepared to address through creative research designs.

Family Programs

Recent research has examined providing early intervention or substance use treatment through programs that actively involve parents. For example, Bry (1988) reports on a program that involved a variant of behavioral family therapy delivered to identified high-risk students. Compared to adolescents receiving only school-based interventions that utilized teachers to track and intervene with behavioral reinforcement strategies, students who participated with their parents in therapy improved grade point averages. Behavioral outcomes revealed that students receiving family therapy maintained current levels of substance use whereas students in the comparison group demonstrated observable increases.

Additional case studies (Liddle *et al.*, 1992; Treadway, 1992) provide documentation about typical methods that are associated with family-involved treatment. A focus of such therapy is to address family systems problems that promote substance use and interfere with positive change, empowering parents to make changes by teaching them skills, dealing with crises.

Insufficient data are available to draw firm conclusions about parent-focused or parent-assisted intervention. Nonetheless, these approaches warrant further research and consideration. Of particular importance may be parental education from the school that instructs parents about special topics. For instance, inhalants and prescription drugs are commonly available in nearly all homes. According to recent national (Edwards, 1993; Johnston *et al.*, 1994) and local (Hansen & Rose, 1995) data, inhalants are among the earliest used substances that might be addressed directly in the home by parents. Information about inhalants and prescription drugs, their storage and potential for misuse and abuse might be directed to parents through school sources.

Twelve-Step Programs

Many approaches for treatment for adolescents have been borrowed from adult treatment strategies. Certainly among the more popular approaches have been 12-step programs modeled after Alcoholics Anonymous and Narcotics Anonymous (Lawson, 1992). This approach is found not only in stand-alone groups, but as part of clinically guided treatment programs. There are two major features of these approaches. The first is the adoption of a 12-step philosophy. The second is a format of meeting that involves a general strategy for social support.

The philosophy of the programs addresses treating the pattern of behavior as a disease, including a belief that the disease is progressive if left untreated. These programs require the addict to admit that he or she is powerless to control the use of the substance. Further, the program requires the participant to commit to never use the substance again. This reflects a belief that once one has become an addict, one never recovers but remains an addict and in a process of recovery throughout life. Part of this approach is the idea of turning oneself over to a "higher power." The philosophy often conceives this higher power as God, but adopts no particular religion's concept of deity. There is a strong belief that within the group, the addict will find the assistance needed. Being free from drugs is clearly stated as being more important than any personal relationship. Because of the uncertainty of causes of relapse and a presumed lack of personal resilience, the threat of relapse is presumed to be constant. Twelve-step programs often adopt a "one day at a time" slogan to represent this concept. Finally, there is a strong belief that only those who are themselves in recovery can help those who are addicted.

Individuals entering 12-step programs are typically assigned a partner to guide them through the steps to recovery. The partner is typically an individual who has previously gone through the steps and is currently abstinent. The partner theoretically works with the new individual until abstinence is attained and the person is living a "straight" life.

Individuals who have gone through 12-step programs tend to become devotees and strongly advocate for this approach. There are many elements of the program that are intuitively appealing. However, 12-step programs have not been evaluated for effectiveness even among adult populations. The effectiveness of the program generally is not known. Group-to-group variability and effectiveness are expected. Some caution in referring all adolescents to these programs must be exercised (Tarter, 1990). At the same time, in many communities, all available brief and outpatient programs may subscribe to a 12-step approach and limited alternatives may be available. Careful monitoring of clients in such settings is highly recommended.

Residential Treatment

Several types of programs involve more intensive treatment that require the person to be removed from the daily environment and housed in a dedicated treatment facility. Most of these programs have primarily addressed the needs of adults and young adults. However, there are facilities that specialize in adolescent care. There are two common types of programs that operate in this manner. The first are hospital or treatment center facilities that primarily address issues of detoxification and "drying out" followed by some form of intensive individual and group therapy. A major focus is on education about addiction. Because of the cost of residential treatment, the stability of these programs has become difficult to predict.

The second type of program is referred to as a "therapeutic community." Often the goal of the latter type of program is to resocialize the individual entirely. Less attention is paid to psychological issues specific to substance abuse. Instead, the individual goes through the process of gaining basic personal and social skills needed to function as a normal individual within society. Often these programs include strict supervision, with freedoms being granted only when responsible behaviors are demonstrated. Therapeutic communities may only accept individuals who are clean from substance use at the time of admission. Requirements for remaining in the community are strictly enforced.

Attempts have been made to evaluate the effectiveness of adolescent treatment. Two national efforts were launched in the 1980s. The first, DARP (Drug Abuse Reporting Program; Simpson & Sells, 1982), included an intake only comparison group. Data from this study were inconclusive about treatment effectiveness and any specific matching between client type and treatment program (Hester & Miller, 1988). The second research project, TOPS (Treatment Outcome Prospective Study; Hubbard, Cavanaugh, Craddock, & Rachal, 1985), was also inconclusive. In these and other studies, the characteristics of enrollees at the initiation of treatment were a good predictor of outcome (Hester & Miller, 1988). This suggests that for all individuals entering any form of treatment, the outcome will be heavily influenced by the extent of abuse already present.

Because the selection criteria for entering therapeutic communities are different than those for entering hospital or clinic settings, comparison of these programs has numerous methodological difficulties. The motivation and drug abuse characteristics of the two samples are not comparable. The intensity of the programs involved also vary greatly.

While there are clearly similarities among both kinds of residential treatment programs, the differences from site to site and, within any given site, from year to year may be profound. Such moving targets create a serious dilemma for researchers who are trying to understand the phenomena. A clear agenda for future research that both researchers and clinicians need to be aware of is the need to make comparisons among programs that account for all of these differences.

In addition to the client's status at the time of enrollment and the structure of treatment, there is an emerging issue relevant to matching treatment with client needs (Hester & Miller, 1988; Tarter, 1990). Underlying causes of substance abuse and underlying response tendencies may both differ in ways that will make some outcomes appear ineffective. Strategies for matching treatment to needs and resources have been advocated. However, little research to guide such decisions is available (Tarter, 1990).

Summary of Treatment Effectiveness

Adolescent drug abuse treatment is clearly needed and is provided in a variety of ways. The available research suggests that various forms of treatment have the potential to be effective tools. However, the research in this area has been relatively sparse and not conclusive. The cost, duration, intensity, format, and availability of treatment for adolescents vary greatly. Selection of programs needs to be made in part on significance of the problem within the individual. In part, program selection will be limited by the availability of affordable programs within the community. Given the current state of research and practice, proven program effectiveness is a less important issue for making decisions about referral.

CONCLUSION

The epidemiology, etiology, prevention, and treatment of substance use among adolescents have generated a sizable body of literature that continues to expand. Nonetheless, the practical problems of effectively preventing and efficiently treating adolescent substance use and abuse remain societal problems. The practical ends will be more readily reached with continued systematic study in which the goal of developing technologies for treatment and prevention are based on scientific evidence and science-based theories. Most theories currently employed have not been critically tested. Most prevention and treatment approaches that are widely available to communities are based on philosophy or untested theory rather than science. However, the number of programs that have been developed from a scientific base and tested empirically is growing. Practitioners and researchers can productively work together to strengthen the field by applying state-of-the-art methods to develop and test treatment and prevention programs, followed by the adoption and dissemination of promising programs.

ACKNOWLEDGMENT. This work was supported in part by Research Grant Nos. DA07030 and DA01411 from the National Institute on Drug Abuse.

REFERENCES

Ajzen, I., & Fishbein, M. (1980). *Understanding attitudes and predicting behavior* (pp. 5–9, 79–91, 260–274). Englewood Cliffs, NJ: Prentice–Hall.

Bachman, J. G., Wallace, J. M., Jr., O'Malley, P. M., Johnston, L. D., Kurth, C. L., & Neighbors, H. W. (1991). Racial/ethnic differences in smoking, drinking, and illicit drug use among American high school seniors, 1976–1989. *American Journal of Public Health, 81,* 372–377.

Bandura, A. (1977). *Social learning theory.* Englewood Cliffs, NJ: Prentice–Hall.

Bangert-Drowns, R. L. (1988). The effects of school-based substance abuse education—A meta-analysis. *Journal of Drug Education, 18,* 243–264.

Becker, M. H. (1974). The health belief model and personal health behavior. *Health Education Monographs, 2,* 324–473.

Bernstein, D. A., & McAlister, A. (1969). The modification of smoking behavior. An evaluative review. *Psychological Bulletin, 71,* 418–440.

Best, J. A., Thomson, S. J., Santi, S. M., Smith E. A., & Brown K. S. (1988). Preventing cigarette smoking among school children. *Annual Review of Public Health, 9,* 161–201.

Botvin G. J., Baker, E., Dusenbury, L., Tortu, S., & Botvin, E. M. (1990). Preventing adolescent drug abuse through a multimodal cognitive-behavioral approach: Results of a 3-year study. *Journal of Consulting and Clinical Psychology, 58,* 437–446.

Botvin, G. J., & Wills, T. S. (1985). Personal and social skills training: Cognitive-behavioral approaches to substance abuse prevention. In C. Bell & R. Battjes (Eds.), *Prevention research: Deterring drug abuse among children and adolescents.* Washington, DC: NIDA, ADAMHA, PHS, DHHS.

Brannon, B. R., Dent, C. W., Flay, B. R., Smith, G., Sussmann, S., Peute, M. A., Johnson, C. A., and Hansen, W. B. (1989). The television, school, and family project. *Preventive Medicine, 18,* 492–502.

Brindis, C., Morales, S. S., McCarter, V., Wolfe, A. L. (1993). An evaluation study of school-based clinics in California: Major findings, 1985–1991. San Francisco: University of California, Center for Reproductive Health Policy Research, Institute for Health Policy Studies.

Brower, K. J., Blow, F. C., Young, J. P., & Hill, E. M. (1991). Symptoms and correlates of anabolic-androgenic steroid dependence. *British Journal of Addiction, 86,* 759–768.

Bruvold, W. H., & Rundall, T. G. (1988). A meta-analysis and theoretical review of school based tobacco and alcohol intervention programs. *Psychology and Health, 2,* 53–78.

Bry, B. H. (1988). Family-based approaches to reducing adolescent substance use: Theories, techniques, and findings. In E. R. Rahdert (Ed.), *Adolescent drug abuse: Analyses of treatment research* (NIDA Research Monograph 77, pp. 39–68).

Edwards, R. W. (1993). Drug use among 8th grade students is increasing. *International Journal of Addictions, 28,* 1621–1623.

Ellickson, P. L., Hays, R. D., & Bell, R. M. (1992). Stepping through the drug use sequence: Longitudinal scalogram analysis of initiation and regular use. *Journal of Abnormal Psychology, 101,* 441–450.

Ennett, S. T., Ringwalt, C., & Flewelling, R. L. (1993). How effective is Project D.A.R.E.? A review and assessment of D.A.R.E. evaluations. University of California, San Diego, San Diego, CA.

Evans, R. I., & Raines, B. E. (1982). Control and prevention of smoking in adolescents: A psychological perspective. In T. J. Coates, A. C. Petersen, & C. Perry (Eds.), *Promoting adolescent health.* New York: Academic Press.

Evans, R. I., Rozelle, R. M., Mittelmark, M. B., Hansen, W. K., Bane, A., & Havis, J. (1978). Deterring the onset of smoking in children: Knowledge of immediate physiological effects and coping with peer pressure, media pressure, and parent modeling. *Journal of Applied Psychology, 8,* 126–135.

Flay, B. R. (1985). Psychosocial approaches to smoking prevention: A review of findings. *Health Psychology, 4,* 449–488.

Flay, B. R., & Petrakis, J. (1995). The theory of triadic influence: A new theory of health behavior with implications for preventive interventions. In G. L. Albrecht (Ed.), *Advances in medical sociology: Vol IV. A reconsideration of models of health behavior change.* Greenwich, CT: JAI Press.

Goodstadt, M. S. (1980). Drug education: A turn on or a turn off? *Journal of Drug Education, 10,* 89–99.

Goodstadt, M. S. (1986). School-based drug education in North America: What is wrong? What can be done? *Journal of School Health, 56,* 278–281.

Gordon, N. P., & McAlister, A. L. (1982). *Adolescent drinking: Issues and research*. New York: Academic Press.

Government Accounting Office. (1993). "Drug Education: Limited Progress in Program Evaluation." Statement of Eleanor Chelimsky before the Subcommittee on Select Education and Civil Rights, Committee on Education and Labor, House of Representatives., GAO/T-PEMD-93-2.

Graham, J. W., Collins, L. M., Wugalter, S. E., Chung, N. K., & Hansen, W. B. (1991). Modeling transitions in latent stage-sequential processes: A substance abuse use prevention example. *Journal of Consulting and Clinical Psychology, 59*, 1–11.

Hansen, W. B. (1988). Theory and implementation of the social influence model of primary prevention, In K. H. Rey, C. L. Gaegre, & P. Lowery (Eds.), *Prevention research findings: 1988*. Rockville, MD: DHHS, PHS, ADAMHA.

Hansen, W. B. (1992). School-based substance abuse prevention: A review of the state of the art in curriculum, 1980–1990. *Health Education Research, 7*, 403–430.

Hansen, W. B., & Graham, J. W. (1991). Preventing alcohol, marijuana, and cigarette use among adolescents: Peer pressure resistance training versus establishing conservative norms. *Preventive Medicine, 20*, 414–430.

Hansen, W. B., & Rose, L. A. (1995). Recreational use of inhalant drugs by adolescents: A challenge for family physicians *Family Medicine, 27*(b), 383–387.

Hansen, W. B., Rose, L. A., & Dryfoos, J. G. (1993). *Causal factors, interventions and policy considerations in school-based substance abuse prevention*. Report submitted to the Office of Technology Assessment, United States Congress.

Hansen, W. B., Uebersax, J. S., & Rose, L. A. Comparison of postulated mediators of school-based substance use prevention in adolescents: A longitudinal examination. Unpublished.

Hawkins, J. D., Catalano, F. R. & Miller, J. Y. (1992). Factors for alcohol and other drug problems in adolescence and early adulthood: Implications for substance abuse prevention. *Psychological Bulletin, 112*, 64–105.

Hester, R. K., & Miller, W. R. (1988). Empirical guidelines for optimal client–treatment matching. In E. R. Rahdert (Ed.), *Adolescent drug abuse: Analyses of treatment research* (NIDA Research Monograph 77, pp. 27–38).

Hirschi, T. (1969). *Causes of delinquency*. Berkeley: University of California Press.

Hubbard, R. L., Cavanaugh, E. R., Craddock, S. G., & Rachal, J. V. (1985). Characteristics, behaviors, and outcomes for youth in the TOPS. In A. S. Friedman & G. M. Beschner (Eds.), *Treatment services for adolescent abusers* (DHHS Publication No. (ADM) 85-1342, pp. 49–65). NIDA Treatment Research Monograph Series. Washington, DC: U.S. Government Printing Office.

Jessor, R., & Jessor, R. (1977). *Problem behavior and psychosocial development*. New York: Academic Press.

Johnston, L. D., O'Malley, P. M., & Bachman, J. G. (1994). *National survey results on drug use from the Monitoring the Future study, 1975–1993. Volume I: Secondary school students* (DHHS Publication No. (NIH) 94-0000) and *Volume II: College students and young adults* (DHHS Publication No. (NIH) 94-0000). Rockville, MD: National Institute on Drug Abuse.

Kandel, D. B. (1978). Convergence in prospective longitudinal surveys of drug use in normal populations. In D. B. Kandel (Ed.), *Longitudinal research on drug use: Empirical findings and methodological issues*. Washington, DC: Hemisphere.

Kandel, D. B., Yamaguchi, K., & Chen, K. (1992). Stages of progression in drug involvement from adolescence to adulthood: Further evidence for the gateway theory. *Journal of Studies on Alcohol, 53*, 447–457.

Kim, S., McLeoad, J. H., Rader, D., & Johnston, G. (1992). An evaluation of prototype school-based peer counseling program. *Journal of Drug Education, 22*, 37–53.

Kleinman, P. H., Tobler, N. S., Morehouse, E. R., Eschbach, & Kleinman (1992). Comprehensive student assistance in residential settings: Outcome evaluation for 1991–92. Unpublished.

Lawson, G. W. (1992). Twelve-step programs and the treatment of adolescent substance abuse. In G. W. Lawson & A. W. Lawson (Eds.), *Adolescent substance abuse: Etiology, treatment, and prevention* (pp. 165–186). Boulder: Aspen Press.

Leventhal, H., & Cleary, P. D. (1980). The smoking problem: A review of the research and theory in behavioral risk modification. *Psychological Bulletin, 88*, 370–405.

Liddle, H. A., Dakof, G., Diamond, G., Holt, M., Aroyo, J., & Watson, M. (1992). The adolescent module in multidimensional family therapy. In G. W. Lawson & A. W. Lawson (Eds.), *Adolescent substance abuse: Etiology, treatment, and prevention* (pp. 165–186). Boulder: Aspen Press.

McGuire, W. (1972). Social psychology. In P. C. Dodwell (Ed.), *New horizons in psychology.* Middlesex: Penguin Books.

Moskowitz, J. M. (1989). The primary prevention of alcohol problems: A critical review of the research literature. *Journal of Studies in Alcohol, 50,* 54–88.

Moskowitz, J. M., Malvin, J., Schaeffer, G. A., & Schaps, E. (1983). Evaluation of a junior high school student primary prevention program. *Addictive Behavior, 8,* 393–401.

Oetting, E. R., & Beauvais, F. (1987). Peer cluster theory, socialization characteristics, and adolescent drug use: A path analysis. *Journal of Counseling Psychology, 34,* 205–213.

O'Malley, P. M., Bachman, J. G., & Johnston, L. D. (1988). Period, age, and cohort effects on substance use among young Americans: A decade of change, 1976–1986. *American Journal of Public Health, 78,* 1315–1321.

Pentz, M. A., Johnson, C. A., Dwyer, J. H., MacKinnon, D. M., Hansen, W. B., & Flan, B. R. (1989). A comprehensive community approach to adolescent drug abuse prevention: Effects on cardiovascular disease risk behaviors. *Annals of Medicine, 21,* 219–222.

Pentz, M. A., MacKinnon, D. P., Dwyer, J. H., Want, E. Y. I., Hansen, W. B., Flay, B. R., & Johnson, C. A. (1989). Longitudinal effects of the Midwestern Prevention Program (MPP) on regular and experimental smoking in adolescents. *Preventive Medicine, 18,* 304–321.

Pollard, J. A., Horowitz, J. E., & Houle, D. M. (1991). *Student Assistant Program Demonstration Project: Process evaluation.* Technical report. Los Alamitos, CA: Southwest Regional Laboratory.

Rohrbach, L. A., Hansen, W. B., & Pentz, M. A. (1992). Strategies for involving parents in drug abuse prevention: Results from the Midwestern Prevention Program. *American Public Health Association Abstracts, 120,* 263.

Rokeach, M. (1968). *Beliefs, attitudes, and values.* San Francisco: Jossey-Bass.

Schaps, E., DiBartolo, R., Moskowitz, J., Palley, C. S., & Churgin, S. (1981). A review of 127 drug abuse prevention program evaluations. *Journal of Drug Issues, 11,* 17–43.

Schinke, S. P., Gilchrist, L. D., & Snow, W. H. (1985). Skills intervention to prevent cigarette smoking among adolescents. *American Journal of Public Health, 75,* 665–667.

Simpson, D. D., & Sells, S. B. (1982). Evaluation of drug abuse treatment effectiveness: Summary of the DARP follow-up research. In *NIDA treatment research report* (DHHS Publication No. (ADM) 85-1209, pp. 1–17). Washington, DC: U.S. Government Printing Office.

Tarter, R. (1990). Decision-tree for adolescent assessment and treatment planning. *American Journal of Drug and Alcohol Abuse, 16,* 1–46.

Thompson, E. L. (1978). Smoking education programs 1960–1976. *American Journal of Public Health. 68,* 250–257.

Tobler, N. S. (1986). Meta-analysis of 143 adolescent drug prevention programs: Quantitative outcome results of program participants compared to a control or comparison group. *Journal of Drug Issues, 16,* 537–567.

Tobler, N. S. (1995). Meta-analysis of adolescent drug prevention programs. Doctoral Dissertation, State University of New York at Albany, June, 1994. *Dissertation Abstracts International, 55* (11a), UMI-Order Number 9509310.

Treadway, D. C. (1992). Hanging on for dear life: Family treatment of adolescent substance abuse. In G. W. Lawson & A. W. Lawson (Eds.), *Adolescent substance abuse: Etiology, treatment, and prevention* (pp. 141–164). Boulder: Aspen Press.

USDHHS. (1993). Substance Abuse and Mental Health Services Administration: National household survey on drug abuse: Main findings, 1992. Bethesda: U.S. Department of Health and Human Services, Public Health Service, National Institutes of Health.

USDOE. (1992). National Center for Educational Statistics. *The Condition of Education 1992.* Washington, DC.

Wallace, J. M., Jr., Bachman, J. G. (1994). Validity of self-reports in student-based studies on minority populations: Issues and concerns. In M. De La Rosa (Ed.), *Drug abuse among minority youth: Advances in research and methodology* (NIDA Research Monograph). Rockville, MD: National Institute on Drug Abuse.

Wallace, J. M., Jr., Bachman, J. G., O'Malley, P. M., & Johnston, L. D. (1995). Racial/ethnic differences in adolescent drug use: Exploring possible explanations. In G. Botvin, S. Schinke, & M. Orlandi (Eds.), *Drug abuse prevention with multi-ethnic youth.* Sage Publications.

Weber, M. D., Graham, J. W., Hansen, W. B., Flay, B. R., & Johnson, C. A. (1989). Evidence for two paths of alcohol use onset in adolescents. *Addictive Behavior, 14,* 399–408.

8

Suicide and Suicidal Behavior

YIFAT COHEN, ANTHONY SPIRITO, and LARRY K. BROWN

INTRODUCTION

From 1950 to 1982, the death rate from suicide among youth (15 to 24 years old) increased dramatically. The costs associated with suicide are considerable and include direct medical costs for treatment prior to death, medicolegal costs for autopsies, police investigations, and treatment for physical and mental health problems in family survivors. It has been estimated that each youth suicide equals $432,000 of lost economic productivity and 53 years of human life (Weinstein & Saturno, 1989). Despite these statistics and general public alarm, the resources that are available for prevention of suicidal behavior in the United States are scant compared to what is available for the prevention of other injuries such as motor vehicle crashes (Diekstra, 1993).

Possible factors hypothesized to account for the dramatic increase in suicide among youth include social disorganization, migration and mobility, family and personal disorganization, diminished moral values, increased use of drugs and alcohol, and the influence of the media including exposure to violence. Thus, suicide is not a singular entity to be captured with singular solutions. The multiple involved factors define the complexity of the phenomenon, but also provide several points of access for study and intervention. Understanding these factors, the interactions between them and the ways in which they exert their influence are a major public health challenge.

Suicidal Behavior: Definitions

Death is but one possible outcome of a suicidal thought or wish. Suicidal behavior thus refers to a continuum of thoughts, motives, and actions. For some, suicide is not a

YIFAT COHEN, ANTHONY SPIRITO, and LARRY K. BROWN • Brown University School of Medicine and Department of Child and Family Psychiatry, Rhode Island Hospital, Providence, Rhode Island 02903.

Handbook of Adolescent Health Risk Behavior, edited by Ralph J. DiClemente, William B. Hansen, and Lynn E. Ponton. Plenum Press, New York, 1996.

single event but a process beginning with passive suicidal ideation and proceeding through stages of active suicide contemplation, active planning and preparation, and, finally, culminating in a suicide attempt and completion (Bonner & Rich, 1987). For others, a suicide attempt can be the result of long-lasting suicidal ideation with the intent to die, an impulsive act carried out with a readily available method at a time of intense emotional distress, or an indirect way of communicating distress (Kreitman, Smith, & Tan, 1970). Despite some similarities in the precursors to a suicide attempt, it is generally concluded that individuals who commit suicide and those who deliberately, but nonfatally, harm themselves are two separate but overlapping populations.

The generic term *suicidal behavior* variously includes completed suicide, suicide attempts, suicidal gestures, self-injury and self-mutilation with or without suicidal intent, suicide threats, and suicidal ideation. There are a number of other terms for attempted suicide used widely in Europe, including *parasuicide* (Kreitman, Philip, Greer, & Bagley, 1969), *deliberate self-poisoning,* and *deliberate self-harm* (Kessel, 1965). For the purpose of this review, the terms *completed suicide, attempted suicide,* and *suicidal ideation* will be used.

EPIDEMIOLOGY

Completed Suicide

Suicide was the third leading cause of death among 15- to 24-year-olds in the United States in 1990 (National Center for Health Statistics, 1993). As shown in Table 1, rates have increased substantially since 1950.

Rosenberg, Smith, Davidson, and Conn (1987) found that between 1950 and 1980, adolescent suicide rates increased 305% for white males, 241% for nonwhite males, 74% for white females, and 20% for nonwhite females. During the 1980s, suicide rates for adolescents remained high. In 1988, a total of 2059 adolescents 15–19 years old committed suicide in the United States, resulting in a suicide rate of 11.3 deaths per 100,000, and accounting for 14% of all of the deaths in this age group (National Center for Health Statistics, 1991).

Statistics on suicide are generally considered to be underestimates of the true inci-

Table 1. Suicide Rates in Preadolescents
and Adolescents in the United States[a]

	10- to 14-year-olds		15- to 19-year-olds	
Year	M	F	M	F
1950	0.5[b]	0.1	3.5	1.8
1960	0.9	0.2	5.6	1.6
1970	0.9	0.3	8.8	2.9
1980	1.1	0.5	13.4	3.2
1987	1.9	0.6	16.9	3.5

[a]From NCHS (1984); CDC (1995).
[b]Per 100,000.

dence because of failure to report and misclassification of unintentional injuries that might be suicides (e.g., single-car crashes). The increase in the rate of suicide among adolescents during the past 30 years may reflect, at least in part, a change in reporting systems and may still be an underrepresentation if failure to report continues to occur. The extent of the underestimation, which is unknown, is considered insignificant by some researchers (Kleck, 1988) and considered very significant by others (Jobes, Berman, & Josselson, 1987). Males (1991) examined the firearms and poisoning death certificates of adolescents from 1953 through 1987 and concluded that underreporting of youth suicide in the past is possible but not dramatic, and that the increase in teen suicide parallels that of adults. Other researchers, such as Smith (1991), believe that there has been a significant increase in teen suicide and that it has risen at over twice the rate of adults. A death is more likely to be reported as a suicide if preceded by mental illness or suicidal threats (Walsh, Walsh, & Whelan, 1975) and suicidal reportage depends to a large degree on the person who certifies the cause of death. The means of death (e.g., gunshot versus single-car crash) might also determine whether the cause of death is classified as intentional (i.e., a suicide) or unintentional·(Walsh et al., 1975; Warshauer & Monk, 1978). Social pressure may also play a role in not certifying deaths as intentional (Monk, 1987). If there has been a true increase, it may be related to the fact that adolescents in a large cohort appear to be at higher risk of suicide than those in smaller cohorts (Holinger & Offer, 1987).

Suicide Attempts

Suicide statistics account only for suicide attempts that result in death. Nonfatal suicide attempts often go unreported and uncounted. Researchers have estimated that for each suicide there are as many as eight suicide attempts (Rosenberg et al., 1987). National rates for adolescent suicide attempts are not available but data are available from cross-sectional surveys. A Gallup telephone poll conducted in late 1990 surveyed a representative sample of 1152 13- to 19-year-olds in the United States and indicated that 60% of the respondents knew a peer who attempted suicide, 15% had considered attempting suicide, and 6% had attempted suicide (cited in Ackerman, 1993). The Youth Risk Behavior Survey (YRBS), used by the Centers for Disease Control to assess the prevalence of certain health risk behaviors, was administered to a representative sample of 11,631 high school students in 1991. Students reported serious suicidal ideation (27.3%), a specific suicidal plan (16.3%), a suicide attempt (8.3%), and an attempt that resulted in the need for medical attention (2%) (Centers for Disease Control, 1991). Holinger (1990) examined 1988 data and estimated that 15,458 adolescents (10–19 years old) who had attempted suicide actually received medical attention.

Only a few studies have been able to calculate rates of suicide attempts seen in emergency departments. The mean annual suicide attempt rate was approximately 140 per 100,000 for 15- to 19-year-olds and 45 per 100,000 for 10- to 14-year-olds between the years 1979 and 1983 in a suburban area near Chicago (Christoffel, Marcus, Sagerman, & Bennett, 1988). A rate of 316.8 per 100,000 was found for suicide attempts in an 18-month period between 1988 and 1989 in a suburban county of Atlanta for adolescents 15–19 years old (Birkhead, Galvin, Meehan, O'Carroll, & Mercy, 1993). In a recent study (Conrad, 1992) that included high school students, 23% of the students reported self-injurious behavior and 6.7% reported suicide attempts. Other studies have found that from 8.4% of high school students in the Midwest (Smith & Crawford, 1986) to 9% in New York City (Harkavy-Friedman, Asnis, Boeck, & DiFiore, 1987) anonymously report having made a suicide attempt. In his recent epidemiologic review, Diekstra (1993) estimates lifetime prevalence of attempted suicide ranging between 2.2 and 20% among adolescents.

Because there are no central registries for suicide attempts like there are for mortality rates, and because there is great variation in obtaining data about suicide attempts in different geographic areas, it is difficult to make meaningful comparisons. Any change in attempt rates over time is thus also difficult to interpret. In summary, these studies suggest that from 6 to 10% of adolescents attempt suicide, but only a small minority of these attempts come to the attention of the medical system.

EPIDEMIOLOGIC RISK FACTORS

Successful prevention of adolescent suicide requires not only a clear picture of its epidemiology but also knowledge about its risk factors.

Suicide and Gender

Information gathered over the last 50 years indicates that males commit suicide five times more frequently than females, while females attempt suicide three to four times more frequently than males (Rosenberg *et al.*, 1987). These trends are valid at all ages and in many countries, with a few exceptions. In India and Southeast Asia, for example, the majority of suicides are committed by women (Shaffer, 1988). Nonetheless, in most countries, suicide accounts for slightly more than 1% of all female deaths and 2% of male deaths (Monk, 1987). In the United States, suicide rates for adolescent males ranged from 13.6 in 1981 to 16.2 in 1987 (National Center for Health Statistics, 1989). For females, the rates ranged from 3.6 in 1981 to 4.2 in 1987. For 19 countries throughout the world, there has been a significant difference in suicide trends between the sexes over the period 1970–1986 (Diekstra, 1993). Suicide rates among men increased in all age groups, with a mean increase of 70% in adolescents and young adults. Among young women (15–29 years old), most countries reported an average increase of 40%. Interestingly, in the United States and Canada there was a decreased rate of suicide in young women in contrast to the substantial increase in the suicide rate among young men. In the YRBS survey that was conducted among high school students, female students reported suicidal ideation, intentions, and suicide attempts significantly more than male students (CDC, 1991), yet there was not a statistically significant difference between the sexes in the rates of suicide attempts that required medical attention (2.5% for females and 1.6% for males). The genders also differ on the methods used for suicide attempt. Males use more lethal methods, such as firearms and hanging, while females use drug ingestion or wrist cutting. Since 1980, however, females have begun to use firearms more frequently as a means for completing suicide (Rich, Kirkpatrick-Smith, Bonner, & Jans, 1992). One explanation for the difference between the sexes in these suicidal behaviors is stereotypic sex role: it is more acceptable for women to express affect and to act on these feelings, while men are expected to control their feelings. Therefore, it has been suggested that men delay expressing their suicidal feelings and, during this time, plan and find the more lethal methods for the suicide attempt (Rosenthal, 1981). This hypothesis was partially supported in a study of 41 male and 161 female adolescents who had attempted suicide seen in a general hospital (Spirito *et al.*, 1993). There were no differences between males and females in precipitating events of the suicide attempt, suicidal ideation, depression, or hopelessness. Males did, however, report more final acts in anticipation of death and a greater degree of planning the attempt than females.

Suicide and Ethnicity

Data on completed suicide over the past 50 years indicate that whites commit suicide three times more than African-Americans (NCHS, 1989). Since 1960, however, the suicide rate has nearly tripled for African-American males and has doubled for African-American females. For adolescents, the rates for white males increased from 14.3 in 1979 to 17.6 in 1987. For adolescent white females, the suicide rates ranged from 3.4 in 1979 to 4.4 in 1987. For African-American adolescent males, the rates varied between 5.5 in 1979 and 8.9 in 1987. For African-American adolescent females, the suicide rate was 2.1 in 1979 and rose to 2.7 in 1987 (NCHS, 1989).

Ethnic-related differences in suicide rate could be related to a reporting artifact or may reflect social class factors that influence suicidality, or may stem from culture-specific attitudes toward suicide (Shaffer, 1988). The risk factors for suicide may differ for African-American and white youth. African-Americans deal more often with poverty, discrimination, frustration, and anger (Gibbs, 1984). In spite of these risk factors, the suicide rates are lower in African-Americans than in the white population. It has been suggested that there are "protective factors" in the African-American population such as strong family ties, the church, fraternal and social organizations, and community schools, all of which increase social cohesion and mutual support (Gibbs & Hines, 1989). However, because proof of masculinity is highly valued for African-American males, they may use more lethal suicide methods (Gibbs & Hines, 1989). African-American males are more frequently killed by other forms of "accidental" deaths such as drowning, drug overdose, and falling from high buildings. Death might actually be the result of suicidal ideation, with behavior aimed at easing the pain of the family. Gibbs and Hines (1989) suggest that life experiences in school, family, and community are generally more negative and problematic for African-American males than for African-American females and thus they tend to be more vulnerable to the development of psychological and behavioral symptoms associated with suicidal risk.

Suicide was the third leading cause of death for Hispanic youth (15 to 24 years old) in 1990 (NCHS, 1993), yet Hispanic youth have a lower rate of suicide than whites. In five Southwestern states between 1975 and 1980, the Hispanic population suicide rate was less than half that found in the Anglo population; birth in Mexico and Catholicism were found to be protective factors among Mexican-Americans (Sorenson & Golding, 1988). Gender differences in suicidal behavior seem to be significantly less marked among Hispanic teenagers (Shaffer, 1988).

The Native American population has a much larger proportion of adolescents and young adults, which inflates the overall suicide rate (Berlin, 1987). Nonetheless, in 1986, the suicide rate for Native American adolescents was estimated at 26.3/100,000 (U.S. Congress, Office of Technology Assessment, 1990). For Native American and Alaska Native tribes living on reservations, the suicide rate varies greatly, ranging from 8 to 120 per 100,000 (McIntosh, 1983–84). Cluster suicides (i.e., a number of suicides occurring in geographic or temporal proximity) appear to have increased in Native American youth (Earls, Escobar, & Manson, 1990). Alcohol has been shown to play a particularly prominent role in the suicides of Alaskan Natives (Hlady & Middaugh, 1988) and those tribes with high adolescent suicide rates (Berlin, 1987).

More detailed information has been collected from certain tribes. For example, the suicide rate among Zuni adolescents has risen steadily (from 5.6 per 100,000 in 1957 to 32.2 per 100,000 in 1989), despite the perception of suicide as a forbidden act (Howard-Pitney, LaFramboise, Basil, September, & Johnson, 1992). A large proportion (30%) of Zuni adolescents have attempted suicide (Howard-Pitney *et al.*, 1992), with typical gender differences noted: girls attempted suicide two to three times more often than boys. Although the Zuni leaders speculated that the youth at risk for suicide were those who were less integrated into the religious life of the pueblo, no such relationship has been found (Howard-Pitney *et al.*, 1992).

Suicide and Religion

Religion has been variously considered a protective factor or a risk factor for suicide. For example, Levav and Aisenberg (1989) found that Israel had the second lowest rate of suicide of countries in Asia, North America, and Europe. However, of persons 25 and older in Israel, Jews have higher rates of suicide than Arabs. One possible explanation for this finding is that Islam (the religion of most of the non-Jewish population in Israel) regards suicide as homicide. It is unclear as to the extent to which religion affects suicidal behavior among adolescents. However, one survey study (Greening & Dollinger, 1993) found parochial school teenagers less likely to report serious suicide risk than public high school students, suggesting that religious communities can affect attitudes about suicide.

Method of Suicide

Among nonfatal suicide attempts, the most common method used in the United States, at all ages, is drug ingestion. Overdoses, however, only account for a minority of completed suicides. In 1985, adolescents (15–19 years of age) used firearms, hanging, and poisoning 60.4, 19.1, and 16.1%, respectively, in suicides (cited in Holinger, 1990). According to the National Center for Health Statistics (1989), suicide by overdose is more common for female (0.9 in 1987) than male (0.4) adolescents, and the rates for both sexes remained essentially unchanged between 1979 and 1987. Rates are slightly higher for whites (0.7 in 1987) than African-Americans (0.6 in 1987). The use of gases and vapors for completed suicide increased between 1979 (0.6 per 100,000) and 1987 (1.4 per 100,000) among white adolescents of both sexes. The rates have remained the same for African-Americans. The rate of hanging as the means of death in the 15- to 19-year-old group has also increased from 1.4 in 1979 to 1.9 in 1987, more so in whites, particularly white males (2.4 to 3.2).

The age-adjusted rates of suicide by firearms increased between 1953 and 1978, while rates of other methods did not change (Sudak, Ford, & Rushforth, 1984). The rate of suicide by handgun did not change among female teenagers (0.3 per 100,000), and increased slightly for males in the same age group, from 0.9 per 100,000 in 1979 to 1.2 in 1987. Interestingly, the rates of suicide by handguns have increased for white males (0.9 to 1.4) but remained the same (0.7) for adolescent males of all other races. The rates of suicide by "other and unspecified firearms" have increased for male adolescents (8.8 to 9.7) of all races between 1979 and 1987, more so for African-American males (3.1 to 5.5) than white males (8.8 to 9.7). Guns are twice as likely to be found in the homes of adolescents who complete suicide relative to the homes of suicide attempters or psychiatric controls (Brent et al., 1991). The method of storing the gun had no effect on suicide in the Brent et al. (1991) study, suggesting that when firearms are accessible, suicidal adolescents will kill themselves at a 75-fold greater rate (Brent et al., 1991; Rosenberg, Mercy, & Houk, 1991).

Exposure to Suicidal Behavior

Exposure may increase the likelihood of suicide through familiarity with the idea of suicide as an acceptable option to life's problems. In their review of five studies of suicidal behavior in the families of suicidal adolescents, Spirito, Brown, Overholser, and Fritz (1989) found that the suicide rates among family members for those who had attempted suicide were always higher than control groups but not consistently higher than nonsuicidal psychiatric controls. Compared to the general population, however, the risk of completing suicide increases with having a family member who has committed suicide (Roy, 1989), and the risk of attempting suicide increases substantially if there is a family history of suicide attempts (Sorenson & Rutter, 1991).

Persons may also be exposed to suicide indirectly (e.g., by newspaper stories or television shows). Prominent news of a suicide in the media leads to an increase in completed suicides, mainly among youth, during the 1–2 weeks following the news (Phillips & Carstensen, 1986; Shaffer, 1988). It is not known whether imitative suicides are different from cases where imitation is not a factor. Exposure to death by all types of violence, not only suicide, increases the likelihood of subsequent suicides among youth in the community (Davidson, 1989). Failure to report the victim's emotional illness, a victim of high status, and death associated with revenge motives contribute to increased imitation (Davidson & Gould, 1989).

Evidence also supports the connection between fictional suicide stories and subsequent imitative suicides. Gould and Shaffer (1986) examined the different rates of suicide 2 weeks before and 2 weeks after showing four TV movies about suicide and concluded that such programs led to an increase in the suicide rates among adolescents in New York. Phillips and Paight (1987), however, were not able to replicate this finding following airing of the same movies in California and Pennsylvania, though in these states the television program was only shown on one station, perhaps limiting the audience and thus the show's impact.

A recent study (Brent, Kolko, *et al.*, 1993) examined the psychiatric sequelae to the suicide of a peer. Although limited by the high percentage of subjects who refused to participate, the study did not find differences in the rates of suicide attempts between adolescents who were exposed to a peer suicide and an unexposed control group. There was an increase in the rates of depression, suicidal ideation, and posttraumatic stress disorder in the exposed group. It is possible that an increased rate of suicide attempts was made by "acquaintances" not involved directly with the victim, that "imitated" suicide attempts are mediated by depression in vulnerable adolescents, or that increased suicidal behavior only becomes evident after a longer interval.

Seasonal Effects

Among adults, holidays are often considered high-risk periods for suicide. Findings of seasonality are less evident for adolescents. For example, in one study winter holidays and start of summer were found to be the times of the highest suicidal activity among adolescents in a suburban area of Chicago (Christoffel *et al.*, 1988). In other surveys of adolescent suicide attempters in emergency departments, January through March had the highest rates of suicidal activity (Garfinkel, Froese, & Hood, 1982; Spirito, Riggs, *et al.*, 1989).

Suicide and Mental Disorders

The incidence of mental disorders among suicide is determined by review of the victim's health records (Hoberman & Garfinkel, 1988) or by a retrospective interview method, "psychological autopsy" (Brent *et al.*, 1988; Shaffer, 1988). For a psychological autopsy, the family of the victim is interviewed regarding the victim's psychiatric history in order to retrospectively establish a diagnosis. Studies indicate a common pattern of diagnoses, including antisocial behavior, depression, and substance abuse (Hoberman & Garfinkel, 1988; Shaffer, Garland, Gould, Fisher, & Trautman, 1988; Shafii, Carrigan, Whittinghill, & Derrick, 1985). Shaffer *et al.* (1988) found that 85% of all adolescent suicides were male and that antisocial behavior was the most frequent risk factor among males, occurring in 67% of the sample. A family history of suicide (41%), substance abuse (37%), major depression (21%), and prior attempt (21%) were also risk factors for males. Among the small number of female suicides ($n = 17$), depression was the most common risk factor (50%), followed by a family history of suicide (33%), a prior attempt (33%), antisocial behavior (30%), and substance abuse (5%). In a Finnish study of 53 adolescent suicides, 51% were diagnosed with affective disorders, 26% with substance abuse, 17% with conduct disorders, 6% with schizophrenia, and 32% with personality disorders (Marttunen, Aro, Henriksson, & Lonnqvist, 1991).

In a study comparing 27 adolescents who committed suicide to 56 psychiatric inpatients who had seriously considered or attempted suicide, Brent *et al.* (1988) found four risk factors to be more prevalent in those who had completed: bipolar disorder, affective disorder with comorbidity (especially attention-deficit disorder, substance abuse, and conduct disorder), lack of previous mental health treatment, and availability of firearms in the home. Blumenthal and Kupfer (1986) believe that coexistence of antisocial and depressive symptoms is a particularly high-risk combination for youth suicide.

As can be seen in the studies reviewed above, substance abuse is often implicated in both adolescent and adult completed suicide. Drug and alcohol abuse is considered to be a significant risk factor for both completed suicide and attempted suicide because it can have multiple effects on different domains such as affective, cognitive, social, familial, and behavioral (Shaffer, 1988). Brent *et al.* (1988) reported that at least 30% of adolescent suicide completers were intoxicated at the time of death. Hawton, Fagg, Platt, and Hawkins (1993) followed up Scottish suicide attempters (15 to 24 years old) over a 20-year period and compared 62 suicides with 124 subjects who did not go on to complete suicide. The best predictors of completed suicide were a history of substance abuse and multiple inpatient psychiatric admissions.

In some studies, a minority of suicide victims with no apparent psychiatric disorder are reported (Apter *et al.*, 1993; Brent, Perper, Moritz, Baugher, & Allman, 1993). Such youngsters are described as perfectionistic and rigid, and seem to be vulnerable at times of change (Apter *et al.*, 1993; Shaffer, 1988). Brent, Perper, Moritz, Baugher, & Allman (1993) found that those who committed suicide with no apparent psychopathology did differ somewhat from community controls. They were more likely to have past suicidal behavior, familial psychopathology, and legal or disciplinary problems. Thus, it is possible that in the other studies, covert major psychopathology was not discovered on interview or was denied by the family.

Prior Suicide Attempts

Although suicide "completers" and suicide "attempters" are believed to constitute two distinct groups with different risk factors and other characteristics, one of the best predictors of successful suicide is previous suicide attempts (Diekstra, 1989; Spirito, Brown, Overhulser, & Fritz, 1989). One-fifth of all male adolescent suicides and one-third of all female adolescent suicide attempters have made a prior suicide attempt (Shaffer *et al.*, 1988). Among adolescents, male suicide attempters are much more likely to complete suicide than girls (Goldacre & Hawton, 1985; Otto, 1972). Other predictor variables include an active method of attempting suicide such as hanging or shooting (Otto, 1972). Because of stringent criteria for hospitalization, adolescent males admitted to a psychiatric hospital following a suicide attempt may be at extremely high risk for completed suicide (Shaffer *et al.*, 1988).

Prior suicide attempts are also a risk factor because every time an adolescent makes a suicide attempt, there is a risk of serious harm and death. Lewinsohn, Rohde, and Seeley (1993) estimate that suicide attempters have an 8.1-fold increased rate of reattempts compared to adolescents who have never made a suicide attempt. Some studies of children and adolescents (e.g., Kosky, Silburn, & Zubrick, 1990) have shown that suicidal ideators and suicide attempters have comparable levels of psychopathology, particularly among males. It is possible that suicidal ideation may be a significant predictor of suicide for males, similar to attempts for females.

Biological Factors

Biological variables have received increasing attention as factors related to suicidal behavior. Most of the research thus far has been conducted with adults. The area is quite complex, and prone to methodological limitations; consequently, it will only be outlined below (for more detailed reviews of this area see Goodwin & Brown, 1989; Rifai, Reynolds, & Mann, 1992; Roy, 1994; van Praag, 1986). Research to date has been most active in three areas: postmortem tissue analyses, brain chemistry, and cerebrospinal fluid and neuroendocrine correlates. The majority of postmortem brain research has been done on the serotonergic system where modest decreases in serotonin and its metabolite 5-hydroxyindoleacetic acid (5-HIAA) in the brain stem have been found, as well as an increase in $5HT_2$ receptors, regardless of diagnosis.

In studies of suicide attempters, the major neurotransmitter that has been consistently related to suicidal behavior is serotonin. Lower levels of serotonin (5-HIAA) and 5-hydroxytryptophan (5-HTP) have been found in samples of suicide attempters and have been related to further suicidal behavior, impulse dyscontrol, and aggression in both depressed and nondepressed samples (Lidberg *et al.,* 1985; Roy, 1994; Traskman-Bendz *et al.,* 1993; van Praag, 1986). The mechanism by which serotonin levels affect suicidal behavior is unknown but likely interacts with environmental/psychological variables because not all persons with low CSF concentrations attempt suicide (Asberg, 1989). Preliminary research on neuroendocrine markers, including a blunted thyroid-stimulating hormone, abnormal dexamethasone suppression test, and increased urinary free cortisol, suggests a possible relationship between these markers and violent suicides (Meltzer & Lowy, 1989).

Other Risk Factors

In addition to the major risk factors described above, there are a number of individual characteristics associated with psychiatric disorders and implicated in suicidal behavior (see Brent & Kolko, 1990; Spirito, Brown, Overholser, & Fritz, 1989, for review). Two of the most significant individual factors are hopelessness and a history of sexual abuse. Hopelessness is often associated with suicidality in adults and a number of studies have shown hopelessness to be a better predictor of eventual completed suicide than depression (Beck, Brown, Berchick, Stewart, & Steer, 1990; Beck, Brown, & Steer, 1989). Studies with adolescents have also found stronger relationships between suicidal behavior and hopelessness than other factors such as family dysfunction or socioeconomic variables (Levy, Jurkovic, & Spirito, 1995) and anxiety or depression (Steer, Kumar, & Beck, 1993).

One stressful life event particularly important for adolescent suicide behavior is sexual/physical abuse. Deykin, Alpert, and McNamara (1985) and Hoberman and Garfinkel (1988) found an association between suicidal behavior and sexual/physical abuse, the latter authors finding it to be particularly significant in girls. In a study of psychiatrically hospitalized adolescents, Shaunesey, Cohen, Plummer, and Berman (1993) found that a history of abuse was significantly correlated with previous suicide attempts and the general severity of suicidal behavior.

Several adolescent subgroups have been identified as being at high risk for attempted or completed suicide. Two of the most prominent are runaway and gay youth. Runaway youth have a very high rate of attempted suicide, ranging from 30% in one study (Stiffman, 1989) to 37% in another study (Rotheram-Borus, 1993). This high rate is confounded by similarly high rates of behavior disorder and substance abuse. Gibson (1989) reviewed several studies indicating that gay youth report suicidal behavior about three times more frequently than other youth and suicide attempts occur at a higher rate (20–35%) among gay adolescents.

PREVENTION

Suicide can be understood as an end product of an interaction among three major factors: social stressors, vulnerabilities of the individual, and availability of methods. Prevention strategies, whether primary or secondary, are directed toward affecting these factors. These strategies include: (1) establishing community services and encouraging their use; (2) providing educational programs designed to improve problem-solving skills and, ultimately, self-esteem; (3) increasing awareness and knowledge about suicide; and (4) restricting access to potential suicide methods. Although there are substantial epidemiologic and clinical data on suicide, as summarized above, the findings only rarely result in prevention and intervention research. To date, very few suicide prevention strategies have been evaluated empirically, and there is no consensus as to the most effective prevention strategy for suicide (Eddy, Wolpert, & Rosenberg, 1987). Thus, many of the prevention recommendations reviewed below await empirical verification.

Establishing Community Services and Encouraging Their Use

Many suicidal individuals do not come to the attention of mental health or health care professionals; they may be hesitant to use mental health services because of the stigma associated with psychiatric care. Consequently, alternative community services need to be available. Yet, little data on the efficacy of community resources exist beyond that concerning telephone crisis lines. About 1000 crisis programs operate in the United States, 200 of which are specifically designated as suicide prevention centers. The majority of these programs serve individuals other than adolescents (Comstock, Simmons, & Franklin, 1989), and 80% of these centers are staffed by nonprofessionals. A recent review suggests that suicide prevention centers do attract populations at high risk for suicide (Dew, Bromet, Brent, & Greenhouse, 1987). But, it is not certain that such centers have an appreciable effect on community suicide rates. Dew et al. (1987) did not demonstrate such an effect in their meta-analysis, while Miller, Coombs, Leeper, and Barton (1984) found suicide rates reduced only for certain types of crisis line users, specifically white females under 24 years of age, suggesting that it may be an effective prevention strategy for adolescent girls.

Shaffer et al. (1988), in their critical review of suicide prevention programs for teenagers, found only two evaluations of crisis services. They concluded that hot lines have limited impact on adolescents for the following reasons: the population at highest risk is not reached, teenagers are less aware of the existence of hot lines than adults (which might be rectified by advertising hot lines in high schools; Slem & Cotler, 1973), and the staff may be limited in knowledge and skills specific to suicidal behavior (Knowles, 1979). Other problems that might limit the benefit of hot lines include the difficulty of building a rapport over the phone, having too little control of the situation, lack of a structured and reliable risk assessment protocol, and confidentiality rules which limit staff actions (Stelmachers, Smith, & Wells, 1990).

Other types of community services in addition to crisis lines might assist in prevention. Establishing community services that will help families to cope with major stressors may also be helpful in suicide prevention. Suicide prevention programs can be developed at community sites where high-risk behaviors and circumstances related to suicide (such as poverty, violent behavior, and substance abuse) are common. Also desirable is designing specific interventions for selected groups such as substance abusers, runaway youth, school dropouts, young delinquents, and adolescents who were exposed to suicidal behavior within their families or their peer group (especially cases of cluster suicides). Community outreach efforts may be useful in encouraging high-risk individuals, particularly school dropouts, to receive appropriate treatment. Collaboration among mental health, medical, educational, and criminal justice programs should be encouraged at these community sites.

Although cluster suicides account for only 1 to 5% of youth suicides (Gould, Wallenstein, Kleinman, O'Carroll, & Mercy, 1990), they might be the most preventable of all suicides if communities are prepared. Surveillance procedures for suicidal behavior allow communities to be ready to intervene quickly in cases of suspected suicide contagion (Rosenberg *et al.*, 1987). The Centers for Disease Control and Prevention have developed guidelines to assist communities in development of a response program to suicide clusters. The recommendations include: plan the response before the onset of a cluster; include all concerned sectors of the community, identify the relevant community; identify and assess high-risk persons; provide accurate, consistent, and appropriate information to the media without disclosing the detailed nature of the suicide methods used; and provide a list of support services in the community (O'Carroll, Mercy, & Steward, 1988).

Improving Diagnosis and Treatment by Health Care Professionals

It is important that primary care physicians be better educated about the problem of adolescent suicide. Hodgman and Roberts (1982) found that only 21% of pediatricians in their survey routinely included questions about suicidal behavior in their interviewing of patients. The use of scales to assess suicidal behavior or risk factors such as depression might be helpful in general practice, as would having a detailed policy in dealing with potentially suicidal adolescents. Educating health care providers should focus on expanding knowledge regarding suicide risk factors such as depression, substance abuse, antisocial behavior, and previous suicidal behavior. Similar education is needed for medical students, residents, pediatricians, family medicine, and emergency medicine (Blumenthal & Kupfer, 1986), as well as nurses (especially school nurses) and other paraprofessionals (Holinger, 1989).

Educating and increasing the number of mental health professionals familiar with the assessment and treatment of suicidal behavior in youth is indicated as a way of preventing suicides associated with psychiatric disorders. Surprisingly, Bongar and Harmatz (1989) found that less than 50% of clinical psychology graduate programs include the subject of suicide in their formal programs. Thus, mental health professionals also need more training in detection and management of potentially suicidal youth (Bongar & Harmatz,

1989). Targeting high-risk youth and designing specific interventions for selected groups such as substance abusers, runaways, and school dropouts might be especially important. Professionals who work with such at-risk adolescents in settings such as detention facilities, runaway shelters, and substance abuse programs should be well educated about suicidal behavior. Such programs have been established and found to be effective at improving clinical skills (Cox, McCarty, Landsberg, & Paravati, 1990).

Increasing Awareness via Education and the Media

A laudable but elusive goal of suicide prevention is to reach individuals prior to the suicidal act. A large proportion of high school students are exposed to peers with suicidal feelings (Nelson, 1988). Thus, adolescents play an important role in prevention via identification and referral. There are a number of approaches to suicide prevention in schools. These include didactic lectures, peer counseling, screening, consultation, school personnel programs, and parent programs (Davis, Sandoval, & Wilson, 1988). Establishing school district policies regarding suicide, and integrating school and community mental health interventions have been advocated (Davis *et al.*, 1988).

Education in schools about emotions, so-called affective education, can help adolescents become aware of potential psychological stresses, be alert to the signs and symptoms that can precede suicide, and teach the steps necessary to identify and help at-risk adolescents. Affective education can sometimes be therapeutic by increasing self-awareness and encouraging a friend's intervention (Rosenberg, Eddy, Wolpert, & Broumas, 1989). Most programs aim to increase awareness of suicide, dispel myths, promote case-finding, provide information about availability of mental health resources, and help others with such feelings. In addition, many programs also teach students methods to deal with their own suicidal feelings. For example, Joan (1986) uses written material, discussion, clarification, nonjudgmental listening, relevant films, role-playing, self-revelation, and "life skills" practice. The goals of this program include helping the students to define their feelings, understanding the ways suicidal thoughts may develop, providing ways to cope with depression and suicidal feelings, stimulating thinking and talking openly about difficult feelings, and encouraging students to seek help.

Despite their intuitive appeal, the efficacy of these suicide prevention programs is, at best, modest. Shaffer, Garland, Underwood, and Whittle (1987) studied the effects of three different school-based prevention programs and did not find an increase in knowledge about risk factors. There was a significant increase in the proportion of students who admitted to personal difficulties, suicidal thoughts, or the need for professional help. Misperceptions about suicide were not changed by the programs and there were no general differences in outcome between programs. One possible reason for the lack of more substantial effects is that these programs were only 3 hours long. A recent study of a 14-hour experimental program in Israel (Orbach & Bar-Joseph, 1992) reported a mild reduction of suicidal feelings and hopelessness. Girls seemed to benefit more than boys, and those students with greater suicidal tendencies improved more than their peers.

Although subject to methodological criticism because they are based on adolescent self-report data, other investigators have also found rather modest results. These studies suggest that knowledge may improve from such educational efforts, but that attitudes about suicide and behavior are largely unaffected immediately following the education (Shaffer *et al.*, 1987; Spirito, Overholser, Ashworth, Morgan, & Benedict-Drew, 1988) and at 18-month follow-up (Vieland, Whittle, Garland, Hicks, & Shaffer, 1991). Shaffer *et al.* (1990) found that suicide awareness programs may be viewed most negatively by adolescents who have made a prior suicide attempt. Final conclusions about the effectiveness of different programs cannot be established until assessment of suicidal behavior and help-seeking behavior is incorporated in future evaluation studies (Garland & Zigler, 1993). To be most helpful, specific programs targeting particular groups of adolescents (e.g., males versus females, attempters versus nonattempters, depressed versus nondepressed) will need to be developed (Overholser, Hemstreet, Spirito, & Vyse, 1989).

Berman and Jobes (1991) suggest that prevention programs that focus on general mental health interventions such as social skills training, problem-solving, crisis management, and anger control may be more beneficial than programs focusing only on suicide. However, Shaffer *et al.* (1988), in their review, found that only a minority of the school-based programs were designed to improve teenagers' coping skills by training in stress management. For adolescents without psychiatric disorders, the examination of maladaptive methods adolescents use when faced with difficult life situations and establishment of programs to improve problem-solving and coping skills may be helpful (Hawton, 1986). Improvement in ability to manage a crisis may result in a decrease of personal vulnerability and prevent the escalation of minor crises (Johnson & Maile, 1987). School-based approaches may include simulation training, providing other options to respond to specific situations, awareness of one's own emotional response patterns, and general stress-reducing techniques. O'Roark (cited in Johnson & Maile, 1987) suggested four skills that should be part of such school curriculum: developing self-esteem, developing efficient communication skills about feelings, building the concept of "positive failure" which stresses the importance of effort and not just accomplishment, and dealing with loss and grief. When these types of programs are widely available, the atmosphere in the schools may contribute to the development of productive social interactions, establish peer group and family networking, and facilitate supportive teacher–student interactions. Such programs still await empirical verification.

As previously discussed, the media may contribute to imitative suicides for adolescents. Media guidelines have been prepared by the Centers for Disease Control (CDC, 1994b; O'Carroll *et al.*, 1988) to decrease media-induced imitative events. The CDC's suggestions include: limiting the description of the suicide method, limiting the amount of media coverage, providing the telephone numbers of crisis centers or mental health agencies as a public service, and establishing a specific mental health liaison with the media (Davidson & Gould, 1989). The media can also be used in a proactive way to inform viewers about health problems that are connected with suicidal behavior and to provide education regarding the importance of early detection of risk factors. Educational programs also may help to decrease the stigma about emotional problems and the use of mental health services. Public service announcements about some health topics are effective, such as crime (O'Keefe & Mendelsohn, 1984), but others may even have an unwanted effect (Plant, Pirie, & Kreitman, 1979). Use of a knowledgeable, identifiable spokesperson focusing on scientific facts; presenting alternatives; repeating the message;

and supplementing all of these efforts through other media have been suggested as ways to increase the efficacy of public service announcements (Flay & Sobel, 1983).

Restricting Access to Methods

Primary prevention of suicide involves reducing access to the means. Examples include building fences around tall buildings and detoxifying domestic gas (Lester, 1990). Firearms were the most commonly used method in completed suicide in 1987, accounting for 7.5/100,000 cases of suicide or 59% of all cases in 1987 (NCHS, 1990). The use of this method has increased dramatically (Boyd, 1983; Saltzman, Levenson, & Smith, 1988). Brent, Perper, Moritz, Baugher, and Allman (1993) examined the characteristics of suicide in adolescents with no apparent psychopathology and found that the presence of a loaded gun in their homes distinguished these suicides from the comparison groups. They concluded that for suicides in which impulsivity is a major determinant, preventing access to methods might be the most beneficial prevention strategy. In two other studies by this group (Brent, Perper, & Allman, 1987; Brent et al., 1991), it was demonstrated that availability of firearms, especially in youth who use alcohol, may increase the risk of suicide.

The extent of the impact of restricting availability of firearms on suicide rates is not clear. Sloan, Rivara, Reay, Ferris, and Kellermann (1990) found lower rates of suicide by firearms in Vancouver, Canada, compared to Washington State where the regulations for possessing guns are less restrictive. Nevertheless, they found higher rates of suicide by other methods in Vancouver in almost all age groups except youth, i.e., 15- to 24-year-olds. Lester and Murrell (1982) also reported increased suicide rates by other methods in areas where the use of firearms was restricted. Rich, Young, Fowler, Wagner, and Black (1990) reported that 5 years after the enactment of Canadian gun control legislation, there was a decrease in the use of guns by suicidal men but an increase in suicide by leaping. However, another study (Loftin, McDowell, Wiersema, & Cottey, 1991) found a reduction in suicide rates by firearms and no increase in suicide rates by other methods in Washington, D.C. after restrictive handgun regulations were implemented in 1976. Thus, restrictive gun regulations may contribute to a reduction of suicide rates in some suicidal youth. There are several possible ways to restrict firearms including a mandatory waiting period, check of backgrounds, possibly even psychiatric history, and licensing of gun holders (Cantor, 1989; Holinger, 1989). Also, parents may be influenced to take more precautions through the dissemination of information about the risk of keeping firearms in the home (Shaffer et al., 1988).

While handguns are the most common means of completed suicide, overdoses are the most common method of suicide attempts and the fourth most common method of completed suicide (NCHS, 1990). In Australia (Oliver & Hetzel, 1972), restricting number of tablets per prescription for sedative-hypnotics resulted in a reduction of suicide rates. Suggestions for reducing or mitigating access to potentially fatal drugs include: restriction of the number of tablets permitted for each prescription (Cantor, 1989), selling antidote or emetic tablets with tricyclic antidepressants in case the person changes his or her mind or is found shortly after overdosing (Holinger, 1990), developing computer networks to record recent medication purchases in order to prevent patients from stockpiling dangerous medications (Holinger, 1990), educating physicians regarding prescribing potentially lethal medications (e.g., tricyclic antidepressants) to high-risk patients (Davidson, 1987), and educating parents about the need to dispose of unused drugs in medicine cabinets.

Estimating the Effectiveness of Prevention Programs

Eddy *et al.* (1987) asked 29 experts to evaluate the effectiveness of six different suicide prevention strategies for youth with three different personality types: depressive, manic-depressive, and "impulsive-aggressive." The strategies included school-based screening, crisis centers and hot lines, affective education, and restriction of access to firearms, medications, and high places. There was a great deal of uncertainty even among experts in terms of prevention effectiveness and none was rated as having a definitive impact. The expected reduction of suicide rate by each of the strategies was between 1 and 16%, and it was estimated that even if all of the programs were used simultaneously, the reduction rate would only be between 15 and 50%. There was no method that was rated significantly more effective than the other and there was no specific basis for choosing which program would be most effective.

The effectiveness of suicide prevention programs is dependent on many factors. There may be a differential response to various prevention strategies based on an individual's specific psychiatric disorder, e.g., depression versus conduct disorder. Similarly, age, race, cultural, and family factors may affect outcomes. Also, as a suicide is often accompanied by a wide variety of other problems, it is difficult to consider it as a unitary phenomenon. Outcome research is made difficult by the mobility of youth, the lack of good surveillance systems, and ethical dilemmas concerning the use of control groups. Nonintervention groups, however, are essential in order to determine the effectiveness of programs.

A major problem in evaluating the efficiency of prevention programs has been the lack of ongoing data collection systems of suicide attempts, which is a major risk factor for completed suicide. Birkhead *et al.* (1993) implemented one of the first active, population-based public health surveillance systems for detecting suicide attempts. Their study included four emergency departments serving a population of 426,000. They concluded that emergency department-based surveillance for attempted suicide is feasible. National surveillance systems would allow trends in suicidal behavior to be monitored, as well as assist in determining the effects of specific local prevention programs. Surveillance systems could be installed in emergency departments, psychiatric hospitals, and private physicians' offices. The data obtained in these different settings could be shared to improve collaboration and quality of prevention and intervention.

In order to improve surveillance, a uniform definition of the different suicidal behaviors is critical. Criteria by Rosenberg *et al.* (1988) have been published to assist coroners and medical examiners on classification of suicide. Systematic training of coroners to ensure better identification of suicide cases would also be helpful. For example, cases of "accidental poisoning" and single-car crashes may be suicides (Monk, 1987). Greater information on the death certificate about psychiatric history is essential. Finally, establishment of community-based registries of suicide attempts would also enhance surveillance (National Committee for Injury Prevention and Control, 1989).

Comstock, Simmons, and Franklin (1989) analyzed the findings from 396 prevention programs for suicidal adolescents including hot lines, school-based programs, walk-in clinics, hospital-based emergency programs, crisis interventions in mental health centers, and support groups for survivors of suicide. They concluded that such programs are generally not centralized, do not keep adequate records to assess outcome, are not visible enough, and lack certification and written standards for the services. Other major problems that were identified included the lack of networking in case coordination and in delivery of services; the need to deal with parents who do not cooperate with their child's need for professional help; and the lack of specific services such as inpatient and residential treatment beds for adolescents. These factors make evaluation extremely complicated and may explain why there are very little empirical data on suicide prevention among youth. The Centers for Disease Control has published a summary of the evidence for the effectiveness of eight different suicide prevention strategies which serves as a useful guide for prevention (CDC, 1994a).

TREATMENT

There are diverse approaches to the prevention of the onset of suicidal behavior, any of which may have some impact. It appears that the more efficacious programs target high-risk individuals and groups. In this section, we focus primarily on interventions with those who have attempted suicide as a high-risk group but also describe some interventions used with other high-risk groups such as those with suicidal ideation, depressed adolescents, and substance abusers.

Because there is a high reattempt rate and because mortality of suicide attempts increases with the number of attempts, suicide attempters are a high-risk group (McIntire, Angle, Wickoff, & Schlict, 1977). Many can be readily located, as they visit emergency rooms, and clinicians do not have to be concerned about introducing the "idea" of suicide in an otherwise nonsuicidal person (Shaffer & Bacon, 1989).

Every adolescent who makes a suicide attempt should receive a thorough evaluation and a therapeutic plan should be formulated with the aid of a family member (Trautman & Shaffer, 1989). Assessment should include the adolescent and his or her family. The home environment should be evaluated carefully for identifying stressors and psychopathology. Direct questioning of the young patient about suicidal thoughts, intentions, and plans is a crucial part of the interview at all ages (Blumenthal, 1988). The immediate goal of the evaluation is to determine whether the young suicidal person requires hospital admission based on persistent suicidal ideation, a major psychiatric disorder that cannot initially be treated as an outpatient, or psychosocial problems that prevent adequate protection of the child. The clinical assessment should also identify the risk factors that are associated with suicidal behavior so they can be the target of therapy. Hawton (1986) outlines nine areas that should be included in an evaluation of a suicide attempter: precipitating events (including whether they are acute or chronic), suicidal intent/reasons for attempt, current problems, psychiatric disorder, family history, previous psychiatric disorder or suicidality, coping strategies/social supports, risk of a reattempt, and attitudes of the adolescent and family toward further treatment. The reader is referred to Hawton (1986) for details regarding the assessment of these important areas. In sum, assessment guides two types of intervention: one addressing the current suicidal behavior in order to prevent another serious suicide attempt, and the other addressing factors that are known to be connected with increased suicide risk, e.g., depression and substance abuse.

If an adolescent who attempts suicide is judged to be in imminent danger for suicide unless monitored in a structured and protected environment, psychiatric hospitalization is necessary. Indications include an inability to maintain a no-suicide contract, a plan for completing suicide, a suicide attempt with high intentionality or lethality, a psychiatric disorder that is associated with increased suicide risk (e.g., psychosis, severe depression, or substance abuse), noncompliance with or failure of prior outpatient treatment, a severe parental psychiatric disorder, and inability or unwillingness of parents to monitor or protect the patient (Brent & Kolko, 1990).

The large majority of adolescents who attempt suicide can be treated as outpatients. Unfortunately, many adolescents and their families will not follow through with outpatient treatment. Trautman and Rotheram-Borus (1987) studied a sample of mostly minority females in a large urban hospital and found that of 76 cases, 14.5% never kept an outpatient appointment, 38% went to one or two appointments, and only 32% were seen three or more times. Spirito *et al.* (1992) followed up 78 adolescents seen in an emergency department and discharged home: 17.5% never attended an outpatient appointment, 11.5% went only once, 2.6% went twice, and 23.1% went to only three or four sessions. The consistency between these two studies demonstrates the significance of treatment nonattendance among adolescent suicide attempters seen in emergency departments. A recent study underscores how problematic treatment compliance is for adolescent suicide attempters. Trautman, Stewart, and Morishima (1993) reported that adolescent suicide attempters and nonsuicidal adolescents with other problems stopped outpatient psychiatric treatment against medical advice at the same rate, i.e., 77%. However, survival analyses indicated that suicide attempters dropped out of outpatient psychotherapy much more quickly than nonsuicidal troubled adolescents (median survival before drop-out: 3 sessions for attempters and 11 sessions for nonsuicidal adolescents). On the other hand, discharged suicide attempters (i.e., cases where there was a mutual decision between therapist and adolescent to terminate psychotherapy) attended significantly more appointments (M = 11.6) than dropouts.

Treatment noncompliance is of particular concern because these adolescents are at high risk. Spirito *et al.* (1992) found a reattempt rate of 6% at 1 month and 10% at 3 months among adolescents seen in an ED following a suicide attempt. The findings on treatment follow-up indicate that it is critical that additional steps be taken by personnel in the ED to facilitate the referral process. Personnel can emphasize the importance of treatment, set a specific date for the follow-up appointment that will be soon after the emergency visit, be clear about the reasons for follow-up as well as about the problems of the patient, and specify the goals of therapy (preferably brief) (Trautman & Rotheram-Borus, 1988). Because of the high rate of noncompliance, development and implementation of brief hospital-based treatment programs for suicide attempters, or intervention with the person who accompanies the suicide attempter has been recommended (Baker, 1989).

Psychotherapy with Adolescent Suicide Attempters

Brief crisis intervention is invariably needed in the beginning of treatment to deal with the suicidal crisis. The initial goal of such intervention is to protect the adolescent from self-harm by restricting access to available means, making a "no-suicide" agreement, decreasing isolation, decreasing perturbation, understanding the goal of the suicidal behavior, and establishing a working alliance (Berman & Jobes, 1991). The most frequent treatment approach for the suicidal adolescent is still individual psychotherapy on an outpatient basis (Berman & Jobes, 1991). The theoretical basis of the therapy depends primarily on the training of the therapist, while the length of treatment depends on therapy orientation, the severity of pathology, the patient's reaction to treatment, and health insurance limitations. Pfeffer (1991) has suggested some general principles for psychotherapy with suicidal youth. These include developing a trustful atmosphere, keeping an empathic but objective concept of the suicidal patient, focusing on the motivation for the suicidal behavior, and discussing new coping strategies. Other factors that are important in therapy include reassurance and modification of hopelessness, alteration of cognitive rigidity, use of indicated pharmacotherapy, and education of the patient and family about suicide (Blumenthal & Kupfer, 1989).

Several specific treatment modalities have been recommended for suicidal adolescents. Cognitive therapy is thought to be suitable for adolescents because it is systematic, highly structured, and didactic (Trautman, 1989). Indeed, several studies have demonstrated the utility of this treatment approach with depressed adolescents (e.g., Reynolds & Coates, 1986). Cognitive distortions, often seen in adolescent suicide attempters, can be addressed directly using this modality. In addition, a systematic approach to teaching problem-solving often is effective for adolescents who define problems as unsolvable and then attempt suicide. Descriptions of the problem-solving approach can be found in Brent and Kolko (1990) as well as Overholser and Spirito (1990). Adding behavioral treatments (e.g., role-playing) to the cognitive techniques may be particularly useful with adolescent suicide attempters in individual psychotherapy (Brent & Kolko, 1990; Hawton, 1986; Overholser & Spirito, 1990). Brent and Kolko (1990) also mention two other specific treatment approaches, the first of which is social skills training, based on the notion that many adolescent suicide attempters have trouble with interpersonal problem-solving and may use a suicide attempt in a coercive manner for interpersonal gain. Second, self-control techniques for affect reduction, especially in the regulation of anger, may be useful.

Although empirical trials of these approaches are under way, almost no data are currently available to support any of these approaches with suicide attempters. Rotheram-Borus, Piacentini, Miller, Graae, and Castro-Blanco (1994) describe a brief (six sessions) cognitive-behavioral treatment for adolescent suicide attempters and their families in an outpatient setting. The treatment consists of a series of structured activities that create a positive family atmosphere, teaches problem-solving strategies, reformulates the family perception of their problems from focusing on difficult individuals to focusing on difficult situations, and builds confidence in the mental health professionals. The therapy uses both behavioral techniques such as behavioral contracting, therapist modeling, and structured role-playing, as well as cognitive techniques such as restructuring and reframing. Preliminary findings suggest a reliable and well-accepted modality but outcome data are still being collected. Several data-based studies with adults are available. Salkovskis, Atha, and Storer (1990) report a randomized intervention trial with adults in which cognitive-behavioral treatment was slightly superior to standard care in reducing repeat suicide attempts over the 6 months of treatment. Patsiokas and Clum (1985) used a similar approach as Salkovskis *et al.* (1990) and found that cognitive-behavioral treatment reduced hopelessness more than nondirective treatment at follow-up but there was no difference between the groups in change of suicidal ideation or intention.

The family should be involved in treatment, whether through formal family therapy or being seen collaterally as part of the adolescent's treatment. Involving parents usually improves compliance, allows opportunity to explore family conflict (often the precipitating factor in adolescent suicide attempts), and helps enlist parents to ensure the safety of the high-risk adolescent (Brent & Kolko, 1990). When parents are seen collaterally, the therapist must be careful to maintain the adolescent's confidentiality and therapeutic alliance. Family therapy shifts the focus of attention from the attempter to the family so that conflictual issues which have presumably contributed to the development of the suicidal behavior can be investigated (Richman, 1979). Specific family training programs in communication skills and problem-solving which have been shown to be effective in reducing family conflict (Robin, 1981) are applicable to work with the families of adolescent suicide attempters.

Psychopharmacology is suggested for psychiatric disorders such as major depression, bipolar affective disorder, and psychosis underlying suicidal behavior. Also, medication should be considered in cases where symptom reduction might help the adolescent to be more accessible and receptive to other modes of therapy (Berman & Jobes, 1991). As with other modalities of treatment, psychopharmacological treatment has not been well studied. In cases where medication is prescribed, careful monitoring of its administration to the suicidal adolescent is essential.

Outcome Studies

Several systematic studies of treatment for adult suicide attempters have been published. Based on reattempt rates, no single treatment has proven superior to the others. Greer and Bagley (1971) found that patients who participated in outpatient therapy were less likely to reattempt suicide than those who did not receive treatment. Welu (1977) reported better compliance with outpatient treatment and fewer repeat attempts by providing outreach following a suicide attempt.

Despite the positive findings reviewed above, other researchers have found no difference in repeat suicide attempts among suicide attempters who did or did not receive intensive outreach (Chowdhury, Hicks, & Kreitman, 1973; Ettlinger, 1975; Gibbons, Butler, Urwin, & Gibbons, 1978). Liberman and Eckman (1981) compared intensive behavior therapy versus insight-oriented therapy during an inpatient stay. The behavior therapy group had significantly fewer suicidal thoughts and threats at follow-up, but the reattempt rate did not differ across the two groups. This was also true of one of the few controlled intervention studies with adolescents. In a nonrandomized intervention trial, Deykin, Hsieh, Joshi, and McNamara (1986) assigned a social worker to adolescent suicide attempters seen in an emergency room. The social worker helped the adolescents keep their follow-up appointments, provided support, and explored potential services available to the adolescent. Adolescents in the experimental group were twice as likely as controls to comply with medical recommendations and less likely to have future visits to the emergency room because of suicidal behaviors. However, there was no effect on repeat suicide attempts after adjustment for prior history of suicidal behavior. Group therapy for psychiatrically hospitalized suicidal adolescents was described by Ross and Motto (1984), who reported no suicides or reattempts during a follow-up period of 2 years. There was no comparison group included in this study, although the successful outcome is in contrast to the other intervention studies reviewed above.

Treatment of High-Risk Groups

There are a number of high-risk subgroups for attempted and completed suicide: gay youth; minority youth; those with suicidal ideation; psychiatrically hospitalized youth; and those with high-risk psychiatric disorders such as depression, substance abuse, conduct disorder, and borderline personality disorder. However, there are only a few examples of interventions with these high-risk groups that have assessed the effects on suicidal ideation or attempts. For example, Rotheram-Borus and Bradley (1991) describe a screening and intervention approach for suicidal runaways seen at community agencies which reduced the number of suicide attempts after implementation. Because of the small number of studies with high-risk groups, both descriptive and data-based studies are reviewed below.

Gay Youth

Although gay youth are apparently at high risk for suicidal behavior, to date there have not been any intervention studies that have specifically examined suicidal behavior in this group. Suggested ways to reduce suicidal risk include change in society's stigmatization of homosexuals, increased acceptance and understanding by families, and access to the same social support systems and recreational activities that other youth have available. Professional counseling that will be sensitive and familiar with the specific needs and problems of this population has also been advocated (Gibson, 1989).

Minority Groups

Because of major differences in social, economic, political, and cultural factors that might influence suicidal behavior, specific programs for minority groups have been recommended. In contrast to the numerous prevention programs developed for different minority groups, there are very few intervention programs and none have been controlled outcome studies.

Intervention programs should be based on the understanding of the cultural values and social structural factors that contribute to suicide (Yu, Chang, Liu, & Fernandez, 1989). In one group of Native Americans, tribal elders have conducted group sessions about leadership for adolescents who have attempted suicide in a boarding school. On another Native American reservation, suicidal adolescents were placed in a residential facility and were trained to perform specific community services (Ward, 1984). There are also examples of specific interventions for Native Americans while in jail, in residential alcohol treatment programs, after apprehension by the police for first-time alcohol abuse, and after dropping out of school (Berlin, 1987; Snyder, 1981). All of these adolescents are at high risk for suicide but suicidal behavior was not specifically examined by the programs.

Research concerning suicide among Asian-American youth is sparse. Specific characteristics that have been suggested to influence suicide among Asian-American youth include a need to excel for the purpose of bringing their parents glory and not shame, the parental pressure for success, identity problems, value discrepancies between the immigrant parents and the large society, and a lack of immediate familial support.

Baker (1989) suggested several intervention strategies regarding suicide among African-American youth including focusing on conflict resolution in the family, helping youth discern the factors they can and cannot control in society which constitute a source of their frustration, and increasing support from the extended family and community groups such as churches and social clubs.

Psychiatrically Hospitalized Youth

A lack of apparent benefit from treatment for suicidal behavior was found by Brent, Kolko, *et al.* (1993), who studied 134 adolescent psychiatric inpatients. Almost 10% of subjects repeated the suicide attempt within 6 months of discharge from the hospitalization despite their receiving treatment during the follow-up period.

Suicide Ideators

Lerner and Clum (1990) compared the effectiveness of social problem-solving therapy to supportive therapy in treating 18 suicidal ideators 18–24 years old. The intervention was based on the assumption that the key deficit in suicidal individuals is poor interpersonal problem-solving skills. The problem-solving therapy group was more effective in reducing depression, hopelessness, and loneliness at 3-month follow-up than the supportive group, but was not significantly different than supportive therapy in reducing suicidal ideation.

Suicidal Youth with Psychiatric Disorders

Because the majority of those who complete suicide have a psychiatric disorder, treating the underlying psychiatric disorder should reduce the risk for suicidal behavior in this population of patients (Brent & Kolko, 1990).

Depressive Disorders

Short-term group therapy combining both a traditional discussion format and social skills training has been described as a treatment for depressed adolescents (Fine *et al.*, 1989). A randomized clinical trial of cognitive-behavioral group treatment for adolescents has been reported by Lewinsohn, Clarke, Hops, and Andrews (1990). Fourteen 2-hour sessions were held over a 20-week period. Compared to wait-list control subjects, the adolescents in the experimental group improved significantly on the depression measures, and these improvements were maintained at the 2-year follow-up period. Suicidal behavior was not assessed as an outcome variable. Antidepressant medication is often prescribed for adolescents, but controversy as to its efficacy exists (Ambrosini, Bianchi, Rabinovich, & Elia, 1993).

Substance Abuse

Specific interventions for young substance abusers who are also suicidal have yet to be described in the literature. Interventions that are considered beneficial for substance-abusing youth include a large specialized service that includes vocational rehabilitation and educational programs for school dropouts (Friedman & Glickman, 1986) or specific cognitive treatment approaches (Kosten, Rounsaville, & Kleber, 1986) that might easily be adapted to include an emphasis on suicidal behavior.

Conduct Disorder

Youth remanded to adult correctional facilities are reported to be at very high risk for suicide and therefore need to be carefully evaluated for suicidal behavior as well as for comorbid disorders such as depression and/or substance abuse (Earls et al., 1990). Although this is a particularly difficult group to treat, certain psychosocial, cognitive-behavioral, and family therapy treatments have been somewhat effective. For example, the effects of problem-solving skills training and parent management training were evaluated in a population of children with severe antisocial behavior (Kazdin, Siegel, & Bass, 1992). Many changes in child and family functioning were reported, but no measure for suicidal behavior was included.

Borderline Personality Disorder

Fine and Sansone (1990) emphasized the need to differentiate between acute and chronic suicidal behavior. In young adults, especially women, chronic suicidal behavior often coexists with borderline personality disorder (BPD). Zich (1984) hypothesized that repeated suicidal behavior among individuals with BPD is a way to control their interpersonal environment by coercive measures (Patterson & Reid, 1970). Based on this model, a major focus of treatment—particularly during hospitalization—should be teaching alternative response styles and help-seeking behaviors, i.e., ways to secure social reinforcement by other than coercive means.

Linehan et al. (1991) developed a cognitive-behavioral therapy for female suicide attempters diagnosed with BPD. Linehan's therapy is based on a biosocial theory that views parasuicide as problem-solving behavior in individuals with emotion dysregulation and an invalidating environment. The therapy involves a combination of individual psychotherapy focusing primarily on suicidal behavior, and group therapy, which is essentially psychoeducational and aims to improve interpersonal effectiveness, regulation of emotion, distress tolerance, and self-management capabilities. The second stage of the therapy focuses on childhood trauma, which is believed to underlie the development of borderline personality disorders in many cases. In a randomized, clinical trial, women with borderline personality disorder who received dialectical behavior therapy over a 1-year period had fewer suicide attempts, fewer psychiatric admissions, and were more compliant with outpatient treatment than a control group of similar patients who received standard treatment in the community; however, there were no differences between groups on depression, hopelessness, or suicidal ideation (Linehan, Armstrong, Suarez, Allmon, & Heard, 1991). It is not clear whether the findings reflect the efficacy of this therapy as opposed to other factors, such as availability and intensity of treatment. This treatment has yet to be empirically evaluated with adolescents.

CONCLUSIONS

Adolescent suicide is a problem of enormous concern which directly or indirectly affects a large proportion of our population. While the rates of death caused by most diseases have decreased, the rate of adolescent suicide has increased dramatically in recent years in the United States. There are significant international differences in adolescent suicide rates which are not fully understood. Attempted suicide is even more frequent than completed suicide and data suggest that many adolescent suicide attempters go unnoticed because they do not seek medical care. An even greater number of teens have seriously contemplated suicide or have a friend who has made an attempt. Reaching adolescents early in this spectrum of suicidality is a priority for our society.

Known risk factors for suicide include gender, ethnicity, family conflict, and mental disorders. Native American adolescent males have the highest rates of completed suicide, followed by white males. In contrast, females of all ethnicities attempt suicide much more frequently than males. Familiarity with suicide as a behavioral option contributes to increase the likelihood of suicidal behavior in times of personal crisis. Thus, suicidal behavior among family and peers constitutes a significant risk factor, as does having made prior suicide attempts. Indirect exposure to suicide through the media also influences suicidal behavior, though to a lesser degree.

Mental disorders that have been significantly associated with suicidal behavior in adolescents are major depression, substance abuse, and conduct disorder. Other suggested risk factors are history of sexual and physical abuse. A thorough clinical assessment is needed to evaluate the presence and importance of each of these risk factors in individual cases.

Major prevention strategies that target suicide risk factors include: establishing community "hot lines" for suicide, creating services for populations at special risk (e.g., depressed adolescents, runaways, substance abusers, delinquents, dysfunctional families with history of suicidal behavior, peers of suicidal adolescents, and dropouts), using the school system and the media to decrease the stigma of psychiatric treatment, improving the quality of assessment and treatment by mental health professionals, adding instruction and self-esteem problem-solving skills to school-based programs, and restricting access to firearms. Empirical studies of prevention programs have been less than conclusive, possibly because of methodological limitations such as lack of reliable definitions for suicidal behavior, lack of control groups, or inadequate sample sizes of subjects. Therefore, the understanding and approach to this symptom must be multifactorial and multidisciplinary. Yet, suicide is the most dangerous symptom among psychiatric symptoms, and actions to intervene and prevent it are urgent.

The major target group for intervention is suicide attempters. The first task is a thorough assessment to evaluate suicidal risk and to determine the level of clinical care that is required. The appropriate modality and setting of therapy are specific to the individual circumstances. Unfortunately, data are lacking to help the clinician justify, based on superior efficacy, the use of any specific therapy. The general effectiveness of all therapies in reducing future suicide attempts also remains controversial.

It is apparent that there is a need for more and better data concerning suicidal behavior in youth, especially in the area of prevention and intervention programs. Ideally, these data will stem from well-designed national and international research projects. Critical elements that will improve our understanding include establishing uniform international definitions of suicidal behavior, developing reliable surveillance systems of suicidal behavior, using data to guide prevention and intervention programs, testing the efficacy of prevention programs using control populations, and focusing on multidisciplinary approaches in our treatment of suicidal youth. Collaboration between researchers and clinicians in the field of suicidal behavior in adolescents could help to achieve a more comprehensive model of suicide that examines the interaction between environmental and individual factors in conjunction with efficacy of prevention and intervention efforts.

REFERENCES

Ackerman, G. (1993). A congressional view of youth suicide. *American Psychologist, 46,* 183–184.

Ambrosini, P., Bianchi, M., Rabinovich, H., & Elia, J. (1993). Antidepressant treatment in children and adolescents. I. Affective disorders. *Journal of the American Academy of Child and Adolescent Psychiatry, 32,* 1–6.

Apter, A., Bleich, A., King, R. A., Kron, S., Fluch, A., Kotter, M., & Cohen, D. J. (1993). Death without warning? A clinical postmortem study of suicide in 43 Israeli adolescent males. *Archives of General Psychiatry, 50,* 138–142.

Asberg, M. (1989). Neurotransmitter monoamine metabolites in the cerebrospinal fluid as risk factors for suicidal behavior. *Report of the Secretary's Task Force on Youth Suicide: Vol. 2. Risk factors for youth suicide* (DHHS Publication No. (ADM)89-1622, pp. 193–212). Washington, DC: U.S. Government Printing Office.

Baker, F. M. (1989). Black youth suicide: Literature review with a focus on prevention. *Report of the Secretary's Task Force on Youth Suicide: Vol. 3. Prevention and interventions in youth suicide.* DHHS Pub. No. (ADM)89-1623. Washington, DC: U.S. Government Printing Office.

Beck, A. T., Brown, G., & Steer, R. A. (1989). Prediction of eventual suicide in psychiatric inpatients by clinical ratings of hopelessness. *Journal of Consulting and Clinical Psychology, 57,* 2, 309–310.

Beck, A. T., Brown, S. M., Berchick, R. J., Stewart, B. L., & Steer, R. A. (1990). Relationship between hopelessness and ultimate suicide: A replication with psychiatric outpatients. *American Journal of Psychiatry, 147,* 190–195.

Berlin, I. N. (1987). Suicide among American Indian adolescents: An overview. *Suicide and Life-Threatening Behavior, 17,* 218–232.

Berman, A. L., & Jobes, P. A. (1991). The treatement of the suicidal adolescent. *Adolescent suicide. Assessment and intervention* (pp. 163–225). Washington, DC: American Psychological Association.

Birkhead, G., Galvin, V., Meehan, P., O'Carroll, P., & Mercy, J. (1993). The emergency department in the surveillance of attempted suicide: Findings and methodological considerations. *Public Health Reports, 108,* 323–331.

Blumenthal, S. J. (1988). Suicide: A guide to risk factors, assessment, and treatment of suicidal patients. *Medical Clinics of North America, 72,* 937–971.

Blumenthal, S. J., & Kupfer, D. J. (1986). Generalizable treatment strategies for suicidal behavior. *Annals of the New York Academy of Science, 487,* 327–340.

Blumenthal, S. J., & Kupfer, D. G. (1989). Overview of early detection and treatment strategies for suicidal behavior in young people. *Report of the Secretary's Task Force on Youth Suicide: Vol. 3. Prevention and intervention in youth suicide* (DHHS Publication No. (ADM)89-1623, pp. 239–252). Washington DC: U.S. Government Printing Office.

Bongar, B., & Harmatz, M. (1989). Graduate training in clinical psychology and the study of suicide. *Professional Psychology: Research and Practice, 20*, 209–213.

Bonner, A., & Rich, R. L. (1987). Concurrent validity of a stress-vulnerability model of suicidal ideation and behavior: A follow-up study. *Suicide & Life Threatening Behavior, 17*, 265–270.

Boyd, J. H. (1983). The increasing rate of suicide by firearms. *New England Journal of Medicine, 308*, 872–874.

Brent, D., & Kolko, D. (1990). The assessment and treatment of children and adolescents at risk for suicide. In S. Blumenthal & D. Kupfer (Eds.), *Suicide over the life cycle: Risk factors, assessment, and treatment of suicidal patients* (pp. 253–302). Washington, DC: American Psychiatric Press.

Brent, D. A., Kolko, D. J., Wartella, M. C., Boylan, M., Moritz, G., Baugher, M., & Zelenak, J. (1993). Adolescent psychiatric inpatients' risk of suicide attempt at 6-month follow-up. *Journal of the American Academy of Child and Adolescent Psychiatry, 32*, 95–105.

Brent, D. A., Perper, J. A., & Allman, C. J. (1987). Alcohol, firearms, and suicide among youth: Temporary trends in Allegheny County, Pennsylvania, 1960–1983. *Journal of the American Medical Association, 257*, 3369–3372.

Brent, D., Perper, J., Allman, C., Moritz, G., Wartella, M., & Zelenak, J. (1991). The presence and availability of firearms in the homes of adolescent suicides: A case–control study. *Journal of the American Medical Association 266*, 2989–2995.

Brent, P. A., Perper, J. A., Goldstein, C. E., Kolko, D. J., Allan, M. J., Allman, C. J., & Zelenak, J. P. (1988). Risk factors for adolescent suicide: A comparison of adolescent suicide victims with suicidal inpatients. *Archives of General Psychiatry, 45*, 581–588.

Brent, P. A., Perper, J. A., Moritz, G., Allman, C., Schweers, J., Roth, C., Balach, L., Canobbio, R., & Liotus, L. (1993). Psychiatric sequelae to the loss of an adolescent peer to suicide. *Journal of the American Academy of Child and Adolescent Psychiatry, 32*, 509–517.

Brent, P. A., Perper, J., Moritz, G., Baugher, M., & Allman, C. (1993). Suicide in adolescents with no apparent psychopathology. *Journal of the American Academy of Child and Adolescent Psychiatry, 32*, 494–500.

Cantor, P. C. (1989). Intervention strategies: Environmental risk reduction for youth suicide. *Report of the Secretary's Task Force on Youth Suicide: Vol. 3. Prevention and interventions in youth suicide* (DHHS Publication No. (ADM)89-1623, pp. 285–293). Washington DC: U.S. Government Printing Office.

Centers for Disease Control. (1991). Attempted suicide among high school students—United States, 1990. *Morbidity and Mortality Weekly Report, 40*, 633–635.

Centers for Disease Control. (1994a). Programs for the prevention of suicide among adolescents and young adults. *Morbidity and Mortality Weekly Report, 43*, 1–7.

Centers for Disease Control. (1994b). Suicide contagion and the reporting of suicide: Recommendations from a national workshop. *Morbidity and Mortality Weekly Report, 43*, 9–18.

Chowdhury, N., Hicks, R. C., & Kreitman, N. (1973). Evaluation of an after-care service for parasuicide (attempted suicide) patients. *Social Psychiatry, 8*, 67–81.

Christoffel, K. K., Marcus, D., Sagerman, S., & Bennett, S. (1988). Adolescent suicide and suicide attempts: A population study. *Pediatric Emergency Care, 4*, 32–40.

Comstock, B. S., Simmons, J. T., & Franklin, J. L. (1989). Community response to adolescent suicide clusters. *Report of the Secretary's Task Force on Youth Suicide: Vol. 3. Prevention and interventions in youth suicide* (DHHS Publication No. (ADM)89-1623, pp. 72–79). Washington, DC: U.S. Government Printing Office.

Conrad, N. (1992). Stress and knowledge of suicidal others as factors in suicidal behavior of high school adolescents. *Issues in Mental Health Nursing, 13*, 95–104.

Cox, J., McCarty, D., Landsberg, G., & Paravati, M. (1990). Local jails and police lockups. In M. J. Rotheram-Borus, J. Bradley, & N. Obolensky (Eds.), *Planning to live: Evaluating and treating suicidal teens in community settings* (pp. 317–332). Tulsa: University of Oklahoma Press.

Davidson, L. (1987). Suicide and violence in the medical setting. In A. Stoudemire & B. Fogel (Eds.), *Principles of medical psychiatry* (pp. 219–235). New York: Grune & Stratton.

Davidson, L. (1989). Suicide clusters and youth. In C. Pfeffer (Ed.), *Suicide among youth: Perspectives on risk and prevention* (pp. 83–99). Washington, DC: American Psychiatric Press.

Davidson, L., & Gould, M. S. (1989). Contagion as a risk factor for youth suicide. *Report of the Secretary's*

Task Force on Youth Suicide: Vol. 2. Risk factors for youth suicide (DHHS Publication No. (ADM)89-1622, pp. 88–109). Washington, DC: U.S. Government Printing Office.

Davis, J. M., Sandoval, J., & Wilson, M. P. (1988). Strategies for the primary prevention of adolescent suicide. *School Psychology Review, 17,* 559–569.

Dew, M. A., Bromet, E. T., Brent, D., & Greenhouse, J. B. (1987). A quantitative literature review of the effectiveness of suicide prevention centers. *Journal of Consulting and Clinical Psychology, 55,* 239–244.

Deykin, E. Y., Alpert, J. J., & McNamara, J. J. (1985). A pilot study of the effect of exposure to child abuse or neglect on adolescent suicidal behavior. *American Journal of Psychiatry, 142,* 1299–1303.

Deykin, E., Hsieh, C., Joshi, N., & McNamara, J. J. (1986). Adolescent suicidal and self-destructive behavior: Results of an intervention study. *Journal of Adolescent Health Care, 7,* 88–95.

Diekstra, R. F. (1989). Suicidal behavior in adolescents and young adults: The international picture. *Crisis, 10,* 16–35.

Diekstra, R. F. (1993). The epidemiology of suicide and parasuicide. *Acta Psychiatrica Scandinavica, 371 (Suppl.),* 9–20.

Earls, F., Escobar, J., & Manson, S. (1990). Suicide in minority groups: Epidemiologic and cultural perspectives. In S. Blumenthal & D. Kupfer (Eds.), *Suicide over the life cycle* (pp. 571–598). Washington, DC: American Psychiatric Press.

Eddy, D. M., Wolpert, R. L., & Rosenberg, M. L. (1987). Estimating the effectiveness of interventions to prevent youth suicides. *Medical Care, 25,* 557–565.

Ettlinger, R. (1975). Evaluation of suicide prevention after attempted suicide. *Acta Psychiatrica Scandinavica, 260(Suppl.),* 5–135.

Fine, M. A., & Sansone, R. A. (1990). Dilemmas in the management of suicidal behavior in individuals with borderline personality disorder. *American Journal of Psychotherapy,, 44,* 160–171.

Fine, S., Gilbert, M., Schmidt, L., Haley, G., Maxwell, A., & Forth, A. (1989). Short-term group therapy with depressed adolescent outpatients. *Canadian Journal of Psychiatry, 34,* 97–102.

Flay, B. R., & Sobel, J. L. (1983). The role of mass media in preventing adolescent substance abuse. In T. J. Glynn, C. G. Leukegeld, & J. P. Ludford (Eds.), *Preventing adolescent drug abuse. Intervention strategies* (NIDA Research Monograph no. 47). Rockville, MD: National Institute on Drug Abuse.

Friedman, A. S., & Glickman, N. W. (1986). Program characteristics for successful treatment of adolescent drug abuse. *Journal of Nervous and Mental Diseases, 174,* 669–679.

Garfinkel, B. D., Froese, A., & Hood, J. (1982). Suicide attempts in children and adolescents. *American Journal of Psychiatry, 139,* 1257–1261.

Garland, A., & Zigler, E. (1993). Adolescent suicide prevention: Current research and social policy implications. *American Psychologist, 48,* 169–182.

Gibbons, J. S., Butler, J., Urwin, P., & Gibbons, M. (1978). Evaluation of a social work service for self-poisoning patients. *British Journal of Psychiatry, 133,* 111–118.

Gibbs, J. T. (1984). Black adolescents and youth: An endangered species. *American Journal of Orthopsychiatry, 54,* 6–21.

Gibbs, J. T., & Hines, A. M. (1989). Factors related to sex differences in suicidal behavior among black youth: Implications for intervention and research. *Journal of Adolescent Research, 4,* 152–172.

Gibson, P. (1989). Gay male and lesbian youth suicide. *Report of the Secretary's Task Force on Youth Suicide: Vol. 3. Prevention and interventions in youth suicide* (DHHS Publication No. (ADM)89-1623, pp. 110–142). Washington, DC: U.S. Government Printing Office.

Goldacre, M., & Hawton, K. (1985). Repetition of self-poisoning and subsequent death in adolescents who take overdoses. *British Journal of Psychiatry, 146,* 395–398.

Goodwin, F., & Brown, G. (1989). Summary and overview of risk factors in suicide: *Report of the Secretary's Task Force on Youth Suicide: Vol. 2. Risk factors for youth suicide* (DHHS Publication No. (ADM)89-1622, pp. 263–270). Washington, DC: U.S. Government Printing Office.

Gould, M. S., & Shaffer, D. (1986). The impact of suicide in television movies: Evidence of imitation. *New England Journal of Medicine, 315,* 690–694.

Gould, M., Wallenstein, S., Kleinman, M., O'Carroll, P., & Mercy, J. (1990). Suicide clusters: an examination of age-specific effects. *American Journal of Public Health, 80,* 211–212.

Greening, L., & Dollinger, S. J. (1993). Rural adolescents' perceived personal risks for suicide. *Journal of Youth and Adolescence, 22,* 211–217.

Greer, S., & Bagley, C. (1971). Effect of psychiatric intervention in attempted suicide. *British Medical Journal, 1,* 310–312.

Harkavy-Friedman, J., Asnis, G., Boeck, M., & DiFiore, J. (1987). Prevalence of specific suicidal behaviors in a high school sample. *American Journal of Psychiatry, 144,* 1203–1206.

Hawton, K. (1986). *Suicide and attempted suicide among children and adolescents.* Beverly Hills, CA: Sage Publications.

Hawton, K., Fagg, J., Platt, S., & Hawkins, M. (1993). Factors associated with suicide after parasuicide in young people. *British Medical Journal, 306,* 1641–1644.

Hlady, W. G., & Middaugh, J. P. (1988). Suicides in Alaska: Firearms and alcohol. *American Journal of Public Health, 78,* 179–180.

Hoberman, H. M., & Garfinkel, B. D. (1988). Completed suicide in children and adolescents. *Canadian Journal of Psychiatry, 33,* 494–506.

Hodgman, C. H., & Roberts, F. (1982). Adolescent suicide and the pediatricians. *Adolescent Medicine, 101,* 118–123.

Holinger, P. C. (1989). Epidemiologic issues in youth suicide. In C. Pfeffer (Ed.), *Suicide among youth: Perspectives on risk and prevention* (pp. 41–62). Washington, DC: American Psychiatric Press.

Holinger, P. C. (1990). The causes, impact, and preventability of childhood injuries in the United States. *American Journal of Diseases of Children, 144,* 670–676.

Holinger, P. C., & Offer, D. (1987). Suicide and homicide in the United States: An epidemiologic study of violent death, population changes, and the potential for prediction. *American Journal of Psychiatry, 144,* 215–219.

Howard-Pitney, B., LaFramboise, T., Basil, M., September, B., & Johnson, M. (1992). Psychological and social indicators of suicide ideation and suicide attempts in Zuni adolescents. *Journal of Consulting and Clinical Psychology, 60,* 473–476.

Joan, P. (1986). *Preventing teenage suicide: The living alternative handbook.* New York: Human Sciences Press.

Jobes, D. A., Berman, A. L., & Josselson, A. R. (1987). Improving the validity and reliability of medical-legal certifications of suicide. *Suicide and Life-Threatening Behavior, 17,* 310–325.

Johnson, S. W., & Maile, L. S. (1987). *Suicide and the schools. A handbook for prevention, intervention and rehabilitation,* Springfield, Ill: Charles C. Thomas.

Kazdin, A. E., Siegel, T., & Bass, D. (1992). Cognitive and problem-solving skills training and parent management training in the treatment of antisocial behavior in children. *Journal of Consulting and Clinical Psychology, 60,* 733–747.

Kessel, N. (1965). Self poisoning. *British Medical Journal, 2,* 1336–1340, 1265–1270.

Kleck, G. (1988). Miscounting suicides. *Suicide and Life-Threatening Behavior, 18,* 219–236.

Knowles, D. (1979). On the tendency for volunteer helpers to give advice. *Journal of Counseling Psychology, 26,* 352–354.

Kosky, R., Silburn, S., & Zubrick, S. (1990). Are children and adolescents who have suicidal thoughts different from those who attempt suicide? *The Journal of Nervous and Mental Disease, 178,* 38–43.

Kosten, T. R., Rounsaville, B. J., & Kleber, H. D. (1986). A 2.5 year follow-up of depression, life crises and treatment effects on abstinence among opioid addicts. *Archives of General Psychiatry, 43,* 733–738.

Kreitman, N., Philip, D. E., Greer, S., & Bagley, C. R. (1969). Parasuicide. *British Journal of Psychiatry* (letter), *115,* 796–797.

Kreitman, N., Smith, P., & Tan, E. (1970). Attempted suicide as language: An empirical study. *British Journal of Psychiatry, 116,* 465–473.

Lerner, M., & Clum, G. (1990). Treatment of suicide ideators: A problem-solving approach. *Behavior Therapy, 21,* 403–411.

Lester, D. (1990). The effects of detoxification of domestic gas on suicide in the United States. *American Journal of Public Health, 80,* 80–81.

Lester, D., & Murrell, M. E. (1982). The preventative effect of strict gun control laws on suicide and homicide. *Suicide and Life-Threatening Behavior, 12,* 131–140.

Levav, I., & Aisenberg, E. (1989). The epidemiology of suicide in Israel: International and intranational comparisons. *Suicide and Life-Threatening Behavior, 19,* 184–200.

Levy, S., Jurkovic, G., & Spirito, A. (1995). A multisystem analysis of adolescent suicide attempts. *Journal of Abnormal Child Psychology,* in press.

Lewinsohn, P., Clarke, G., Hops, H., & Andrews, J. (1990). Cognitive-behavioral treatment for depressed adolescents. *Behavior Therapy, 21,* 385–401.

Lewinsohn, P., Rohde, P., & Seeley, J. (1993). Psychosocial characteristics of adolescents with a history of suicide attempt. *Journal of the American Academy of Child and Adolescent Psychiatry, 32,* 60–68.

Liberman, R., & Eckman, T. (1981). Behavior therapy vs. insight oriented therapy for repeated suicide attempters. *Archives of General Psychiatry, 38,* 1126–1130.

Lidberg, L., Tuck, J. R., Asberg, M., Scalia-Tomba, G. P., & Bertilsson, L. (1985). Homicide, suicide and CSF 5-HIAA. *Acta Psychiatrica Scandinavica, 71,* 230–236.

Linehan, M. M. (1986). Suicide people, one population or two? *Annals of the New York Academy of Sciences, 487,* 16–33.

Linehan, M. M., Armstrong, H. E., Suarez, A., Allmon, D., & Heard, H. L. (1991). Cognitive-behavioral treatment of chronically parasuicidal borderline patients. *Archives of General Psychiatry, 48,* 1060–1064.

Loftin, C., McDowall, D., Wiersema, B., & Cottey, T. J. (1991). Effects of restrictive licensing of handguns on homicide and suicide in the District of Columbia. *New England Journal of Medicine, 325,* 1615–1620.

McIntire, M. S., Angle, C. R., Wickoff, R. L., & Schlict, M. L. (1977). Recurrent adolescent suicidal behavior. *Pediatrics, 60,* 605–608.

McIntosh, J. (1983–84). Suicide among Native Americans: Further tribal data and considerations. *Journal of Death and Dying, 14,* 215–229.

Males, M. (1991). Teen suicide and changing cause of death certification, 1953–1987. *Suicide and Life-Threatening Behavior, 21,* 245–259.

Marttunen, M., Aro, H., Henriksson, M., & Lonnqvist, T. (1991). Mental disorders in adolescent suicide. *Archives of General Psychiatry, 48,* 834–839.

Meltzer, H., & Lowy, M. (1989). The neuroendocrine system and suicide. *Report of the Secretary's Task Force on Youth Suicide: Vol. 2. Risk factors for youth suicide* (DHHS Publication No. (ADM)89-1622, pp. 235–246). Washington, DC: U.S. Government Printing Office.

Miller, H. L., Coombs, D. W., Leeper, J. D., & Barton, S. N. (1984). An analysis of the effects of suicide prevention facilities on suicide rates in the United States. *American Journal of Public Health, 74,* 340–343.

Monk, M. (1987). Epidemiology of suicide. *Epidemiologic Reviews, 9,* 51–69.

National Center for Health Statistics. (1989). *United States 1979–87.*

National Center for Health Statistics. (1990). *Final mortality statistics, 1987.* Washington, DC: U.S. Government Printing Office.

National Center for Health Statistics. (1991). Vital statistics of the United States. Vol. 2. *Mortality—Part A (for the years 1966–1988).* Washington, DC: U.S. Government Printing Office.

National Center for Health Statistics. (1993). Advance report of final mortality statistics, 1990. *Monthly Vital Statistics Report, 41,* 7, 1–44.

National Committee for Injury Prevention and Control. (1989). Suicide. *Injury prevention: Meeting the challenge* (pp. 252–260). London: Oxford University Press.

Nelson, F. L. (1988). A research note on knowledge of youth suicide among high school students. *Journal of Community Psychology, 16,* 241–243.

O'Carroll, P., Mercy, J., & Steward, J. (1988). CDC recommendations for a community plan for the prevention and containment of suicide clusters. *Morbidity and Mortality Weekly Reports, 37* (Suppl. 5–6), 1–12.

O'Keefe, G. J., & Mendelsohn, J. (1984). *"Taking a bite out of crime." The impact of a mass media crime prevention campaign.* Washington, DC: U.S. Department of Justice, National Institute of Justice.

Oliver, R. G., & Hetzel, B. S. (1972). Rise and fall of suicide rates in Australia: Relation to sedative availability. *Medical Journal of Australia, 2,* 919–923.

Orbach, I., & Bar-Joseph, H. (1992). The impact of a suicide prevention program for adolescents on suicidal tendencies, hopelessness, ego identity, and coping. *Suicide and Life-Threatening Behavior, 23,* 120–129.

Otto, U. (1972). Suicidal acts by children and adolescents. *Acta Pediatrica Scandinavica, 233(Suppl.),* 7–123.

Overholser, J. C., Hemstreet, A., Spirito, A., & Vyse, S. (1989). Suicide awareness programs in the schools.

Effects of gender and personal experience. *Journal of the American Academy of Child and Adolescent Psychiatry, 28,* 925–930.

Overholser, J., & Spirito, A. (1990). Cognitive-behavioral treatment of suicidal depression. In E. Feindler & G. Kalfus (Eds.), *Adolescent behavior therapy handbook* (pp. 211–231). Berlin: Springer.

Patsiokas, A., & Clum, G. (1985). Effects of psychotherapeutic strategies in the treatment of suicide attempters. *Psychotherapy, 22,* 281–290.

Patterson, G. R., & Reid, J. (1970). Reciprocity and coercion: Two facets of social systems. In C. Neuringer & J. Michael (Eds.), *Behavior modification in clinical psychology.* New York: Appleton–Century–Crofts.

Pfeffer, C. R. (1991). Attempted suicide in children and adolescents: Causes and management. In M. Lewis (Ed.), *Child and adolescent psychiatry: A comprehensive textbook.* Baltimore: Williams & Wilkins.

Phillips, D. P., & Carstensen, L. L. (1986). Clustering of teenage suicides after television news about suicide. *New England Journal of Medicine, 315,* 685–689.

Phillips, D., & Paight, D. (1987). The impact of televised movies about suicide: a replicative study. *New England Journal of Medicine, 317,* 809–811.

Plant, M. A., Pirie, F., & Kreitman, N. (1979). Evaluation of the Scottish Health Education Unit's 1976 campaign on alcoholism. *Social Psychology, 14,* 11–24.

Reynolds, W., & Coates, K. (1986). A comparison of cognitive-behavioral therapy and relaxation training for the treatment of depression in adolescents. *Journal of Consulting and Clinical Psychology, 54,* 653–660.

Rich, A. R., Kirkpatrick-Smith, J. K., Bonner, R. L., & Jans, F. (1992). Gender differences in the psychosocial correlates of suicidal ideation among adolescents. *Suicide and Life-Threatening Behavior, 22,* 364–373.

Rich, C. L., Young, J. G., Fowler, R. C., Wagner, J., & Black, J. W. (1990). Guns and suicide: Possible effects of some specific legislation. *American Journal of Psychiatry, 147,* 342–346.

Richman, J. (1979). The family therapy of attempted suicide. *Family Process, 18,* 131–142.

Rifai, A., Reynolds, C., & Mann, J. J. (1992). Biology of elderly suicide. *Suicide and Life-Threatening Behavior, 22,* 48–61.

Robin, A. L. (1981). A controlled evaluation of problem-solving communication training with parent–adolescent. *Behavior Therapy, 12,* 593–609.

Rosenberg, M. L., Eddy, D. M., Wolpert, R. C., & Broumas, E. P. (1989). Developing strategies to prevent youth suicide. In C. R. Pfeffer (Ed.), *Suicide among youth: Perspectives on risk and prevention* (pp. 203–225). Washington, DC: American Psychiatric Press.

Rosenberg, M. L., Mercy, J. A., & Houk, V. N. (1991). Guns and adolescent suicides. *Journal of the American Medical Association, 266,* 3030.

Rosenberg, M. L., Davidson, L. E., Smith J. C., Berman, A., Buzbee, M., Gantner, G., Gay, G., Moore-Lewis, B., Mills, D., Murray, D., O'Carroll, P., & Jobes, D. (1988). Operational criteria for the determination of suicide. *Journal of Forensic Science, 32,* 1445–1455.

Rosenberg, M. L., Smith, J. C., Davidson, L., & Conn, J. (1987). The emergence of youth suicide: An epidemiologic analysis and public health perspective. *Annual Review of Public Health, 8,* 417–427.

Rosenthal, M. (1981). Sexual differences in the suicidal behavior of young people. *Adolescent Psychiatry, 9,* 422–442.

Ross, C., & Motto, J. (1984). Group counseling for suicidal adolescents. In H. Sudak, A. Ford, & N. Rushforth (Eds.), *Suicide in the young.* Littleton, MA: John Wright PSG.

Rotheram-Borus, M. (1993). Suicidal behavior and risk factors among runaway youth. *American Journal of Psychiatry, 180,* 103–107.

Rotheram-Borus, M., & Bradley, J. (1991). Triage model for suicidal runaways. *American Journal of Orthopsychiatry, 61,* 122–127.

Rotheram-Borus, M. J., Piacentini, J., Miller, S., Graae, F., & Castro-Blanco, D. (1994). Brief cognitive-behavioral treatment for adolescent suicide attempters and their families. *Journal of the American Academy of Child and Adolescent Psychiatry, 33,* 508–517.

Roy, A. (1989). Genetics and suicidal behavior. In C. R. Pfeffer (Ed.), *Suicide among youth: Perspectives on risk and prevention* (pp. 247–262). Washington, DC: American Psychiatric Press.

Roy, A. (1994). Recent biological studies on suicide. *Suicide & Life-Threatening Behavior, 24,* 10–14.

Salkovskis, P., Atha, C., & Storer, D. (1990). Cognitive-behavioral problem-solving in the treatment of patients who repeatedly attempt suicide. *British Journal of Psychiatry, 157,* 871–876.

Saltzman, L. E., Levenson, A., & Smith, J. C. (1988). Suicides among persons 15–24 years of age, 1970–1984. *Morbidity and Mortality Weekly Reports, 37,* 61–68.

Shaffer, D. (1988). The epidemiology of teen suicide: An examination of risk factors. *Journal of Clinical Psychiatry, 49,* 36–41.

Shaffer, D., & Bacon, K. (1989). A critical review of preventive intervention efforts in suicide with particular reference to youth suicide. *Report of the Secretary's Task Force on Youth Suicide: Vol. 3. Prevention and interventions in youth suicide* (DHHS Publication No. (ADM)89-1623, pp. 31–61). Washington, DC: U.S. Government Printing Office.

Shaffer, D., Garland, A., Gould, M., Fisher, P., & Trautman, P. (1988). Preventing teenage suicide: A critical review. *Journal of the American Academy of Child and Adolescent Psychiatry, 27,* 675–687.

Shaffer, D., Garland, A., Underwood, M., & Whittle, B. (1987). *An evaluation of three youth suicide prevention programs in New Jersey.* Report prepared for the New Jersey State Department of Health and Human Services.

Shaffer, D., Vieland, V., Garland, A., Rojas, M., Underwood, M., & Busner, C. (1990). Adolescent suicide attempters: Response to suicide prevention programs. *Journal of the American Medical Association, 264,* 3151–3155.

Shafii, M., Carrigan, S., Whittinghill, J. R., & Derrick, A. (1985). Psychological autopsy of completed suicide in children and adolescents. *American Journal of Psychiatry, 142,* 1061–1064.

Shaunesey, K., Cohen, J. L., Plummer, B., & Berman, A. (1993). Suicidality in hospitalized adolescents: Relationship to prior abuse. *American Journal of Orthopsychiatry, 63,* 113–119.

Slem, C. M., & Cotler, S. (1973). Crisis phone services: Evaluation of hotline programs. *American Journal of Community Psychology, 1,* 219–227.

Sloan, J. H., Rivara, F. P., Reay, D. T., Ferris, J. A., & Kellermann, A. L. (1990). Firearm regulations and rates of suicide: A comparison of two metropolitan areas. *New England Journal of Medicine, 322,* 369–373.

Smith, K. (1991). Comments on "Teen suicide and changing cause-of-death certification, 1953–1987." *Suicide and Life-Threatening Behavior, 21,* 260–262.

Smith, K., & Crawford, S. (1986). Suicidal behavior among "normal" high school students. *Suicide and Life-Threatening Behavior, 14,* 215–242.

Snyder, R. (1981). The first offender program: Children and our future. In I. N. Berlin (Ed.), *The International Year of the Child, 1979–1980.* Albuquerque: University of New Mexico Press.

Sorenson, S. B., & Golding, J. (1988). Prevalence of suicide attempts in a Mexican-American population: Prevention implications of immigration and cultural issues. *Suicide and Life-Threatening Behavior, 18,* 322–333.

Sorenson, S. B., & Rutter, C. M. (1991). Transgenerational patterns of suicide attempt. *Journal of Consulting and Clinical Psychology, 59,* 861–866.

Spirito, A., Bond, A., Kurkjian, J., Devost, L., Bosworth, T., & Brown, L. (1993). Gender differences among adolescent suicide attempters. *Crisis: International Journal of Suicide and Crisis Studies, 62,* 464–468.

Spirito, A., Brown, J., Overholser, J., & Fritz, G. (1989). Attempted suicide in adolescence. A review and critique of the literature. *Clinical Psychology Review, 9,* 335–363.

Spirito, A., Overholser, J., Ashworth, S., Morgan, J., & Benedict-Drew, C. (1988). Evaluation of a suicide awareness curriculum for high school students. *Journal of the American Academy of Child and Adolescent Psychiatry, 27,* 705–711.

Spirito, A., Plummer, B., Gispert, M., Levy, S., Kurkjian, J., Lewander, W., Hagberg, S., & Devost, L. (1992). Adolescent suicide attempts: Outcomes at follow-up. *American Journal of Orthopsychiatry, 62,* 464–468.

Spirito, A., Riggs, S., Lewander, W., Bond, A., Fritz, G., & Simon, P. (1989). Surveillance of adolescent suicide attempts in the Rhode Island Hospital Pediatric Emergency Department. *Rhode Island Medical Journal, 72,* 401–405.

Steer, R., Kumar, G., & Beck, A. (1993). Self-reported suicidal ideation in adolescent psychiatric inpatients. *Journal of Consulting and Clinical Psychology, 61,* 1096–1099.

Stelmachers, Z., Smith, M., & Wells, J. (1990). Suicide prevention community services. In A. E. Berman (Ed.), *Suicide prevention case consultations* (pp. 56–79). New York: Springer Publications.

Stiffman, A. R. (1989). Suicide attempts in runaway youth. *Suicide and Life-Threatening Behavior, 19,* 147–159.

Sudak, H. S., Ford, A. B., & Rushforth, N. B. (1984). Adolescent suicide: An overview. *American Journal of Psychotherapy, 38,* 350–363.

Traskman-Bendz, L., Alling, C., Alsen, M., Regnell, G., Simonsson, P., & Ohman, R. (1993). The role of monamines in suicidal behavior. *Acta Psychiatrica Scandinavica, Suppl. 371,* 45–47.

Trautman, P. D. (1989). Specific treatment modalities for adolescent suicide attempters. *Report of the Secretary's Task Force on Youth Suicide: Vol. 3. Prevention and interventions in youth suicide* (DHHS Publication No. (ADM)89-1623, pp. 253–263). Washington, DC: U.S. Government Printing Office.

Trautman, P. D., & Rotheram-Borus, M. J. (1987). *Referral failure among adolescent suicide attempters.* Poster presented at the Annual Meeting of the American Academy of Child and Adolescent Psychiatry, Los Angeles.

Trautman, P. D., & Rotheram-Borus, M. J. (1988). Cognitive therapy with children and adolescents. In A. J. Frances & R. E. Hals (Eds.), *Review of psychiatry* (Vol. 7, pp. 584–607). Washington, DC: American Psychiatric Press.

Trautman, P. D., & Shaffer, D. (1989). Pediatric management of suicidal behavior. *Pediatric Annals, 18,* 134–143.

Trautman, P. D., Stewart, N., & Morishima, A. (1993). Are adolescent suicide attempters noncompliant with outpatient care? *Journal of the American Academy of Child and Adolescent Psychiatry, 32,* 89–94.

U. S. Congress, Office of Technology Assessment. (1990). *Indian adolescent mental health* (OTA-H-446). Washington, DC: U.S. Government Printing Office.

van Praag, H. M. (1986). Biological suicide research outcome and limitations. *Biological Psychiatry, 21,* 1305–1323.

Vieland, V., Whittle, B., Garland, A., Hicks, R., & Shaffer, D. (1991). The impact of curriculum based suicide prevention programs for teenagers: An 18-month follow-up. *Journal of the American Academy of Child and Adolescent Psychiatry, 30,* 811–815.

Walsh, B., Walsh, P., & Whelan, B. (1975). Suicide in Dublin. II. The influence of some social and medical factors on coroners' verdicts. *British Journal of Psychiatry, 126,* 309–312.

Ward, J. A. (1984). Preventive implications of a Native Indian mental health program: Focus on suicide and violent death. *Journal of Preventive Psychiatry, 2,* 371–385.

Warshauer, M. E., & Monk, M. (1978). Problems in suicide statistics for whites and blacks. *American Journal of Public Health, 68,* 383–388.

Weinstein, M. C., & Saturno, P. J. (1989). Economic impact of youth suicide and suicide attempts. *Report of the Secretary's Task Force on Youth Suicide: Vol. 4. Strategies for the prevention of youth suicide* (DHHS Publication No. (ADM)89-1624, pp. 82–93). Washington, DC: U.S. Government Printing Office.

Welu, T. C. (1977). A follow-up program for suicide attempters. *Suicide and Life-Threatening Behavior, 7,* 17–30.

Yu, E., Chang, C. F., Liu, W. T., & Fernandez, M. (1989). Suicide among Asian American youth. *Report of the Secretary's Task Force on Youth Suicide: Vol. 3. Prevention and interventions in youth suicide* (DHHS Publication No. (ADM)89-1623, pp. 157–176). Washington, DC: U.S. Government Printing Office.

Zich, J. M. (1984). A reciprocal control approach to the treatment of repeated parasuicide. *Suicide and Life-Threatening Behavior, 14,* 36–51.

9

Unintentional Injury

ILANA LESCOHIER and
SUSAN SCAVO GALLAGHER

Young people are thoughtless as a rule.
—Homer

Youth is perpetual intoxication; it is a fever of the mind.
—La Rochefoucauld

The ripeness of adolescence is prodigal in pleasures, skittish, and in need of a bridle.
—Plutarch

The right way to begin is to pay attention to the young, and make them just as good as possible.
—Socrates

INTRODUCTION

Viewing adolescent behavior as reckless, in need of restraint and modification, is not new. Whereas earlier generations of thinkers and educators were concerned with building character, a growing segment of their counterparts today are couching the discussion in terms of health. Expressions such as *youthful recklessness, problem behaviors, excessive* or *deviant risk-taking, health-compromising behaviors,* and *behavioral misadventures* are being used not only to describe adolescent behavior, but also to explain adverse health

ILANA LESCOHIER • Injury Control Center, Harvard School of Public Health, Boston, Massachusetts 02115.   SUSAN SCAVO GALLAGHER • Children's Safety Network, Education Development Center, Inc., Newton, Massachusetts 02158-1060.
Handbook of Adolescent Health Risk Behavior, edited by Ralph J. DiClemente, William B. Hansen, and Lynn E. Ponton. Plenum Press, New York, 1996.

outcomes in this population. A review of the current literature on adolescent behavior and health reveals a repeated theme of attributing ill health in this age group primarily to risk-taking behavior. Injuries, as the major contributor to adolescent death and disability, are being used as a principal example of such a link.

Until about the middle 1960s, public health professionals shared the popular perception that most injury events are direct consequences of aberrant behavior, human error, ignorance, or stupidity. The public health response was conceived as efforts to educate people about adopting safe behaviors. In a personal reminiscence, Julian Waller (1994) reflects on the reasons for the persistence of this orientation. Waller, who has been involved in injury control activities for more than 30 years, and knew key players in this field, suggests that one reason has to do with the ethos of the frontier society which placed major emphasis on individual responsibility for coping with the environment. Another reason is associated with the emergence of the field of psychiatry which emphasized the influence of emotional and subconscious antecedents on life events. More importantly, a third reason involves the difficulty many professionals have understanding the conceptualization of injury events as a complex interplay between human and environmental factors, triggered by several causes.

Needless to say, it was in the interest of consumer goods manufacturers to reinforce the prevailing perception of personal responsibility for injury as a way of protecting themselves against liability by deflecting attention from the role of products in injury events. Things have changed dramatically since that time in the automobile industry, for example. Improvements in design have contributed to safety. Recalls of models with faulty components have become common. Yet, even today the earlier perception still prevails, as exemplified by the campaign slogan of the gun lobby: "Guns don't kill people, people kill people." But, as engineers like to point out, products "talk" to people through their design concepts: Hold me, Push this lever, Open this door, Pull this trigger. Injury may occur under a variety of scenarios such as when the product is used correctly but perhaps not as intended (a young child pulls the trigger of a loaded gun), when the product is faulty (incorrect wiring in electrical appliances, defective auto brakes), or related to poor design and design that conveys a wrong message (vehicles that roll over, chemicals in containers that resemble those for beverages).

Unlike most of the topics addressed in this volume, this chapter on unintentional injury will deviate from a primary focus on risk-taking behavior. Instead, we will refer to risk as an epidemiological term to denote the probability that an injury, or a specific level of injury severity, will occur during the use of a given product or participation in a given activity (Robertson, 1992). Measures of risk are usually derived from rates, although risk is an estimate of future events while a rate describes the relative frequency of past occurrences. Risk estimators can generally be divided into two classes: measures of occurrence which quantify the risk for disease or injury (e.g., incidence, prevalence), and measures of association which contrast risk/rate estimators from two different groups (e.g., risk ratio, odds ratio). A related concept, which is crucial for the understanding and interpretation of risk in descriptive epidemiology, is the concept of exposure. Since injury rates are expressed as the product of frequency of occurrence (numerator) per specified units of exposure (denominator), the nature and quality of measures of exposure will affect the interpretation of risk estimates.

For example, between 1950 and 1990, the annual number of traffic fatalities in the United States increased by 33%. During the same period, the number of licensed drivers increased almost threefold; the number of registered vehicles, fourfold; and the number of vehicle miles driven, almost fivefold. The traffic fatality rate, measured as the number of traffic fatalities per 100 million vehicle miles driven was cut by almost 72% (Graham, 1993). In comparison, the overall motor vehicle death rate per 100,000 population has not shown such major changes during the past half century (Baker, O'Neill, Ginsburg, & Li, 1992). Many indicators of exposure to risk have some limitations, and may be more useful for some purposes than for others. Such indicators can include behaviors such as alcohol use, legal violations, and failure to use motor vehicle restraints and other protective gear. These behaviors will be discussed in this chapter as part of a range of factors that contribute to elevated risk of injury.

The concept of exposure is also important for understanding injuries associated with specific age groups. Throughout the life cycle people change the type, and frequency, of their activities. The nature of activity, its location and intensity, as well as age-associated physiological and mental attributes, all have bearing on the level of risk and its interpretation. Thus, the pattern of injury among adolescents who, as a group, have a high level of participation in sports and recreational activities, is expected to differ from that of older people. Similar differences would be expected between younger and older teenagers who become active as drivers and workers. These issues are discussed in greater detail in other sections of this chapter.

Injury is the leading cause of death, hospital admission, emergency department visits, and emergency medical transport for adolescents in the United States (Schwarz, 1993). Injury mortality rates of children and adolescents in the United States are higher than rates in other industrial countries. Much of the difference in these rates is explained by motor vehicle injuries and homicide, with the excess mortality in this country largely attributable to deaths among preschool children and adolescents (Williams & Kotch, 1990). Unintentional injury accounts for more than 60% of all injury deaths of teenagers (NCHS, 1994), and has a higher ratio of nonfatal events for each death than injuries caused by violence (Guyer, Lescohier, Gallagher, Hausman, & Azzara, 1989).

The phrase *unintentional injury* represents a grouping of diverse conditions that can be classified by several dimensions such as external cause (e.g., motor vehicle collisions, falls, drowning, fire, poisonings); type of activity (work, sport, informal recreation); location of activity (e.g., school, farm, home); product involved (e.g., firearm, snowmobile, gym equipment, meat-cutting machine); mechanism of injury (blunt, penetrating, burn); nature of injury (e.g., fracture, laceration, contusion); body region affected (e.g., head, chest, abdomen, extremities); and levels of injury severity. Injury severity can be assessed by specific scaling systems, including the Injury Severity Score and Glasgow Coma Scale, or through proxy measures of patient outcome (death versus nonfatal) and use of medical resources (inpatient admission versus emergency department visit).

The patterns of injury classified on these dimensions differ by population characteristics: age, sex, race, residence, socioeconomic status. Thus, the development of effective interventions to reduce unintentional injury among adolescents, requires efforts to identify patterns of injury in this population and elucidate both the unique and common features revealed by an analysis across facets. Our objectives for this chapter are more modest. In the section on epidemiology we focus on two aspects: the difference between injury patterns in early (10–14 years) versus late (15–19 years) adolescence, and the difference in patterns of mortality versus morbidity in these age groups. The segment dealing with prevention will describe a science-based model for the study of injury events and their control, using examples from motor vehicle crashes, sports, and work-related injuries. Under the part devoted to treatment, we will raise system-related issues associated with acute care and rehabilitation of the adolescent patient.

EPIDEMIOLOGY

Although the general public may view injuries as random, chance events, injuries are predictable, preventable, and can be studied using scientific tools and principles. In fact, the epidemiological model of disease causation (host, agent, environment) can be applied to injury. Patterns of injury can be identified the same way epidemiologists analyze an outbreak of malaria, by looking at who is at risk and how they were exposed. The analogy is thus: for malaria, the agent is a mosquito and the exposure event is a mosquito bite; in the case of a fractured skull, the agent is kinetic energy transferred by a motor vehicle and the exposure event is a crash.

There are distinct patterns of injury for different age groups. Several challenges confront the reviewer of data on the epidemiology of injury in adolescents. First, there seems to be no agreement about the definition of adolescence in terms of age. This poses a particular problem for those who wish to study health status indicators in this population. For example, Crockett and Petersen (1993), when discussing adolescent development and its implications for health promotion, divide the adolescence decade into three phases: early adolescence (11–14), middle adolescence (15–17), and late adolescence (18–20). But few, if any, reports—whether from routine sources or special studies—present data in this fashion. Second, there is a lack of consistency in age groupings used by the various sources of data that collect information on injury, making it difficult to select and present data relevant to adolescents (Paulson, 1988). In addition, unlike information about deaths, which is routinely collected, population-based data on nonfatal injury are limited. In this section we review the epidemiology of unintentional injury for youth aged 10 through 19 years, and compare data for two subgroups labeled younger (10–14) and older (15–19) adolescents. When no comparable data are available, other age groupings will be used.

Mortality

A 1966 report to Congress described injury as "the neglected disease of modern society" (NAS/NRC, 1970). Injury had begun to receive more attention by the public health community as other causes of death, particularly infectious diseases among the young, showed marked decline in the first half of this century. As deaths from natural causes were continuing to drop, the order of leading causes among adolescents reversed (Figure 1). Among adolescents 15–19 years of age, this reversal occurred earlier and resulted in a larger gap between natural causes and injury, as death rates from disease continued to decline while injury rates tended to rise. In younger adolescents, age 10–14 years, both disease and injury rates have been decreasing consistently throughout the

Age 10-14

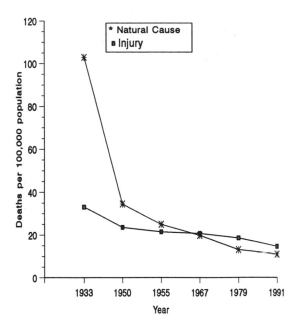

Age 15-19

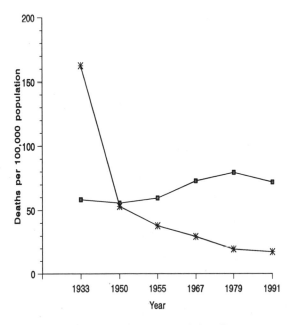

Figure 1. Death rates per 100,000 due to natural causes versus injury: By age group, selected years. Source: NCHS (1993, 1994) and Fingerhut (1989).

period, and in a parallel fashion for more than two decades. Consequently, between 1955 and 1979, injury as a proportion of all deaths in adolescence increased from 46 to 57% among the younger age groups, and from 61 to 81% among older teens (Fingerhut, 1989). The proportions in 1991 were similar to those in 1979.

In 1991, 14,955 adolescents ages 10 through 19 years died as a result of injury. Of these deaths, 8856 were classified as unintentional injury deaths. The proportion of injury deaths attributed to unintentional events differs by age. Almost three out of four injury deaths in 10- through 14-year-olds were unintentional as compared with 56% among their older counterparts. Black females in the younger age group had the highest proportion of violent injury deaths. Among white females, violence accounted for less than one in four injury deaths throughout the teenage years. This relationship was reversed for black males in the 15–19 age group for whom 75% of injury deaths resulted from violence.

Figure 2 depicts unintentional injury death rates by age, sex, and race groups in 1991. Overall, a 15- to 19-year-old was almost four times more likely to be killed by an unintentional injury as a 10- to 14-year-old. Male-to-female ratios in the young and older adolescent groups were 2.2:1 and 2.3:1, respectively, among whites. Among blacks, these ratios were higher (3.2:1 and 4:1, respectively). Unintentional injury death rates in the 10–14 age group were highest among black males. The rate in older black male adolescents was also high, although somewhat lower than the rate for white males in this age group. Residential fires, drowning, and pedestrian deaths account for the higher rate of unintentional injuries in black males (Onwuachi-Saunders & Hawkins, 1993).

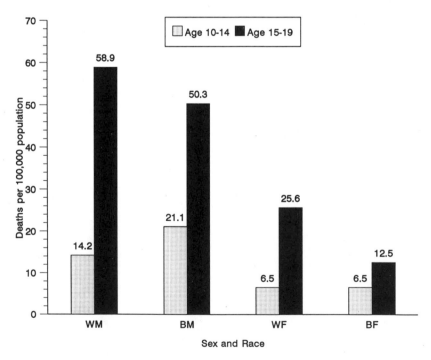

Figure 2. Unintentional injury death rates per 100,000: By age, sex, and race. Source: NCHS (1994).

Between 1979 and 1991, unintentional injury death rates declined more than 30% among both young and older adolescents (NCHS, 1993). Examination of the trends reveals declining rates for both males and females in the two age groups. However, rates for black adolescents, particularly older adolescents, did not follow this pattern and have actually risen. The additional burden of unintentional injury among black adolescents is particularly worrisome given the disproportionately high homicide rates in this group.

Traffic-related fatalities are the leading cause of unintentional injury death through-out adolescence, followed by drowning and unintentional firearm events (Figures 3 & 4). However, further examination of motor vehicle deaths shows that children ages 10–14 die most often as passengers, pedestrians, or bicyclists. Of all motor vehicle-related deaths in this age group in 1991, 38% were pedestrians or bicyclists. In comparison, teens ages 15–19 die most often as drivers and passengers (Figure 4). Only 8% of motor vehicle-related deaths in older adolescents were pedestrians and bicycle riders.

Motor Vehicle Crashes

Motor vehicle death rates vary greatly in the general population by age and sex, with a peak in the late teenage years and early twenties. By type, bicyclist death rates peak at age 14, occupant rates at age 18, and motorcyclist rates at age 21. Pedestrian death rates are highest among the elderly, followed by young children and older adolescents age 18–21 (Baker *et al.*, 1992).

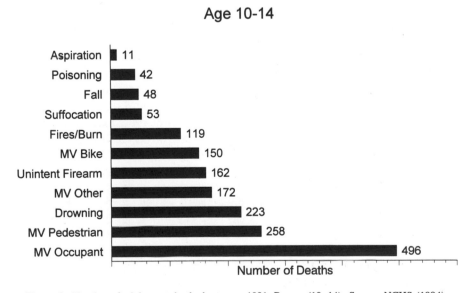

Figure 3. Number of adolescent deaths by cause, 1991: By age (10–14). Source: NCHS (1994).

Age 15-19

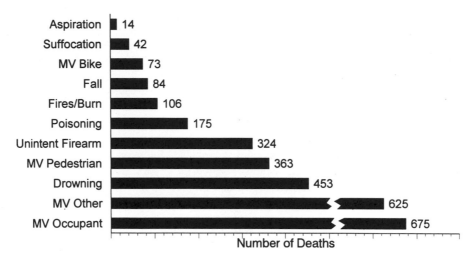

Figure 4. Number of adolescent deaths by cause, 1991: By age (15–19). Source: NCHS (1994).

The pattern of motor vehicle injury among adolescents over age 15 reflects several factors generally associated with higher risk of collision and injury: driving at night and on the weekend, drinking and driving, speeding and other traffic violations, and driving smaller cars. More than half (59%) of all teenage motor vehicle deaths occurred on weekends. About half of teenage motor vehicle deaths occur between 9 p.m. and 6 a.m. Both female and male 16- to 19-year olds were three to four times more likely to be involved in nighttime fatal crashes per 100 million miles traveled than drivers 30–54 years old (IIHS, 1991). Alcohol is an important contributing factor to the high rate of nighttime and weekend motor vehicle-related deaths. Alcohol involvement in crashes peaks at night and is higher on weekends than weekdays.

Alcohol affects driving ability at even very low blood alcohol concentrations (BAC). The probability of a crash begins to increase significantly at 0.05% BAC and climbs rapidly after about 0.08% (IIHS, 1991). In the last quarter of 1991, alcohol was identified in 46% of all teenage traffic fatalities, and 29% of teenage drivers involved in fatal crashes (CDC, 1992c). Although adults have higher rates of alcohol involvement as well as higher BAC, the rate of alcohol-involved deaths per average driving mileage is much higher among adolescents. Thus, Runyan and Gerken (1989) conclude that while adolescents are less likely than adult drivers to drive after drinking, those who do are at a higher risk of being in a crash, even with drinking less alcohol. These findings have led 19 states to lower the legal BAC limits for adolescent drivers to 0.05% or less. Alcohol is also involved in a significant proportion of pedestrian fatalities among older adolescents (34%) and young adults (50%) (NHTSA, 1994).

In response to telephone surveys, teenage drivers were significantly more likely than adult drivers to report that they speed, run red lights, make illegal turns, do not wear safety belts, drive after heavy drinking, drive after marijuana use, and ride with intoxicated drivers. Many of these driving behaviors, known to be associated with fatal and nonfatal crashes, disproportionately cluster in the same adolescent drivers (Hingson & Howland, 1993). For example, in 1990 adolescents made up only 10% of the driving population but were involved in 20% of fatal crashes involving speeding. Nevertheless, between 1979 and 1991, death rates from motor vehicle crashes declined 26% among the 10–14 age group, and 30% among teenagers 15–19 (NCHS, 1993).

Drowning

Drowning is the third most common cause of unintentional injury death; it is among the top five causes of injury mortality through age 30. It ranks second in terms of potential years of life lost before age 65 due to injury (National Safety Council, 1991). Rates of drowning vary substantially by state, locality, and age as a result of different exposure to pools, natural bodies of water, and climate. For the period 1980–1985, drowning rates among children under age 15 ranged from 0.8/100,000 per year in Rhode Island to 6.8 in Alaska. California, Oregon, and Utah were among the states with significantly higher rates of drowning deaths, although they did not have significantly higher childhood death rates for most other causes (Waller, Baker, & Szocka, 1989). Among adolescents and young adults, drowning occurs most often during swimming or boating activities. The extent of this problem may be unappreciated because drowning deaths related to boats, even small recreational craft, are classified as water transport deaths and are often excluded from official drowning statistics. The death rate from drowning peaks in late adolescence and is highest among 18-year-old males. The male-to-female ratio is 10:1 among 15- to 19-year-olds, and black youth are three times more likely to drown than their white counterparts. Alcohol is involved in 40% of adolescent drowning and is believed to increase the risk of drowning by influencing judgment, reducing dexterity, and increasing the likelihood of aspiration of water on immersion (Schwarz, 1993). Like motor vehicle crash deaths, death rates from drowning also declined between 1979 and 1991. There was a 46% decline among younger adolescents, and 41% decline among 15- to 19-year-olds.

Firearms

Unintentional firearm injury resulted in 486 deaths in teens ages 10–19 during 1991. Using an alternative ranking scheme for causes of deaths, Fingerhut (1993) found that firearms, irrespective of injury intent, are the second leading cause of death (after motor vehicle injury fatalities) for children 10–14 years of age, teenagers 15–19 years of age, and young adults. This analysis illustrates the importance of looking at specific vectors of injury across causes or circumstances since "intent" may often be unclear while issues related to exposure to guns are similar. Runyan and Gerken (1989) report findings of studies that documented the availability of firearms among youth. In Baltimore, Maryland, half of the males reported that they had carried a handgun to high school and 60% knew someone who was threatened by a gun. In rural North Carolina, 75% of teenagers reported having guns of some type in their home, with 55% of males owning a personal weapon. Another study in North Carolina, mentioned by Paulson (1988), found that the unintentional firearm death rate was highest among 15- to 19-year olds, that the largest percentage of deaths (28%) were hunting-related, and that one-fifth were related to "fooling around." Data from the North American Association of Hunter Safety Coordinators also show that adolescents aged 10–19 contributed the greatest number of both fatalities and overall firearm-related hunting injuries (Schwarz, 1993).

Socioeconomic and Geographic Differences

Unintentional injury death rates differ considerably among socioeconomic groups and between geographic locations. National data show that the death rate for unintentional injury varies inversely with per capita income of the area of residence of those who died; that both motor vehicle and non-motor-vehicle unintentional injury death rates are highest in rural areas; and that these rates tend to be high in the West and South (Baker *et al.*, 1992). Although comparable national analyses for the adolescent age group are not readily available, studies that explored deaths throughout the continuum of childhood and adolescence have demonstrated social, economic, and geographic disparities. For example, a study of childhood death and poverty in Maine showed that children who were participating in social welfare programs at the time of death were at higher risk for unintentional injury death than other children (2.6:1), and that the disparity in rates was highest for deaths from fire and drowning (Nersesian, Petit, Shaper, Lemieux, & Naor, 1985). The inverse relationship between income and childhood mortality from all injuries, and from non-vehicle-related unintentional injuries was also reported for Massachusetts (Lescohier, Shapiro, Guyer, & Wise, 1988). An analysis of national mortality data regarding unintentional firearm-related fatalities among children and teenagers shows substantial differences by region of residence. Children and teenagers living in the South were three times more likely to die from an unintentional gunshot wound than those living in the Northeast (CDC, 1992a). Socioeconomic status may explain some of the differences in mortality rates observed by race (Onwuachi-Saunders & Hawkins, 1993).

Morbidity

Most injury studies focus on fatal events, but mortality does not tell the whole story. Deaths account for less than one-tenth of 1% of all injuries (Guyer & Gallagher, 1985). Among teenagers 13–19 years old, for every unintentional injury death there are 41 hospitalizations and 1132 emergency department visits for unintentional injury (Gallagher, Finison, Guyer, & Goodenough, 1984). Moreover, the causes of injury morbidity present a different pattern than the causes of mortality. This section will briefly review unintentional injury morbidity and focus on frequent, but overlooked injuries to teens, namely, sports injuries and work-related injuries. While the morbidity rates presented here are somewhat old, they remain the best age-specific data available.

In the United States in 1991, an estimated 10.4 million adolescents ages 10–19 received an injury serious enough to require inpatient or outpatient treatment at a hospital. More than 90% of these nonfatal injuries to teens were classified as unintentional compared to only 59% of fatal injuries. The proportion of nonfatal injuries attributed to unintentional events differed only slightly by age. Almost 98% of injuries in 10- to 14-year-olds were unintentional as compared with 93% in older teens (Malek, Chang, Gallagher, & Guyer, 1991).

The overall unintentional injury rate for adolescents is 2718 per 10,000 and males have twice the rate of females (Gallagher *et al.,* 1984). Unlike mortality, traffic-related injuries do not predominate. Younger teens are injured most often from sports (25%), falls (21%), being struck by an object (16%) (which includes striking against an object, being hit by a falling object, slamming a finger in a door, and striking head on furniture), cutting and piercing instruments such as hand tools, knives, and sharp objects (12%), and as bicyclists (6%). Older teens are injured most often from sports (21%) cutting and piercing (14%), struck by object (14%), falls (11%), and as motor vehicle occupants (10%) (Malek *et al.,* 1991).

Differences in risk by age group are presented in Table 1. These rates indicate the likelihood of a specific injury occurring to an adolescent in a given year and should be interpreted as 1 out of X number of adolescents will sustain a particular cause of injury requiring hospital admission or emergency department treatment annually. One out of every 16 teenagers requires hospital treatment for a sports injury annually. One out of every 32 older teens will be injured as a motor vehicle occupant each year. The most common poison ingestions were related to alcohol or drug abuse. Burns to teenagers often were work-related and involved contact and flame burns, occurred on the leg while riding a motorcycle, or were chemical burns received during automotive maintenance and repair (e.g., battery acid). For traffic-related incidents, children ages 10–14 are most often

Table 1. Incident Ratios for Adolescents Rank Ordered by External Cause and Age[a]

External cause	Age 10–14	External cause	Age 15–19
Sports	1:17	Sports	1:16
Falls	1:21	Struck by object	1:24
Struck by object	1:27	Cutting and piercing	1:24
Cutting and piercing	1:35	Other[b]	1:26
Other[b]	1:40	Falls	1:30
Bicyclist	1:72	Motor vehicle occupant	1:32
Motor vehicle occupant	1:192	Assault/undetermined	1:59
Assault/undetermined	1:222	Foreign body[c]	1:145
Foreign body[c]	1:410	Burns	1:157
Pedestrian	1:459	Bicyclist	1:222
Burns	1:495	Other motor vehicle[d]	1:275
Poisonings	1:893	Poisonings	1:313
Other motor vehicle[d]	1:1282	Suicide attempts	1:379
Suicide attempts	1:1961	Pedestrian	1:505
Unintentional firearms	1:2500	Unintentional firearms	1:1667

[a]Source: Malek *et al.* (1991).
[b]Other includes near drowning, overexertion, machinery, rides on animals, other environmental exposures.
[c]Foreign body includes objects in the eye or in an orifice and objects inhaled.
[d]Other motor vehicle includes motorcycles and off-road vehicles (e.g., ATVs, snowmobiles, dirt bikes).

injured as bicyclists, occupants, and pedestrians. Older teens are most often injured as occupants, bicyclists, and from other means such as motorcycles and off-road vehicles.

The largest proportion of injuries were less severe ones such as lacerations, contusions, sprains, followed by fractures and dislocations to the upper and lower extremities. More serious injuries included traumatic brain injuries (20–27% of admissions) and injuries to the chest, trunk, abdomen, and pelvis (7–9% of admissions).

The locations where teens were most frequently injured varied by age. Among the 10- to 14-year-olds, nonfatal injuries are more likely to occur in outdoor areas (32%), at school (28%), or at home (21%). Among older teens, nonfatal injuries occur most often at work (28%), in a motor vehicle (21%), or an outdoor area (18%). Similar proportions (12%) occurred at home and in school (SCIPP, 1994).

Trends over time and rates by race, ethnicity, and socioeconomic status are not available for nonfatal, unintentional injuries.

Sports

We have chosen to highlight sports injuries because of their high incidence, high medical costs, and the relative lack of attention paid to their prevention.

While the number of adolescents who die playing competitive sports is small, an estimated 2.6 million sports injuries requiring treatment at an emergency department occur to children and adolescents in the United States every year. Another 92,000 hospitalizations occur in the same population (Guyer & Ellers, 1990). One in every 16 younger teens and one in every 17 older teens will suffer a sports-related injury in a given year (Malek *et al.*, 1991). Sports injuries are, in fact, the most frequent cause of both emergency department visits and hospitalizations for an injury for both older and younger teens.

Studies of sports injuries are almost exclusively focused on a single sport like football or baseball, competitive sports in schools, or the high school age population (Gallagher, 1993). Studies that produce statistics on the full range of sports injuries and age groups, so that the risk of injury in different sports can be compared, are rare. In one such study, the overall rate of sports injuries was 584 per 10,000 for 10- to 14-year-olds and 607 per 10,000 for 15- to 19-year-olds (Malek *et al.*, 1991). The overall male-to-female ratio in this study was about 2:1, but the sex differential increased and rose to nearly 3:1 as adolescents got older. Although the largest proportion of sports injuries in teens are mainly from well-known, organized team sports—football (20%), basketball (17.4%), rollerskating (13.4%), and baseball (9.4%)—nonorganized and/or individual sports such as soccer, ice hockey, sledding, skiing, horseback riding, skateboarding, and track and field are more serious as evidenced by a higher ratio of injuries that require hospital admission (Gallagher, 1993). In fact, in this study, a contact team sport like football had a relatively small share of concussions (2.6%) than many individual activities like track and field (7.1%), ice skating (4.2%), or even horseback riding (4.5%).

The majority of sports injuries were caused by falls (42%), being struck by an object (28%), or from overexertion (10%). The most frequent types of injuries were fractures of the extremities. Hospitalizations for sports injuries account for 16% of all injury discharges with an average length of stay of 3.8 days. The largest number of sports-related hospitalizations occur for younger teens aged 10–14 with a peak rate at ages 14 and 15.

Despite the fact that 55% of all sports-related hospitalizations occur for younger teens, this age group has not been well studied for risks of injury from sports.

Risk and exposure have not been adequately addressed in sports injuries because of the difficulty in determining the total number of youth participants and hours of play or practice for each sport in a community. In addition, many studies of sports only document the rate of severe injuries. Yet, less severe injuries from overuse may result in chronic problems with a profound effect in later years.

Work-Related Injuries

Employment is a significant and often essential factor in the lives of many adolescents. Benefits include money for personal or family use, enhanced feelings of competence and independence, and acquisition of new skills. Families usually express approval and pride when teens enter the workforce. There may also be a false sense of security with the notion that the teen is off the street and out of potential trouble.

Yet, U.S. adolescents, especially those living on family farms, are at high risk of work-related injuries. In 1992 an estimated 64,100 teenagers ages 14–17 were treated in emergency departments for a work-related injury (Layne, Castillo, Stout, & Cutlip, 1994). Overall, males accounted for nearly two-thirds of the cases. The industries in which adolescents were most likely to be injured were the retail trades (54%), where they sustain lacerations and burns within eating and drinking establishments, services industries (20%), especially within the health sector, amusement, recreation, and educational services, and agriculture (7%). In agriculture, teens are likely to sustain lacerations related to running machinery or equipment. A greater proportion of injuries to 14- and 15-year-olds occurred in agriculture (40%) compared to other industries (12%) and to males in agriculture (88%) compared to other industries (64%). Almost 40% of workplace injuries occur during the first year of work (Bureau of Labor Statistics, 1994).

Clearly, these and other estimates of such injuries are conservative given the problems of underreporting (Suruda & Halperin, 1991; Parker, Clay, Mandel, Gunderson, & Salkowicz, 1991; Brooks, Davis, & Gallagher, 1993; Banco, Lapidus, & Braddock, 1992; Fingar, Hopkins, & Nelson, 1992) and an inability to determine an accurate number of younger teens in the workforce by industry. Regardless of the source of the data, recent studies indicate that working minors are at very high risk for occupational injury (Castillo, Landen, & Layne, 1994; Suruda & Halperin, 1991; Glor, 1989; Banco et al., 1992; Belville, Pollack, Godbold, & Landrigan, 1993; Heyer, Franklin, Rivara, Parker, & Haug, 1992). Both the number and proportion of injuries attributed to work increase sharply with age of the adolescent (Brooks et al., 1993). The estimated annual rate of occupational injuries treated at emergency departments rises from 3.7 per 1000 teens for 14- to 15-year-olds (or 1 out of every 270) to 44.7 per 1000 for 17-year-olds (or 1 out of every 22 teens). Work-related injuries rose from 2% of all injuries seen in the emergency department among 14-year-olds to 26% among 17-year-olds.

Given that not all children work, and those who do, work only part time or seasonally, injury rates based on actual hours worked are much higher, with reported ranges of 5.8 per 100 full time equivalents (FTEs) (Layne et al., 1994) to 16 per 100 FTEs (Brooks et al., 1993). Applying the national estimates on youth employment to one

Massachusetts study, yielded an injury rate of 22 per 100 FTEs for 16- to 17-year-old males (Brooks *et al.,* 1993). This rate is significantly greater than the national rate for adults of 8.9 per 100 FTEs (Bureau of Labor Statistics, 1993), or the Healthy People 2000 goal of 6 per 100 FTEs (PHS, 1991).

Disability

Population-based data on disability resulting from injury are not readily available. The National Pediatric Trauma Registry (NPTR) collects data from selected hospitals on the causes, treatment, and outcomes of hospitalized pediatric trauma patients. The NPTR data depository included 12,720 records of adolescents 10 years of age or older. Of this group, 48% were diagnosed, on discharge from the acute care setting, with at least one impaired function in activity of daily living, cognition, or behavior. One out of four adolescent patients was discharged with three or more impairments (NPTR, 1994).

Disability resulting from injuries treated at the outpatient setting was examined in a population of children and adolescents who belonged to a health maintenance organization in Seattle, Washington (Rivara, Thompson, Thompson, & Calonge, 1991). Overall, 55% in this population had limitations in their usual activities during the week following injury. Adolescents 10–19 years of age had more functional impairments than younger children. Injuries occurring in organized sports resulted in proportionately more restrictions in physical activity than any other cause. The study estimated that trauma presenting to the primary care settings resulted in 558 days of restricted activity per 1000 children annually.

Physical limitations are not the only sequelae of acute injury. A follow-up study of trauma patients found that 6 months after the injury, 54% of 15- to 34-year-old patients suffered pain, 19% had psychologic impairment, and 17% were suffering mental impairment (Maurette *et al.,* 1992).

Cost

A 1989 report to Congress estimated the total lifetime cost of injury in the United States at $158 billion (Rice, MacKenzie, & Associates, 1989). These costs include medical expenses as well as loss of earnings related to death or disability. Information was not presented by the age groupings used in this paper. But the lifetime cost of injury for 15- to 24-year-olds was estimated at $39 billion, one-quarter of cost for all age groups combined. Direct cost for medical care, rehabilitation, and nonmedical care directly related to the injury, accounted for 23% of total cost in this age group. Morbidity and mortality costs of lost productivity resulting from injury-related illness and disability, or death, accounted for 40 and 37%, respectively, of total cost.

A study that combined injury incidence data from the Massachusetts Statewide Childhood Injury Prevention Project with insurance claims data, estimated annual cost for initial medical care of injury to adolescents aged 10–19 at $3.5 billion in 1987 dollars (Malek *et al.,* 1991). The study only included costs for initial hospitalizations and emergency department care because information on incidence and charges at primary care settings is not available. Table 2 presents the estimated medical care costs for adolescents by age, selected causes, and treatment setting.

Table 2. Estimated Initial National Medical Cost of Injury by Age, Cause of Injury Group, and Treatment Setting (in Millions of 1987 Dollars)[a]

Cause	Age group (years)			
	10–14		15–19	
	Inpatient	Outpatient	Inpatient	Outpatient
Motor vehicle injury—occupant/unspecified	$ 23.4	$13.9	$416.6	$103.3
Pedal cycle	76.1	37.9	41.7	13.4
Motor vehicle injury—pedestrian	25.4	5.4	25.7	5.8
Other vehicle injury	20.1	1.3	81.7	10.3
Falls	120.3	132.6	116.5	109.3
Burns	6.7	4.4	26.9	15.3
Poisonings	7.9	1.7	25.3	7.5
Foreign body/suffocation	2.5	4.9	5.1	16.8
Struck by object	36.5	99.7	67.9	140.3
Cutting/piercing	21.0	68.3	40.6	139.7
Unintentional firearms	3.9	0.8	19.0	1.5
Suicide	6.4	0.7	71.9	4.3
Assault/undetermined	14.7	12.6	126.2	56.1
Sports	141.8	165.7	228.1	196.7
Other	8.2	70.1	78.1	135.0
Total	541.8	620.3	1371.1	955.2
Mean cost	4546.0	172.0	6159.0	185.0

[a]Source: Malek *et al.* (1991).

Because of both a higher injury incidence and a greater mean cost per injury, the projected initial cost of injuries to teenagers 15–19 years old was much higher than that of younger children, accounting for 46% of total cost in the 0–19 age group. Among younger teenagers, the highest medical care costs were generated by sports injuries followed by falls. Sports injuries were the second leading cause of estimated total costs (after motor vehicle occupant injury) in older adolescents.

PREVENTION

The term *injury control* is currently being used to describe a comprehensive approach that includes strategies to counter the injury process at several stages. There are three levels of injury control where such strategies can be employed:

- *Prevention*—where we aim to prevent, reduce, or modify hazards or events that cause injury
- *Acute care*—when we begin to counter the damage already done by the hazard and move to stabilize and repair the damage; and
- *Rehabilitation*—efforts made to restore the functioning of injured patients to preinjury levels

In the past four decades the scientific base of injury prevention has made dramatic progress. This progress drew on the work of experts in disciplines such as epidemiology, medicine, ergonomics, engineering, and biomechanics. Landmark scientific developments by injury prevention pioneers such as De Haven, McFarland, Gordon, and Haddon have been described in several publications (National Committee for Injury Prevention and Control, 1989; Baker *et al.*, 1992; Waller, 1994). Examples of how these scientists tackled the injury problem are instructive.

Hugh De Haven, a World War I combat pilot who survived an airplane crash, subsequently studied individuals who fell from heights of 50 to 150 feet without sustaining serious injury. He determined how structural provisions could help reduce impact and distribute the forces of energy over the body in automobile and airplane crashes. His ideas were later translated into "crash packaging" design concepts—safety belts, airbags, collapsible steering assemblies, and dashboard padding—that adapt the structure of cars to enhance survival.

One of the first researchers in the field of ergonomics—the study of how people respond to and interact with the environment—was Ross McFarland. He applied concepts from the field of human factors to highway safety by showing how the design and placement of the gear shift in trucks prevented taller drivers from moving their legs quickly from the accelerator to the brake.

Another early researcher, Harvard epidemiologist John Gordon, suggested in 1949 that methods used to analyze patterns of infectious diseases be directed to the study of injury. He observed that each injury, like each disease outbreak, was the product of at least three sources: the host, the agent, and the environment in which the host and agent find themselves. One problem with this model was that, given the diversity of products, objects, and substances associated with injury, the list of potential agents was almost limitless.

The problem of how to define the agent of injury was solved by James Gibson, an experimental psychologist, who wrote that injury to a living organism can be produced only be some energy interchange. In the early 1960s, Dr. William Haddon, Jr., an engineer and public health physician, took Gibson's and Gordon's analyses further and developed a conceptual model that is the basis of our current understanding of injury events. Haddon concluded that the five forms of physical energy (mechanical, chemical, thermal, electrical, and radiation) are the agents of injury, and that these agents are transmitted to the body through vectors, or vehicles (e.g., cars, guns, hot liquids). Further, Haddon developed a matrix that looks at risk factors for injury associated with the host, the vector, and the physical environment. These factors are related to three phases in the injury process: before, during, and after an injury event takes place. This approach helps to identify the elements that need to be modified in order to prevent an injury or reduce its severity and sequelae.

Haddon, and later his students, placed an emphasis on modifying vectors and the physical environment—a radical shift from previous injury prevention efforts directed at changing individual behavior through education. At present, there is a growing interest in studying the role of human behavior in injury, and in evaluating the effects of economic, social, and political strategies on modifying behavior. Table 3 depicts a modified Haddon Phase–Factor Matrix using a motor vehicle occupant injury as an example. The matrix suggests that interventions may be applied in one or several cells, but it does not predict

Table 3. A Modified Haddon Matrix: Example of Factors Related to the Likelihood of Motor Vehicle-Associated Injury and Its Outcome[a]

Phase	Host (human)	Vector (vehicle)	Physical environment	Socioeconomic environment
		Factors		
Precrash	Driver vision	Brakes, tires	Visibility of hazards	Attitudes about alcohol
	Alcohol intoxication	Center of gravity	Road curvature and gradient	Laws related to impaired driving
	Experience and judgment	Jackknife tendency	Surface coefficient of friction	Enforcement of speed limits
	Amount of travel	Speed of travel	Divided highways	Laws: teens driving
	Night and weekend	Ease of control	Intersections, access control	
	Traffic violations		Signals	
Crash	Safety-belt use	Speed at impact	Recovery areas	Attitudes about safety-belt use
	Age	Vehicle size	Guard rails	Laws about safety-belt use
	Sex	Automatic restraints	Characteristics of fixed objects	
		Airbag	Median barriers	
		Type of contact surface	Roadside embankments	
		Rollover	Speed limits	
Postcrash	Age	Fuel system integrity	Emergency transport system	Support for trauma care systems
	Physical condition		Quality of EMS	Skill of EMS personnel
	Severity of injury		Distance to trauma center	Law and attitudes re: disability
	Body region injured		Rehabilitation programs	School integration

[a]Source: Adapted from the National Committee for Injury Prevention and Control, 1989.

the extent of benefit that may accrue from these interventions. In order to evaluate the relative effects of various types of prevention efforts we review briefly 40 years of progress in traffic safety.

Progress in Preventing Motor Vehicle Crash Injuries

In explaining the progress made in highway safety between 1950 and 1980, Graham (1993) suggests that the declining fatality rates can be traced to a handful of key factors in highway design, vehicular design, and improvements in the delivery of emergency medical services. He notes that the single most important factor was the development of the

Interstate Highway System, which incorporates safety features such as divided traffic streams, controlled access, few dangerous curves, highly visible traffic signs, wide roadside shoulders, and forgiving roadside fixtures. These design features influence crash rates and help explain why the fatality rate on interstate highways is one-third of the rate on rural highways. In 1990, 29% of all deaths in motor vehicle crashes involved roadside hazards which are more common on roads other than superhighways, including trees, utility poles, sign posts, light supports, and other poles and posts (IIHS, 1991). Federal safety standards regulating vehicle design have also resulted in reductions in traffic fatalities.

Less clear are the reasons for the progress during the 1980s, when reductions in the number and rate of fatalities exceeded those achieved in the earlier three decades. Two areas of increased prevention efforts during the 1980s are of particular relevance to the adolescent age group. These include the campaign against drunk driving, and strategies to increase safety belt use.

Drinking and Driving

Between 1980 and 1990, the proportion of fatally injured drivers with BAC $\geq 0.10\%$ declined systematically from 53% in 1980 to 40% in 1990 (IIHS, 1991). A similar trend has been observed with respect to all traffic-related fatalities. Of all age groups, the reduction in alcohol-related fatalities was largest among adolescent drivers under 21 years of age (National Safety Council, 1990). In 1991, the number of alcohol-related traffic fatalities continued to decline and was the lowest since more complete alcohol-related fatal crash data became available in 1982. Again, the largest 1990 to 1991 declines in total alcohol-related traffic fatalities (13%) and among alcohol-involved drivers (15%) were observed in the 15–20 age group (CDC, 1992c).

A combination of legal strategies and grass roots community efforts have been cited as important factors in reducing drunk driving deaths among adolescents as well as adults. Raising the legal drinking age to 21, adopted by all states as of 1988, was accompanied by a 10–15% reduction in fatal crashes in the age group targeted by these laws. Other laws, not specifically directed at adolescents, also had an effect. These include criminal laws that intend to deter drunk driving regardless of traffic violations, and administrative laws that permit license suspension between the time of arrest and trial.

These legislative changes were partly achieved as a result of well-organized campaigns by groups such as Mothers Against Drunk Driving (MADD) and Remove Intoxicated Drivers (RID). Other information and educational strategies such as the "designated driver," Students Against Drunk Driving (SADD), and other alcohol education programs may have contributed to changes in social norms about drinking and driving but the extent of beneficial effects of these efforts has not been established (Graham, 1993; Hingson & Howland, 1993).

Other approaches that do not rely on a direct appeal to the adolescent driver include increasing the price of alcoholic beverages, an economic measure that has been shown to decrease availability to the young and thus lower the risk of alcohol-related injury in this population (Saffer & Grossman, 1987). Alcohol server interventions to increase compliance on the part of servers with laws prohibiting the sale of alcoholic beverages to minors and intoxicated patrons, and liberalization of liability laws allowing third parties injured in alcohol-related collisions to recover damages from those who served the alcohol, are more recent approaches with potential to reduce drinking and driving.

Safety-Belt Use

Low safety-belt use has frequently been cited as a prime example of risk-taking behavior among adolescents. The concern over occupant restraints is well placed because use of lap and shoulder belts is known to reduce the risk for fatal injury by 40–50% and the risk for moderate to critical injury by 45–55% (NHTSA, 1984). Since the early 1980s there has been a consistent rise in safety-belt use and in states' laws mandating such use: from 14% in 1984 when only one state had a mandatory use law, to 54% in 1991 with 41 states having such laws (Datta & Guzek, 1991). According to the most recent data released by the National Highway Traffic Safety Administration, the national use rates rose to 66% in 1993. By 1994, only two states (Maine and New Hampshire) did not have mandatory belt use laws. Whereas national usage rates reported by the National Highway Traffic Safety Administration arc based on observational studies, data about the prevalence of safety-belt use among adolescents have relied primarily on self-reported surveys. For example, in a periodic school-based survey conducted through the CDC's Youth Risk Behavior Surveillance System, a representative sample of students in grades 9–12 are asked how often they use safety belts when riding in a car or truck driven by someone else. In the 1991 survey, 28% of students said they "always" wore seat belts (CDC, 1992b).

While students' responses indicate a low rate of seat-belt use, it is difficult to correlate these findings with the observational data cited earlier except to say that in both methods large variations in usage rates were found among states and jurisdictions. Few studies have compared seat-belt use among adolescents and adults using the same methods and controlling for local variations, although there is an association between observed safety-belt use and demographic and socioeconomic indicators (Shinar, 1993). One study that did employ similar observational methods for teenagers and other drivers in the community, in order to evaluate the effect of New York's seat-belt use law, found that teenagers have responded to the law with substantial increase in belt use: from 14% prior to adoption of the law to 63% 5 months later. The study also found that both before and after the law, teenage belt use was similar to, but typically lower than, belt use in the community in which the school was located (Preusser, Williams, & Lund, 1987).

Indeed, laws have been found to be more effective in increasing the rate of seat-belt use than other programs, although all interventions seem to have a positive effect (Johnston, Hendricks, & Fike, 1994). Further, states with primary laws that permit police to stop motorists solely for not wearing seat belts, have higher usage rates than states with secondary laws. As national efforts are being mounted to reach the goal of 75% seat-belt use by 1997, the relationship of trends in the general population and among adolescents in given communities requires further study. Some argue that to realize the actual lifesaving benefits of occupant restraints, the increase in seat-belt use rate has to be substantial because those who comply first are usually safe drivers. Others suggest a possible adverse effect of such increase among drivers who, perceiving better personal protection by the belt, will assume other unsafe practices such as speeding. These issues are particularly pertinent to young drivers and should also attract further research.

Summary

The example of progress in motor vehicle safety illustrates how a combination of approaches can improve adolescent health status. This age group has gained primarily from injury countermeasures directed at all vehicle occupants such as improvements in the design of cars and roads, speed limit, seat belt and alcohol-related laws, and better systems for the transport and care of the critically injured. Specific measures aimed at modifying adolescent behavior, such as increase in the legal drinking age, have also made a contribution. Although the effectiveness of education and persuasion efforts in changing individual behavior may be limited when conducted in isolation, public education and well-organized grass roots advocacy can lead to change in community norms as well as increased demand for safety measures.

Injury Countermeasures

Earlier we discussed the Haddon Matrix, a framework for analyzing injury events and the interaction among factors that lead to their occurrence. Similarly, there was a need for a conceptualization of approaches that interfere with the injury process. During the 1960s, Haddon developed and refined a list of ten measures that can be applied to the prevention and control of many types of injury. Baker *et al.* (1992) used sports injuries to illustrate Haddon's ten basic strategies. Because sports injuries are the leading cause of morbidity and costs among adolescents, we will do the same, relying on some of their examples and focusing on those that are particularly relevant to youth.

The ten strategies are the following:

1. *Prevent the creation of the hazard.* This can be done either by banning the manufacture and sale of specific products that are inherently unsafe, or by prohibiting activities. An example of the first approach is the 1987 ban on three-wheeled all-terrain vehicles (ATVs) in the United States. These unstable recreational vehicles, favored by adolescents, were responsible for an estimated 85,900 emergency department admissions in 1985, and 12 times more deaths than caused by bicycles (Runyan & Gerken, 1989). Another example, mentioned by Baker *et al.* (1992), relates to trampolines, an important source of spinal cord injuries. It seemed impossible to introduce changes to this sport that would reduce the incidence of serious injuries. A 60% drop in the number of hospital-treated head and neck injuries caused by trampolines was reported after the American Academy of Pediatrics recommended, in 1977, a ban on the use of trampolines in schools. An example of the second approach, to prohibit specific activities, is the 1976 ruling that eliminated spearing in both high school and college football. Spearing, using the helmet as the point of contact to block an opponent while tackling, places axial loading on the spine and is associated with neck and spinal cord injuries. A decline in the incidence of permanent quadriplegia from 35 cases in 1971 to an annual average of less than 10 by 1986, has been attributed to the 1976 ban (Runyan & Gerken, 1989). Still, in 1988 there

were six deaths directly attributed to high school football, and in the 1989 season, four high school football players in Louisiana sustained cervical spine injuries resulting in quadriplegia, suggesting that the practice continues (Widome, 1991).

2. *Reduce the amount of the hazard.* The National Committee for Injury Prevention and Control (1989) has recommended that children and young adults should be discouraged from participating in boxing because this sport is likely to cause brain damage. They also urge schools and community groups not to sponsor youth boxing programs. Sponsoring alternative sports that offer similar conditioning opportunities but little risk of head injury is one example of limiting participation and reducing risk. Other examples include prohibiting participation of players who use alcohol and drugs, postponing games or practice sessions during inclement weather, and replacing leather soccer balls (which become waterlogged and very heavy) with synthetic nonabsorbent balls during wet playing conditions.

3. *Prevent the release of a hazard that already exists.* The U.S. Hunter Education Association recorded 139 fatal and 1132 nonfatal hunting injuries in 1992, of which 31% were self-inflicted (National Safety Council, 1994). Short of a total ban, weapon redesign is one way to reduce injury (Hemenway & Weil, 1990). Design suggestions include a safety mechanism that prevents the gun from discharging unintentionally, and a color-coded display to indicate whether there is ammunition in the chamber. Another example relates to movable soccer goals that can tip over and cause injury. The Consumer Product Safety Commission reported 18 deaths and 14 serious injuries since 1979 resulting from soccer goal tipovers. Injuries could be prevented if portable goals are securely anchored or counterweighted at all times.

4. *Modify the rate of spatial distribution of the hazard.* Many injuries are caused when baseball and softball players collide with fixed bases while sliding. The introduction of detachable bases, designed to break away from their mooring posts, has reduced the rate and severity of sliding injuries. Based on a study in Michigan, the CDC estimated that exclusive use of breakaway bases would reduce injuries by 96% and medical costs by 99% (Janda, Wojtys, Henkin, & Benedict, 1988).

5. *Separate, in time or space, the hazard from that which is to be protected.* Approximately 1000 diving-related spinal cord injuries occur each year and most victims are adolescents and young adult males. The injury usually occurs in shallow waters when the diver's head hits the bottom. An increasing number of spinal cord injuries result from swimmers diving off starting blocks in pools. A review of a series of 25 such cases revealed that every one of these injuries occurred in water of 4 feet or less. This hazard can be reduced by moving starting blocks to locations where the minimum depth of the water is 6 feet (Gabrielson & Shulman, 1990).

6. *Separate the hazard from that which is to be protected by a material barrier.* Protective eyewear to prevent ocular injury during sports activity is a good example for this strategy. In Canada, where ice hockey is the leading cause of sports-related eye injury, required eye protection for amateur players has reduced eye injuries significantly. Sports are the leading cause of eye injury in the 11–15 age group, where they account for 40% of all such injuries. Among children, sports lead to over 20% of penetrating and about 40% of blunt eye trauma (Widome, 1991). Blunt eye trauma is associated with many ball games and racket sports. Shattered glass from prescription eyeglasses is also a cause of

sports-related injury. Based on laboratory experiments, Vinger (1994) suggests that although eye protection devices are available on the market, some of them do not meet the necessary standards to withstand real-world situations. As a practicing ophthalmologist, Winger notes that another barrier to reducing eye injury among children and adolescents is the reluctance of both ophthalmologists and optometrists to prescribe polycarbonate lenses for individuals who participate in sports and other recreational activities. Unlike glass and conventional plastic, polycarbonate lenses that meet ASTM standards tend to bend rather than shatter. One of the reasons for this reluctance may be the rigid character of the material, which makes it more difficult to fashion and adjust. The higher cost for consumers may also make providers hesitant to offer this choice.

7. *Modify relevant basic qualities of the hazard.* A consensus meeting of medical experts, convened by the National Youth Sports Foundation for the Prevention of Athletic Injuries (1994), recommended the adoption of softer baseballs by coaches and youth leagues nationwide. Baseball has the highest fatality rate of any youth sport with the least amount of safety equipment mandated. Softer balls can reduce the incidence and severity of head injury and soft tissue injury among children and adolescents. The balls, called RIF for reduced injury factor, have foam cores inside stitched leather exteriors, as opposed to the wound fiber cores of conventional hardballs. Both balls weigh about the same and go about as far when hit. Results of a 1993 analysis of youth league games in Michigan were reported at a press conference held in Boston by sports medicine physicians and researchers. It showed that youth team players were three times more likely to be seriously hurt if they were playing with the harder ball (*Boston Globe,* 1994). Lyle Micheli, director of sports medicine at Children's Hospital in Boston, and chairman of the consensus panel, reported at the same meeting that impact from the traditional hardball typically used in youth league games, caused the majority of deaths and injuries in the sport.

8. *Make what is to be protected more resistant to damage from the hazard.* Gymnastics appears to pose the greatest injury risk among sports with high female participation. Musculoskeletal conditioning to build strength and preserve agility is particularly important in this sport. Too often, however, a secondary injury occurs because initial injuries were not allowed to heal completely before the student returns to practice. In addition, practice sessions for sports with a limited number of competitive athletes include students with a variety of skill levels, which may increase risk of injury for those less fit. Baker *et al.* (1992) note that grouping students by skill, physical fitness, and physical maturity rather than age has reportedly reduced injury rates.

9. *Begin to counter the damage already done by the hazard.* Proper emergency response to the injured adolescent depends on prompt recognition of the injury and its nature. It is important to identify life-threatening injuries and injuries with neurological involvement that require attention by skilled emergency medical personnel and timely transport to appropriate facilities. Immobilization of the patient with spinal cord injuries and airway management in patients with head injuries are important first steps in preventing disabling sequelae. The development of emergency medical services for the pediatric population has lagged behind the system for adults (IOM, 1993). Many schools lack protocols for responding to injury emergencies. Training of school personnel, athletic trainers, and sports coaches in how to identify emergencies, provide first aid, and access the EMS system can improve injury outcomes.

10. *Stabilize, repair, and rehabilitate the object of the damage.* The outcome of injury can be improved if definitive care facilities are available for the treatment of the injured child and adolescent. A study in Pennsylvania found that rural trauma centers have a higher pediatric mortality than urban centers. A possible explanation was that the difference was related, in part, to longer prehospital transport in rural areas (Nakayama, Copes, & Sacco, 1992). Early and well-integrated rehabilitative care can also promote recovery. Haller and Beaver (1989) report that among children receiving such coordinated care, 88% recovered without major motor or intellectual deficits.

Maintaining Diversity of Preventive Strategies

Injury prevention is based on a combination of efforts to alter unsafe behaviors, change social norms, convince policymakers to take action through education, make the physical environment and consumer products less hazardous through engineering and design techniques; and regulate compliance with safety standards through passage of legislation and enforcement (Haddon & Baker, 1981). In the injury control field, notable successes have been achieved through passive countermeasures that require little action on the part of the individual (e.g., airbags) as opposed to active countermeasures that require repeated attention to behavior (e.g., buckling up every time you travel in a motor vehicle) (Robertson, 1984). Although passive measures are often touted as more effective by injury control "gurus," extensive educational efforts are required to create the demand for passive measures and their implementation. There has been a lengthy debate in the injury control field about the merits of each of these approaches. In reality, providing effective protection for adolescents requires a mix of strategies. Although knowledge to implement many strategies exists, the political will to do so has not been marshalled. Work-related injuries among youth offer a good example of insufficient progress in implementing preventive strategies.

- A 15-year-old female working at a supermarket suffered a crushed hand after it became caught in a juice maker. She was told by the employer to clean the juicer while the machine was still on.
- A 15-year-old female restaurant worker suffered second- and third-degree burns when a pot of boiling soup she was carrying spilled on her when bumped by a customer. She had been hired to work in a restaurant where alcohol was sold. She worked more than 20 hours per week. The restaurant had failed to obtain written consent allowing the minor to work on school nights.
- A student working at a print shop as part of her school work-study program suffered the amputation of two fingers when a power lock on a paper cutting machine failed to work. The shop did not have workers compensation insurance and her mother had signed a waiver for the school.
- A 17-year-old male student died from compression asphyxiation after being crushed in a manufacturers baling machine. He was pulled into the baler when attempting to remove clogged paper. No one was on hand who knew how to operate the machine. There were no warnings or instructions on stopping the machine or removing something from the baler.

- A 16-year-old male industrial worker cleaning a meat mixer suffered the amputation of four toes and required three surgeries when his coat got caught in a chain and he was pulled toward the machine. A co-worker had removed the safety guard on the mixer and another co-worker who didn't see him had switched on the machine.

These are but a sample of cases brought to trial. The circumstances that surrounded these injuries reflect a wide range of possible failures that could be attributed to machine design, safety features, job training by the employer, supervision, level of skill or risk behavior by the teen worker, and aspects of child labor laws and their enforcement.

The first federal child labor laws were created in 1938 to avoid putting children at risk. The Federal Fair Labor Standards Act sets age, time, and hour restrictions on employing youth as well as specifying permitted and prohibited occupations and activities for teens ages 14–15 and those 16–17. However, federal child labor laws exempt family farms, represent a minimum level of protection, and do not cover many hazardous situations. As a result, teens are often injured even while under full compliance with the laws (Pollack, Landrigan, & Mallino, 1990).

Better public information and education about child labor laws and their limitations could help parents assess employment risks for their teens. It could also create public pressure for amendments of the laws, and increase enforcement.

The passage of the federal School to Work Opportunities Act in 1994 is one example of a recent initiative that could provide an important opportunity for health and safety education in the workplace. Thus far, 8 states and 15 localities have been funded to develop systems that will build partnerships between schools and employers, and will increase the number of youth in school-sponsored, work-based learning programs. However, comprehensive health and safety education for participants is not an essential component of this Act. Federal and state agencies themselves need understanding of, and education on, this issue so that health and safety language is included in new requests for proposals related to school-to-work implementation.

Despite the existence of child labor laws, adolescent employees use unsafe equipment, work more than the legal number of hours, and engage in prohibited occupations. Relaxation of federal enforcement of child labor laws is one of three factors cited in the reemergence of unsafe practices (Landrigan, 1993). Reported child labor violations, including work hour violations, minimum age violations, and hazardous order violations, have increased from 8731 in 1984 to 22,312 in 1989 (Treanor & Goldnor, 1990). A three-day enforcement effort in 1990 ordered by former U.S. Secretary of Labor, Elizabeth Dole, discovered 15,000+ youth working under illegal conditions, bringing into question the level of enforcement during the 1980s.

Enforcement at the state level has also been lax (Beyer, 1993). Three states (Florida, Texas, and Wyoming) no longer have any child labor investigators. Instead, they refer complaints to the U.S. Department of Labor. A notable exception is New York State, which uses a proactive, multifaceted child labor program, as well as the usual "by complaint" enforcement. Still, in 1992, illegal child labor practices were found in 60% of sites visited in the state (Beyer, 1993). These practices included operating hazardous machinery, exposure to toxic chemicals and pesticides, driving delivery vans when under age, working in construction site excavations, and exceeding maximum hours of employment. Another study of adolescent deaths at work indicated that 86% of the fatalities in one state (North Carolina) appeared to have involved activities in violation of federal child labor laws (Dunn & Runyan, 1993). In addition to better enforcement, child labor laws need to be updated and modified to reflect new technology in the workplace.

Technological solutions to identified problems, and changes in equipment and job design, seldom incorporate the characteristics of the young worker. Design changes could be enhanced by pairing ergonomic specialists with child and adolescent development specialists. A recent analysis of work-related injuries among minors in Connecticut resulted in the implementation of an alternatively designed, safer, cutting tool in a supermarket chain (Banco *et al.*, 1992).

TREATMENT

Once an injury has occurred, the purpose of treatment is to prevent unnecessary death and restore patients to the highest possible level of functioning. Advances in trauma care, and improved survival, have resulted from several processes. Within the past century, surgeons have made phenomenal strides in the understanding of the body's response to injury. Advances in technology have also made important contributions to the science of trauma care (ACS/COT, 1993). The development of formal emergency medical services (EMS) systems in the United States in the early 1970s followed experience in the Korean and Vietnam wars. The rate of survival of wounded soldiers evacuated to medical facilities was higher than in earlier wars. The drop in death rates was a result of decrease in the time from injury to definite surgical care, accomplished through a well-organized system of medical personnel and transport capabilities.

Indeed, it is now recognized by both clinicians and policymakers that the treatment of injury requires an organized approach. Both the American College of Surgeons Committee on Trauma and the American College of Emergency Physicians have developed guidelines for a comprehensive system to deal with injury (ACS/COT, 1993; ACEP, 1987). To promote development at the state level, Congress passed the Trauma Care Systems Planning and Development Act in 1990. This legislation (PL 101-590) formed the foundation for a grant program to encourage states to follow the principles outlined in the Model Trauma Care System Plan developed at the federal level (HRSA, 1992).

Trauma care systems are locally coordinated approaches to swift identification of injured persons and their subsequent transport to optimal care. A model trauma care system links prehospital, hospital, and rehabilitation services in order to provide prompt response and the optimal care commensurate with the seriousness of the injury. At the prehospital stage, the injury needs to be recognized and emergency services notified, the severity of injury assessed, emergency care to stabilize the patient provided, and the person transported to a facility equipped for the care of trauma patients. Major trauma patients, who constitute a small proportion of all injured patients, require care in a designated trauma center, a facility with more comprehensive capabilities than other hospitals. Rehabilitation services should start at the acute care phase and continue after discharge. An optimal trauma care system integrates prevention efforts and advocacy, training of personnel, research, and system evaluation into all levels of clinical patient care.

Although there are only few comprehensive and coordinated trauma systems in the United States, many localities have at least some components in place. Evaluations of regionalized systems have demonstrated their effectiveness in reducing the frequency of preventable deaths and suboptimal care (West, Williams, Trunkey, & Wolferth, 1988; Shackford, Hollingworth-Fridlund, Cooper, & Eastman, 1986). These findings have provided further impetus for system implementation efforts.

Yet, at the same time that these systems were evolving, advocates for children were asking whether the needs of children are being met by the existing structures for delivering emergency response and trauma care services. An examination of this question by several national committees (Haller, 1989; Seidel & Henderson, 1991; IOM, 1993) reached several conclusions.

First, there is a consensus that the emergency and acute care needs of children and youth differ from those of adults. Children differ from adults in their anatomy, physiology, and developmental status. They have special psychological and emotional support needs. In addition to employing different techniques in the management of pediatric patients, including special equipment and medication doses, the care of children also requires an understanding of their psychosocial needs. Yet, the development of subspecialties to care for the injured child (such as pediatric surgery and pediatric emergency medicine) lagged behind. These delays were related in part to the need to integrate knowledge from both pediatrics and the specialty area, a long process. For example, the American College of Emergency Physicians (ACEP) was formed in 1968, but its section on Pediatric Emergency Medicine was not approved until 1989.

Second, there are indications that the emergency and acute care needs of children have been neglected in a system that was built for treating adult patients. Gaps in the system may differ from state to state but there are some common features: The majority of children and youth in the United States who may benefit from pediatric critical care services do not receive them. Curricula for prehospital and emergency care providers offer little or no pediatric training. Protocols for field triage, treatment, transport, and interfacility transfers often lack criteria relevant for children. Experience with pediatric trauma centers, as compared with designated trauma centers for adults, is limited because they are newer and fewer in number. Specialized pediatric rehabilitation services are not available throughout much of the United States.

Third, there is no uniform national data collection system to evaluate emergency and trauma care services offered to pediatric patients. Data systems that do exist have many deficiencies. Often they lack crucial information about the location of injury event, mode of transport to the hospital, time from injury to admission, patient status at admission, measures of injury severity, mechanism, or external cause of injury, and morbidity outcomes at discharge. Without these data, it is difficult to assess the effectiveness of the acute care system, plan for appropriate rehabilitation services, and target effective prevention efforts at the community level.

The catalyst for addressing some of these gaps was provided by professional organizations in the early 1980s. With leadership by the American Academy of Pediatrics and the American College of Emergency Physicians, curricula were developed for training prehospital and critical care providers in the care of the acutely ill and injured child. Throughout the 1980s, sections on pediatric emergency and critical care were formed by several medical societies and nursing associations (IOM, 1993). Federal involvement started in 1985 after Congress established the Emergency Medical Services for Children (EMS-C) program through the 1984 legislation on preventive health services (PL 98-555).

From 1986 through 1994, the federal EMS-C program, administered by the Maternal and Child Health Bureau, has funded 38 states to implement EMS-C projects and an additional 4 states received planning grants (Athey, 1995). Initially, funding was given for demonstration projects designed to improve knowledge that can be applied to improving the pediatric care capabilities of existing emergency medical systems around the country (NCEMCH, 1992). More recently, the program shifted its focus from a demonstration to an implementation phase. Since 1991, funding has been directed at projects to improve state resources for the emergency care of children by applying knowledge gained since the inception of the EMS-C program.

Although progress has been made in acquiring new knowledge and in stimulating professional attention to the unique care needs of children and youth, the EMS-C program is still in its initial stage. The 1993 Institute of Medicine report on this topic concludes: "The needs of children must be more widely recognized and made a genuine priority for policymakers at national, state, and local levels, particularly those in a position to influence the future directions of EMS and EMS-C" (IOM, 1993, p. 334).

One issue requiring further attention is the place of older adolescents within the system of acute care and rehabilitation. The lack of consensus about the age at which childhood ends and adulthood begins is reflected in the variation found in field practice. In a survey of state EMS agencies, Seidel (1991) found that among the 12 states that set an age limit for pediatric patients, the age used ranged from 14 to 21 years. Practice among hospitals that provide pediatric tertiary care also varies. In a discussion on this topic among pediatric surgeons, Barlow (1989) argues for excluding older adolescents from the pediatric unit, particularly in urban centers, because of the violent nature of their injuries and concomitant behavior.

In outlining the hospital resources required for the care of pediatric trauma patients, Tepas (1993) includes adolescents but does not set a specific age limit. He notes that older adolescents are especially difficult to manage because they combine the psychological requirements of a child with the physical needs of an adult. The recovery of adolescents from traumatic injury may benefit from the care of providers with training in pediatric and adolescent medicine. Issues of self-image, particularly following disfiguring injuries such as burns, demand special understanding of this age group. Pain management in the adolescent patient, and worries about lost status in school and sport activities, also need to be addressed by providers with the appropriate skills.

The proportion of severely injured adolescents who are treated at trauma centers with pediatric capabilities is currently unknown. However, evaluations of trauma system performance in Maryland and Massachusetts have shown that young people over age 14, with severe injuries requiring trauma center care, are less likely to receive such care than their younger counterparts (MacKenzie, Steinwachs, & Ramzy, 1990; Lescohier, 1994).

The needs of adolescents in the transition from the acute care setting to rehabilitation, and school reentry following injury, have also received insufficient attention. Savage

(1987) notes that while the number of high-school-aged students suffering traumatic brain injuries has been increasing, rehabilitation programs have focused primarily on the adult head-injured population. As a result, many youth return home and to school with minimal support services and little information for families and schools about intervention strategies that can help these students to succeed in school. Collaboration of specialists from medicine, rehabilitation, and education, and a team approach that involves the family, are essential for successful reentry into schools (Savage & Wolcott, 1994).

CONCLUSIONS

The epidemiology of adolescent unintentional injury exhibits certain patterns by age, sex, race, place of residence, and socioeconomic status. Among these patterns we would like to focus attention on the differences in type of injuries sustained by younger versus older adolescents, and the different profile of unintentional injury reflected in morbidity versus mortality data.

First, comparison of both mortality and morbidity data for the two age groups examined in this chapter (ages 10–14 and 15–19) indicates that developmental stage and its ensuing behaviors alone cannot explain differences in injury patterns. Rather, exposure, such as the rate of participation in specific activities, as well as the character and the location of such activities, have a great deal to do with the incidence, nature, and cause of injury. For example, younger teens, who are not permitted to drive motor vehicles, are more likely to die as bicyclists and pedestrians than their older counterparts. Older teens, who gradually become more active in the world of work, sustain a much higher rate of occupational injuries than younger youth, for whom employment is restricted.

Second, whereas a great deal of discussion about the adverse health effects of risk-taking behavior in adolescence has relied on examples from injury mortality, little attention has been paid to implications presented by morbidity data. Mortality from unintentional injury is a relatively infrequent event, which reveals only the "tip of the iceberg" of the injury problem. Nonfatal unintentional injuries are at least 1000 times more common than deaths, and represent an enormous burden to individuals and society. Sports injuries, falls, and injuries sustained by being struck by, or cut with, objects rank higher in their incidence ratio than motor vehicle occupant injuries. A significant number of nonfatal injuries among older adolescents are work-related. Involvement in sports and work activities is both expected and encouraged in adolescence. Adults often perceive participation in these activities as signs of wholesome life-style and growing maturity. A high level of commitment to sport practice and employment responsibilities on the part of youth is admired. The resultant injuries have been overlooked by many professionals.

One of the reasons for this state of affairs is the paucity of data on nonfatal injury. Data on the incidence and causes of injury deaths have been routinely collected through vital statistics systems available at the state, national, and international levels. In contrast, information on the incidence of nonfatal injuries is estimated based on a combination of sources including periodic surveys, hospital discharge summaries, insurance data, and local studies. Future research in this field would benefit a great deal from the implementation of population-based injury surveillance systems with emphasis on morbidity. Surveillance is critical for reducing morbidity and mortality from injuries. A well-designed system can provide data to evaluate the extent of the problem, set priorities for interventions, develop sound policies, and monitor and evaluate prevention strategies. Appropriate denominator measures coupled with information about the circumstances, location, nature and severity of injury, and use of protective devices are some of the important features to be included in a data-gathering system.

The section on prevention described the science base of injury control measures and noted areas where progress has been made. The example of consistent declines in motor vehicle occupant injuries underscores the benefits of a combination of preventive approaches applied in addressing this problem: engineering and design modifications, legislation and enforcement, and public education. At the same time, there are today effective prevention measures that have not been uniformly applied in areas of particular relevance to adolescents such as sports and employment. The question arises, therefore, whether we, as a society, have done what can be done to implement safety strategies such as enforcement of child labor laws and adoption of recommended safety measures in youth sport and recreation. Pless (1994) suggests that continued progress will be proportional to the extent to which injury control is perceived as a health problem, and that health and public health agencies need to take a primary responsibility for injury prevention.

Yet, a 1992 assessment of injury prevention efforts under way in state maternal and child health agencies found that adolescents, the age group with the highest injury rate, are less frequently targeted than younger children. Few interventions are in place to prevent those injury causes that take a large toll on adolescents, such as sports (two states), workplace/job-related (two states), motor vehicles (six states), assaults (seven states), and suicide (four states) (Miara, Gallagher, & Dana, 1992). As maternal and child health agencies increase their collaboration with schools, school-based clinics, and other youth-serving programs, more emphasis must be placed on adolescents and the prevention of adolescent injuries.

Work-related injuries provide a good example. The opening of the federal child labor laws to amendment for the first time in 30 years sets the stage for substantial public policy debate around the commonly overlooked, but high-risk area for teens—the work environment. This is not enough. Also needed are model, community-based projects designed to increase safe practices among employers and teen workers alike, and a major effort to promote interagency collaboration among health, labor, and education agencies. To be successful, such efforts need to be based on a clear understanding of the role each agency plays in promoting teen health and safety on the job, and reach an effective balance of education, enforcement, and engineering approaches.

Further, much of the research effort in injury control has focused on preventing unintentional injuries to young children of preschool age. In the past, burns, poisonings, and motor vehicle occupant injuries have been investigated more often than other causes in response to the availability of funding sources. Future research needs to focus on teenagers, a population neglected in the injury control field. Such research should address causes of fatal and nonfatal injury relevant to this population and amenable to prevention.

Another area of prevention where research is lacking relates to assessment of behavior and its modification in teenagers within the context of their communities. Few studies have compared the effects of injury control intervention on different age groups in the same localities. Teasing out the contribution of the socioeconomic environment, as well as local norms, to safe behavior among teens would help in devising more effective interventions strategies.

The increasing fascination and attention given to violence, and injuries associated with violence, raises questions about the future of research in unintentional injury. Will research on violence syphon funding resources, and researchers, away from unintentional injury? Will we return to an era with primary focus on individual behavior as a cause of injury, so prominent at the early part of this century? Or can we learn from the progress made in reducing motor vehicle occupant injuries and other causes of unintentional injury, which combined multiple approaches, and apply it to violence as well?

Although clinical management of the trauma patient has advanced substantially, coordinated systems for the care of the injured are still in the developmental stage in the United States. These systems for emergency response, acute care, and rehabilitation have been conceived with the adult patient in mind. The special needs of children and youth within these systems have only recently been recognized. Programmatic initiatives to address gaps in the emergency care system with respect to the pediatric population only began a decade ago. Standards of care and treatment protocols at the prehospital, acute care, and postacute settings must be developed for this population. Providers need to be trained in appropriate response to pediatric trauma emergencies. Currently, care for the older adolescent is not well defined as a result of uncertainty about their place in the spectrum from childhood to adulthood. This area needs further exploration by professionals with interest and experience in the care of adolescents.

Research should assess the effectiveness of emergency response and rehabilitation interventions on children and youth of various ages. Evaluation of the performance of the EMS and trauma care systems with respect to youth is an important goal. System evaluation should be conducted periodically to examine the effectiveness of measures being taken to address the needs of children. Little information is currently available about the long-term consequences of traumatic injuries and their effect on functional status throughout adolescence. Much of the available literature on this topic focuses on head injury and its sequelae while extracranial injuries, such as fractures to the upper and lower extremities, are often overlooked. The extent of functional limitations and need for rehabilitation services that result from extracranial injuries must be studied. These injuries are relatively frequent among youth. Also needed are studies about successful methods of returning adolescents to school after severe injury.

Finally, one of the most apparent conclusions of this chapter is that progress in injury control is accomplished through the efforts of many diverse individuals and groups. We need to continue and expand collaboration among professionals and practitioners from multiple disciplines, and between the professional community and the public, in order to gain a better insight about promising approaches for improving the well-being of our children.

REFERENCES

ACEP (American College of Emergency Physicians). (1987). Guidelines for trauma care systems. *Annals of Emergency Medicine, 16,* 459–463.
ACS/COT (American College of Surgeons/Committee on Trauma). (1993). *Resources for optimal care of the injured patient.* Chicago: American College of Surgeons.

Athey, J. (1995). Personal communication with Jean Athey, Bureau of Maternal and Child Health, January.

Baker, S. P., O'Neill, B., Ginsburg, M. J., & Li, G. (1992). *The injury fact book: Second edition*. London: Oxford University Press.

Banco, L., Lapidus, G., & Braddock, M. (1992). Work-related injury among Connecticut minors. *Pediatrics, 89*, 957–960.

Barlow, B. (1989). Discussion. In J. A. Haller, Jr. (Ed.), *Emergency medical services for children. Report of the 97th Ross Conference on Pediatric Research* (pp. 15–17). Columbus, OH: Ross Laboratories.

Belville, R., Pollack, S. H., Godbold, J. H., & Landrigan, P. J. (1993). Occupational injuries among working adolescents in New York State. *Journal of the American Medical Association, 269*, 2754–2759.

Beyer, D. (1993). Current trends in state child labor legislation and enforcement. *American Journal of Industrial Medicine, 24*, 347–350.

Boston Globe, April 21, 1994.

Brooks, D. R., Davis, L. K., & Gallagher, S. S. (1993). Work-related injuries among Massachusetts children: A study based on emergency department data. *American Journal of Industrial Medicine, 24*, 313–324.

Bureau of National Affairs, Inc. (1993). Job related injuries increase; OSHA vows better enforcement standards. *Occupational Safety and Health Reporter, 23*(30), 867–868.

Bureau of National Affairs, Inc. (1994). Sprains, strains lead other injury types; repetitive motion cases detailed in BLS survey. *Occupational Safety and Health Reporter, 23*(43), 1659–1660.

Castillo, D. N., Landen, D. D., & Layne, L. A. (1994). Occupational injury deaths of 16- and 17-year-olds in the United States. *American Journal of Public Health, 84*, 646–649.

CDC (Centers for Disease Control). (1992a). Unintentional firearm-related fatalities among children and teenagers—United States, 1982–1988. *Morbidity and Mortality Weekly Report, 41*, 442–445.

CDC. (1992b). Behaviors related to unintentional and intentional injuries among high school students—United States, 1991. *Morbidity and Mortality Weekly Report, 41*, 760–765, 771–772.

CDC. (1992c). Factors potentially associated with reductions in alcohol-related traffic fatalities—United States, 1990 and 1991. *Morbidity and Mortality Weekly Report, 41*, 893–899.

Crockett, L. J., & Petersen, A. C. (1993). Adolescent development: Health risks and opportunities for health promotion. In S. G. Millstein, A. C. Petersen, & E. O. Nightingale (Eds.), *Promoting the health of adolescents: New directions for the twenty-first century* (pp. 13–37). London: Oxford University Press.

Datta, T. K., & Guzek, P. (1991). *Restraint systems use in 19 U.S. cities—1990 annual report*. U.S. Department of Transportation Report DTNH22-89-C-070034. Washington, DC: U.S. Department of Transportation.

Dunn, K. A., & Runyan, C. W. (1993). Deaths at work among children and adolescents. *American Journal of Diseases in Children, 147*, 1044–1047.

Fingar, A. R., Hopkins, R. S., & Nelson, M. (1992). Work-related injuries in Athens County 1982 to 1986: A comparison of emergency department and worker's compensation data. *Journal of Occupational Medicine, 34*, 779–787.

Fingerhut, L. A. (1989). *Trends and current status in childhood mortality, United States, 1900–1985*. Vital and Health Statistics. Series 3. Washington, DC: U.S. Government Printing Office.

Fingerhut, L. A. (1993). *Firearm mortality among children, youth, and young adults 1–34 years of age, trends and current status: United States, 1985–1990*. Advance Data from Vital and Health Statistics. No. 231. Washington, DC: U.S. Government Printing Office.

Gabrielson, M. A., & Shulman, S. M. (1990). *Starting blocks: The etiology of 25 spinal cord injuries as a result of dives made from starting blocks, with recommendations*. Detroit: Foundation for Spinal Cord Injury Prevention.

Gallagher, S. S. (1993). Massachusetts: A case study of how surveillance systems work. In *Injuries in youth: Surveillance strategies. Workshop proceedings* (NIH Publication No. 93-3444, pp. 33–39). Bethesda: National Institutes of Health.

Gallagher, S. S., Finison, K., Guyer, B., & Goodenough, S. (1984). The incidence of injuries among 87,000 Massachusetts children and adolescents: Results of the 1980–1981 statewide injury prevention program surveillance system. *American Journal of Public Health, 74*, 1340–1347.

Glor, E. D. (1989). Survey of comprehensive accident and injury experience of high school students in Saskatchewan. *Canadian Journal of Public Health, 80*, 435–440.

Graham, J. D. (1993). Injuries from traffic crashes: Meeting the challenge. *Annual Review of Public Health, 14*, 515–543.

Guyer, B., & Ellers, B. (1990). Childhood injuries in the United States. *American Journal of Diseases in Children, 144,* 459–652.

Guyer, B., & Gallagher, S. S. (1985). An approach to the epidemiology of childhood injuries. In J. J. Alpert & B. Guyer (Eds.), *Pediatric clinics of North America, 32,* 5–15.

Guyer, B., Lescohier, I., Gallagher, S. S., Hausman, A., & Azzara, C. V. (1989). Intentional injuries among children and adolescents in Massachusetts. *New England Journal of Medicine, 321,* 1584–1589.

Haddon, W., & Baker, S. P. (1981). Injury control. In D. Clark & B. MacMahon (Eds.), *Preventive and community medicine.* Boston: Little, Brown.

Haller, J. A., Jr. (Ed.). (1989). *Emergency medical services for children. Report of the 97th Ross Conference on Pediatric Research.* Columbus, OH: Ross Laboratories.

Haller, J. A., Jr., & Beaver, B. (1989). A model: Systems management of life threatening injuries in children for the State of Maryland, USA. *Intensive Care Medicine, 15,* S53–S56.

HRSA (Health Resources and Services Administration). (1992). *Model trauma system plan, September 30, 1992.* Rockville, MD: U.S. Department of Health and Human Services, Public Health Service.

Hemenway, D., & Weil, D. (1990). Phasers on stun: The case for less lethal weapons. *Journal of Policy Analysis and Management, 9,* 94–98.

Heyer, N. J., Franklin, G., Rivara, F. P., Parker, P., & Haug, J. A. (1992). Occupational injuries among minors doing farm work in Washington State: 1986 to 1989. *American Journal of Public Health, 82,* 557–560.

Hingson, R., & Howland, J. (1993). Promoting safety in adolescents. In S. G. Millstein, A. C. Petersen, & E. O. Nightingale (Eds.), *Promoting the health of adolescents: New directions for the twenty-first century* (pp. 305–327). London: Oxford University Press.

IIHS (Insurance Institute for Highway Safety). (1991). *Facts, 1991 Edition.*

IOM (Institute of Medicine). (1993). *Emergency medical services for children,* J. S. Durch & K. N. Lohr (Eds.). Washington, DC: National Academy Press.

Janda, D. H., Wojtys, E. M., Henkin, F. M., & Benedict, M. E. (1988). Softball sliding injuries—Michigan, 1986–1987. *Morbidity and Mortality Weekly Report, 37,* 169–170.

Johnston, J. J., Hendricks, S. A., & Fike, J. M. (1994). Effectiveness of behavioral safety belt interventions. *Accident Analysis and Prevention, 26,* 315–323.

Landrigan, P. J. (1993). Child labor: A reemergent threat. *American Journal of Industrial Medicine, 24,* 267–268.

Layne, L. A., Castillo, D. N., Stout, N., & Cutlip, P. (1994). Adolescent occupational injuries requiring hospital emergency department treatment: A nationally representative study. *American Journal of Public Health, 84,* 657–660.

Lescohier, I. (1994). *Patterns of pediatric trauma hospitalizations in Massachusetts: Final report.* Boston: Harvard Injury Control Center.

Lescohier, I., Shapiro, E., Guyer, B., & Wise, P. (1988). *Staying alive: Preventing child death; The Massachusetts child death study.* Boston: Massachusetts Department of Public Health.

MacKenzie, E. J., Steinwachs, D. M., & Ramzy, A. I. (1990). Evaluating performance of statewide regionalized systems of trauma care. *Journal of Trauma, 30,* 681–688.

Malek, M., Chang, B., Gallagher, S., & Guyer, B. (1991). The cost of medical care for injuries to children. *Annals of Emergency Medicine, 20,* 997–1005.

Maurette, P., Masson, F., Nicaud, V., Cazaugade, M., Garros, B., Tiret, L., Thicoipe, M., & Erny, P. (1992). Posttraumatic disablement: A prospective study of impairment, disability, and handicap. *The Journal of Trauma, 33,* 728–736.

Miara, C., Gallagher, S. S., & Dana, A. (1992). *Injury prevention outlook: An assessment of injury prevention in state maternal and child health agencies.* Newton, MA: Education Development Center, Inc. & Children's Safety Network.

Nakayama, D. K., Copes, W. S., & Sacco, W. (1992). Differences in trauma care among pediatric and nonpediatric trauma centers. *Journal of Pediatric Surgery, 27,* 427–431.

NAS/NRC (National Academy of Sciences/National Research Council). (1970). *Accidental death and disability: The neglected disease of modern society* (PHS Publication No. 1071-A-13) (Sixth Printing). Washington, DC: U.S. Government Printing Office.

NCEMCH (National Center for Education in Maternal and Child Health). (1992). *Emergency medical services for children: Abstracts of active projects FY 1992*. Arlington, VA: Author.

NCHS (National Center for Health Statistics). (1993). Death rates for 282 selected causes, by 5-year age groups, color, and sex: United States, 1979–1991, printed per special request, March, 1994.

NCHS. (1994). Data from the National Vital Statistics System, compiled by L. A. Fingerhut per special request, March, 1994.

National Committee for Injury Prevention and Control. (1989). *Injury prevention: Meeting the challenge*. Published by Oxford University Press as a supplement to the *American Journal of Preventive Medicine*, Volume 5, Number 3, 1989. London: Oxford University Press.

NHTSA (National Highway Traffic Safety Administration). (1984). *Final regulatory impact analysis. Amendment of FMVSS No. 208-passenger car front seat occupant protection*. Washington, DC: U.S. Department of Transportation.

NHTSA. (1994). *Traffic safety facts: Pedestrians 1993*. Washington, DC: Department of Transportation.

NPTR (National Pediatric Trauma Registry). (1994). Special data request on adolescent injuries and impairments, compiled by Carla DiScala, March, October, 1994. Boston: NPTR, Research and Training Center in Rehabilitation and Childhood Trauma, Tufts University School of Medicine.

National Safety Council. (1990). *Accident facts, 1990 edition*. Chicago: Author.

National Safety Council. (1991). *Accident facts, 1991 edition*. Chicago: Author.

National Safety Council. (1994). *Accident facts, 1994 edition*. Itasca, IL: Author.

National Youth Sports Foundation for the Prevention of Athletic Injuries. (1994). *Proceedings of consensus meeting on the merits of using softer baseballs and softballs to reduce injuries, January 15, 1994*. Needham, MA: Author.

Nersesian, W. S., Petit, M. R., Shaper, R., Lemieux D., & Naor, E. (1985). Childhood death and poverty: A study of all childhood deaths in Maine, 1976 to 1980. *Pediatrics, 75*, 41–50.

Onwuachi-Saunders, C., & Hawkins, D. F. (1993). Black–white differences in injury: Race or social class? *Annals of Epidemiology, 3*, 150–153.

Parker, D. I., Clay, R. L., Mandel, J. H., Gunderson, P., & Salkowicz, L. (1991). Adolescent occupational injuries in Minnesota. A descriptive study. *Minnesota Medicine, 74*, 25–28.

Paulson, J. A. (1988). The epidemiology of injuries in adolescents. *Pediatric Annals, 17*, 84–96.

Pless, I. B. (1994). Editorial: Unintentional injury—where the buck should stop. *American Journal of Public Health, 84*, 537–539.

Pollack, S. H., Landrigan, P. J., & Mallino, D. L. (1990). Child labor in 1990: Prevalence and health hazards. *Annual Review of Public Health, 11*, 359–375.

Preusser, D. F., Williams, A. F., & Lund, A. K. (1987). The effect of New York's seat belt use law on teenage drivers. *Accident Analysis and Prevention, 19*, 73–80.

PHS (Public Health Service). (1991). *Healthy people 2000: National health promotion and disease prevention objectives*. Washington, DC: U.S. Government Printing Office.

Rice, D. P., MacKenzie, E. J., & Associates (1989). *Cost of injury in the United States: A report to Congress*. San Francisco: Institute for Health & Aging, University of California, and Injury Prevention Center, Johns Hopkins University.

Rivara, F. P., Thompson, R. S., Thompson, D. C., & Calonge, N. (1991). Injuries to children and adolescents: Impact on physical health. *Pediatrics, 88*, 783–788.

Robertson, L. S. (1984). *Injuries: Causes, control strategies, and public policy*. Lexington, MA: Lexington Books.

Robertson, L. S. (1992). *Injury epidemiology*. London: Oxford University Press.

Runyan, C. W., & Gerken, E. A. (1989). Epidemiology and prevention of adolescent injury. *Journal of the American Medical Association, 262*, 2273–2279.

Saffer, H., & Grossman, M. (1987). Beer taxes, the legal drinking age, and youth motor vehicle fatalities. *Journal of Legal Studies, 16*, 351–374.

Savage, R. C. (1987). Educational issues for the head-injured adolescent and young adult. *Journal of Head Trauma Rehabilitation, 2*, 1–10.

Savage, R. C., & Wolcott, G. F. (1994). *Educational dimensions of acquired brain injury*. Austin, TX: PRO-Ed Pub.

Schwarz, D. (1993). Adolescent trauma: Epidemiologic approach. *Adolescent Medicine: State of the Art Reviews, 4,* 11–22.

Seidel, J. S. (1991). Emergency medical services and the adolescent patient. *Journal of Adolescent Health, 12,* 95–100.

Seidel, J. S., & Henderson, D. P. (Eds.). (1991). *Emergency medical services for children: A report to the nation.* Washington, DC: National Center for Education in Maternal and Child Health.

Shackford, S. R., Hollingworth-Fridlund, P., Cooper, G. F., & Eastman, A. B. (1986). The effect of regionalization upon the quality of trauma care as assessed by concurrent audit before and after institution of a trauma system. *Journal of Trauma, 26,* 812–820.

Shinar, D. (1993). Demographic and socioeconomic correlates of safety belt use. *Accident Analysis and Prevention, 25,* 745–755.

SCIPP (Statewide Comprehensive Injury Prevention Program). (1994). Unpublished data from the SCIPP surveillance project. Boston: Massachusetts Department of Public Health.

Suruda, A., & Halperin, W. (1991). Work-related deaths in children. *American Journal of Industrial Medicine, 19,* 739–745.

Tepas, J. J., III. (1993). Pediatric trauma care. In ACS/COT, *Resources for optimal care of the injured patient* (pp. 57–62). Chicago: American College of Surgeons.

Treanor, B., & Goldnor, L. (1990). *Working America's children to death.* Washington, DC: American Youth Work Center and the National Consumers' League.

Vinger, P. (1994). Eye injuries: A mostly preventable health hazard. Seminar March 21, 1994, at Harvard Injury Control Center, Boston.

Waller, A. E., Baker, S. P., & Szocka, A. (1989). Childhood injury deaths: National analysis and geographic variations. *American Journal of Public Health, 79,* 310–315.

Waller, J. A. (1994). Reflections on a half century of injury control. *American Journal of Public Health, 84,* 664–670.

West, J. C., Williams, M. J., Trunkey, D. D., & Wolferth, C. C., Jr. (1988). Trauma systems: Current status–future challenges. *Journal of the American Medical Association, 259, 3597–3600.*

Widome, M. D. (1991). Pediatric injury prevention for the practitioner. Current Problems in Pediatrics, 21, 428–469.

Williams, B. C., & Kotch, J. B. (1990). Excess injury mortality among children in the United States: Comparison of recent international statistics. *Pediatrics, Supplement,* 1067–1073.

10

Delinquency

DENISE C. GOTTFREDSON, MIRIAM D. SEALOCK, and CHRISTOPHER S. KOPER

INTRODUCTION

Delinquency is a broad term covering a variety of antisocial acts committed by juveniles. It includes such diverse acts as robbery, sexual assault, drug use, vandalism, and underage drinking. Many delinquent acts are illegal for both adults and juveniles. Status offenses, in contrast, are acts that are only illegal for juveniles. Examples of the latter include underage drinking, skipping school, and running away from home. From a behavioral point of view, delinquency proneness is best conceived of as a general characteristic that youths have to a greater or lesser degree (Farrington, 1987). Serious delinquents engage in a variety of crimes and status offenses rather than specialize in any one type (Farrington, 1992; M. Gottfredson & Hirschi, 1990). This chapter summarizes information describing the nature and extent, prevention, and treatment of delinquent behavior.

EPIDEMIOLOGY: COSTS, NATURE, AND EXTENT OF DELINQUENCY

Costs of Delinquency

Delinquency imposes many costs both on society and on the individuals engaged in delinquent acts. One of these is the cost of institutionalization in a variety of types of secure institutions and community-based facilities, including detention centers, training schools, shelters, camps, diagnostic centers, and halfway houses. In the United States in

DENISE C. GOTTFREDSON, MIRIAM D. SEALOCK, and CHRISTOPHER S. KOPER • Department of Criminal Justice and Criminology, The University of Maryland, College Park, Maryland 20742; *present address for C. S. K.:* Crime Control Institute, Washington, D.C.
Handbook of Adolescent Health Risk Behavior, edited by Ralph J. DiClemente, William B. Hansen, and Lynn E. Ponton. Plenum Press, New York, 1996.

1988, there were 619,181 admissions to public juvenile facilities and 141,463 admissions to private juvenile facilities (Maguire, Pastore, & Flanagan, 1993). A population day count of public and private juvenile facilities taken in 1989 revealed these facilities held 93,945 juveniles, representing a rate of 367 institutionalized juveniles per 100,000 juveniles age 10 and over (Maguire *et al.*, 1993). Some of these institutionalized youths are being sheltered because they were abused or neglected, but the majority are held for criminal or status offenses. The operating expenditures of these facilities totaled over $2.8 billion in 1989 (Maguire *et al.*, 1993). Adult jails and prisons also hold a small number of juvenile offenders. Society also bears the costs for community supervision of juvenile offenders who are sentenced to probation rather than residential institutions, not to mention costs for running juvenile courts.

Police costs must also be considered. Nationally, over $31.8 billion was spent on police protection services in 1990 (Maguire *et al.*, 1993). Not all police expenditures are related to crimes committed by juveniles, but teenagers, having higher rates of offending than any other age group, contribute more than their share to police costs.

Over 18.9 million crimes against persons and over 15.7 million crimes against households were committed in the United States in 1991 (Maguire *et al.*, 1993). Costs to victims for these crimes are difficult to quantify and estimate. Victims may experience financial and property losses, medical costs related to physical injuries, lost wages from missed work time, and/or suffer psychological trauma which lowers their quality of life and their productivity. Losses from theft and property damage alone total in the billions of dollars each year (Maguire *et al.*, 1993). Further, Lindgren (1988) points out that even people who are not directly victimized can suffer indirectly, as when their property values are lowered because of crime rates in their neighborhoods.

Finally, delinquency endangers the well-being of delinquents. In addition to being disproportionately involved in offending, young people are disproportionately the victims of crime. To illustrate, youths in the 12–19 age range have higher personal victimization rates than any other age group with the exception of 20- to 24-year-olds (Maguire *et al.*, 1993). Moreover, criminological research shows that people who engage in deviant lifestyles are more likely to become involved in crime both as offenders and as victims (Kennedy & Baron, 1993; Sampson & Lauritsen, 1990). Injury and homicide are outcomes of delinquency that are serious health concerns. Delinquent youths also risk arrest and incarceration; may receive a variety of informal sanctions including shaming, rejection, or differential treatment by parents, teachers, friends, and employers; and may have lowered lifetime earnings.

Measurement of Delinquency

Delinquency is typically measured using official records, self-report, and victim surveys. Each method has its own strengths and weaknesses. Criminologists look for consistencies in findings across methods to obtain the most accurate portrait of delinquency and its correlates. The most frequently used official report data consist of police and court records. Crimes reported to police and arrest data include many offenses that never reach the court and are used more often in criminological research than are court records (Farrington, 1987). The major drawback to official data is that much crime simply goes undetected by authorities. Surveys indicate that about 60% of crimes are not reported to police. Even for serious crimes like robbery, individual victims (as opposed to commercial victims) only report about 50% of their victimizations (Bastian, 1993). Differences in reporting practices by law enforcement agencies may further distort offense and arrest statistics, and official measures may be contaminated by offense seriousness, race, sex, or class bias in criminal justice processing.

Self-reports of one's own crimes are also used in delinquency research. Surveys ask respondents whether or not they have committed various criminal acts within a given time period and how often they have engaged in these acts. Some of the limits to the self-report method include inaccurate recollections, untruthful responses, and nonresponse bias (the last problem concerns the fact that certain types of people are less likely to be surveyed and less likely to cooperate). Whereas official records cover relatively serious offenses, self-reports can also provide more data on less serious acts (e.g., minor fights and thefts, underage drinking, cheating on tests).

Victimization surveys ask respondents about their experience as victims of crime. Victimization surveys suffer from some of the same problems as do self-reports such as inaccurate recall and nonreporting (as when one does not wish to or fears to reveal victimization by a family or household member). Another problem with using victimization surveys for delinquency research is that many victims never actually see their victimizers. When they do, we have to rely on the victims' judgment as to the characteristics of the offenders.

Despite these drawbacks, research suggests all three methods are useful and complement one another. Delinquency researchers primarily use official records and self-reports. Self-reports give us a better idea of the amount of overall delinquency occurring, while official records perhaps provide better data on serious offending (Farrington, 1987).

Delinquency Prevalence and Incidence

Delinquency prevalence is the *proportion of juveniles* in the population who engage in delinquency during a certain time period (lifetime, a year, a month, etc.). Delinquency incidence is the *number of offenses* committed by juveniles during the time period. More serious offenses are less prevalent than less serious offenses. For example, U.S. studies with official records indicate that the percentage of males having some kind of nontraffic arrest or police contact prior to their 18th birthday ranges from around 25 to over 45% (Blumstein, Cohen, Roth, & Visher, 1986). Yet when examining arrests for "index offenses" (defined here as murder and nonnegligent manslaughter, forcible rape, robbery, aggravated assault, burglary, larceny-theft, and motor vehicle theft), prevalence estimates from official records drop to about 15%. Similarly for incidence estimates, studies based on official reports (covering more serious offenses) often yield higher incidence rates than studies based on self-reports covering less serious offenses (Farrington, 1987).

Self-report studies also show more serious crime to be less prevalent. A 1976 survey of a national random sample of youths ages 11–17 (the National Youth Survey) revealed that 76% of the males had engaged in some type of "general delinquency" in the previous year (this scale included a number of offenses ranging in seriousness from aggravated assault to hitting students) while 29% reported having committed acts comparable to index

offenses in the previous year (Elliott, Huizinga, & Menard, 1989). The higher delinquency rates found in self-reports than official reports reflect the fact that not all offenders are
caught. To illustrate, studies of two youth cohorts born in Racine, Wisconsin, in 1942 and
1949 revealed that 95% of the 1942 cohort males and 94% of the 1949 cohort males stated
that they either had been stopped by the police or had done things for which they could
have been stopped. However, only 64% of the 95% and 71% of the 94% actually showed
up in the police records for a police contact before reaching 18 (Shannon, 1991).

Both self-report and official sources indicate that a relatively small percentage of
offenders are responsible for a disproportionate number of offenses. Six percent of the
boys in a Philadelphia study were responsible for 52% of the police contacts found for the
entire study population (Wolfgang, Figlio, & Sellin, 1972). Likewise, researchers analyzing the National Youth Survey identified a subset of the sample as "serious" offenders.
These youths reported having engaged in three or more index offenses in the previous
year. In 1976, the serious offenders accounted for 8.6% of the total sample, yet were
responsible for 62% of all general offenses reported and over 75% of the reported index
offenses (Elliott *et al.*, 1989).

SOCIODEMOGRAPHIC CHARACTERISTICS AND DELINQUENCY

Age and sex are strong correlates of offending. Though the associations between
these factors and crime may appear to vary somewhat across types of offenses, it is
generally true that younger people and males are disproportionately involved in crime.
Offending rates are also somewhat higher for urban residents and members of certain
minority groups.

Age

National figures for 1992 indicate that arrest rates for index offenses were highest for
people ages 15 through 18 and reached their peak at age 16 (Federal Bureau of Investigation, 1993a). Statistics for most criminal offenses show that offending rates begin increasing during the early teenage years (15 to 17), peak in the middle to late teenage years, and
decline thereafter. This phenomenon is observed for both males and females (Farrington,
1987). Figure 1 shows the association of age and crime for the violent index crimes
(murder, forcible rape, robbery, and aggravated assault) for 1992. The peak age for these
crimes is slightly higher than for crimes in general. The age distributions for different
offenses differ somewhat in terms of their peak ages and rate of decline, but all offenses
follow the pattern of a rise, peak, and decline. Whereas the *proportion* of teenagers
engaging in crime is higher than that of other age groups, teenage offenders do not commit
a greater *number* of offenses than their adult counterparts.

Gender

Males are disproportionately involved in offending across age groups and for virtually all criminal offenses. A study of males and females born in Philadelphia in 1958

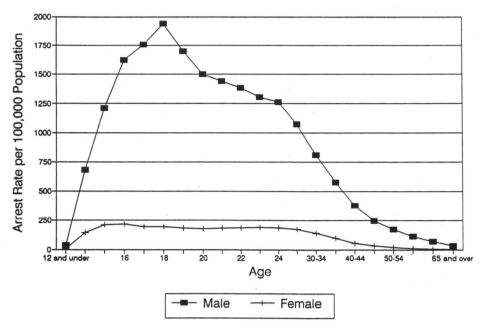

Figure 1. Age-specific violent crime arrest rates, 1992. Source: U.S. Department of Justice, Federal Bureau of Investigation. (1993). *Age-specific arrest rates and race-specific arrest rates for selected offenses, 1965–1992.* Washington, DC: U.S. Government Printing Office.

found that 33% of males and 14% of females had at least one nontraffic police contact before age 18 (Tracy, Wolfgang, & Figlio, 1985). However, the magnitude of the gender gap varies somewhat across factors like offense type, age, and race (Smith & Visher, 1980). Male predominance appears to be greatest for more serious crimes like robbery and auto theft for which female arrests account for about 7% of all arrests, and less for offenses like larceny theft and forgery for which female arrests account for 34 and 29% of all arrests (Wilson & Herrnstein, 1985; Smith & Visher, 1980). Male predominance for more serious offending appears to be greatest during the teenage and early adult years based on official data (Federal Bureau of Investigation, 1993a). Yet, Smith and Visher's (1980) analysis of 44 studies showed that when offense type was taken into account, the gender gap in crime was less for juveniles than for adults. This gender gap applies to both the prevalence and the incidence of delinquency.

Race

Nonwhite persons, especially African-Americans, are disproportionately involved in delinquency. For persons under 18, the respective ratios of nonwhite-to-white arrest rates for index, violent, and property offenses in 1992 were 1.94, 4.23, and 1.65 (Federal Bureau of Investigation, 1993a). Most of the research on race and delinquency has compared white and black Americans, although there is also evidence that Hispanics are disproportionately involved in crime and that Asian-Americans are least involved in crime. The comments below focus on white and black delinquency.

Official statistics have long shown that African-Americans are overrepresented among criminal offenders. Although African-Americans constitute less than 15% of the U.S. population, they were responsible for 35% of all index offense arrests and 45% of all violent crime arrests in 1992 (Federal Bureau of Investigation, 1993b). Such figures were challenged by early (late 1960s and early 1970s) self-report studies which suggested that white and black delinquency levels were not substantially different. Some attributed the overrepresentation of African-Americans in official statistics to bias in criminal justice processing. But, later studies indicated that the discrepancies between early self-reports and official statistics stemmed from the former's overreliance on minor acts. After taking into account the different behavioral domains tapped by official statistics and self-reports, the two sources show general agreement in the demographic characteristics of offenders (Hindelang, Hirschi, & Weis, 1979). There is evidence of criminal justice discrimination in certain social contexts [Hagan & Bumiller (1983); see also, for example, Sampson (1986) and Smith (1986) on police behavior], but the greater representation of African-Americans in official data is also related to their disproportionate involvement in serious offenses which are more likely to appear in official statistics. This conclusion has also been supported by analysis of offender race in victimization surveys (Hindelang, 1978).

African-Americans also self-report higher prevalence rates for the more serious acts. For example, National Youth Survey figures from 1976 indicated that 4.3% of white and 8.5% of black respondents had admitted to committing robbery in the previous year (Elliott *et al.*, 1989). Such prevalence differences exist for both males and females but may be greater for females (Farrington, 1987). Based on a sample of Seattle youths, Hindelang, Hirschi, and Weis (1981) estimated that 28% of white males and 47% of black males in Seattle had official records of delinquency. The difference between Seattle's white and black females was somewhat greater: 9% of white females and 26% of black females were estimated to have official records of delinquency. In contrast, there do not appear to be substantial race differences in the incidence of offending (Blumstein *et al.*, 1986).

Urban Residence

Area of residence is another important correlate of delinquency (Braithwaite, 1989). Victimization surveys indicate that personal and household victimization rates for various crimes are consistently higher in central cities than in suburban and nonmetropolitan areas (Bastian, 1993). Direct evidence that urban residents engage in more crime comes from the National Youth Survey. In the 1976 sample 26.4% of urban and 15.9% of rural youths admitted to having committed index offenses within the previous year (Elliott *et al.*, 1989). Incidence was 6.9 index offenses per year for urban offenders and 3.2 index offenses per year for rural offenders. The relationship between urban residence and delinquency is confirmed in official data. A study of three youth cohorts in Racine, Wisconsin, revealed " . . . reasonably systematic declines from the inner city and interstitial areas to the suburban fringe in the incidence and prevalence of delinquency and crime, in the seriousness of offenses, and in the seriousness of delinquent and criminal careers" (Shannon, 1991, p. 13).

Temporal Trends

In the years since World War II, crime rates have increased in most countries for which data are available (Braithwaite, 1989). Historical examination of crime trends suggests that crime rates in industrial nations have followed a U-shaped curve (perhaps better described as a reversed J shape at this point in time), falling during the later 1800s and early 1900s and then increasing during the later part of this century (Lane, 1992; Wilson & Herrnstein, 1985). Official statistics and victimization data show that crime levels reached a recent peak during the late 1970s and early 1980s (Bastian, 1993).

Figure 2 shows evidence, however, that violent crime has been rising since the mid-1980s (Bastian, 1993; Federal Bureau of Investigation, 1993b). Moreover, homicide rates among persons 15 to 19 years of age have recently risen as a result of increases in firearm homicides among this group (Fingerhut, Ingram, & Feldman, 1992).

The overall increases in crime since the middle of this century have been attributed in large measure to the changing age structure of the population (Wilson & Herrnstein, 1985). During this time period, the cohorts of the postwar baby boom generation passed through the peak offending ages. Nevertheless, this change in the population's age structure cannot alone account for all of the change in crime levels (Wilson & Herrnstein, 1985; see also Cohen & Felson, 1979).

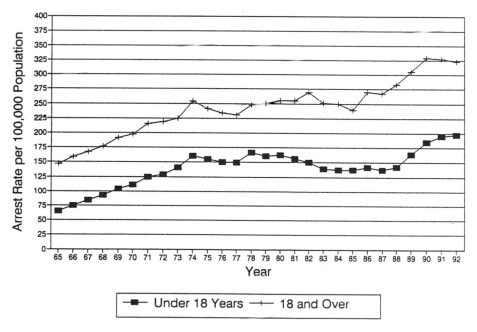

Figure 2. Violent crime arrest rates, by age group, 1965–1992. Source: U.S. Department of Justice, Federal Bureau of Investigation (1993). *Age-specific arrest rates and race-specific arrest rates for selected offenses, 1965–1992.* Washington, DC: U.S. Government Printing Office.

In sum, delinquency is general rather than specialized among adolescents, i.e., people who engage in one form of delinquent behavior are likely also to engage in other forms. Engaging in one type of crime as a juvenile does not seem to lead to other types of crime, i.e., seriousness does not steadily increase over successive arrests (Visher, 1991). A high proportion of all juveniles engage in crime, but a relatively small population of high-rate offenders account for a large fraction of all crimes. Offending rates increase during the adolescent years and then decline, and crime is more likely to be committed by males than females. Urban residents and blacks are also overrepresented among offenders.

PREVENTION

Traditionally, prevention has been defined as those activities aimed at stopping or slowing the initiation into delinquent behaviors. Treatment has been defined as those activities aimed at reducing the frequency or seriousness of delinquent behaviors already established. This distinction is difficult to maintain because it does not map well into what is known about the nature of delinquent behavior, i.e., that it is more continuous than categorical. The distinction between preventing one from "becoming delinquent" and reducing delinquent behavior among delinquents is tenuous at best. It is more useful to define any effort to prevent upward movement along the continuum of delinquency seriousness or frequency as delinquency prevention. This section discusses precursors of delinquency and strategies aimed at altering those precursors. The next section discusses the correctional treatment of juveniles.

Precursors of Delinquency

Effective prevention practices are likely to include those most directly affecting the experiences, characteristics, beliefs, attitudes, or behaviors causally linked to delinquency. Research has uncovered dozens of factors related to delinquency. These include characteristics of the community and school environments and many individual factors describing family process, school-related experiences and attitudes, peer group experiences, personal values, attitudes, and beliefs. Community factors include laws and norms proscribing criminal behavior; availability of weapons and opportunities for criminal activity; and social disorganization. School factors include lack of clarity and consistency of rule enforcement. Family-related factors include criminal parents, excessively severe, lax, or inconsistent discipline styles, poor communication, conflict, abuse, neglect, and low levels of attachment. School-related experiences and attitudes include poor school performance, low attachment to school, and low commitment to schooling. Peer-related experiences include rejection by peers and exposure to or association with delinquent peers. And individual factors include early problem behavior, impulsivity or low levels of self-control, rebellious attitudes, beliefs favoring law violation, and low levels of social competency skills such as identifying likely consequences of actions and alternative solutions to problems, taking the perspective of others, and correctly interpreting social cues.

Not all of these factors are likely to be causal. Some may be consequences of delinquency and others may represent spurious associations. For example, attitudes may become more favorable to law-violating behaviors as part of a rationalization process following the commission of crimes. Or, youths who lack self-control may have difficulty succeeding in academic ventures and they may commit more crimes. The common reliance on self-control may completely account for the association between academic performance and delinquency. Targeting prevention activities at variables whose associations with delinquency are not causal will not necessarily reduce delinquency.

It seems useful to trim the long lists of "risk factors" to arrive at a smaller set of factors whose causal status is more certain. Evidence for a causal association would require more than a simple association. It would also show that (1) the causal factor occurred temporally prior to the delinquent behavior (as might be established in longitudinal studies) and (2) that the association cannot be explained by common reliance on other factors. Evidence of causality ideally comes from experimental manipulations of the factors, but may also be gleaned from carefully controlled studies. Among the many factors known to be associated with delinquency, a few stand out as particularly likely to be causal in nature. These are summarized below.

Low Self-Control

Several studies have demonstrated that individuals who possess a traitlike constellation of characteristics that might be called low self-control (including defiance, poor impulse control, and aggression) are at greater risk for later problem behaviors, including delinquency. These traits—whether measured at a very early age, age 3 and 4 (Block, Block, & Keyes, 1988), grade 1 (Kellam, Brown, & Fleming, 1981), in middle childhood, ages 7 through 11 (Shedler & Block, 1990; Spivack & Cianci, 1987), in early adolescence, grades 7 and 8 (Smith & Fogg, 1978), or in later adolescence, grade 10 (Conger & Miller, 1966)—are predictive of later problem behaviors. These personality characteristics predict a wide range of problem behaviors (e.g., drug use, delinquency, drop-out, poor work performance, and mental health problems) measured in a variety of ways (e.g., self-reports, official records, behavior ratings by others).

This set of personality characteristics is often reflected in reduced social competency skills. For example, individuals with low levels of self-control may find it more difficult to control impulses to act in self-gratifying but socially unacceptable ways and concentrate on goal-directed activities such as those required for successful school performance. These incompetent behaviors increase the likelihood of peer rejection and teacher judgments of incompetence (Dodge, Pettit, McClaskey, & Brown, 1986; McFall, 1982; Rubin & Krasnor, 1986). Self-control, or its lack, is a stable trait and is therefore a plausible target for early, prevention-oriented, as well as later, treatment-oriented, interventions.

Family Functioning

Research consistently shows that parenting practices and family interactions are associated with delinquent behavior (Glueck & Glueck, 1968; McCord, 1978). In a review of predictors of male delinquency, Loeber and Dishion (1983) found family management practices to be the earliest and most efficient predictor of delinquency. The important elements of family management include lax, neglectful, erratic, inconsistent, overly harsh or punitive discipline practices; interactions that emphasize coldness and rejection, lack of involvement with the child, passivity and neglect, lack of shared leisure time; and low parental awareness of the child's peer associates, free time activities, and physical whereabouts (Snyder & Patterson, 1987). Evidence suggests that these characteristics are predictive of initiation as well as maintenance of delinquent behavior, and they predict several forms of delinquent behavior, including aggressive crimes, property crimes, and drug use.

School Performance and Attitudes

Academic failure is one of the largest and most consistently found predictors of later drug and alcohol use, delinquent behavior, teenage pregnancy, and school dropout (Bachman, Green, & Wirtanen, 1971; G. Gottfredson, 1981, 1987a; Grissom & Shepard, 1989; Jessor & Jessor, 1977; Kandel, Kessler, & Margulies, 1978; Lloyd, 1978; Loeber & Dishion, 1983; Smith & Fogg, 1978; West & Farrington, 1973). Low commitment to conventional goals and attachment to prosocial others also predict delinquency (Bachman, O'Malley, & Johnston, 1978; G. Gottfredson, 1987a; Jessor & Jessor, 1977; Smith & Fogg, 1978). Low commitment to school is generally measured by low levels of effort expended on schoolwork and by low educational and occupational aspirations. Low attachment to school, on the other hand, is usually measured by low liking for school or the people in school. These factors are thought to weaken the "social bond" which provides an effective restraint against engaging in proscribed behaviors (Hirschi, 1969). Children who are not motivated to succeed in their endeavors are less likely to be constrained to behave in socially acceptable ways because they have relatively little to lose by misbehaving.

Although the association of these school-related factors with later delinquency has been established in longitudinal studies, some evidence suggests caution in interpreting the association as causal. Grades in school are influenced by students' social competencies as well as their academic performance (Bowles & Gintis, 1976; Porter, 1974), and teacher and peer ratings of earlier behavior problems predict later academic performance as well as problem behavior (Feldhusen, Thurston, & Benning, 1973; Spivack & Cianci, 1987; Ullmann, 1957). A recent study explicitly testing the alternative causal pathways linking academic performance and later delinquency (Tremblay & Masse, 1993) concludes that the association is primarily explained by the reliance of both variables on early and persistent behavior problems. Academic performance at grade 10 does not predict delinquency net of behavior problems measured in kindergarten. Another recent study shows that being held back has no effect on later rebellious behavior when earlier characteristics that predispose individuals to both delinquency and school failure are controlled (D. Gottfredson, Fink, & Graham, 1994). More research is needed to clarify the causal path.

Association with Delinquent Peers

Children who associate with peers who engage in delinquent activities are much more likely to engage in such behaviors themselves. This is one of the most consistent predictors research has identified (Elliott, Huizinga, & Ageton, 1985; Glueck & Glueck, 1950; Jessor & Jessor, 1977). Social learning theory explanations of the association

(Akers, Krohn, Lanza-Kaduce, & Radosevich, 1979) suggest that delinquent peers influence others through associative learning. Delinquent peers model behaviors for others to imitate and strengthen the behaviors through reward and the avoidance of punishments. In addition, people learn valuative definitions (norms, attitudes, orientations) of behavior as good or bad through association with groups. The more individuals define a behavior as good or at least justified, the more likely they are to perform it.

Delinquents also have histories of being actively disliked by peers (Conger & Miller, 1966; Cowen, Pederson, Babigian, Izzo, & Trost, 1973; Havighurst, Bowman, Liddle, Matthews, & Pierce, 1962; Roff & Sells, 1968). It is not clear whether peer rejection increases the likelihood of delinquency or is merely another marker for youths headed for delinquency, but some evidence shows that youths sort themselves into friendship groups on the basis of aggressive personality (Cairns, Cairns, Neckerman, Gest, & Gariepy, 1988; Patterson & Dishion, 1985)—a mechanism that, according to social learning theory, should increase delinquency through differential association. Early child socialization scholars (Kupersmidt, Coie, & Dodge, 1990) have suggested that rejection from the mainstream social groups may deprive rejected children of important opportunities for social interaction with peers which promote healthy adaptational behaviors. These children, already deficient in social skills, may learn more maladaptive behaviors in association with other rejected children, and these maladaptive behaviors may be reinforced in association with other aggressive children.

Environmental Constraints

Features of the environment also promote or inhibit delinquent behavior. Environments that limit opportunities to engage in undesired behaviors and those in which norms proscribing certain behaviors are clear and well-communicated experience less undesired behavior. On the individual level, persons who perceive drugs as being readily available in their community or school environment (Dembo, Farrow, Schmeidler, & Burgos, 1979; G. Gottfredson, 1988) use more drugs. At the aggregate level, the density of firearms (supposedly a measure of availability) in a city is positively related to its homicide rate (McDowall, 1991).

The environment closest in time and place to the adolescent problem behavior is most likely to have the most direct effect on the behavior. Characteristics of the classroom and school environments (e.g., strong academic mission, clarity about behavioral norms, predictability, consistency and fairness in applying consequences for behaviors, and climate of emotional support; G. Gottfredson & Gottfredson, 1985; Office of Educational Research and Improvement, 1992) are more likely to *directly* affect problem behavior which occurs *in* school rather than the more serious delinquent behaviors which occur primarily outside of the school. But school and classroom environments are likely to *indirectly* affect delinquency through their effect on individual-level characteristics and school-related experiences which directly influence delinquency.

Prevention Strategies

The research investigating the causes of delinquency suggests that effective prevention approaches will enhance adaptive interpersonal behaviors, improve family functioning, increase academic performance and favorable attitudes toward conventional pursuits, and reduce association with delinquent peers. Prosocial outcomes are also likely to be enhanced through environmental changes that clarify norms and expectations for prosocial behavior, limit opportunities for engaging in misbehavior, and consistently sanction misbehavior. The following section describes approaches aimed at altering these likely causal factors.

Increasing Socially Competent Behaviors

Social competency promotion strategies focus on developing a range of skills necessary to adapt and integrate feelings, thinking, and actions to achieve specific goals (Kendall, 1991). Emotional skills targeted in these programs include identifying and labeling feelings, expressing feelings, and controlling impulses. Cognitive skills include using steps for problem-solving and decision-making, understanding the perspective of others, and interpreting social cues. Behavioral skills include communicating effectively both verbally and nonverbally, and resisting negative pressures.

Effective programs to teach these skills have been developed and tested for all ages from preschool through adolescence and are marketed both as general skill-building programs (e.g., Spivack & Shure, 1974) and as programs targeting specific problem behaviors (e.g., Prothrow-Stith, 1987). Many programs are available. Some of these are: *Interpersonal Cognitive Problem Solving* (ICPS), available from Hahnemann University (Spivack & Shure, 1974), *Think Aloud,* available from Research Press (Camp & Bash, 1985), *Social Decision-Making Skills,* available from Maurice Elias at Rutgers University (Elias & Clabby, 1989), and *Social Problem Solving,* available from Roger Weissburg at the University of Illinois at Chicago (Weissburg, Caplan, & Sivo, 1989). Examples of targeted programs are *All Stars,* available from William Hansen at Tanglewood Research in Clemmons, North Carolina (Hansen, 1994), *Life Skills Training,* available from Gilbert Botvin at Cornell University Medical College (Botvin, Baker, Renick, Filazzola, & Botvin, 1989) for substance abuse, and the *Violence Prevention Curriculum* (Prothrow-Stith, 1987) published by Education Development Center in Newton, Massachusetts.

Social competency promotion is a cornerstone of both prevention and treatment because the behaviors targeted by the programs are consistently related to all kinds of problem behaviors, for all age groups. Social competency promotion programs are found in family-based programs for preschoolers as well as for adjudicated delinquents and drug-users, in client-based settings for troubled youngsters of all ages, and in school settings from preschool through high school. Different modalities are also used, ranging from individual and family therapy, to coaching, to classroom instruction.

Classroom-based social competency promotion programs generally teach children how to solve problems of an interpersonal nature. They focus on increasing youths' self-confidence in their ability to solve problems, recognizing when problems exist, identifying the feelings that accompany problems and the perspectives of others, assessing the alternative solutions available and the likely consequences of each, choosing the best solution and enacting it, self-monitoring, and self-adjusting. Different programs emphasize different segments of the process. The pioneering work of Spivack and Shure showed that young children (ages 4 and 5) can learn problem-solving skills, and that the acquisition of these skills results in more positive teacher ratings of behavior. Results from several subsequent studies (Weissberg & Allen, 1986) are not as consistently positive. The research, taken as a whole, suggests that children can acquire social skills, but the application of these skills is not always generalized to the settings where the skills are most needed. Social competence promotion programs do not always improve adjustment in broader domains.

Strategies that focus more on behavioral than on cognitive development have proven effective for reducing conduct problems in school-based programs—e.g., *The Good Behavior Game* (Barrish, Saunders, & Wolf, 1969) and other behavior modification techniques (O'Leary & O'Leary, 1977)—and in programs that involve parents in reinforcing school behaviors—e.g., *Home-Based Reinforcement* (Atkeson & Forehand, 1979; Barth, 1979). While cognitively oriented approaches focus on improving cognitive processing, behaviorally oriented ones address the behavior directly through modeling, practice, feedback, and reinforcement. The cognitive and behavioral approaches are compatible, and research (Michelson, 1987) demonstrates that their combination is more effective than either one alone.

Improving Family Functioning

Consistent with the evidence about family practices related to delinquency, evidence from family-based prevention activities suggests that programs that teach parents to use consistent but not harsh discipline strategies, interact positively with the child, and supervise the child are effective for reducing children's problem behavior. Early work to develop and test *Functional Family Therapy* (FFT) by Alexander and Parsons (1973) showed that families of 13- to 16-year-old delinquents (mostly status offenders) referred to a family clinic by the juvenile court could be taught to communicate more clearly, negotiate solutions to problems, and use contingency contracting. Families were randomly assigned to a behavioral intervention (FFT), two other types of family treatment, or a no-treatment control group. Youths of families in the FFT group had substantially lower recidivism rates 6 to 18 months following treatment than those assigned to any other condition.

Decades of work by researchers at the Oregon Social Learning Center (OSLC) have shown that parents can be helped to use positive reinforcement, mild punishment, negotiation, contingency contracting, and other methods based on social learning principles to reduce their children's problem behavior. The original program developed by Patterson and his staff focused on helping families of predelinquent boys to use social learning principles to recognize, track, record, and reinforce their childrens' behavior. This program, demonstrated successful in reducing antisocial behavior at least in the short run (Patterson, Chamberlain, & Reid, 1982), was made available in the form of programmed textbooks (Patterson, 1975, 1976) and cassette tapes (Patterson & Forgatch, 1975, 1976) which have been revised over time to reflect new learnings and elaborations to different target problems and different populations. The most recent version of the program, the *Adolescent Transitions Program* (also available from OSLC), combines training for parents (12 two-hour sessions employing videotapes) with training for adolescents aimed at the same goals.

Although clearly a prevention mainstay, the full value of programs like the OSLC program depends in part on improving their ability to reach hard-to-reach families. A review of parent training research (McAuley, 1982) suggests that stable, well-adjusted families respond better to programs like the OSLC program, while multiproblem families respond less well.

Enhancing Academic Performance and Positive School Attitudes

As noted above, it is not clear that poor school performance *per se* increases one's probability of engaging in delinquent behavior. Both poor school performance and delinquent behavior may stem from behavioral and cognitive deficits that both make it difficult to succeed academically and to control one's impulses to engage in behaviors such as theft and fighting. But the behaviors are intertwined, and some evidence (Coie & Krehbiel, 1984) suggests that interventions to improve one's academic standing (e.g., tutoring) can improve peer acceptance at least as much as interventions aimed at enhancing social skills. Because early acceptance by peers may lessen the likelihood of later association with deviant peers, strategies aimed at improving academic skill deserve attention.

Efforts aimed at building success experiences in school should begin even before the child enrolls in school. Many children fail in the first grade (Jackson, 1975). Such early school failure experiences may set in motion a series of educational decisions that limit youths' opportunities to learn and interact with prosocial peers (such as placement in special education classes) and alter childrens' self-perceptions of academic competence.

Parents can help prepare students to succeed in school by providing a language-enriched home environment—pointing out letters, signs, and labels, giving the child opportunities to read, spell, and print words, talking with and reading to their children. Programs such as the Mother–Child Home Program of the Verbal Interaction Project (Levenstein, O'Hara, & Madden, 1983) encourage mother–child play sessions by using trained "toy demonstrators" to help mothers use specially designed materials to stimulate verbal interaction. This program was aimed at improving the child's language skills and positive interaction between child and mother, and helping the parent support the child's social and emotional development.

Structured models of early language development implemented in preschool and kindergarten settings also increase success experiences. One such program, available from the Johns Hopkins University, is *STaR—Story Telling and Retelling* (Karweit, 1989)—in which children listen to a story, respond to questions about it, and then retell it in pairs and groups. Instructional innovations such as one-on-one tutoring, frequent assessment and feedback about performance, and cross-grade grouping have been shown to improve academic learning in the early grades, even in populations at high risk for failure (Slavin, Madden, Karweit, Dolan, & Wasick, 1992).

The same self-control skills that help children solve social problems also help them succeed at academic tasks. Programs that teach children cognitive self-management skills such as goal-setting, linking effort with task success, self-monitoring, self-evaluating, and self-reinforcement have been shown to increase self-perception of competencies and academic success experiences (Manning, 1988; Meichenbaum & Goodman, 1971; Schunk, 1984, 1986). The interpersonal problem-solving skills strategies described above in the context of behavioral adjustment have also been applied with young children and their parents and teachers in an academic context. These programs use parents or teachers to teach and reinforce self-control mechanisms in children by playing specially developed games. Programs developed and tested for younger children include the *Think Aloud* program (Camp & Bash, 1985) and the *Interpersonal Cognitive Problem Solving* program (Spivack, Platt, & Shure, 1976). These programs, which also encourage verbal interaction between adult and child, have been shown to enhance both behavioral and academic performance in the early school years. Principles of cognitive self-instruction have recently been incorporated into a prevention program for middle school-aged youths. This program is currently being evaluated in an urban middle school (G. Gottfredson, 1994).

Decreasing Association with Delinquent Peers

Little is known about how to reduce association with delinquent peers or to limit the learning that takes place within these social groups. Although association with delinquent peers is the single largest correlate of delinquent behavior, changing peer associations once patterns of association have been established presents a challenge. Because youths sort themselves into peer groups on the basis of similarity at a fairly young age, changing patterns of peer influence during adolescence seems to require much earlier efforts to alter peer interactions. We have only sketchy evidence related to the success of such efforts. Nevertheless, social competence promotion efforts appear at least worthy of consideration as strategies to reduce negative peer associations.

Coaching-type social competency promotion programs teach socially isolated or rejected elementary-school children skills such as communication, cooperation, participation, and validation/support and provide opportunities to practice these skills. Some of these programs focus solely on individual behavior by providing coaching individually or in small groups to socially rejected or neglected children (e.g., Coie & Krehbiel, 1984). Others embed the intervention into the natural classroom context by training teachers to structure opportunities for exhibiting and reinforcement for displaying social skills (e.g., Hops, 1982). These coaching interventions improve the sociometric status of children, but the generalizability of the findings to diverse groups and their long-term effects remain unclear.

Coie and Koeppl (1990) argue that interventions to promote social acceptance by peers would be more effective if they were targeted more precisely at the specific source of the peer rejection. For aggressive children, interventions that directly alter the contingencies for the display of aggressive behaviors are likely to be effective. When the source of the peer rejection is disruptive, disorderly behavior rather than overt aggression, effective solutions include reinforcing on-task behavior (O'Leary & O'Leary, 1977) or increasing the cost of off-task behavior (Barrish *et al.*, 1969).

Other strategies with potential for reducing influence by negative peers include increased parental supervision during the adolescent years to limit the association of children with negative peers. The parenting skills programs described earlier include an emphasis on enhancing parental skill to recognize and provide consequences for undesirable behavior. Associating with negative peers can be defined in these programs as itself a problem behavior. Peer mediation and conflict resolution programs have become popular in recent years as strategies for reducing disruptive behavior in school. These programs involve students in helping other students to think before they act impulsively when faced with a potentially explosive situation. Although we know little about the success of these programs for reducing negative peer influence or problem behavior, the idea of engaging youth in promoting prosocial responses has a certain appeal.

Changing the Environment

Research summarized above suggests that efforts aimed at reducing availability of drugs and opportunities for crime in the environment, and changing norms to be less accepting of deviant behavior should reduce adolescent problem behavior. Changing community environments is a difficult undertaking, as is conducting rigorous research on them. Research on the efficacy of community intervention programs is sparse and provides mixed results. Studies of the effects of developing *Neighborhood Watch* programs suggest that they have the potential to reduce crime (Bennett & Lavrakas, 1989; Pennell, Curtis, Henderson, & Tayman, 1989), but they are most difficult to organize in the highest crime neighborhoods and might result in increased fear (Rosenbaum, 1987; Skogan, 1989).

One impressive line of research to limit conflict in schools has been undertaken in Norway (Olweus, 1991, 1992; Olweus & Alsaker, 1991). Olweus noted that certain adolescents, called "bullies," repeatedly victimized other adolescents. Typically bullies were characterized as displaying an "aggressive reaction pattern combined (in the case of boys) with physical strength" and as representing "a more general conduct disordered, antisocial and rule-breaking behavior pattern." Olweus also noted that the victims of bullying tended to be neglected by the school. Although they were known to be targets of harassment, the problem was largely ignored by adults who failed to actively intervene and thus providing tacit acceptance of the bullying.

A program was devised to alter environmental norms regarding bullying. A campaign directed communication to redefining the behavior as wrong. A booklet was directed to school personnel, defining the problem and spelling out ways to counteract it. Parents were sent a booklet of advice. A video illustrating the problem was made available. And questionnaire surveys to collect information and register the level of the problem were fielded. Information was fed back to personnel in 42 schools in Bergen, Norway. Reassessment implied that the problem had declined.

Efforts focused on specific drug-related outcomes also appear successful. The Midwestern Prevention Program developed a community coordinating structure to implement changes in mass media programming, a school-based normative reeducation and skill-building curriculum, parent organization and education, and health policy change. Youths in the target communities were found to have lower prevalence of cigarette, alcohol, and marijuana use than youths in control communities (Pentz *et al.*, 1989). Limiting the availability of alcohol to adolescents by increasing the minimum drinking age and increasing the price of alcohol reduces alcohol-related traffic accidents (Grossman, Coate, & Arluck, 1987; Mosher, 1985). Efforts focused even more narrowly on reducing drinking under certain conditions, such as responsible beverage server programs which teach alcohol licensees to institute practices that limit heavy drinking in their establishments, also appear promising (Saltz, 1987).

Efforts to alter the school environment have met with some success. D. Gottfredson (1986) reported the results of a comprehensive school improvement intervention—*Project PATHE*—that altered the organization and management structures in seven secondary schools. The broad-based structural changes (e.g., changes in the discipline and management of the school, testing practices, and amount and kinds of activities available to staff and students) targeted the entire population and were effective for increasing attachment to school and perceived fairness and clarity of rules, decreasing alienation, and reducing disorder.

D. Gottfredson (1987b) reported the results of a similar effort—*The Effective Schools Project*—in a difficult Baltimore City junior high school. Organization development (OD) methods were used to plan and implement changes to instructional and discipline practices. The OD method, Program Development Evaluation (available from Gottfredson Associates, Inc. in Ellicott City, Maryland; G. Gottfredson, 1984; G. Gottfredson, Rickert, Gottfredson, & Advani, 1984), helps organizations define problems and set goals, specify theories of action on which to base improvement efforts, define measurable objectives based on the theory, select interventions with a high likelihood of achieving those objectives, identify and plan to overcome the obstacles to implementation of the interventions selected, and develop detailed implementation standards to serve as blueprints for each intervention. Researchers and practitioners collaborate to develop and implement programs using the method. A spiral of improvement is created as evaluative data are continuously fed back to the practitioners for program refinement. Using the method, major classroom management and instructional innovations and a number of less potent interventions were undertaken. Indicators of organizational health (e.g., staff morale, cooperation and collaboration between faculty and administration, and staff involvement in planning and action for school improvement) improved dramatically, and significant reductions in delinquency were observed.

More recently, D. Gottfredson, G. Gottfredson, and Hybl (1993) demonstrated that a school-based program (*Project BASIS*, available from D. Gottfredson at the University of Maryland)—designed to increase clarity of school rules and consistency of rule enforcement, improve classroom organization and management, increase the frequency of communication with the home regarding student behavior, and increase reinforcement of appropriate behavior—was successful in improving student conduct. An important component of this schoolwide program was a classroom management module developed and tested by Emmer, Evertson, Sanford, Clements, and Worsham (1984). These researchers demonstrated a reduction in classroom disorder using a teacher training intervention focusing on increasing clarity of communication, styles of monitoring and responding to student behavior, extent of student responsibility and accountability for work, and methods of organizing instruction. Materials for training are provided in the Emmer *et al.* (1984) book.

This research, taken together, provides support for the efficacy of reducing problem behavior through changes in the organization and management of the environment. Larger effects seem to be associated with more focused efforts.

In sum, delinquent behavior may be preventable. But even the strongest prevention strategies are only modestly effective, and their effects diminish over time. In order to enhance prevention effectiveness, we need to (1) create multicomponent strategies by combining moderately successful components; (2) string components together over the life course to provide continuous preventive intervention; (3) target services at individuals or environments most at risk; and (4) enhance the capacity of organizations to faithfully implement the strategies.

TREATMENT

Though the debate continues as to the proper role that treatment plays in the lives of adjudicated adult offenders, treatment of some kind has traditionally been recognized as crucial for adjudicated juveniles because they are considered to be less rooted in a criminal life-style and to have a greater potential of being made a productive member of society. The strategies summarized in this chapter are intended, unless otherwise noted, to reduce recidivism among youths who are already officially adjudicated delinquents.

Treatment Settings: Institutional Treatment versus Community-Based Treatment

Institutional treatment services are provided in institutional environments, such as training schools, hospitals, detention centers, work camps, and, more recently, boot camps. Such services can vary greatly in type (i.e., group or individual therapy, social skills training, academic or vocational education) and theoretical approach by which the treatment is justified. Several research summaries have assessed the efficacy of institutional correctional treatment. Izzo and Ross (1990) conducted a meta-analysis* of 46 studies. Focusing on recidivism, they found that treatment setting was an important variable in a program's effectiveness, and that most effective programs were conducted in community rather than institutional settings. Whitehead and Lab (1989) examined 50 studies appearing in professional journals between 1975 and 1984 and compared five different broad categories of treatment in terms of recidivism: nonsystem diversion, system diversion, community corrections (including probation and parole), institutional/residential treatment programs, and novel/specialty programs (i.e., Scared Straight and Outward Bound). Despite their generous standard of significance, they found no treatment that had overwhelmingly positive results, but concluded that institutional/residential treatment programs appeared to have more negative effects than the community corrections programs. Desiring to retest these findings, Andrews *et al.*, (1990) conducted a meta-analysis that included most of the studies used by Whitehead and Lad. They found that community-based settings had stronger positive effects than residential/institutional settings. Institutional/residential settings, in fact, appeared to decrease the positive effects of some treatments and increase the negative effects of others. When institutional treatment is compared with no treatment or specific and inconsistent community-based treatment, however, institutionalized youths recidivate less than comparison youths.

A relatively new form of institutional treatment that has enjoyed popular support is the shock incarceration, or "boot camp" concept. These camps, usually designed for young, male offenders convicted of nonviolent offenses, are modeled after military boot

---

*A meta-analysis is a "statistical analysis of a large collection of analysis results from individual studies for the purpose of integrating findings" (Glass, 1976, p. 3).

camp training. They involve military drill and ceremony, physical training, and hard labor. Beyond this basic core of military-style training, programs vary considerably on dimensions such as the extent of rehabilitative programming, intensity of supervision on release, and type of aftercare services. Boot camp evaluation studies suggest that they are no panacea. MacKenzie and Souryal (1994) show that the programs generally have no effect on the future recidivism of offenders, but they provide a less expensive alternative to other forms of institutional treatment and have the potential to reduce prison over-crowding.

Community-based treatment is provided in a community environment. It includes nonresidential day programs and residential services provided in places that are located in the community and generally smaller and less secure than institutions. Following the 1974 Juvenile Justice and Delinquency Prevention Act, there was a great push for the deinstitu-tionalization of juvenile offenders and, correspondingly, a tremendous growth in community-based treatment for them. It was hoped that community-based treatment would provide an environment more conducive to treatment while avoiding some of the problems of institutional treatment. Community-based treatment itself may range from minimal supervision of the youth to residential placements, which may be in reality quite similar to institutional placement in terms of atmosphere and community access. Some common types of community treatment include differential parole treatment, guided group interaction counseling techniques, foster-home care, group-homes, and residential youth centers (Wright & Dixon, 1977). As with institutional treatment, a heterogeneous assortment of activities is labeled "community-based treatment," and it is difficult to disentangle the effect of the content of the program from the setting in which it is delivered. Broadly speaking, community-based treatments are guided by the belief that treating youth in an institutional environment will not facilitate the transference of the skills the youth has learned in the isolated institutional environment to his home environ-ment. These treatments are intended to keep the youth either at home or in a home-type environment in order to ease his adjustment and, potentially, decrease the chances of recidivism. Furthermore, community treatment has often been used simply to avoid sending youths to a correctional facility (Wright & Dixon, 1977).

Gottschalk, Davidson, Gensheimer, and Mayer (1987) performed a meta-analysis of community-based programs' efficacy in treating adjudicated delinquents. Their research included both residential and nonresidential community-based programs. They looked not only at recidivism, but also at behavioral (e.g., academic performance and social behav-ior) and attitudinal (e.g., cognitive measures and self-esteem) outcomes. They found that the effects of community-based treatment, although in the positive direction for virtually all outcomes, were not statistically significant. A majority of the studies examined suf-fered from a weak application of the treatment and/or severe methodological problems. Gottschalk et al. noted that positive effects of treatment are more likely to emerge from a strong treatment that has been carefully implemented as designed. The importance of a strong theoretical base, a solid treatment program, a consistent and competent application of the program elements, and a willing and receptive clientele appears to be a common-ality between institutional and community-based treatment programs.

Although community-based treatment has potential for reducing the cost of juvenile treatment, it often involves less intensive supervision than institutional programs, and therefore has the potential to *increase* recidivism relative to more secure programs. Barton and Butts (1990), for example, compared three in-home, intensive supervision programs with commitment to the state's Department of Social Services which usually resulted in placement at a public or private institution. The supervision programs used behavioral supervision and individual counseling, and frequently school placement assistance and social skills training. The intensive probation programs cost about one-third as much as institutional commitment.

The results showed that the intensive probation group had higher levels of repeat offending than the training school group during the 2 years following random assignment. The differences could mostly be accounted for by greater opportunity to reoffend: The intensive probation group spent 7.6 more months "at large" during the follow-up period than did the incarcerated group. Once these differences in time-at-large were taken into consideration, the offending level of the intensive probation group was only slightly higher than that of the institutionalized group. When only criminal charges were considered, the group differences were not significant. The study showed that community-based interventions can be cost-effective alternatives to incarceration. But weak and inconsistent community-based treatments may well increase recidivism by reducing supervision levels.

Treatment Modalities

Most treatments can be applied in either an institutional or community-based setting. While treatment setting might very well be an important factor in the efficacy of a particular treatment, it appears more valuable to instead examine the effectiveness of the individual treatments, regardless of setting.

Garrett's (1985) meta-analysis grouped treatment modalities into the following four categories: psychodynamic (which included individual, group, and family therapies), behavioral (which included such treatments as contingency management, cognitive-behavioral, guided group interaction/positive peer culture, and milieu therapy), life skills (which included treatments designed to enhance skills thought to be related to successful everyday functioning such as drug/alcohol training and academic, vocational, and outdoor experience), and "other" (which included music therapy, multivitamin treatment, and undifferentiated "skills"). The following summary is organized around these categories.

Therapy-Oriented Approaches

Psychodynamic therapy is a popular form of treatment, particularly in residential settings. It has not demonstrated its effectiveness among adjudicated youth (Mulvey, Arthur, & Reppucci, 1993; Lipsey, 1992; Greenwood, 1986). Some studies have declared that individual and group therapies in a residential setting appear to have little impact on recidivism (Mulvey *et al.*, 1993), while others have declared it helpful in reducing recidivism in both institutional and community settings (Lipton, Martinson, & Wilks, 1975). In Garrett's (1985) analysis of various modes of treatments, individual and group therapy produced relatively small effects. Gordon and Arbuthnot (1987) found that individual psychotherapy does not consistently reduce recidivism because it aims for "global cognitive changes such as insight and new understanding of the causes of behavior, against the backdrop of a warm, supportive relationship" (p. 295). In other words, vague treatment goals and loose treatment patterns do not lend themselves well to the client's long-term engagement in desired behaviors. This assessment was confirmed by Lipsey (1992), who found that less structured and focused treatments such as counseling had lower levels of effectiveness than more structured and focused treatments. Lipton *et al.* (1975) suggest that therapy that emphasizes immediate, real-life issues might prove more effective in reducing recidivism.

Family therapy, on the other hand, appears effective (Garrett, 1985). The Functional Family Therapy model involving behavioral contracting and communication techniques described in the prevention section of this chapter (Alexander & Parsons, 1973) was effective for reducing recidivism among delinquents. Geismar and Wood (1985) found no effect for nonbehavioral family therapy.

One variation on personalized therapy is casework and individual counseling. Lipton *et al.* (1975) suggested that casework specifically tailored to each youth will have a greater effect on recidivism than will casework that is designed to be implemented in a more general manner. In general, however, casework and counseling in both institutional and community settings produce mixed results in terms of recidivism. Gordon and Arbuthnot (1987) found that casework does not appear to affect recidivism for the same reasons that individual psychotherapy does not, i.e., because treatment goals are global and vague.

Cognitive-Behavioral Approaches

Consistent with the material summarized in the prevention section, cognitive-behaviorally oriented treatments that focus on social skills deficits demonstrate the greatest success of any category of treatment in terms of reducing recidivism (Garrett, 1985; Lipsey, 1992). As in prevention research, these programs can be subdivided into primarily behavioral and primarily cognitive orientations. The Teaching Family Model is a primarily behavioral treatment approach that has been implemented in community residential group home settings such as Achievement Place. In Teaching Family homes, a trained couple lives with about six chronic delinquents. These "Teaching Parents" administer a systematic behavioral system of points and privileges to guide the youths' behavior (Phillips, 1968). Evaluations of this model indicate that it reduces delinquent behavior while youths are in the program; the behavioral differences disappear once youths leave. Izzo and Ross (1990) concluded that programs that included a cognitive component (e.g., some element that targeted the offender's thinking, including problem-solving, negotiation skills training, interpersonal skills training, rational-emotive therapy, role-playing and modeling, or cognitive behavior modification) were more than twice as effective as programs that did not. But Gordon and Arbuthnot (1987) warn that while the cognitive ability to see something from another's point of view may be valuable in reducing antisocial behavior, affective abilities such as the ability to empathize with another person's emotions are also important. When Garrett (1985) examined specific, ungrouped treatments while taking methodological rigor into account, cognitive-behavioral approaches appeared to be the most successful.

Not all assessments of cognitive-behavioral therapy types have been positive, however. Whitehead and Lab's (1989) meta-analysis concluded that behavioral interventions are no more effective than any other type of intervention in reducing recidivism, and, in fact, may have a negative effect. And Granziano and Mooney (1984) suggest that behavioral approaches have not successfully exhibited a positive effect on youth behavior outside of the confines of the treatment program itself.

Academic, Vocational, and Life Skills Programs

Garrett's (1985) meta-analysis showed positive effects for academic programs. An example of such a program is the CASE II project (Contingencies Applicable to Special Education; Mulvey *et al.*, 1993; Cohen & Filipczak, 1971). This program used behavior modification techniques to reinforce academic goals, with schedules of reinforcements for individual success. The youths in the program were rewarded with points for successful completion of elements of the program, and the points could be traded for money and goods. The youths exhibited immediate academic improvement, as measured by a standardized test, and within the first year a decreased rate of recidivism (two-thirds that of a control group). The difference in recidivism waned by the end of 3 years, suggesting the necessity for sustained treatment.

Vocational and skill development programs aim to teach responsibility and goal setting. Such programs also help youths gain a sense of accomplishment on completion of a project and are often combined with regular schooling, particularly for school-aged youth. The effects of such programs on recidivism are not yet clear.

A different type of life skills programs is outdoor experience treatment, which includes such modalities as Outward Bound and wilderness camping programs. Such programs use the natural stresses and situations of the wilderness to encourage individual development and group cooperation. Mulvey *et al.* (1993) report the results of an analysis conducted by Roberts and Schervish (1988) which finds that wilderness programs have a relatively high ratio of effectiveness to risks and costs. Garrett's (1985) analysis suggested that outdoor experience programs have a fairly positive overall effect. But most of the studies looking at wilderness programs and Outward Bound have been plagued by methodological difficulties and inconclusive results. So far, claims as to their effectiveness have been mainly subjective in nature. No systematic evaluations of such programs have been conducted (Greenwood, 1986; Mulvey *et al.*, 1993).

Treatment effectiveness research parallels prevention effectiveness research in suggesting that treatment can reduce delinquency but that it has not yet reached an optimal level of effectiveness. Treatment research favors behavioral/cognitive approaches and approaches that build commitment to conventional goals. Regardless of whether they were implemented in an institutional or community-based setting, all treatment modalities appear to share a common deficiency: a program does not effect a long-term change in delinquent youth once the program has terminated. This indicates the need for follow-up or aftercare treatment. The design of the treatment and the strength and integrity with which it is delivered appear to be major issues in treatment effectiveness. Often treatments with the same label (e.g., "boot camp") have vastly different designs and are implemented with very different levels of strength and integrity. The greater the strength and integrity of the implementation, regardless of setting, the more effective the treatment is.

CONCLUSION

In order to increase the effective prevention and treatment of delinquency, we must (1) improve the design of prevention and treatment strategies, (2) improve the rigor and the appropriateness of program evaluations, and (3) enhance the strength and fidelity of program implementation. Program designs can be strengthened by focusing programs more on the plausible causal factors summarized under the prevention section of this chapter and increasing the duration and intensity of programs. It is encouraging that the research on causal factors corresponds with the findings of meta-analyses of prevention and treatment effectiveness. Lipsey's (1992) meta-analysis of treatment programs, for example, found that interventions of longer duration, involving more structured and focused treatments (e.g., behavioral, skill-oriented) and multimodal treatments were more effective than less structured and focused approaches (e.g., counseling). Research on the causes of delinquency also point to the importance of behavior and cognitive skill deficits in explaining delinquency, and to the multiple causes of delinquency. Evaluations of prevention programs aimed at enhancing cognitive and behavioral skill deficits suggest that these approaches are among the more promising prevention strategies, and the effectiveness of this approach in a variety of different modalities (e.g., family, school, and residential facilities) suggests the efficacy of multimodal treatment.

Complementary programs should be designed to address the causal factors from several different angles simultaneously and to provide *continuous* services. Such programs might contain, for example, a school-based curriculum component aimed at teaching cognitive self-management skills, a school climate component aimed at increasing the clarity and consistency of school rule enforcement, *and* a parenting skills component aimed at increasing supervision and discipline management. The ideal program would provide for services over a several-year period, particularly for high-risk youths.

Unfortunately, prevention and treatment as typically practiced fall short of this continuous, multimodal ideal. An evaluation of 17 delinquency prevention programs funded by the Office Of Juvenile Justice and Delinquency Prevention (D. Gottfredson, 1987a) reported on the diverse prevention services offered: alternative schools with environments ranging from regimented and military-style to caring but permissive; alternative classrooms within the regular school setting using a variant of the law-related education curriculum; vocational training job readiness skill building; after-school programs offering recreational activities; remedial education featuring individualized education; peer culture development or other forms of group counseling offered in semester-long classes; music lessons; counseling and academic assistance offered as extra services during the school day to high-risk youths; and school climate improvement. Many of the ideas were viable and, indeed, several produced positive effects, at least in the short run. But most were offered on a short-term basis (i.e., for a semester or a school year), and most provided services in only one setting.

The programs included in this evaluation, like many others described in the published literature, have the benefit of dedicated staff and (often) researcher collaboration made possible by adequate funding. More typically, prevention activities are funded sporadically and at relatively low levels. Many prevention activities are funded through federal block grant monies which are divided up among a large pool of prevention providers. Activities funded through this mechanism seem more subject to influence by fads and tend often to be of the "one-shot" variety.

Perhaps the most pressing need for improving the efficacy of delinquency prevention and treatment concerns the strength and fidelity with which the activity is implemented. Even programs with ideal designs often fail at the implementation stage. If the activity is strong and implemented as designed, the likelihood of positive effects emerging is greater (Gottschalk *et al.*, 1987). Lipsey (1992) also found that program effectiveness was related to more careful service delivery.

The problem of poor quality of implementation plagues all efforts to change existing practices, but is especially acute in those settings and for those populations most in need of services. The factors that contribute to low-level implementation are often embedded within the culture of the implementing organization. Teacher morale, teacher–administration cooperation and communication, the presence of decision-making structures that foster teacher involvement in planning and action to solve problems, clear school rules and reward structures, and unambiguous role definitions are related to the school's capacity to initiate and maintain an innovation (Corcoran, 1985; D. Gottfredson, 1987b; G. Gottfredson & Gottfredson, 1985; D. Gottfredson *et al.*, 1993). The conditions that hinder effective innovation are more likely to exist in greater degrees in troubled communities whose resources are often diverted to crisis management (D. Gottfredson, Fink, & Gottfredson, 1993) or which have difficulty recruiting and retaining competent staff.

Characteristics of the target population also contribute to lowered implementation strength. For example, the promising parent training intervention strategies summarized in this chapter are known to be least effective with the most dysfunctional families, i.e., with families in which the mother is socially isolated, in coercive entrapment with other adults, and at socioeconomic disadvantage (Wahler & Dumas, 1987). Attrition rates are much higher among this population than among more functional families. Issues of treatment population recruitment and retention are likely to plague any prevention or treatment activities targeting high-risk populations.

Finally, program evaluations must be strengthened. Without strong program evaluations we will be unable to amass evidence of program effectiveness. Most attempts to reduce delinquency are not studied, and most evaluations that are conducted suffer from one or more weaknesses that limit confidence in the study results. It is difficult to meld research ideals to real-world conditions, and evaluations often suffer accordingly. The salient evaluation issues differ somewhat depending on the focus of the program. In prevention research, studies of the effectiveness of community-based prevention are particularly difficult to undertake. In treatment research, issues related to subject attrition are more pressing because of difficulties in controlling the flow of juveniles through the juvenile justice system. In both areas, controlling the effects of extraneous variables in order to obtain an unambiguous reading of program effectiveness is a key issue requiring the identification of appropriate comparison groups.

Another common research problem is the failure to measure program implementation. All treatments are not delivered uniformly, and it is important to correlate the actual level of program implementation with observed outcomes rather than assuming that the program was in fact implemented with adequate integrity. Indeed, Garrett (1985) concludes that those studies supporting the conclusion that "nothing works" tends to employ a "ballot-box" technique which simply discerns whether or not a statistically significant result was obtained without reference to what was actually implemented. When research controls for variation across programs in level of implementation, results are more encouraging. In short, it is necessary now to increase the rigor of program evaluations and to tailor them better to the specific outcomes sought and activities undertaken in the program, in order to eventually improve practice.

Delinquency appears amenable to treatment and prevention activities, but we are not yet close to an effective solution to this problem. Efforts now need to focus on redesigning programs to make better use of what is known about the causes of delinquency, and improving the strength and integrity of program implementation.

ACKNOWLEDGMENTS. We appreciate Gary D. Gottfredson's editorial assistance and Julie Marshall's clerical help.

REFERENCES

Akers, R. L., Krohn, M. D., Lanza-Kaduce, L., & Radosevich, M. (1979). Social learning and deviant behavior: A specific test of a general theory. *American Sociological Review, 44,* 636–655.

Alexander, J. F., & Parsons, B. V. (1973). Short-term behavioral intervention with delinquent families: Impacts on family process and recidivism. *Journal of Abnormal Psychology, 81,* 219–225.

Andrews, D. A., Zinger, I., Hoge, R. D., Bonta, J., Gendrea, P., & Cullen, F. T. (1990). Does correctional treatment work? A clinically relevant and psychologically informed meta-analysis. *Criminology, 28,* 369–404.

Atkeson, B. M., & Forehand, R. (1979). Home-based reinforcement programs designed to modify classroom behavior: A review and methodological evaluation. *Psychological Bulletin, 86,* 1298–1308.

Bachman, J. G., Green, S., & Wirtanen, I. D. (1971). *Youth in transition: Vol. 3. Dropping out—Problem or symptom?* Ann Arbor: University of Michigan Institute for Social Research.

Bachman, J. G., O'Malley, P. M., & Johnston, L. (1978). *Adolescent to adulthood: Change and stability in the lives of young men.* Ann Arbor: University of Michigan Institute for Social Research.

Barrish, H. H., Saunders, M., & Wolf, M. M. (1969). Good behavior game: Effects of individual contingencies for group consequences on disruptive behavior in a classroom. *Journal of Applied Behavior Analysis, 2,* 119–124.

Barth, R. (1979). Home-based reinforcement of school behavior: A review and analysis. *Review of Educational Research, 49,* 436–458.

Barton, W. H., & Butts, J. A. (1990). Viable options: Intensive supervision programs for juvenile delinquents. *Crime and Delinquency, 36,* 238–255.

Bastian, L. D. (1993). *Criminal victimization 1992.* Washington, DC: Bureau of Justice Statistics, U.S. Department of Justice.

Bennett, S. F., & Lavrakas, P. J. (1989). Community-based crime prevention: An assessment of the Eisenhower Foundations's Neighborhood Program. *Crime and Delinquency, 35,* 345–364.

Block, J., Block, J. H., & Keyes, S. (1988). Longitudinally foretelling drug usage in adolescence: Early childhood personality and environmental precursors. *Child Development, 59,* 336–355.

Blumstein, A., Cohen, J., Roth, J., & Visher, C. (1986). *Criminal careers and career criminals.* Washington, DC: National Academy Press.

Botvin, G., Baker, E., Renick, N., Filazzola, A., & Botvin, E. (1984). A cognitive behavioral approach to substance abuse prevention. *Addictive Behaviors, 9,* 137–147.

Bowles, S., & Gintis, H. (1976). *Schooling in capitalist America.* New York: Basic Books.

Braithwaite, J. (1989). *Crime, shame, and reintegration.* London: Cambridge University Press.

Cairns, R. B., Cairns, B. D., Neckerman, H. J., Gest, S. D., & Gariepy, J. L. (1988). Social networks and aggressive behavior: Peer support or peer rejection? *Developmental Psychology, 24,* 815–823.

Camp, B. W., & Bash, M. S. (1985). *Think aloud: Increasing social and cognitive skills—A problem-solving program for children.* Champaign, IL: Research Press.

Cohen, H. L., & Filipczak, J. (1971). *A new learning environment.* San Francisco: Jossey–Bass.

Cohen, L. E., & Felson, M. (1979). Social change and crime rate trends: A routine activity approach. *American Sociological Review, 44,* 588–608.

Coie, J. D., & Krehbiel, G. (1984). Effects of academic tutoring on the social status of low-achieving, socially rejected children. *Child Development, 55,* 1465–1478.

Coie, J. D., & Koeppl, G. (1990). Adapting intervention to the problems of aggressive and disruptive rejected children. In S. R. Asher & J. D. Coie (Eds.), *Peer rejection in childhood* (pp. 275–308). London: Cambridge University Press.

Conger, J. J., & Miller, W. C. (1966). *Personality, social class, and delinquency.* New York: Wiley.

Corcoran, T. B. (1985). Effective secondary schools. In R. M. J. Kyle (Ed.), *Reaching for excellence: An effective schools sourcebook.* Washington, DC: U.S. Government Printing Office.

Cowen, E. L., Pederson, A., Babigian, H., Izzo, L. D., & Trost, M. A. (1973). Long-term follow-up of early detected vulnerable children. *Journal of Consulting and Clinical Psychology, 41*(3), 438–446.

Dembo, R., Farrow, D., Schmeidler, J., & Burgos, W. (1979). Testing a causal model of environmental influences on early drug involvement of inner city junior high youths. *American Journal of Drug and Alcohol Abuse, 6,* 313–336.

Dodge, K. A., Pettit, G. S., McClaskey, C. L., & Brown, M. M. (1986). Social competence in children. *Monographs of the Society for Research in Child Development, 51*(2, Serial No. 213).

Elias, M. J., & Clabby, J. F. (1989). *Social decision-making skills: A curriculum guide for the elementary grades.* Rockville: Aspen.

Elliott, D. S., Huizinga, D., & Ageton, S. S. (1985). *Explaining delinquency and drug use.* Beverly Hills: Sage.

Elliott, D. S., Huizinga, D., & Menard, S. (1989). *Multiple problem youth: Delinquency, substance use, and mental health problems.* Berlin: Springer-Verlag.

Emmer, E. T., Evertson, C. M., Sanford, J. P., Clements, B. S., & Worsham, M. (1984). *Classroom management for secondary teachers.* Englewood Cliffs, NJ: Prentice–Hall.

Farrington, D. P. (1987). Epidemiology. In H. C. Quay (Ed.), *Handbook of juvenile delinquency.* (pp. 33–61). New York: Wiley.

Farrington, D. P. (1992). Explaining the beginning, progress, and ending of antisocial behavior from birth to adulthood. In J. McCord (Ed.), *Advances in criminological theory: Vol. 3. Facts, frameworks, and forecasts.* New Brunswick: Transaction Publishers.

Federal Bureau of Investigation. (1993a). *Age-specific arrest rates and race-specific arrest rates for selected offenses, 1965–1992.* Washington, DC: U.S. Government Printing Office.

Federal Bureau of Investigation. (1993b). *Crime in the United States 1992.* Washington, DC: U.S. Government Printing Office.

Feldhusen, J. F., Thurston, J. R., & Benning, J. J. (1973). A longitudinal study of delinquency and other aspects of children's behavior. *International Journal of Criminology and Penology, 1,* 341–351.

Fingerhut, L. A., Ingram, D. D., & Feldman, J. J. (1992). Firearm and nonfirearm homicide among persons 15 through 19 years of age: Differences by level of urbanization, United States, 1979 through 1989. *Journal of the American Medical Association, 267,* 3048–3053.

Garrett, C. J. (1985). Effects of residential treatment on adjudicated delinquents: A meta-analysis. *The Journal of Research in Crime and Delinquency, 22,* 287–308.

Geismar, L. L., & Wood, K. M. (1985). *Family and delinquency: Resocializing the young offender.* New York: Human Sciences Press.

Glass, G. V. (1976). Primary, secondary, and meta-analysis of research. *Review of Educational Research in Education, 5,* 3–8.

Glueck, S., & Glueck, E. T. (1950). *Unraveling juvenile delinquency.* Cambridge, MA: Harvard University Press.

Glueck, S., & Glueck, E. T. (1968). *Delinquents and non-delinquents in perspective.* Cambridge, MA: Harvard University Press.

Gordon, D. A., & Arbuthnot, J. (1987). Individual, group, and family interventions. In H. C. Quay (Ed.), *Handbook of juvenile delinquency* (pp. 290–324). New York: Wiley.

Gottfredson, D. C. (1986). An empirical test of school-based environmental and individual interventions to reduce the risk of delinquent behavior. *Criminology, 24,* 705–731.

Gottfredson, D. C. (1987a). Examining the potential of delinquency prevention through alternative education. In H. Hurst (Ed.), *Today's delinquent* (Vol. 6, pp. 87–100). Pittsburgh: National Center for Juvenile Justice.

Gottfredson, D. C. (1987b). An evaluation of an organization development approach to reducing school disorder. *Evaluation Review, 11,* 739–763.

Gottfredson, D. C., Fink, C. M., & Gottfredson, G. D. (1993). *Making prevention work by improving program integrity: A field trial.* Paper presented at the annual meeting of the American Society of Criminology.

Gottfredson, D. C., Fink, C. M., & Graham, N. (1994). Grade retention and problem behavior. *American Educational Research Journal, 31*(4), 761–784.

Gottfredson, D. C., Gottfredson, G. D., & Hybl, L. G. (1993). Managing adolescent behavior: A multi-year, multi-school experiment. *American Educational Research Journal, 61,* 179.

Gottfredson, G. D. (1981). Schooling and delinquency. In S. E. Martin, L. B. Sechrest, & R. Redner (Eds.), *New directions in the rehabilitation of criminal offenders.* Washington, DC: National Academy Press.

Gottfredson, G. D. (1984). A theory-ridden approach to program evaluation: A method for stimulating researcher–implementer collaboration. *American Psychologist, 39,* 1101–1112.

Gottfredson, G. D. (1987a). American education: American delinquency. *Today's Delinquent, 6,* 5–70.

Gottfredson, G. D. (1987b). Peer group interventions to reduce the risk of delinquent behavior: A selective review and a new evaluation. *Criminology, 25,* 671–714.

Gottfredson, G. D. (1988). *Issues in adolescent drug use.* Unpublished final report to the U.S. Department of Justice. Johns Hopkins University, Center for Research on Elementary and Middle Schools, Baltimore.

Gottfredson, G. D. (September, 1994). *Multi-Model School-Centered Prevention Demonstration Progress Report No. 9.* Unpublished report available from Gottfredson Associates, Inc., Ellicott City, MD.

Gottfredson, G. D., & Gottfredson, D. C. (1985). *Victimization in schools.* New York: Plenum Press.

Gottfredson, G. D., Rickert, D. E., Gottfredson, D. C., & Advani, N. (1984). Standards for program development evaluation plans. Ms. No. 2668. *Psychological Documents, 14,* 32.

Gottfredson, M. R., & Hirschi, T. (1990). *A general theory of crime.* Stanford: Stanford University Press.

Gottschalk, R., Davidson, W. S., Gensheimer, L. K., & Mayer, J. P. (1987). Community-based interventions. In H. C. Quay (Ed.), *Handbook of juvenile delinquency* (pp. 266–289). New York: Wiley.

Granziano, A. M., & Mooney, K. C. (1984). *Children and behavior therapy.* Chicago: Aldine.

Greenwood, P. W. (Ed.). (1986). *Intervention strategies for chronic juvenile offenders.* New York: Greenwood Press.

Grissom, J. B., & Shepard, L. A. (1989). Repeating and dropping out of school. In L. A. Shepard & M. L. Smith (Eds.), *Flunking grades: Research and policies on retention.* New York: Falmer Press.

Grossman, M., Coate, D., & Arluck, G. M. (1987). Price sensitivity of alcoholic beverages in the United States: Youth alcohol consumption. In H. Holder (Ed.), *Advances in substance abuse: Behavioral and biological research: Supplement 1. Control issues in alcohol abuse prevention: Strategies for states and communities* (pp. 169–198). Greenwich, CT: JAI Press.

Hagan, J., & Bumiller, K. (1983). Making sense of sentencing: A review and critique of sentencing research. In A. Blumstein, J. Cohen, S. E. Martin, & M. H. Tonry (Eds.), *Research on sentencing: The search for reform* (Vol. 2). Washington, DC: National Academy Press.

Havighurst, B. J., Bowman, P. H., Liddle, G. P., Mathews, C. V., & Pierce, J. V. (1962). *Growing up in River City.* New York: Wiley.

Hindelang, M. J. (1978). Race and involvement in common law personal crimes. *American Sociological Review, 43,* 93–109.

Hindelang, M. J., Hirschi, T., & Weis, J. G. (1979). Correlates of delinquency: The illusion of discrepancy between self-report and official measures. *American Sociological Review, 44,* 995–1014.

Hindelang, M. J., Hirschi, T., & Weis, J. G. (1981). *Measuring delinquency.* Beverly Hills: Sage.

Hirschi, T. (1969). *Causes of delinquency.* Berkely: University of California Press.

Hops, H. (1982). Social skills training for socially isolated children. In P. Karoly & J. Steffen (Eds.), *Enhancing children's competencies.* Lexington, MA: Lexington Books.

Izzo, R. L., & Ross, R. R. (1990). Meta-analysis of rehabilitation programs for juvenile delinquents. *Criminal Justice and Behavior, 17,* 134–142.

Jackson, G. (1975). The research evidence on the effects of grade retention. *Review of Educational Research, 45,* 613–635.

Jessor, R., & Jessor, S. L. (1977). *Problem behavior and psychosocial development: A longitudinal study of youth.* Boulder: University of Colorado Institute of Behavior Science.

Kandel, D. B., Kessler, R. C., & Margulies, R. S. (1978). Antecedents of adolescent initiation into stages of drug use: A developmental analysis. *Journal of Youth and Adolescence, 7,* 13–40.

Karweit, N. L. (1989). *The effects of a story reading program on the vocabulary and story comprehension skills of disadvantaged prekindergarten and kindergarten students* (Report No. 39). Baltimore: The Johns Hopkins University, Center for Research on Elementary and Middle Schools.

Kellam, S. G., Brown, C. H., & Fleming, J. P. (1981). The prevention of teenage substance use: Longitudinal research and strategy. In T. J. Coates, A. C. Peterson, & C. Perry (Eds.), *Promoting adolescent health: A dialogue on research and practices.* New York: Academic Press.

Kendall, P. C. (1991). Guiding theory for therapy with children and adolescents. In P. C. Kendall (Ed.), *Child and adolescent therapy: Cognitive-behavioral procedures.* New York: Guilford Press.

Kennedy, L. W., & Baron, S. W. (1993). Routine activities and a subculture of violence: A study of violence on the street. *Journal of Research in Crime and Delinquency, 30*(1), 88–112.

Kupersmidt, J. B., Coie, J. D., & Dodge, K. A. (1990). The role of poor peer relationships in the development of disorder. In S. A. Asher & J. D. Coie (Eds.), *Peer rejection in childhood* (pp. 274–305). London: Cambridge University Press.

Lane, R. (1992). Urban police and crime in nineteenth-century America. In M. Tonry & N. Morris (Eds.), *Modern policing.* (pp. 1–50). Chicago: University of Chicago Press.

Levenstein, P., O'Hara, J., & Madden, J. (1983). The Mother–Child Home Program of the Verbal Interaction Project. In Consortium for Longitudinal Studies, *As the twig is bent: Lasting effects of preschool programs* (pp. 237–264). Hillsdale, NJ: Erlbaum.

Lindgren, S. A. (1988). The cost of justice. In *Report to the Nation on Crime and Justice* (2nd ed.). (pp. 113–127). Washington, DC: Bureau of Justice Statistics, U.S. Department of Justice.

Lipsey, M. W. (1992). Juvenile delinquency treatment: A meta-analytic inquiry into the variability of effects. In T. D. Cook, H. Cooper, D. S. Covolray, H. Hartman, L. V. Hedges, R. V. Light, T. A. Louis, & F. Mosteller (Eds.), *Meta-analysis for explanation* (pp. 83–127). Beverly Hills: Sage.

Lipton, D., Martinson, R., & Wilks, J. (1975). *The effectiveness of correctional treatment.* New York: Praeger.

Lloyd, D. N. (1978). Prediction of school failure from third-grade data. *Educational and Psychological Measurement, 38,* 1193–1200.

Loeber, R., & Dishion, T. J. (1983). Early predictors of male delinquency: A review. *Psychological Bulletin, 93,* 68–99.

McAuley, R. (1982). Training parents to modify conduct problems in their children. *Journal of Child Psychology and Psychiatry, 23,* 335–342.

McCord, J. (1978). Some child rearing antecedents of criminal behavior in adult men. *Journal of Personality and Social Psychology, 9,* 1477–1486.

McDowall, D. (1991). Firearm availability and homicide rates in Detroit, 1951–1986. *Social Forces, 69*(4), 1085–1101.

McFall, R. M. (1982). A review and reformulation of the concept of social skills. *Behavioral Assessment, 4,* 1–35.

MacKenzie, D. L., & Souryal, C. (1994). *Multi-site evaluation of shock incarceration: Final report to the National Institute of Justice.* College Park, MD: Department of Criminal Justice and Criminology.

Maguire, K., Pastore, A. L., & Flanagan, T. J. (Eds.), (1993). *Sourcebook of criminal justice statistics 1992.* Bureau of Justice Statistics, U.S. Department of Justice. Washington, DC: U.S. Government Printing Office.

Manning, B. H. (1988). Application of cognitive behavior modification: First and third graders' self-management of classroom behaviors. *American Educational Research Journal, 25,* 193–212.

Meichenbaum, D., & Goodman, J. (1971). Training impulsive children to talk to themselves: A means of developing self-control. *Journal of Abnormal Psychology, 77,* 115–126.

Michelson, L. (1987). Cognitive-behavioral strategies in the prevention and treatment of antisocial disorders in children and adolescents. In J. D. Burchard & S. N. Burchard (Eds.), *Prevention of delinquent behavior* (pp. 275–311). Beverly Hills: Sage.

Mosher, J. F. (1985). Alcohol policy and the nation's youth. *Journal of Public Health Policy, 6,* 295–299.

Mulvey, E. P., Arthur, M. W., & Reppucci, N. D. (1993). The prevention and treatment of juvenile delinquency: A review of the research. *Clinical Psychology Review, 13,* 133–167.

Office of Educational Research and Improvement. (1992). *Review of research on ways to attain goal six.* Washington, DC: U.S. Department of Education, Office of Educational Research and Improvement.

O'Leary, K. D., & O'Leary, S. G. (1977). *Classroom management: The successful use of behavior modification* (2nd ed.). New York: Pergamon.

Olweus, D. (1991). Bully/victim problems among schoolchildren: Basic facts and effects of a school based intervention program. In D. J. Pepler & K. H. Rubin (Eds.), *The development and treatment of childhood aggression* (pp. 411–448). Hillsdale, NJ: Erlbaum.

Olweus, D. (1992). Bullying among schoolchildren: Intervention and prevention. In R. D. Peters, R. J. McMahon, & V. L. Quincy (Eds.), *Aggression and violence throughout the life span*. Beverly Hills: Sage.

Olweus, D., & Alsaker, F. D. (1991). Assessing change in a cohort-longitudinal study with hierarchical data. In D. Magnusson, L. R. Bergman, G. Rudinger, & B. Torestad (Eds.), *Problems and methods in longitudinal research: Stability and change* (pp. 107–132). London: Cambridge University Press.

Patterson, G. R. (1975). *Families*. Champaign, IL: Research Press.

Patterson, G. R. (1976). *Living with children*. Champaign, IL: Research Press.

Patterson, G. R., Chamberlain, P., & Reid, J. B. (1982). A comparative evaluation of parent training procedures. *Behavior Therapy, 13,* 638–649.

Patterson, G. R., & Dishion, T. J. (1985). Contributions of families and peers to delinquency. *Criminology, 23*(1).

Patterson, G. R., & Forgatch, M. (1975). *Family living series. Part 1*. Five cassette tapes to be used with *Living with children and families*. Champaign, IL: Research Press.

Patterson, G. R., & Forgatch, M. (1976). *Family living series. Part 2*. Three cassette tapes to be used with *Living with children and families*. Champaign, IL: Research Press.

Pennell, S., Curtis, C., Henderson, J., & Tayman, J. (1989). Guardian Angels: A unique approach to crime prevention. *Crime and Delinquency, 35,* 378–400.

Pentz, M. A., Dwyer, J. H., MacKinnon, D. P., Flay, B. R., Hansen, W. B., Wang, E. Y. I., & Anderson-Johnson, C. (1989). A multi-community trial for primary prevention of adolescent drug abuse: Effects on drug use prevalence. *Journal of the American Medical Association, 261,* 3259–3266.

Phillips, E. L. (1968). Achievement Place: Token reinforcement procedures in a home style rehabilitation setting for "predelinquent" boys. *Journal of Applied Behavior Analysis, 1,* 213–219.

Porter, J. N. (1974). Race, socialization, and mobility in educational and early occupational attainment. *American Sociological Review, 39,* 303–316.

Prothrow-Stith, D. (1991). *Violence prevention curriculum for adolescents*. Newton, MA: Education Development Center.

Quay, H. C. (1987). Institutional treatment. In H. C. Quay (Ed.), *Handbook of juvenile delinquency* (pp. 244–265). New York: Wiley.

Roberts, A. R., & Schervish, P. (1988). A strategy for making decisions and evaluating alternative juvenile offender treatment programs. *Evaluation and Program Planning, 11,* 115–122.

Roff, M., & Sells, S. B. (1968). Juvenile delinquency in relation to peer acceptance–rejection and socioeconomic status. *Psychology in Schools, 5,* 3–18.

Rosenbaum, D. P. (1987). The theory and research behind Neighborhood Watch: Is it a sound fear and crime reduction strategy? *Crime and Delinquency, 33,* 103–134.

Rubin, K. H., & Krasnor, L. R. (1986). Social cognitive and social behavioral perspectives on problem solving. In M. Perlmutter (Ed.), *Minnesota symposium on child psychology* (Vol. 18, pp. 1–68).

Saltz, R. F. (1987). The roles of bars and restaurants in preventing alcohol-impaired driving: An evaluation of server intervention. *Evaluation and the Health Professions, 10*(1), 5–27.

Sampson, R. J. (1986). Effects of socioeconomic context on official reaction to juvenile delinquency. *American Sociological Review, 51,* 876–885.

Sampson, R. J., & Lauritsen, J. L. (1990). Deviant lifestyles, proximity to crime, and the offender–victim link in personal violence. *Journal of Research in Crime and Delinquency, 27,*(2), 110–139.

Schunk, D. H. (1984). Self-efficacy perspective on achievement behavior. *Educational Psychologist, 19,* 48–58.

Schunk, D. H. (1986). Verbalization and children's self-regulated learning. *Contemporary Educational Psychology, 19,* 199–218.

Shannon, L. W. (1991). *Changing patterns of delinquency and crime: A longitudinal study in Racine*. Boulder, CO: Westview Press.

Shedler, J., & Block, J. (1990). Adolescent drug use and psychological health: A longitudinal inquiry. *American Psychologist, 45,* 612–630.

Skogan, W. G. (1989). Communities, crime and neighborhood organization. *Crime and Delinquency, 35,* 437–457.

Slavin, R. E., Madden, N. A., Karweit, N. L., Dolan, L., & Wasick, B. (1992). *Success for all: A relentless approach to prevention and early intervention in elementary school.* Arlington, VA: Educational Research Service.

Smith, D. A. (1986). The neighborhood context of police behavior. In A. J. Reiss, Jr., & M. Tonry (Eds.), *Communities and crime.* (pp. 313–342). Chicago: University of Chicago Press.

Smith, D. A., & Visher, C. A. (1980). Sex and involvement in deviance/crime: A quantitative review of the empirical literature. *American Sociological Review, 45,* 691–701.

Smith, G. W., & Fogg, C. P. (1978). Psychological predictors of early use, late use and non-use of marijuana among teenage students. In D. Kandel (Ed.), *Longitudinal research on drug use: Empirical findings and methodological issues.* (pp. 101–113). Washington, DC: Hemisphere–Wiley.

Snyder, J., & Patterson, G. (1987). Family interaction and delinquent behavior. In H. C. Quay (Ed.), *Handbook of juvenile delinquency.* (pp 216–243). New York: Wiley.

Spivack, G., & Cianci, N. (1987). High-risk early behavior pattern and later delinquency. In J. D. Burchard & S. N. Burchard (Eds.), *Prevention of delinquent behavior* (pp. 44–74). Beverly Hills: Sage.

Spivack, G., Platt, J. J., & Shure, M. B. (1976). *The problem-solving approach to adjustment.* San Francisco: Jossey–Bass.

Spivack, G., & Shure, M. B. (1974). *Social adjustment of young children.* San Francisco: Jossey–Bass.

Tracy, P. E., Wolfgang, M. E., & Figlio, R. M. (1985). *Delinquency in two birth cohorts: Executive summary.* Washington, DC: Office of Juvenile Justice and Delinquency Prevention, U.S. Department of Justice.

Tremblay, R. E., & Masse, L. C. (1993). *Cognitive deficits, school achievement, disruptive behavior and juvenile delinquency: A longitudinal look at their developmental sequence.* Paper presented at the Annual Meeting at the American Society of Criminology, Phoenix, Arizona. Canada: University of Montreal.

Ullmann, C. A. (1957). Teachers, peers and tests as predictors of adjustment. *The Journal of Educational Psychology, 48*(5), 257–267.

Visher, C. (1991). Career offenders and selective incapacitation. In J. F. Sheley (Ed.), *Criminology: A contemporary handbook.* Belmont, CA: Wadsworth Publishing.

Wahler, R. G., & Dumas, J. E. (1987). Stimulus class determinants of mother–child coercive interchanges in multidistressed families: Assessment and intervention. In J. D. Burchard & S. N. Burchard (Eds.), *Prevention of delinquent behavior* (pp. 190–219). Beverly Hills: Sage.

Weissberg, R. P., & Allen, J. P. (1986). Promoting children's social skills and adaptive interpersonal behavior. In B. A. Edelstein & L. Michelson (Eds.), *Handbook of prevention* (pp. 153–175). New York: Plenum Press.

Weissberg, R. P., Caplan, M. Z., & Sivo, P. J. (1989). A new conceptual framework for establishing school-based competence promotion programs. In L. A. Bond & B. E. Compas (Eds.), *Primary prevention and promotion in the schools: Vol. 12. Primary prevention of psychopathology* (pp. 225–296). Beverly Hills: Sage.

West, D. J., & Farrington, D. P. (1973). *Who becomes delinquent?* London: Heinemann.

Whitehead, J. T., & Lab, S. P. (1989). A meta-analysis of juvenile correctional treatment. *Journal of Research in Crime and Delinquency, 26,* 276–295.

Wilson, J. Q., & Herrnstein, R. J. (1985). *Crime and human nature.* New York: Simon & Schuster.

Wolfgang, M. E., Figlio, R. M., & Sellin, T. (1972). *Delinquency in a birth cohort.* Chicago: University of Chicago Press.

Wright, W. E., & Dixon, M. C. (1977). Community prevention and treatment of juvenile delinquency. *Journal of Research in Crime and Delinquency, 14,* 35–67.

11

Adolescent Violence

ARLENE RUBIN STIFFMAN, FELTON EARLS, PETER DORE, RENEE CUNNINGHAM, and SHARON FARBER

RODNEY CARTER: A STORY OF U.S. YOUTH VIOLENCE

Born: 10-8-77. Shot to death: 3-16-93. Age: 15.

Rodney was chatting with friends near Fairground Park one evening in mid-March when he made the casual remark that would kill him.

Referring to one youth, Rodney turned to a girl and quipped: "Hey, you're picking them real young these days."

The youth became angry, walked around the corner and returned with a gun. He fired four shots at Rodney.

"This is one of those homicides that get to you because the victim was a good kid," said Homicide Detective Sgt. Joe Beffa. "This was a clean-cut young man who had a lot going for him. His death truly was senseless."

Rodney lived with his twin brother, Robert, an 8-year-old sister, and his mother, Janet Carter, in a neat town-house in the 4200 block of North Florissant Avenue. Police call it a high-crime area.

"I constantly question God as to 'Why?'" said Carter, a housekeeper at St. Anthony's Medical Center.

ARLENE RUBIN STIFFMAN, PETER DORE, RENEE CUNNINGHAM, and SHARON FAR-BER • George Warren Brown School of Social Work, Washington University, St. Louis, Missouri 63130.   FELTON EARLS • Department of Behavioral Science, Harvard University School of Public Health, Boston, Massachusetts 02113.
Handbook of Adolescent Health Risk Behavior, edited by Ralph J. DiClemente, William B. Hansen, and Lynn E. Ponton. Plenum Press, New York, 1996.

Rodney was a ninth-grader at Rockwood South Junior High School, where he starred in basketball. Relatives described him as an outgoing young man.

"Three girls were crying over his casket consoling each other at the funeral," Carter said. "Then they found out he was seeing them all at the same time."

Homicide detectives arrested a 15-year-old for Rodney's murder. He has been charged as an adult and is awaiting trial.

"They say kids are our future," Janet Carter said. "I can't see us having a future if they keep killing each other like this."

—Bryan and Bell (1993)

INTRODUCTION

Why does violence occupy our daily consciousness—in the newspapers, on television, and as a topic of discussion between neighbors? Although it has become a theme of modern American society, the myriad manifestations of violence make it difficult to define. In this chapter we define violence as a behavioral act that results in physical injury. Although most violent behavior produces relatively minor injuries, long-term disability and death are also frequent consequences. In fact, throughout history the two leading causes of mortality have been infectious diseases and violence (Rosenberg & Fenley, 1991). Of the current five leading causes of death, two, suicide and homicide, are the results of violent acts, and violence has become the leading cause of death for young black males. There is also convincing evidence that the rate of violence in the United States is distinctly higher than in most other developed countries.

Before turning to the focus of this chapter, which relates specifically to adolescent violence in the United States, a brief overview sets the stage. We know a great deal about how to locate violence, at least the most serious consequences of it as reflected in homicides and violent crimes, such as forcible rape, assault, robbery, and murder (Earls, Cairns, & Mercy, 1993). We know that groups at high risk for engaging in and being victimized by these problems are marked by low socioeconomic status, residence in large urban centers, and being minority and male (Reiss & Roth, 1993). The heavy use of alcohol, even more than illicit drugs, is another correlate. We know further that the proliferation of handguns has contributed to increasing severity of injury associated with violence. But beyond these facts, there is a great deal that we do not know. How have changes in the structure and functioning of modern families, the deteriorating social organization of urban neighborhoods, or centuries of racism contributed to a culture that yields high levels of violence? How has exposure to violence in the media contributed to violent behaviors? How can we reduce and even prevent violence?

Over the past decade violence has become a key issue on the federal agenda. In response to the rising tide of violence, the Centers for Disease Control and Prevention began a violence epidemiology program about a decade ago that has now fully matured as an administrative and scientific unit (Rosenberg & Fenley, 1991). This program will not only track violence but will also conduct interventions and measure their impact within community context throughout the nation (Rosenberg & Fenley, 1991). Dr. C. Everett

Koop, a former U.S. surgeon general, was the first to publish a report stating that violence was a major cause of youth injury and death. This report called for health efforts to prevent violence and to reduce its attendant morbidity and mortality. This call served to frame violence as an item on the public health agenda (Rosenberg & Fenley, 1991).

Recently the U.S. government has identified federal priorities concerning violence (Silverman *et al.*, 1988). Furthermore, four of the objectives in *Healthy People 2000* (USDHHS, 1990) relate to violence and abusive behavior. These actions reflect the current consensus concerning the menace of violence, and the need for more information and action in this area.

We cannot dismiss violence as only a problem of individual behavior or as only a social problem. Violence is associated with an entire social and economic structure, a particular youth's community and family environment, and the particular youth's mental health. That association immediately implies that prevention or intervention cannot be focused just on the individual's behavior but must also address larger social issues. This chapter addresses issues of knowledge and issues of action. Our knowledge about violence is a strength. Because of excellent epidemiological data, we are able to identify both individual youths who are at risk for violent behavior and those general populations that are at risk for violence. We can do this by understanding the general environment and the other behavior problems of the youths in those environments.

Counterpointing the strengths in our knowledge are weaknesses in theories that should serve as a bridge between that knowledge and our own actions. The lack of broad inclusive theories of causality interferes with the mounting of coherent preventive interventions. Although a number of existing theories purportedly address the causes of violence, many of them fail to account for the wide range of contributing variables and the interactive relationships between these variables in causing violent behavior.

Two problems occur: theories that do not include elements of our knowledge about violence have led to interventions that ignore critical environmental causes and are, therefore, inappropriate for those populations most at risk; or the theories incorporating concepts of environment have not defined the concepts in such a way that they can be incorporated into interventions, so that interventions based on those theories largely leave the environmental components out.

Despite the gap between knowledge and action, this chapter reports good news and bad news about the state of the art of prevention and treatment of violent behavior. The bad news is that existing interventions are fragmented. In general, most interventions are not related to theory. They most often focus on punishment or removal of the individual from society. When treatment is mounted, it is largely focused on a narrow behavioral approach that attempts to intervene with the individual, and to focus on hypothetical interim behavior rather than violent behavior while ignoring that individual's environment. Only recently have interventions focused on the issue of access through the gun buy-back or trade-in programs.

The good news about current interventions concerns an increasing recognition of the inadequacies of past actions and the need for future effective action. Recently, a spate of publications reviewed the evaluations of interventions for violence. Also, recently, governmental, health, education, and juvenile justice fields have all called for more extensive intervention and cooperation between services. Prompted by the dramatically increasing rates of violence, both the government and the public health sector have jointly called for mobilization and coordination of comprehensive efforts to intervene in youth violence. This call for mobilization has been echoed by the health sector, the medical sector, the educational sector, the religious sector, and the media. Also, a recent major shift in attitude has taken place with recognition by leaders of those ethnic minority communities most afflicted by youth violence that communities must take responsibility for the behavior of their own youth and promote interventions within their own community (Urban League, 1994).

EPIDEMIOLOGY OF VIOLENCE

Data concerning violence are collected for many purposes, including purely epidemiological reasons, public health surveillance, risk group identification, or risk factor identification (Rosenberg & Fenley, 1991). Many data collection and surveillance systems in the United States provide information about violence and violent deaths, but all of these surveillance systems have common problems. Reported rates of violence may be very different from actual rates. For instance, the number of rapes reported may very well depend on the social/historical context in which they are reported. This context may concern one's definition of rape (e.g., as including date rape or acquaintance rape) or the prevailing atmosphere of blaming the victim. Also, data on violent deaths may be particularly inaccurate since they depend heavily on coroners' decisions. In many locales, coroners are political appointees, sometimes without medical backgrounds. Cultural expectations concerning deaths among Caucasians versus African-Americans may impact the recorded rate of violence.

In reporting some selected trends that particularly impact on adolescents, we have focused on two sources of data: one is from Statistical Abstracts of the United States, the other is from a longitudinal study of inner-city youths that we began conducting in 1984 (Earls, Robins, Stiffman, & Powell, 1989).

National data can be somewhat misleading and confusing. In part this is related to the change in reporting methods. In 1980, national data were reported for youths 15 to 24 years old. In 1990, they were reported separately for youths 15 to 19 and 20 to 24 years old. Figure 1 reports death rates from homicide. Reading from left to right for each gender/race category reveals that homicide rates have increased only slightly for white males, not at all for white females, almost doubled for black males (to almost 2 in 1000 such youths), but only increased slightly for black females. Figure 2 shows the same pattern for firearm death rates.

Of importance are not only changes in rates of violence within the United States, but also how rates of violence in the United States compare with rates in other countries. The startling fact is that homicide rates among 15- to 24-year-olds in the United States are higher than those in any of the other 21 developed countries that maintain such statistics (Prothrow-Stith, 1991).

In addition to looking at national trends in death rates, it may prove useful to examine what young people themselves are reporting about violent behavior. Since 1984, the authors have been following a group of 2787 youths who were recruited at inner-city

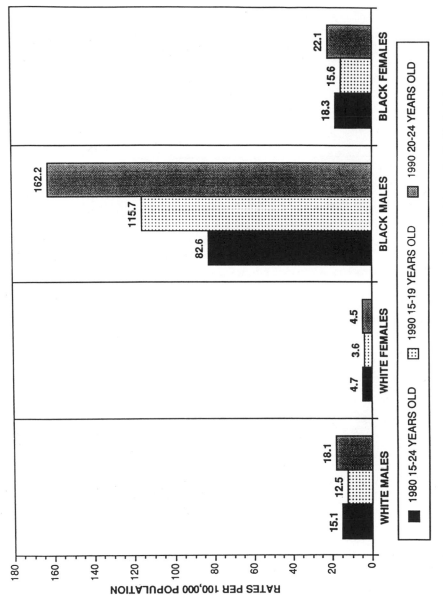

Figure 1. Homicide death rates: 1980 and 1990. Sources: CDC, National Center for Health Statistics.

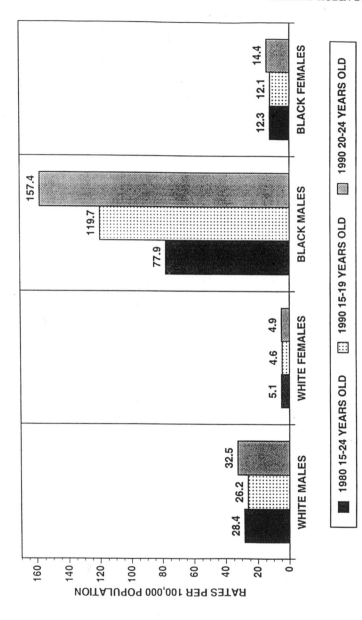

Figure 2. Firearm death rates: 1980 and 1990. Sources: CDC, National Center for Health Statistics.

public health clinics. This study, funded by the Robert Wood Johnson foundation, was originally designed as an evaluation of clinics in ten cities. The youths were selected in the order of their attendance at these clinics for face-to-face interviews in 1984–1985 and again in 1986–1987. Of the adolescents interviewed, nearly 70% were nonwhite and nearly 70% were female. They ranged in ages from 13 to 18, and their average age in 1984 was 16.2 years.

The interviews covered several psychosocial areas, including demographics, health and mental health symptoms, behavior problems, criminal justice involvement, family structure and dynamics, and drug and sexual behavior. Within those contexts we obtained extensive information about the violent acts the youths had committed and the violence they had experienced as victims. A violent act was considered as one in which there was physical struggle, injury, beating, or an attempt to injure another person or animal.

A remarkably high percentage of youths reported that they had committed acts of violence during their adolescence. Table 1 describes the extent of violence in our sample. Over 85% of males, whether white or nonwhite, reported that they had committed an act of violence. Although lower in percentage, almost two-thirds of females, regardless of race, had committed an act of violence. [White males engaged in twice as many violent behaviors as nonwhite males (6.4 versus 3.2)]. Similarly, white females, despite engaging in fewer acts of violence than males of either race, engaged in almost twice as many such acts as nonwhite females (2.1 versus 1.5).

The self-report data that we gathered from our study of inner-city youths are echoed by other data collected through the CDC's Youth Risk Behavior Surveillance System (CDC, 1992); however, our data show rates of violence that are nearly twice as high as those shown by their data. According to the CDC self-report data, approximately 42% of teen students who were surveyed admitted to being in at least one physical fight during the 12 months preceding the survey. Furthermore, male students were more likely than females to have been in such a fight. No racial differences were reported.

Table 1. Violence Committed by Inner-City Adolescents (N = 2787)

	Number committing a violent act[a]
Males	
White	88.8%
Black	85.9
Females	
White	65.2%
Black	60.0

[a]$p < 0.0001$.

Risk Identification

One of the purposes of obtaining epidemiological data concerning violence is to identify those factors that would put an individual at risk for engaging in violence. In this respect, our knowledge is excellent, as all studies have shown consistent association. The consistencies are particularly noteworthy for homicide.

Race/Socioeconomic Status

In the United States it is difficult to separate community differences in violence rates from racial and socioeconomic status differences. There is ample evidence that low socioeconomic status and minority status contribute to violence. Individuals in many minority communities face an extraordinarily high risk of death or injury from violent behavior (*Public Health Reports,* 1991a).

Racism and poverty, both forms of social violence, are known to contribute to individual violence. In part this may be because the poor in our society, who are disproportionately of minority status, do not have equal access to criminal justice, health, or educational systems, and may be markedly less well off economically and socially (*Public Health Reports,* 1991b).

Race and socioeconomic status are associated both with homicidal violence and with other nonfatal violence and suicides. In fact, the Secretary of Health's national report on black and minority health recently noted that many, if not most, homicide victims tend to have prior involvement in other serious violence (Silverman *et al.,* 1988).

Community

There is some evidence that the community in which an individual lives might be a very important contributor to risk for violent behavior. It is interesting to note a distinct geographical variation in the rates of youth homicide. In five states in the United States the homicide rates for young black males exceed 100 per 100,000 population. Those five states and Washington, D.C. account for more than half of all homicides among 15- to 24-year-old males in the United States (Roper, 1991). Although we know that such differences exist, we do not know if the differences are related to community/neighborhood characteristics that influence participation in delinquency and crime. We also do not know how the community differences are connected with other social and individual differences.

The community differences in violence rates are likely to be attributable to the larger social context in which violence occurs. Violent behavior seems to be associated with a range of economic, environmental, political, cultural, educational, and behavioral factors (Belloni *et al.,* 1991). Among the community issues related to violence are the presence of gangs, the degree of underemployment or unemployment, the availability of illicit drugs, and the availability of sophisticated weapons within a community (Earls, 1991b). Some of the social factors associated with violence concern the distribution of wealth and resources. Also, within communities, conflictual situations occurring in and between families and in and between small groups may also engender violence (Earls, 1991b). In addition, cultural explanations indicate that tolerance toward violent behavior may encourage such violence.

Family

Family environment is an important factor in a youth's becoming homicidal. It appears that juvenile murderers learn aggression during early childhood through living in criminally violent families and through experiencing child abuse (Zager, Arbit, Sylvies, Busch, & Hughes, 1990). A study of convicted murderers found that two-thirds had experienced "continuous, remorseless brutality during childhood" (Mason, 1991). The genesis of violent behavior is thought to have had its roots early in childhood through physical abuse, observation of violence in their families, and observation of violence in the community (Roper, 1991).

Access to Means

A large body of literature attributes the increase in homicide rates, particularly among young black males, to access to firearms (e.g., see Cook *et al.*, 1991). To illustrate the magnitude of the problem, in 1986 and 1987, more people died from firearm injuries in the United States than during the Vietnam War, which lasted more than 8 years (Rosenberg & Fenley, 1991). Nevertheless, it is very difficult to show the exact direction of the association between firearms and homicide. Some studies have found that the strictness of handgun statutes is unrelated to homicide rates but is associated with suicide rates, while other studies have shown that the extent of actual gun ownership is the factor that is most strongly related to homicide rates (e.g., see Lester, 1988).

Multiple Predictors from Our 1984 Longitudinal Study

It is interesting to see how our study of inner-city youths compares to others' findings concerning the correlates and causes of violence. As Table 2 shows, if the youths are experiencing symptoms of mental health problems such as depression, suicidality, substance misuse, or posttraumatic stress symptoms, they are more likely to act violently toward others.

Our data also support other reports (e.g., see Reiss & Roth, 1993) that factors in the youth's environment contribute to violence. Early family conditions and mental health problems are significantly related to committing violent acts during adolescence. Table 3 shows that regardless of the race or gender of the youths, being reared in a family situation characterized by disruption (resulting from parental separation, divorce, or early parent death), being physically or sexually abused as a child, or having a family member with a serious mental illness increases a youth's likelihood of being violent. Also, constant ongoing stressors or having experienced traumatic events (such as witnessing someone murdered) were both significantly related to a youth being a perpetrator of violence. Finally, violent behavior was associated with neighborhood murders and with local rates of unemployment.

Risk Factors

Risk factors may be considered both the cause of the problem and the focus of the potential solution to the problem. There has been a great deal of speculation about what

Table 2. Violence Committed by Inner-City Youths.
Personal and Environmental Correlates from
Bivariate Linear Regressions: Controlling
for Race and Sex Differences

Variable	F	r^2
Personal correlates		
Depressive symptoms	113.4	0.04[a]
Suicidal symptoms	93.0	0.03[a]
Substance misuse symptoms	192.7	0.06[a]
Posttraumatic stress symptoms	59.8	0.02[a]
Environmental correlates		
Family mental illness	56.3	0.02[a]
Family instability	4.5	0.001[b]
Child abuse	28.0	0.04[c]
Traumatic events	77.2	0.02[a]
Stressful events	169.2	0.05[a]
Murders in neighborhood	25.2	0.01[a]
Rates of unemployment	21.4	0.01[c]

[a] $p < 0.0001$.
[b] $p < 0.05$.
[c] $p < 0.001$.

causes violence. Some have speculated that violent behavior is part of the instinctual
nature of humans and that the tendency to violence may be inherited (DiLalla & Gottesman, 1991), while others have strongly argued against inheritance but for a physiological
contribution to risk for violence (Mednick, Brennan, & Kandel, 1988). Although a
number of identifiable risks for violence have been uncovered, it is difficult to separate the
biological, psychological, social, communal, and economic risk factors to distinguish

Table 3. Three-Pronged Intervention
for Violence

Personal
    1. Intra- and interpersonal skills training
        a. Problem-solving
        b. Anger control
    2. Changing cognitions
        a. Goal setting
        b. Job training
    3. Substance abuse treatment
Societal
    1. Reduce acceptability of violence
    2. Reduce access to weapons
    3. Increase opportunities
Postvention
    1. Elimination of family violence
    2. Elimination of community violence
    3. Targeting early offenders

their relative influence. Associated with these issues are questions concerning how aggressive behaviors sequence and develop over the life span, what determines the variation in rates of violence across communities, and how violence is transmitted from one generation to the next (Earls, 1991a).

The literature reveals some consistent factors that need to be considered in planning any intervention. First of all, we note that there are individual differences that may be present from the very beginning of life. Nevertheless, these biological and psychological characteristics have been ignored as causes or as potential avenues of intervention (Earls & Tonry, 1989).

One of the areas strongly associated with violence, and obviously a factor amenable to potential intervention, has been poor parenting practices, including modeling violent behavior, punitive disciplinary practices, and child abuse (Earls & Tonry, 1989). The consistent finding that those engaging in violence or delinquency have had problems in school indicates the potential for looking at school factors in determining causality and in focusing interventions. Nevertheless, poor experiences in school and school failures have not been found to be either a necessary or sufficient cause of violence (Earls & Tonry, 1989). It could be that both the school problems and violence are symptoms of the root problems. Peer influences are also mentioned frequently in the literature as being associated with violence. We do know that violent youths are more likely to come from violent communities, associate with other violent youths, and belong to violent gangs (Earls & Tonry, 1989).

Understanding violence requires an awareness of the differences between those youths who engage in sporadic violent behaviors and then desist, and those who develop criminal careers, marked by continuing violence. This pattern of criminal career is still relatively understudied. Although we know that only a small percentage of active offenders commit most of the acts of violence, we still do not know how to predict the level of dangerousness of a particular individual (Earls & Tonry, 1989).

Finally, although we know that the community may have a strong influence on the individual, we still do not understand how that community interacts with the rest of the individual's personal world to contribute to violence (Earls & Tonry, 1989). Until we can understand this, we cannot begin to develop any targets of preventive intervention.

Risk Factor Theories

Current theories applicable to violent behavior are usually found as theories of antisocial or risk behavior. These can be categorized into three major groupings: those theories that emphasize the person and motivation; those theories that emphasize the environment and control; and those theories that focus on aspects of both person and environment. Among theories that emphasize the person, some theorists suggest that violence or criminality is an outcome of the strain between individuals' aspirations and their low expectations (Oetting & Beauvais, 1987). Still others emphasize the genetic/biological/chemical aspect of violent behavior (see DiLalla & Gottesman, 1991).

The environmental or control approaches focus on the social conditions or processes that weaken informal or formal social controls (Janis & Mann, 1977). Jessor and Jessor (1977) emphasize the failure of conventional bonding to the family, the school, and community systems. In the absence of this conventional bonding, peer bonding to deviant peer subgroups may occur. Other theorists emphasize violence and criminality as survival strategies for the urban underclass who are economically deprived (Liebow, 1967). Still other theorists look at the combination of a tolerant social environment and the availability of behavior models (Dembo, Blount, Schmeidler, & Burgos, 1986). In a similar vein, disorganization theory (Gartner, 1990; Merton, 1957) emphasizes the disorganization that accompanies crime-ridden neighborhoods.

There are a number of approaches that focus on both the person and the environment. Social cognitive theory posits that behavior, personal determinants (cognitive, affective, and biological), and environmental influences all function as interacting determinants of each other (Bandura, 1986), although the major emphasis is on the person and his or her cognitions (Lochman, 1992).

The sociocultural model (Rodriguez & Zayas, 1990) incorporates the ideas of self-concept, bonding, disadvantage, antisocial environment, and acculturation. In doing so, it is particularly applicable to minority or immigrant populations, though it does not deal with concepts related to skills or motivation.

The Opportunity Model approach focuses on the person in terms of motivation, and on the environment in terms of controls that hinder and opportunities that engender violent activities (Cohen & Land, 1987; Devine, Shelley, & Smith, 1988; Fiala & LaFree, 1988). In this model, disadvantage, low income, discrimination, and an environment that tolerates violence lead to the personal problems of weaker bonding, stronger deviant bonding, and strains between aspirations and expectations. The combination of disadvantage and tolerance provides a causal model for the development of violent behavior.

Within the person/environment approach, the Developmental Model (Earls, 1991b) adds to the above models by holding that there is a chain of events and experiences, perhaps beginning as early as the prenatal period, which accumulate over the first two decades of life to help determine the probability of violence. This theory also includes biological factors such as temperament in addition to factors included by the other theories. Some of the chain of events and experiences relate to environment focused theories (such as social motivation, social control, and social opportunity). The Developmental Model also attempts to incorporate what is known from many other behavioral theories. These include attachment theory, temperament theory, social learning theory, social control theory, network theory, and social disorganization theory. In some ways the developmental approach attempts to explain violent behaviors in terms of the interaction between the individual and the community (Earls, 1991b). Nevertheless, the developmental approach runs the danger of being so inclusive as to remove itself from the ability to be studied or acted on.

PREVENTION

Any discussion of prevention can focus on either of two levels: primary prevention or secondary prevention. Primary prevention is designed to avoid the start of specific problems (U.S. Congress, OTA, 1991). Any such effort implies an understanding of the causes of the condition and the ability to modify it. Secondary prevention, on the other hand, is intended to keep high-risk populations from developing the problem and to delay or prevent the recurrence of a problem (U.S. Congress, OTA, 1991).

We wish we could report here about successful programs that have been based on knowledge about the causes and correlates of violence; however, very few intervention attempts have been implemented and no good outcome research exists (Wilson-Brewer, Cohen, O'Donnell, & Goodman, 1991). Most prevention programs have not even been evaluated in terms of their impact on violence. Therefore, under the topic of "prevention," we must, of necessity, focus on attitudes toward prevention and promising directions taken in response to calls for action.

Instead of specific prevention programs, what we can report is a series of calls for action by individuals or consortiums trying to review the state of the art in violence prevention. Among the actions taken recently have been papers sponsored by the Office of Technology Assistance through the United States Congress on Prevention of Violence, the conference on youth violence in minority communities sponsored by the Centers for Disease Control and minority Health Professions, the document *Healthy Nation 2000*, and a review of the state of the art in violence prevention sponsored by the Carnegie Council (Cohen & Wilson-Brewer, 1991; Wilson-Brewer *et al.*, 1991).

The Centers for Disease Control (CDC) of the Public Health Service and the Minority Health Professions Foundation sponsored the Forum on Youth, Violence and Minority Communities: Setting the Agenda for Prevention (*Public Health Reports,* 1991a). The primary focus of their work was to develop youth violence prevention programs. The CDC soon recognized that the state of knowledge concerning effectively preventing death and injuries from youth violence was not well advanced; they found that knowledge about prevention had not been assembled in a coordinated way and thus was not useful for the development of further prevention programs within communities. (*Public Health Reports,* 1991a). Therefore, rather than developing violence programs, the forum resulted in recommendations derived from the recognized present lack of services.

Governmental involvement changed the direction of violence prevention activities. Previously, approaches to prevention and treatment were largely in the hands of the police, the courts, and the penal system. However, since former Surgeon General C. Everett Koop decided to focus on the prevention of violence, violence has become the province of public health (Rosenberg & Fenley, 1991). The United States Congress developed a National Public Health Agenda for Prevention of Violence to promote mental health and lower the violence rates in the general population (U.S. Congress, OTA, 1991). This Agenda influenced the development of the publication *Healthy Nation 2000,* which includes calls for reduction of homicides and weapon-related deaths (USDHHS, 1990).

Historically, various sectors dealing with violence prevention functioned separately; therefore, the clearest way to review efforts is by sector. We discuss, in turn, violence prevention efforts of the criminal justice, health, educational, and communal sectors.

Criminal Justice Sector

Many of the best-known and most widely implemented preventive interventions have involved secondary prevention through the criminal justice sector. Traditionally, violent youths were removed from society to either residential treatment programs or institutions.

The criminal justice approach to crime and violence was supposed to involve both deterrence and incapacitation (Rosenberg & Fenley, 1991). Despite their extensive use over many years, however, the approach was never particularly effective in solving juvenile crime (e.g., Romig, 1978). For instance, recidivism rates for juvenile institutions have been high (Scarpitti & Stephenson, 1971). Also, the rising rates of violence in communities tell us that this approach to deterrence has not worked. The rising rates of violence indicate that although incarceration may work for some individuals, it does not work at the community level. As one individual engaging in violent behavior is removed from the community to an institution, others are left in the community and the general rate continues to increase (Mayer, Gensheimer, Davidson, & Gottschalk, 1986). The Carnegie Council, for instance, identified only one violence prevention program by the criminal justice sector as having an evaluation component (Wilson-Brewer *et al.*, 1991). That program concerned stress management and drug education for institutionalized youths; unfortunately, violent behavior was not measured as an outcome.

Although institutionalization has apparently failed as a preventive intervention, a different criminal justice approach has been associated with lower rates of violence. This approach focuses on access to means of violence and concerns local restrictions on firearm sales and lengthened sentences when firearms are involved in crimes (Cook *et al.*, 1991).

Incarceration alone has shown disappointing results for the juvenile justice sector and has led to a number of recommendations. Despite the poor record, a few recommendations still focus on increasing deterrence and incapacitation for criminal and physical assaults among family members, intimates, and acquaintances; and on increasing police training. Other recommendations are more innovative. But the lack of success of the criminalization approach has elicited calls for coordinating social service responses with police responses (Rosenberg & Fenley, 1991). Some recommendations call for increasing limitations on access by limiting the possession and use of weapons; improving security and safety of communities, neighborhoods, and homes; requiring firearm safety courses; banning the most destructive weapons and ammunition; promoting product liability litigation against gun manufacturers; and cracking down on illegal trafficking in firearms (Cook *et al.*, 1991).

Health Sector

Violence has only recently been conceptualized as a province of health services. So far, many papers have been written with extensive recommendations for preventive interventions but few have been implemented and virtually none evaluated. The only health sector program that was evaluated was actually a communal program that involved many sectors (see our discussion under the Communal Sector) (Wilson-Brewer *et al.*, 1991). Therefore, the state of violence prevention within the health sector lies solely in recommendations for interventions. Obviously, to mount preventive interventions in the health sector would first require identifying violent youths and involving medical personnel. Second, it would require decreasing financial barriers to violence-focused health care. For health services to be effective in violence intervention, the services must network with both the criminal justice and educational arenas. Then, through the network, health personnel could develop employment programs for high-risk adolescents, mount alcohol and drug misuse prevention programs, teach conflict resolution skills, increase family life and child-rearing education, and support families within the community (Rosenberg & Fenley, 1991).

Educational Sector

The school system has mounted the majority of violence prevention programs outside of the criminal justice sector (Boruch *et al.*, 1991). These programs vary widely in their focus. Some concentrate only on violence, some on education about risk or about conflict resolution. Many are actually generic life skills training programs that are focused only on skills or interim behaviors thought to be associated with later violence (see Wilson-Brewer *et al.*, 1991). A few take a holistic approach and address the complex interacting factors associated with violence, such as low academic achievement, drug use, and so forth. School programs are likely to include a combination of life skills training, mentoring, tutoring, and various prevention education (Boruch *et al.*, 1991; Wilson-Brewer *et al.*, 1991). All assume that violence is a learned behavior that therefore can be changed and prevented (Belloni *et al.*, 1991). All such programs most often target youths from dysfunctional families. Currently, programs focus on managing anger, fostering self-esteem, and accepting responsibility. Often the programs include mentoring, academies for promising youths, or programs such as the National Youth Service (Cairns *et al.*, 1991). Many of them are based on aspects of social cognitive theory (Lochman, 1992).

Life skills training often emphasizes nonviolent approaches, interpersonal problem-solving skills, and social skills training. These programs have been mounted for preschool and primary school children, and their outcome has been measured in terms of reducing aggression (Cahn *et al.*, 1991). Data show limited behavioral affects within the school setting (Lochman, 1992), however, and there is no information about how the reduction of aggression within an early school setting carries over to violence within the community as a whole (Wilson-Brewer *et al.*, 1991).

A few programs have been directed at helping parents reduce antisocial behavior of preadolescent children (Cahn *et al.*, 1991). These programs have been found effective in reducing antisocial behavior, but there are several problems with such programs: once again, violent behavior in adolescence and young adulthood has not been measured; and many of the most violent youths lack parents who would be interested in or capable of participating in such programs.

Despite the lack of data concerning preventive interventions within the educational system, there is a wealth of anecdotal records and experience. Records do document positive immediate effects on behaviors known to be associated with violence (Lochman, 1992). Since school attendance is mandatory, educational interventions, by law, have the opportunity to involve each and every youth. While youths can avoid going for health care, and can avoid getting involved with the criminal justice system, they cannot avoid becoming involved in the education system (Boruch *et al.*, 1991). Thus, the educational sector is arguably the best vehicle for violence prevention interventions that must reach *all* youths.

Communal Sector

The Carnegie Council's review of violence prevention efforts uncovered two communal approaches which had an evaluation component (Wilson-Brewer *et al.*, 1991). The Violence Prevention Project of the Boston Department of Health and Hospitals involved health, educational, social service, and communal sectors, as well as a media campaign.

Although the evaluation produced evidence of attitudinal changes, the program was unable to document changes in behavior or in neighborhood violence.

Because of the known connection between violence and social environment and culture, recommendations related to the communal sector include a focus on decreasing cultural acceptance of violence, decreasing the social violence of racial and gender discrimination, and supporting more positive male role models (Rosenberg & Fenley, 1991). These communal sector recommendations are based also on the presumed notion that inequity in resource and justice distribution, and high tolerance toward violent behavior contribute to violence when they combine with a sense of powerlessness and lack of control (Belloni *et al.*, 1991).

Because of the association of violence with minority status, many prevention programs have focused on minority communities (*Public Health Reports*, 1991a), but the focus needs to expand to all communities as violence increasingly permeates all of society.

Communal prevention always begins with recommendations for careful planning, forming partnerships, developing resources, involving all participants, setting goals, approaching problems from multiple directions, hiring qualified personnel, and evaluating programs (Belloni *et al.*, 1991). Unfortunately, at this point, we have very little information on how effective any community programs have been.

In summary, all groups attempting to deal with violence prevention have noted the need for integration of services. There is a general consensus that agencies need better linkage and communication, and that the media should be involved in preventive interventions (Boruch *et al.*, 1991). Violence prevention is a concern of public health, health care, mental health, criminal justice, social service, education, and the media. All systems impacting the youth, such as family, community, education, and employment, must be included in violence prevention strategies (USDHHS, 1990). Violence is the manifestation of very complex economic, environmental, political, cultural, educational, and behavioral factors. Therefore, preventative interventions must echo that same complexity through coordination of services and foci of responses (Belloni *et al.*, 1991).

Because of the analyses and recommendations of the above-cited working groups, consensus has been reached that the first step in implementing preventive intervention should be the development of effective working partnerships among different public areas and among communities in the public and private sectors. Specifically, we need a national plan that will enable individual communities, minority and nonminority, to develop and coordinate prevention programs (Boruch *et al.*, 1991).

TREATMENT

Treatment approaches for violence target those individuals who are at risk (which we discuss under prevention), those individuals who are already violent, or communities with high levels of violence (Cairns *et al.*, 1991).

Individual-Level Interventions

Treatment programs for the already violent individual include some of the same elements as prevention programs for high-risk youths. These include (Cairns *et al.*, 1991):

- Conflict resolution and anger management training
- Peer counseling
- Job corps training or military-style camps
- Outward Bound and similar programs designed to promote self-esteem, healthy risk-taking, and cooperation
- Mentoring
- Diversion from juvenile justice into public service
- Psychological counseling

Treatment approaches for the individual have been developed from three different psychological approaches: the psychodynamic/psychoanalytic approach, the humanistic/nondirected approach, and the behavior modification approach. All three share the concept that violent behavior is related to some lack within the individual and all three assume that, if this lack were compensated, effective and healthy behavior would be the result (Goldstein, 1986). Unfortunately, a number of reviews of those interventions that have an evaluative component have failed to demonstrate the clear superiority of any approach (Kazden, 1987; Wilson-Brewer *et al.*, 1991). Nevertheless, several authors state that overall, the results of repeated evaluation studies concerning the three different psychological approaches tend to support the effectiveness of behavioral or social learning approaches (Blakely & Davidson, 1982; Braukman, Fixsen, Phillips, & Wolf, 1975; Nietzel, Winett, MacDonald, & Davidson, 1977; Redner, Snellman, & Davidson, 1982; Mayer *et al.*, 1986).

Within the social learning approach, the techniques of conflict resolution, anger management, and skills training treat the individual as lacking skills rather than as needing therapy. The focus is on teaching the individual those skills that will lead to effective and satisfying personal interactions without resorting to violence (Goldstein, 1986). Results have shown that aggressive youths can learn a whole range of psychosocial skills, including interpersonal skills, aggression and anger management, and emotion control (Goldstein, 1986). But given the roots of violent behaviors, which include family violence and abuse, we know that such an approach is not enough. Although such skills training has been evaluated widely by a variety of investigators through many different methods, and the research does support the short-term effectiveness of such training, the major deficit or problem appears to be the difficulty in obtaining transfer of the behavior to the youth's normal environment, particularly if that environment is marked by frequent violence (Goldstein, 1986).

Programs in three different cities illustrate the use of social learning approaches:

- Fulton County, Georgia, has a program in their high schools that paired African-American and Amerasian boys in order to reduce the high violence within and between the two groups and the high dropout rate of the two groups (Jenkins, 1991).
- Kansas City, Missouri, has a project run through the health department that consists of training and conflict resolution and anger control over five 2-hour sessions (Mitchell, 1991).
- The Boston Department of Health and Hospitals is sponsoring a health promotion program for urban youth that provides both outreach and education. The education aspect supports a violence prevention program used in Boston high schools. This

program teaches conflict resolution skills, provides information about violence and homicide, and tries to create a nonviolent classroom environment (Prothrow-Stith, 1991).

Reviews of mental health services indicate that most services target intermediate behaviors rather than violent acts themselves (Mayer *et al.*, 1986). Some of the behaviors targeted are alcohol and drug abuse and gang-related behaviors (USDHHS, 1990; Ostos, 1991). Frequently, alcohol and drug abuse treatment and violence prevention are linked.

Community-Level Interventions

Some approaches target not the individual but the community itself. As discussed in the epidemiology section of this chapter, we know that those adolescents who are exposed to violence in their community have more of a tendency to engage in violence themselves. Furthermore, poorer communities are likely to have higher rates of violence. Treatment programs targeted for communities in which there are high levels of violence include the following:

- Street-level intervention efforts
- Mobilizing community members
- School programs
- Job placement programs
- Recreational programs
- Coordinated mental health, drug abuse, and social service programs (Cairns *et al.*, 1991)
- Provision of role models
- Family interventions
- Neighborhood projects
- Education and job training (Greene, 1993)

Many violent individuals have difficulty functioning as community members. As such, they need a different approach to services and to mental health services. For these individuals the following changes must occur:

- Enhancing local mental health services
- Increasing the financing for mental health services
- Training mental health professionals
- Increasing research (U.S. Congress, 1991)

One major community approach has been to remove violent youth from society through residential treatment or incarceration. Unlike incarceration, the purpose of residential treatment is to provide the residents with individual treatment. Unfortunately, many residential services are ill-equipped for violent youths. Their behavior may tax the resources of the staff and place nonviolent residents at risk. Staff often have a problem in both managing and treating the behavior of violent youths within an institutional setting. For those reasons, few programs are willing to accept violent youth, who are therefore often shuffled from one program to another until they end up in adult jails (Agee,1986).

In summary, treatment approaches to violence have the same major problems as do preventive approaches. There is a basic lack of community responsiveness and lack of coordination between services (USDHHS, 1990). Work groups who have consulted on this topic have recommended that the government provide leadership, and that the first step in this leadership be to listen to those people who speak for affected populations. The lack of responsiveness and coordination is complicated by underfunding for treatment. Interestingly enough, although the government pays the total cost for the juvenile justice system, 52% of preventive and treatment programs have had to rely on foundation funding. Only one-third of projects have been funded by federal, state, or local governments (Green, 1991).

DISCUSSION

In this chapter we have been very free with criticisms of existing programs. It is one thing to criticize programs and quite another to say what should be done. That speculation is by far the most difficult. Let us pretend first that we have unlimited funds and unlimited power. What could and should be done? The literature, research, and experience quite clearly point to the necessity of multifaceted intervention. The authors would propose a three-pronged intervention (Table 3): one prong would focus on prevention at the personal level; one would focus on prevention at a societal level; and one on "postvention."

Prevention on a Personal Level

What are the most effective ways of treating violent behavior on the individual level? One way is skills training. It seems quite clear that the skills of problem-solving and anger control are lacking in many youths who find themselves caught up in violent behavior. We also know from prior experience that it is possible to teach these skills, particularly at a very early age.

A second effective personal intervention involves changing cognitions through goal setting and/or career/job training. Many youths involved in violent behavior see no future for themselves. They have no goals, and cannot visualize themselves respectably and gainfully employed. Therefore, one personal-level intervention would be to change the individual youth's perception of his or her future, and preparation for that future. It is financially easier to influence the sense and perception that opportunities exist than it is to influence the exact actual opportunities. In addition to influencing the perception that opportunities exist, however, it is also possible to influence the preparation that youths have undergone to take advantage of existing opportunities.

The third effective personal intervention is treatment for addiction. A lot of violent behavior revolves around the world of alcohol and drugs, which has the double problem of disinhibition for the users and violence associated with the illicit dealers. Drug treatment and alcohol treatment should be made universally available.

One of the difficulties is intervening on the personal level while recognizing that these youths may come from problematic environments. They may have an incarcerated parent, a drug-using parent, and/or an unstable and violence-filled home. They may lack adequate food and shelter, supervision, and schooling. The list goes on and on. Unless intervention on the personal level also includes consideration of the youth's environment, skill development, goal-setting, and influencing perception and self-esteem are likely to fail.

Prevention on a Societal Level

The second prong of our ideal intervention would deal directly with the youth's social world—their environment. On the wider social level, it would be appropriate to reduce the acceptability of violent behavior, both in the media and on the street. The concern is to balance issues about censorship, the profit-making motive of the media, societal welfare, and individual freedom. We have managed to do something concerning the use of cigarettes. Why can we not reduce the social acceptability of violence in the same manner? The attack on cigarette smoking first came through control of the media and later it became socially acceptable to limit smoking areas, and finally it is becoming increasingly socially unacceptable to smoke. The same kind of approach could be taken with violence.

The second social intervention would be to reduce access to weapons that, when handled by a violent or angry youth, are likely to kill rather than just injure. We know that in those places where access to guns is limited, rates of homicide go down. It is just as important to reduce the lethality of violent acts as it is to reduce the number of violent acts. Here we have two concerns, one with legal issues and one with the cyclical nature of attack and defense. The legal concern is a political one; one must balance the National Rifle Association's outcry that the Constitution guarantees the right to bear arms with the need to protect the population. We need public outcry to balance politicians' concern with pleasing the NRA lobbyists. The cyclical concern relates to the issue that guns beget guns in many community areas. The more violence there is in an area, the more likely people are to have guns in order to protect themselves. This cycle has to be broken.

The third major social intervention revolves around opportunities. Positive opportunities must be increased for activities that will reduce the likelihood of violence, while negative opportunities, which allow violent behavior to flourish, must be decreased. The positive opportunities concern the enhancement of *real* possibilities for gainful employment, and for adequate, effective, and appropriate education. Opportunities available to youths may be very limited. Many gender- and ethnicity-specific mentor and role-model programs have already been instituted. These programs must also provide the educational, financial, and social support youths need to emulate the models.

In many areas where the violence rates are highest, the most common employment opportunities are through an underground illicit economy that allows the growth of gangs, turf wars, and other violent behaviors. Is the solution through cracking down on such illegal behavior or legalizing drugs and prostitution? Certainly the violence rates around alcohol distribution dropped after Prohibition was repealed. Whether the same thing would happen with drug use is not known, but maybe the situation is desperate enough that it is worth a try.

Violence often occurs during idle moments when groups of youths are unsupervised and get carried away. Many programs are already trying to increase opportunities for filling idle time in a constructive manner. Midnight basketball leagues try to do this. So do various programs at churches and community centers, such as sports activities or choir activities.

Postvention

The third prong of violence intervention involves "postvention" of violent behaviors that have been tolerated or ignored. Violence must be stopped before it serves as a model of behavior. Youths are most likely first exposed to violence in the family. As a society, we tolerate an extraordinary degree of domestic violence. Until spouses are prevented from engaging in violent behavior, and parents stopped from engaging in violent forms of discipline, children will be socialized to be violent. We also need to stop community-sanctioned violence. Police violence is an accepted fact of life. Many school systems still allow corporal punishment. Sports heroes become violent during games. Any acceptance of violence is likely to engender future involvement in violence. Finally, offenders need to be stopped early in their careers: not by incarceration, but by giving them skills so that they will not *have* to resort to violence, and by providing opportunities for a bright future so that they will not *want* to resort to violence.

The reality is that such a three-pronged multifaceted approach will never be implemented. It involves too much manipulation of arenas where there are political and financial investments and it would be too costly. So, given the unlikelihood of ever having unlimited funds and unlimited power, what would be the most important kind of interventions to mount? The authors posit that two interventions would be important: (1) to reduce the social acceptability of violence by obtaining cooperation of the media and (2) to increase both the real opportunities for positive future life and the perception that those opportunities exist.

The events of the next few years will be very interesting, as we will see how society mobilizes to take action on an increasingly dangerous and extensive problem. This chapter has been written at the start of a new era in violence intervention. We have awakened to the recognition that violence is like a cancer growing within our society and is posing a threat to the whole fabric of our way of life. If we wish to continue that analogy, we can relate our collective reaction to the stages of grief. As a society we have gone through the periods of denial and blame and are now ready for a period of self-awareness and mobilization for action.

ACKNOWLEDGMENTS. Research for this project was funded by the Robert Wood Johnson Foundation and National Institute of Mental Health grants 1RO1MH45119-10 and 1R24MH50857-01A1.

REFERENCES

Agee, V. L. (1986). Institutional treatment programs for the violent juvenile. In S. J. Apter & A. P. Goldstein (Eds.), *Youth violence: Programs and prospects* (pp. 75–88). New York: Pergamon Press.

Bandura, A. (1986). *Social foundations of thought and action: A social cognitive theory.* Englewood Cliffs, NJ: Prentice–Hall.

Belloni, J., Blumenthal, D., Bracy, P., Braithwaite, R., Cohen, S., Goodman, R. H., Green, L. W., Hausman, A. J., Ketto, C., Kreuter, M. W., Sterling, E. E., Walter, J., & Wilson-Brewer, R. (1991). Application of principles of community intervention. *Public Health Reports, 106,* 244–247.

Blakely, C., & Davidson, W. S. (1982). Behavioral approaches to delinquency: A review. In P. Karoly (Ed.), *Adolescent behavior disorders* (pp. 241–272). New York: Pergamon Press.

Boruch, B., Coleman, D., Doria-Ortiz, C., Girouard, S., Goodman, A., Hudson, L., Kraus, J., Maseru, N., Prothow-Sith, D., Rugg, D. L., Stark, E., Stephens, R. D., & Sterling-Scott, R. (1991). Violence prevention strategies targeted at the general population of minority youth. *Public Health Reports, 106,* 247–250.

Braukman, C. J., Fixsen, D. O., Phillips, E. L., & Wolf, M. M. (1975). Behavioral approaches to treatment in crime and delinquency. *Criminology, 13,* 299–331.

Bryan, B., & Bell, K. (1993). The young lives that street violence stole. *St. Louis Post-Dispatch* (pp. 1, 11).

Cahn, K., Chamberlain, B., Old Dog Cross, P., Daro, D., Eron, L. D., Froehlke, R. G., Galter, J. L., Guerra, F. A., Hammett, M., Hill, H., Ostos, T., Parron, D., Saltzman, L., Slaby, R. G., Sorenson, S. B., Vince, C. J., & Widom, C. S. (1991). Interventions in early childhood. *Public Health Reports, 106,* 258–263.

Cairns, R., Coleman-Miller, B., Greenwood, P., Hewitt, W. W., Jenkins, E., Jenkins, R., Maccannon, G., Mitchell, M., Napper, D., Reiss, A. J., Sciammarella, E., Valdivia, S. D., & Warren, R. C. (1991). Violence prevention strategies directed toward high-risk minority youths. *Public Health Reports, 106,* 250–254.

Centers for Disease Control. (1992). *Morbidity and Mortality Weekly Report, 41,* 1–33.

Cohen, L. E., & Land, K. (1987). Age structure and crime: Symmetry versus asymmetry and the projection of crime rates through the 1990s. *American Sociological Review, 52,* 170–183.

Cohen, S., & Wilson-Brewer, R. (1991). *Violence prevention for young adolescents: The state of the art of program evaluation.* New York: Carnegie Corporation.

Cook, P., Juarez, P., Lee, R., Loftin, C., Marshall, O. A., Maurrain, W. A., Roth, J. A., Ryan, J., Smith, G. K., Spivak, H., Teret, S. P., Walker, M., & Wintermute, G. J. (1991). Weapons and minority youth violence. *Public Health Reports, 106,* 254–258.

Dembo, R., Blount, W. R., Schmeidler, J., & Burgos, W. (1986). Perceived environmental drug use risk and the correlates of drug use and non-use among inner-city youths: The motivated actor. *International Journal of the Addictions, 21,* 977–1000.

Devine, J. A., Shelley, J., & Smith, M. D. (1988). Macroeconomic and socio-control policy influences on crime rate changes, 1948–1985. *American Sociological Review, 53,* 401–420.

DiLalla, L. F., & Gottesman, I. (1991). Biological and genetic contributors to violence—Widom's untold tale. *Psychological Bulletin, 109*(1), 125–129.

Earls, F. (1991a). Not fear, nor quarantine, but science: Preparation for a decade of research to advance knowledge about causes and control of violence in youths. *Journal of Adolescent Health, 12,* 619–629.

Earls, F. (1991b). A developmental approach to understanding and controlling violence. In H. E. Fitzgerald, B. M. Leister & M. W. Yoguray (Eds.), *Theory and research in behavioral pediatrics* (Vol. 5, pp. 61–87). New York: Plenum Press.

Earls, F., Robins, L. N., Stiffman, A. R., & Powell, J. (1989). Comprehensive health care for high-risk adolescents: An evaluation study. *American Journal of Public Health, 79,* 999–1005.

Earls, F., & Tonry, M. (1989). Program on human development and criminal behavior: Proposed research agenda. Submitted to John D. and Catherine T. MacArthur Foundation. Harvard University Mimeograph.

Earls, F., Cairns, R., & Mercy, J. (1993). The control of violence and the promotion of nonviolence in adolescents. In S. Millstein, A. Petersen, & E. Nightengale (Eds.), *Adolescent Health Promotion* (pp. 285–304). New York: Oxford University Press.

Fiala, R., & LaFree, G. (1988). Cross-national determinants of child homicide. *American Sociological Review, 53,* 432–435.

Gartner, R. (1990). The victims of homicide: A temporal and cross-national comparison. *American Sociological Review, 55,* 92–106.

Goldstein, A. P. (1986). Psychological skill training and the aggressive adolescent. In S. J. Apter & A. P. Goldstein (Eds.), *Youth violence: Programs and prospects* (pp. 89–119). New York: Pergamon Press.

Green, L. W. (1991). Establishing a public–private partnership. *Public Health Reports, 106,* 242–243.

Greene, M. B. (1993). Chronic exposure to violence and poverty: Interventions that work for youth. *Crime and Delinquency, 39,* 106–124.

Janis, L. W., & Mann, L. (1977). *Decision making: A psychological analysis of conflict, choice and commitment.* New York: Free Press.

Jenkins, R. S. (1991). New way of fighting. *Public Health Reports, 106,* 240.

Jessor, R., & Jessor, S. L. (1977). *Problem behavior and psycho-social development: A longitudinal study of youth.* New York: Academic Press.

Kazden, A. E. (1987). Treatment of antisocial behavior in children: Current status and future directions. *Psychological Bulletin, 102,* 187–203.

Lester, D. (1988). Gun control, gun ownership, and suicide prevention. *Suicide and Life Threatening Behavior, 18,* 176–180.

Liebow, E. (1967). *Tally's Corner: A study of Negro street corner men.* Boston: Little, Brown.

Lochman, J. F. (1992). Cognitive-behavioral intervention with aggressive boys: Three-year follow-up and preventive effects. *Journal of Consulting and Clinical Psychology, 60,* 426–432.

Mason, J. O. (1991). Prevention of violence: A public health commitment. *Public Health Reports, 106,* 265–268.

Mayer, J. P., Gensheimer, L. K., Davidson, W. S., & Gottschalk, R. (1986). Social learning treatment within juvenile justice: A meta-analysis of impact in the natural environment. In S. J. Apter & A. P. Goldstein (Eds.), *Youth violence: Programs and prospects* (pp. 24–38). New York: Pergamon Press.

Mednick, S. A., Brennan, P., & Kandel, E. (1988). Predisposition to violence. *Aggressive Behavior, 14,* 25–33.

Merton, R. K. (1957). *Social theory and social structure.* New York: Free Press.

Mitchell, M. (1991). The Kansas City Project. *Public Health Reports, 106,* 237.

Nietzel, M. T., Winett, R. A., MacDonald, M. L., & Davidson, W. S. (1977). *Behavioral approaches to community psychology.* New York: Pergamon Press.

Oetting, E. R., & Beauvais, F. (1987). Common elements in drug abuse: Peer clusters and other psychological factors. *Journal of Drug Issues, 17*(1 & 2), 133–151.

Ostos, T. (1991). Alternatives to gang membership: The Paramount plan. *Public Health Reports, 106,* 241.

Prothrow-Stith, D. (1991). Boston's Violence Prevention Project. *Public Health Reports, 106,* 237–239.

Public Health Reports. (1991a). Background of the forum. *106,* 237–239.

Public Health Reports. (1991b). The necessity of social change in preventing violence. *106,* 227–277.

Redner, R., Snellman, L., & Davidson, W. S. (1982). A review of behavioral methods in the treatment of delinquency. In R. J. Morris & T. Kratochwill (Eds.), *Practice of therapy with children: A textbook of methods* (pp. 193–220). New York: Pergamon Press.

Reiss, A. J., Jr., & Roth, J. A. (Eds.). (1993). *Understanding and preventing violence.* Washington, DC: National Academy Press.

Rodriguez, O., & Zayas, L. H. (1990). Hispanic adolescents and antisocial behavior: Sociocultural factors and treatment implications. In A. R. Stiffman & L. E. Davis (Eds.), *Ethnic issues in adolescent mental health* (pp. 147–171). Beverly Hills: Sage Publications.

Romig, V. A. (1978). *Justice for our children.* Lexington, MA: Health.

Roper, W. L. (1991). Prevention of minority youth violence must begin despite risks and imperfect understanding. *Public Health Reports, 106,* 229–231.

Rosenberg, M. L., & Fenley, M. A. (Eds.). (1991). *Violence in America: A public health approach.* London: Oxford University Press.

Scarpitti, F., & Stephenson, R. M. (1971). Juvenile court dispositions. *Crime and Delinquency, 17,* 142–151.

Silverman, M. M., Lalley, T. L., Rosenberg, M. L., Smith, J. C., Parron, D., & Jacobs, J. (1988), Control of stress and violent behavior: Mid-course review of the 1990 health objectives. *Public Health Reports, 103,* 38–48.

Urban League. (1994). *The state of black America: 1994.* New York: National Urban League.

U.S. Congress, Office of Technology Assessment. (1991). Background and the effectiveness of selected prevention and treatment. *Adolescent health services* (Vol. II, OTA-H-466). Washington, DC: U.S. Government Printing Office.

U.S. Department of Health and Human Services. (1990). *Healthy People 2000: National health promotion and disease prevention objectives.* Washington, DC: U.S. Government Printing Office.

Wilson-Brewer, R., Cohen, S., O'Donnell, L., & Goodman, I. (1991). *Violence prevention for young adolescents: A survey of the state of the art.* Washington, DC: Carnegie Council.

Zagar, R., Arbit, J., Sylvies, R., Busch, K. G., & Hughes, J. R. (1990). Homicidal adolescents: A replication. *Psychological Reports, 67,* 1235–1242.

12

Adolescent Pregnancy

CATHERINE STEVENS-SIMON
and ELIZABETH R. McANARNEY

INTRODUCTION

During the past three decades, adolescent pregnancy has become a source of increasing social, economic, and political concern in the United States. Bearing children during adolescence has profound health and social consequences for most young parents and their children (Furstenberg, Brooks-Gunn, & Morgan, 1987; Stevens-Simon & White, 1991; Moore & Waite, 1977; Card & Wise, 1978). The results of studies conducted over the past 30 years suggest that adolescent pregnancy limits the educational achievements and the vocational opportunities of adolescent females. Additionally, it contributes to the impoverishment of one of the most socioeconomically disadvantaged segments of our society, and promotes the intergenerational transmission of poverty (Furstenberg et al., 1987; Stevens-Simon & White, 1991; Moore & Waite, 1977; Card & Wise, 1978). After an extensive review of the literature, a panel established by the National Research Council reached the following conclusion: "Women who become parents as teenagers are at greater risk of social and economic disadvantage throughout their lives than those who delay childbearing until their twenties. They are less likely to complete their education, to be employed, to earn high wages, and to be happily married, and they are more likely to have larger families and to receive welfare" (Hayes, 1987).

School failure and welfare dependence are the two most frequently reported and serious long-term sequelae of adolescent childbearing (Furstenberg et al., 1987; Stevens-Simon & White, 1991). Current data suggest that parous teenagers are more likely than are nulliparous teenagers to drop out of high school and less likely to return to high school

CATHERINE STEVENS-SIMON • Division of Adolescent Medicine, University of Colorado Health Science Center, The Children's Hospital, Denver, Colorado 80218. ELIZABETH R. McANARNEY • Department of Pediatrics, University of Rochester Medical Center, Rochester, New York 14642.
Handbook of Adolescent Health Risk Behavior, edited by Ralph J. DiClemente, William B. Hansen, and Lynn E. Ponton. Plenum Press, New York, 1996.

and graduate after having dropped out (Furstenberg *et al.,* 1987; Miller, 1992, 1993; Furstenberg, 1992). In one study that traced the timing of three critical events—first birth, high school drop-out, and high school graduation—in the lives of a sample of 14-year-old high school students (Upchurch & McCarthy, 1990). Five percent of the young women became pregnant while they were enrolled in high school. Thirty-nine percent of the parous teenagers dropped out of school, and only 30% of those who dropped out subsequently returned to school and graduated. By contrast, only 19% of the nulliparous teenagers dropped out of school (compared to 39% of the parous teenagers), and 85% of the nulliparous young women who dropped out subsequently returned to school and graduated, compared to only 30% of their parous peers who dropped out.

In addition to poorer education prospects associated with teen pregnancy, the economic burden that teen pregnancy places on society is enormous. In terms of Aid to Families with Dependent Children, Medicaid, and food stamps, the cost of births to adolescents in 1985 was estimated to be $6.65 billion. These estimates do not take into consideration the additional costs of social services, protective services, special education or job-related education for the young mother. The public cost for a single cohort of infants born to adolescent mothers followed over 20 years was estimated at $5.16 billion (Hardy & Zabin, 1991). These figures included the costs associated with social, education, and health services for the child from birth to 20 years of age, but failed to account for the opportunity costs associated with the loss of labor force productivity.

Further evidence of the detrimental economic effects of early childbearing is found in the results of two recently conducted studies (Furstenberg *et al.,* 1987; Hoffman, Foster & Furstenberg, 1993). These studies demonstrate that, on average, young women who begin childbearing during their teens complete one year less schooling and are less likely to earn greater than $25,000 a year than are sociodemographically similar women who have their first child after 20 years of age. This is related to the fact that these young women are less likely to complete high school and are less likely to take post-secondary school courses (Furstenberg *et al.,* 1987).

The high incidence of medical and social problems noted among the infants and children of adolescent mothers is another consequence of adolescent pregnancy. During the neonatal period (the first 28 days of life), these children are at increased risk for morbidity and mortality because they are smaller and more often premature than are children born to older mothers (Stevens-Simon & White, 1991). Even when birth weight is controlled, however, these infants remain at increased risk for the medical and social problems. Evidence from a variety of sources indicates that the children of adolescent mothers are more likely to die of sudden infant death syndrome and other causes during the neonatal period, to be evaluated for accidental and nonaccidental trauma, to exhibit behavioral problems, to score lower on intellectual tests, and to repeat a school grade than are the children of socioeconomically similar adult mothers (Stevens-Simon & White, 1991; Stevens-Simon & Reichert, 1994; Babson & Clarke, 1983; Shapiro, McCormick, Starfield, Krischer, & Bross, 1980; Taylor, Wadsworth, & Butler, 1983; Strobino, Ensminger, Nanda, & Young, 1992).

While teen pregnancy is not unique to the United States, we have by far the highest rates of pregnancy, childbirth, and elective abortion among our teenagers than other

Westernized countries (Hardy & Zabin, 1991). We are the only Westernized country in which the rate of pregnancy per 1000 teenage females has not decreased substantially in recent years. Researchers cite poor contraceptive use as the primary reason for high pregnancy rates, with 18% of U.S. adolescents sexually active before age 15 and 66% active by age 19, but only one-third report using contraceptives.

Following sections describe the epidemiology of teenage pregnancy, its consequences, prevention strategies, and treatment alternatives.

EPIDEMIOLOGY

Teen pregnancy is epidemic: every 31 seconds an adolescent becomes pregnant in the United States and every 2 minutes a teen gives birth. Each year approximately 1 million women under the age of 20 become pregnant (Hardy & Zabin, 1991); just under one-half of these women are younger than 18. Approximately 500,000 of these youth give birth and another 400,000 obtain elective abortions. The remainder experience a spontaneous abortion or later fetal death.

Trends in Adolescent Pregnancy

The interpretation of the trends pertaining to adolescent childbearing is complex. The overall rate of adolescent childbearing in the United States dropped through the late 1970s and leveled off in the 1980s. Since 1988, however, the rate has shown slight increases (Hardy & Zabin, 1991). These overall trends can be misleading as reductions in the numbers of births to adolescents tend to coincide with declines in the U.S. adolescent population. Between 1980 and 1984, the number of adolescents who were 15 to 19 years old declined by 11.4% (Hardy & Zabin, 1991). Therefore, adjusting for the U.S. adolescent birth rate, the overall pregnancy rates among 15- to 19-year-olds actually increased from 94/1,000 in 1972 to 109/1,000 in 1984. Examination of pregnancy rates among sexually active teenage females shows a modest decline, from 272/1000 in 1972 to 233/1000 in 1984. Much of this reduction has been attributed to the increased use of contraceptives. While the proportion of teenage pregnancies that resulted in a live birth decreased from 66.2% in 1972 to 46.7% in 1982, this was concurrent with the legalization of abortion in 1973. Therefore, adolescent birth rates as well as advances in reproductive technology must be considered when interpreting trends in adolescent pregnancy.

Sexual Activity and Contraceptive Use

The percentage of females 15 to 19 years of age who report having had sexual intercourse has increased dramatically over the past two decades. In 1970, 26.6% reported having had sexual intercourse, by 1975 increased to 36.4%, and rose to 42% in 1980, to 44.1% in 1985, and to 51.5% in 1988 (Hardy & Zabin, 1991). The largest increases in the percentage of adolescent females who report sexual activity have occurred among 15-year-olds: from 4.6% in 1970 to 25.6% in 1988. While the rate of contraceptive use has increased over the past decade, it has not kept pace with the numbers of young people who engage in sexual intercourse. In 1988, 78.8% of 15- to 19-year-olds reported use of a contraceptive method, compared with 71% of the same age group in 1982.

Sociodemographic Characteristics of Adolescent Mothers

The sociodemographic characteristics of adolescents who become mothers have changed markedly over the past decade. The number and rate of nonmarital births to adolescent mothers increased dramatically between 1980 and 1988 [from 271,801 (49%) of the 562,330 births to adolescents in 1980 to 322,406 (66%) of the 488,941 births to adolescents in 1988] (Moore, 1990). Moreover, greater than 90% of births among black adolescents occurred outside of marriage compared with about half of the births to white adolescents. While the number of births to teenagers, overall, has declined, births to black teenagers 18 and 19 years old have declined less than those for other ages. Additionally, in 1986, repeat pregnancies were more common among black teens—30% compared with 22% for their white peers. Among teenage mothers in the United States, 61% of whites and 65% of blacks had 12 or more years of education at the time of delivery in 1985 (Hardy, 1991). While 12.7% of all births in 1985 were to teenage mothers, only 3% of all U.S. fathers in 1985 were teenagers, reflecting the fact that the great majority of fathers were considerably older (on average 2 to 4 years) than the mothers.

Correlates of High-Risk Sexual Behavior and Pregnancy

Numerous developmental, social, behavioral, emotional, and psychological factors have been associated with high-risk sexual behavior and pregnancy (Stevens-Simon & White, 1991; Zabin & Clark, 1981; Stevens-Simon & Reichert, 1994; Stevens-Simon, Beach, & Eagar; 1993; Brooks-Gunn & Chase-Lansdale, 1991; Zabin, Stark, & Emerson, 1991; Abrahamse, Morrison, & Waite, 1988; Elster, Ketterlinus, & Lamb, 1990; McAnarney & Schreider, 1984; Levinson, 1986; DuRant & Jay, 1989; Smith & Udry, 1985; Winter, 1988; Rainey, Stevens-Simon, & Kaplan, 1993; Zabin, Astone, & Emerson, 1993; Matsuhashi, Felice, Shragg, & Hollingsworth, 1989; Kelly, Stevens-Simon, Singer, & Cox, 1994; Jessor, 1991; Gabriel & McAnarney, 1983). Factors such as having older boyfriends, school failure or drop-out, having a history of physical or sexual abuse, engaging in other high-risk behaviors (such as drug and alcohol abuse), denial, and having many friends, mothers, sisters, and/or other relatives who are or were teen parents are factors associated with having a higher-than-average risk for conception. Another important factor associated with unprotected sexual intercourse and pregnancy is physical maturity. Young adolescent females who appear more mature than their peers are at greater risk of sexual intercourse and pregnancy as these adolescents may initiate sexual activity before they develop sufficient cognitive maturity to think about the future consequences of their behavior (Stevens-Simon & White, 1991; Card & Wise, 1978; Stevens-Simon & Reichert, 1994; Stevens-Simon et al., 1993; Brooks-Gunn & Chase-Lansdale, 1991; Zabin et al., 1991; Abrahamse et al., 1988; Elster et al., 1990; McAnarney & Schreider, 1984; Friede et al., 1986; Cox, Emans, & Bithoney, 1993).

Developmental Influences

There are a variety of plausible explanations for the increased risk of conception among these young women and girls. For example, current data suggest that the endocrinologic events associated with the development of adult reproductive capacity, and the psychosocial events associated with the development of an adult sexual identity have the potential to affect the likelihood of conception during adolescence both directly (by increasing sexual arousal and fecundity) and indirectly (by fostering new standards for socially acceptable heterosexual behavior and by widening the gap between adolescent physiologic and psychosocial maturity) (Udry, 1988; Stevens-Simon & White, 1991). Asynchrony between reproductive and psychosocial maturity is particularly problematic for young people who mature physically more rapidly than their peers (Gross & Duke, 1980). Since direct mechanisms alone do not explain the tremendous cultural variation observed in the timing of the first pregnancy, it seems probable that within certain social groups, the outward, physically mature appearance of early developing adolescents alters adult expectations for their behavior and makes it possible for them to engage in social relationships for which they are cognitively and psychologically unprepared (Udry, 1988; Stevens-Simon & White, 1991).

Social Sexual Influences

Other studies suggest that the former victims of childhood sexual abuse are at increased risk for adolescent pregnancy, in part, because similar personal and societal conditions predispose young people to abuse during childhood and early conception (e.g., dysfunctional, substance-abusing families in which the parents communicate poorly and/or have many unmet emotional needs), and, in part, because the experience of childhood sexual abuse fosters concerns about fecundity and enhances the desire for conception (Stevens-Simon & Reichert, 1994).

Social Influences

There is evidence suggesting that adolescent females who dropped out of school, who come from disadvantaged families and neighborhoods, and who have many friends and relatives who are or were teen-parents and adolescents who are themselves already teen parents are more likely to become pregnant. The lack of opportunities for personal advancement may lead to a lack of motivation to avoid pregnancy as early parenthood entails little in the way of lost opportunities and may be both culturally and socially acceptable (Moore, 1988; Stevens-Simon & White, 1991; Miller, 1992; Furstenberg, 1992; Klerman, 1993). For these adolescent females, early childbearing is neither an isolated act of rebellion against parental authority nor a part of a complex of socially deviant behaviors (Moore, 1988; Stevens-Simon & White, 1991; Miller, 1992; Furstenberg, 1992; Klerman, 1993). Rather, adolescent pregnancy and childbearing are deeply embedded in the fabric of their lives, activities that are often supported, consciously or unconsciously, by family members and friends, and which enable many young women to join the sisterhood of adult women and to feel closer to the emotionally significant women in their lives. Indeed, there is evidence suggesting that some of the young girls and women who grow up in communities where adolescent childbearing is considered normative worry that others will wonder about their fertility and their ability to attract male partners if they elect to postpone pregnancy (Rainey *et al.*, 1993).

Current data suggest that for some teenagers pregnancy is a rite of passage, part of the process of becoming an adult. This sentiment appears to be particularly common among female adolescents who are doing poorly in school and/or living in impoverished social environments in which adolescent pregnancy is rampant and adult roles other than parenthood are perceived to be inaccessible (Stevens-Simon & White, 1991; Zabin & Clark, 1981; Stevens-Simon & Reichert, 1994; Stevens-Simon *et al.*, 1993; Brooks-Gunn & Chase-Lansdale, 1991; Zabin *et al.*, 1991, 1993; Abrahamse *et al.*, 1988; Elster *et al.*, 1990; McAnarney & Schreider, 1984; Levinson, 1986; DuRant & Jay, 1989; Smith & Udry, 1985; Winter, 1988; Rainey *et al.*, 1993; Matsuhashi *et al.*, 1989; Kelly *et al.*, 1994; Jessor, 1991; Gabriel & McAnarney, 1983).

Emotional Influences

It has been hypothesized that with time, as the frequency of sexual relations increases and romantic relationships deepen, feeling of closeness legitimize sexual activity and enable adolescents to think cognitively about their sexual behavior and make conscious choices about sexual activity and contraception (DuRant & Jay, 1989). While the results of most studies demonstrate that both contraceptive use and the consistency of contraceptive use increase in relation to age and the duration of sexual activity (Newcomer & Baldwin, 1992; Leigh, Morrison, Trocki, & Temple, 1994), the findings are less consistent with regard to the relationship between the duration of individual romantic relationships and the consistency of contraceptive use (Rainey *et al.*, 1993). At least one study suggests that as the duration of a romantic relationship increases, feelings of closeness legitimize latent desires for childbearing and/or foster fertility concerns which actually deter, rather than promote, consistent contraceptive use (Rainey *et al.*, 1993). In fact, several studies have suggested that many teens seek pregnancy because they want something or someone to love, and to know that there is someone who will always love them. Furthermore, studies of the sequence of adolescent sexual relations suggest that within many adolescent subcultures the tempo of progression from hand-holding to sexual intercourse is very rapid (Smith & Udry, 1985). Thus, many young women could become pregnant before they have time to develop the types of romantic interpersonal relationships that foster a positive sexual self-concept and promote future-oriented planning and regular contraceptive use (Smith & Udry, 1985; Winter, 1988).

While only a minority of young Americans actually state that they wish to become pregnant, many more are clearly ambivalent about their desire to postpone childbearing (Rainey *et al.*, 1993; Zabin *et al.*, 1993; Matsuhashi *et al.*, 1989). The results of a recently conducted study of 200 never-pregnant teenagers in Denver, Colorado, revealed that even though only 10% of the young women seeking routine health care in the city's teen clinics openly admitted that they wanted to get pregnant, an additional 40% said they "wouldn't mind being pregnant" (Rainey *et al.*, 1993). Other investigators have also found that many female American teenagers have ambivalent feelings about postponing childbearing (Zabin *et al.*, 1993; Matsuhashi *et al.*, 1989). The results of these studies are of concern because they have consistently shown that young women who have ambivalent feelings about postponing childbearing are significantly less likely than their peers to use contraceptives and are, therefore, at higher risk for conception (Rainey *et al.*, 1993; Zabin *et al.*, 1993; Matsuhashi *et al.*, 1989). Indeed, we recently reported that the most common reply that adolescents who are in the third trimester of pregnancy give to the question "Why weren't you using birth control before you got pregnant?" is not "I just didn't get around to it," but rather, "because I didn't mind getting pregnant" (Kelly *et al.*, 1994). This response was followed closely in frequency by "I wanted to get pregnant" or "My boyfriend wanted me to get pregnant." Since approximately 40% of the respondents gave answers suggesting that their pregnancies were wanted and/or planned or, at least, not entirely unwanted and unplanned at the time of conception, it is imperative that we gain a better understanding of why so many American teenagers "don't mind" or "want to" get pregnant.

Reasons Why Adolescents Delay Obtaining Contraceptives

One area that has been extensively studied is adolescents' rationale for delay in seeking contraceptives. When investigators first pose the question, "Why did you delay seeking contraception?" to young people attending urban family planning and school-based clinics, the most common response is, "I just didn't get around to it" (Zabin & Clark, 1981; Zabin *et al.*, 1991). The next set of responses include fear (of side effects, of parental discovery, of the physical examination) and an unwillingness to make conscious decisions about sexual activity ("I was waiting for a closer relationship with my boy-friend" or "I wasn't planning to have sex") (Zabin & Clark, 1981; Zabin *et al.*, 1991). Other reasons are cited far less frequently and indicate a lack of knowledge about the need for contraceptives ("I thought I was too young to get pregnant") and/or how to obtain and utilize contraceptives ("I was too embarrassed to buy contraceptives").

These responses clearly indicate that lack of knowledge and lack of access are less serious deterrents to contraceptive use than are attitudinal and perceptual barriers. This finding illustrates one of the most important shortcomings of traditional knowledge-based sex education classes and access-based contraceptive programs. It is imperative that health care providers attempt to learn more about the reasons why so many young people "just don't get around to" using contraceptives and/or fail to appreciate their ongoing need for contraceptives despite their statements that they aren't "planning to have sex."

Many American teenagers describe their first sexual encounter as something that "just happened" because they "got carried away" (Levinson, 1986). This suggests that one reason why so many young women in this country don't "get around" to obtaining contraceptives is that they are denying their sexual behavior and, as a consequence, avoiding the concomitant decisions around issues of self-protection. It seems probable that the guilt that most young Americans experience when they initially violate social taboos prohibiting nonmarital sexual intercourse makes it easier for them to deny their reproductive and contraceptive knowledge than to utilize it (Levinson, 1986). Young people who do not believe they should or can control their sexual and contraceptive behavior may unwittingly minimize their need for contraceptives and exaggerate the logistical problems associated with obtaining them. This, in turn, results in inconsistent or nonexistent contraceptive use and a relatively high frequency of unprotected sexual intercourse (Levinson, 1986).

The data presented thus far suggest that most female teenagers in the United States delay seeking contraceptives and become pregnant either because they are unwilling or unable to make conscious decisions about their sexual and contraceptive behavior, or because they do not mind becoming pregnant. Thus, enhancing regular contraceptive use among sexually active adolescents requires that they believe that they can become pregnant and that using prescription contraceptives is safe and the only way to prevent pregnancy. In addition, they must have access to reliable, affordable contraceptive agents and must have a positive sexual self-concept which allows them to make conscious decisions about their sexual and contraceptive behavior. Finally, they must want to postpone childbearing.

PRIMARY PREVENTION OF ADOLESCENT PREGNANCY

This section examines the strengths and weaknesses of various strategies for preventing adolescent pregnancy in light of the minimal requirements for regular contraceptive use listed in Table 1.

During the 1960s and 1970s, adolescent pregnancy prevention programs focused primarily on the first minimal requirement (Kirby, 1992). Believing that increasing knowledge about the consequences of unprotected sexual activity and contraception would be enough to prevent adolescent pregnancy, policymakers expanded school-based sex education programs to include information about sexually transmitted diseases, contraception, and pregnancy (Kirby, 1992). While there is now an extensive body of literature documenting the positive effect that these early, knowledge-based sex education programs had on student understanding of reproductive physiology, sex, and contraception, there is little evidence that these programs affected adolescent sexual or contraceptive behavior or adolescent pregnancy rates (Kirby, 1992; Stout & Rivara, 1989; Zellman, 1982; Miller, 1993). This is in part because, to date, only a minority of investigators have actually evaluated the effect of sex education on adolescent sexual and contraceptive behavior, and, in part, because most of the studies that have utilized behavioral outcomes have not been randomized (Zellman, 1982). Thus, while there is little evidence that sex

Table 1. Minimal Requirements for Regular Contraceptive Use
among Sexually Active Adolescents

- Belief that pregnancy is possible and that prescription contraceptives are safe and the only way to prevent pregnancy
- Access to affordable contraceptive agents
- Positive sexual self-concept which enables conscious decision-making about sexual and contraceptive behavior and communication with a male partner about childbearing
- Desire to postpone childbearing

education classes entice students toward earlier sexual activity or promote nonmarital sexual activity among middle and high school students, there is also no clear evidence that traditional knowledge-based sex education programs have a significant effect on adolescents' use of contraceptives and even less evidence that they influence the rate of adolescent pregnancies (Kirby, 1992; Stout & Rivara, 1989; Zellman, 1982; Miller, 1993).

During the 1980s the failure of knowledge-based sex education programs to change adolescent pregnancy-related behavior was attributed to the difficulty that developmentally younger, concrete-operational teenagers have with anticipating future events and applying knowledge they possess cognitively in real life situations (Kirby, 1992). Thus, the next generation of sex education programs included "values clarification" and "decision-making" components (Kirby, 1992). Some of these new sex education classes were linked to general-purpose school-based health care facilities with the anticipation that eliminating traditional access barriers would make teenagers more willing to obtain and utilize contraceptives (Kirby, 1992). The efficacy of this approach to the prevention of adolescent pregnancy is still being evaluated. The results of published studies indicate that programs that emphasize specific values (e.g., "Just say NO") strengthen those values and may influence concomitant sexual behavior in the short run (Miller, 1993; Olsen, Weed, Ritz, & Jensen, 1991; Roosa & Christopher, 1990; Thiel & McBride, 1992). However, values-based sex education programs appear to have little or no long-term effect on adolescent pregnancy-related behavior (Miller, 1993; Olsen et al., 1991; Roosa & Christopher, 1990, Thiel & McBride, 1992). Similarly, there is little evidence that comprehensive school-based clinics have had a measurable effect on student contraceptive behavior (Kirby, 1992; Zellman, 1982; Kirby, Waszak, & Ziegler, 1991). While the consensus in the family planning literature is that aggressive family planning programs are an effective way to reduce pregnancy rates in most populations (Anderson & Cope, 1987), only a few school-based clinics have been able to provide their students with focused reproductive health services because most parents and many teachers in this country still fear that the increased availability of contraceptives would be misinterpreted as approval of nonmarital sexual relationships (Kirby, 1992). Therefore, despite the apparent success of one school-based family planning program in Baltimore (Zabin, Hirsch, Smith, Streett, & Hardy, 1986), there are minimal data for evaluating the efficacy of this approach to the prevention of adolescent pregnancy.

By the late 1980s the consensus was that traditional knowledge-based sex education programs, even those that included "values clarification" components and were linked to general-purpose school-based clinics, had failed to bridge the gap between reproductive knowledge, childbearing attitudes, and contraceptive behavior (Kirby, 1992). Studies suggest that this may have occurred because during the time these programs were being implemented in middle and high schools across the country, only a minority of teenagers were telling their health care providers that they had delayed seeking contraceptives because they lacked knowledge of their need for them, feared the side effects of prescription methods, or did not know how or where to obtain them (Zabin & Clark, 1981; Zabin et al., 1991). Thus, even if these programs had been entirely successful at changing the contraceptive behavior of those students who thought "they were too young to get pregnant" or were "having sex too infrequently to get pregnant," it seems unlikely that knowledge-based sex education classes would substantially reduce the number of adolescent pregnancies in this country as most adolescents fail to use contraceptives for other, more complex psychosocial reasons (Zabin *et al.*, 1991; Kelly *et al.*, 1994). The failure of the early knowledge-based and access-based sex education programs to change the pregnancy-related behavior of most American teenagers is not a unique experience. Indeed, the results of international studies indicate that inconsistencies between what women state their childbearing preferences to be and what their sexual and contraceptive behavior actually is result in a large number of seemingly untimely pregnancies in all parts of the world (Kirby, 1992; Miller, 1993; Bongaarts, 1991).

Ultimately, the rising rates of adolescent sexual activity and adolescent pregnancy, and the growing evidence that physical and knowledge barriers are far less significant deterrents to regular contraceptive use than are attitudes and perceptions, focused attention on the third minimal requirement for regular contraceptive use listed in Table 1, a sexual self-concept that enables individuals to make conscious decisions about their sexual and contraceptive behavior.

To this end, the third generation of sex education classes and pregnancy prevention programs were based on social learning theory (Kirby, 1992; Miller, 1993). Their premise was that young people engage in high-risk behaviors such as unprotected sexual intercourse because of societal influences (Kirby, 1992; Miller, 1993). Within this theoretical framework, it seemed unlikely that classroom courses would be able to change sexual behavior in a direction that was in opposition to the sexual world as portrayed by the media, parents, and peers. Thus, the directors of social learning theory-based sex education classes and pregnancy prevention programs attempted to counteract prevailing social forces by helping students identify the origins of pressures to engage in high-risk sexual behaviors and to develop the skills that would enable them to respond effectively and to avoid them. By providing a forum in which young people are encouraged to apply cognitive decision-making process to their own sexual lives, these programs assist teenagers to overcome the guilt they may experience over sexual feelings which are in conflict with their parental or religious values, thus enabling them to take responsibility for controlling their sexual lives (Levinson, 1986; Stout & Rivara, 1989; Miller, 1993).

The recently published evaluations of two social learning theory-based sex education programs, "Postponing Sexual Involvement" and "Reducing the Risk," suggest that this approach to the prevention of adolescent pregnancy may be more effective than its predecessors (Howard & McCabe, 1990; Gilchrist & Schinke, 1983). The results of these studies indicate that programs that teach decision-making skills and give students practice applying these skills in personally difficult situations have the potential to delay the initiation of sexual intercourse among participants who have not already become sexually active, and to decrease the frequency of unprotected sexual activity among participants who initiated sexual activity after they had been exposed to the program (Howard & McCabe, 1990; Gilchrist & Schinke, 1983). This approach does not appear to decrease the frequency of sexual intercourse or to increase the use of contraceptives among teenagers who have initiated sexual intercourse prior to the program (Howard & McCabe, 1990; Gilchrist & Schinke, 1983). These findings emphasize the importance of reaching young people before they become sexually active and before they join an adolescent subculture which does not perceive pregnancy and parenthood to be negative life-course events.

Most recently, the failure of social learning theory-based sex education programs to change the pregnancy-related behavior of sexually active teenagers and the growing evidence that many adolescent pregnancies are planned or at least not entirely unplanned have focused attention on the fourth minimal requirement for regular contraceptive use listed in Table 1, a desire to postpone childbearing.

To this end the fourth generation of sex education classes and pregnancy prevention programs have included "life options" components (Stout & Rivara, 1989; Miller, 1993). These programs are based on the premise that teenagers need motivations and opportunities as much as they need abstinence values or contraceptive services to avoid pregnancy (Miller, 1993). High-risk behaviors such as unprotected sexual intercourse are not treated as random behaviors that are engaged in whimsically but, rather, as functional, purposeful, goal-directed activities that have both positive and negative consequences for adolescent development. Realizing that young people are not apt to abandon behaviors that meet their developmental needs if there are no alternatives, the directors of these new programs have attempted to give adolescents career options that are more attractive than is parenthood (Miller, 1993; Field, Widmayer, Greenberg, & Stoller, 1982). Acknowledging the prominence of the personal myth, "It can't happen to me," in adolescent thinking (Elkind, 1974; Stevens-Simon, 1993), life options-based pregnancy prevention programs have been designed to simultaneously discourage high-risk sexual behaviors and to promote protective behaviors (e.g., activities that enable impoverished young people to discover new ways to meet their developmental needs). Since the rewards that life options programs promise participants tend to be somewhat intangible (e.g., improved self-esteem) and distant (e.g., better job opportunities), some program directors have incorporated shorter-term, tangible incentives.

One of the best publicized examples of this approach is the Dollar-A-Day Program (Dolgan & Goodman, 1989). This program is based on the premise that impoverished adolescent parents require immediate, tangible rewards for behaviors that do not result in pregnancy. Program participants meet weekly to collect seven dollars (one dollar for each nonpregnant day in the week) and to share snacks and converse about common problems and concerns and educational goals and objectives in a supportive group environment. Initially the monetary and food incentives serve as motivators and central organizing features for the group, rewards intended to mitigate against or counterbalance the strong environmental pressures to conceive. As the group and its members mature, participation and recognition of personal achievements by peers and adults become their own rewards and the need for external rewards for pregnancy-preventing behaviors is replaced by an internal desire to delay further childbearing and to pursue careers other than parenthood. The initial clinical trials of the Dollar-A-Day Program produced very encouraging results (Dolgan & Goodman, 1989). Interpretation of these findings is difficult, however, because of the lack of an adequate control group and because group assignment was not random. The efficacy of the life options and incentive approaches to the prevention of adolescent pregnancy remains uncertain; these types of programs are still being evaluated (Miller, 1993).

An innovative approach to reducing adolescent pregnancy is through a community-based program. In 1982, such a program was developed in the western portion of a South Carolina county. The goal of the School/Community Program for Sexual Risk Reduction Among Teens was to reduce the occurrence of unintended pregnancies among unmarried adolescents. Intervention messages were targeted at parents, teachers, ministers and representatives of churches, community leaders, and children enrolled in the public school system. The messages emphasized development of decision-making and communication skills, self-esteem enhancement, and understanding human reproductive anatomy, physiology, and contraception. The estimated rate of pregnancy (live births plus fetal deaths plus induced abortions/1000 female population) for females aged 14 to 17 years in the county's western portion declined significantly from 67.1 in 1982 to 25.1 in 1985; comparison communities failed to demonstrate a decline in their estimated rate of pregnancy. Conclusions from this investigation suggest that pregnancy prevention programs need adequate funding to recruit professional personnel and to allow enough time to implement and fine-tune a program, target a receptive intervention population made more responsive through appropriate information dissemination strategies, ánd include the entire community in the educational process of the program (Vincent, Clearie, & Schluchter, 1987).

Thus, in summary, the findings presented in this section suggest that to be maximally effective, pregnancy prevention programs should address all four of the minimal requirements for regular contraceptive use listed in Table 1 early in a child's life. Parents also need to become knowledgeable in order to be able to educate their children. Discussions about these topics should continue throughout the elementary school years; comprehensive education programs that link the classroom to community family planning and jobs programs should be included during the middle school years. As a result, young people would enter high school with a clear sense that their future holds opportunities that are more attractive than parenthood, and they are equipped with the knowledge, means, and attitudes that make them willing and able to postpone childbearing. However, replicating communitywide programs such as the School/Community Program may be more effective in reducing adolescent pregnancy on a larger scale.

SECONDARY PREVENTION OF ADOLESCENT PREGNANCY

Diagnosis of Pregnancy

Secondary prevention refers to early detection and interventions to reverse, halt, or at least retard the progress of a condition. Tertiary prevention refers to the minimization of the effects of a condition. Pregnancy is not an illness *per se,* and thus it does not fit in neatly with the nomenclature of secondary or tertiary prevention. However, in this chapter we will consider secondary prevention of adolescent pregnancy as the early recognition of pregnancy and the provision of adequate prenatal care. The early diagnosis of pregnancy is very important so that adolescents can enter obstetric care early (McAnarney & Hendee, 1989). Diagnosis often follows the arousal of suspicion in a professional consulted about an unexplained secondary amenorrhea. Pregnant adolescents may not give a history of secondary amenorrhea, however, because they may experience vaginal spotting at the time of implantation, which they misinterpret as menses. These adolescents may complain of other symptoms, such as fatigue, morning vomiting, abdominal discomfort, headache, lightheadedness, dizziness, or syncope. Even if the history is not positive for sexual intercourse or is not highly consistent with pregnancy, a pregnancy test would be performed if the clinician suspects pregnancy.

The serum immunoassay for the beta subunit of human chorionic gonadotropin is the most accurate laboratory test for diagnosis of pregnancy. Results are positive approximately 7 to 10 days after conception. If the test result is not positive and pregnancy is still a possibility, repeated pregnancy testing in 1 week is suggested.

Once a diagnosis of pregnancy is made, discussions between the pregnant adolescent and the physician about pregnancy options should be initiated immediately. In addition, an estimate of the gestational week of pregnancy should be made to facilitate counseling the adolescent about her options. The pregnant adolescent has three options: (1) continuing the pregnancy and keeping the infant, (2) continuing the pregnancy and placing the infant for adoption, and (3) having an abortion.

Provision of Adequate Prenatal Care

Early and consistent comprehensive prenatal care should be initiated immediately if the adolescent decides to continue her pregnancy. Studies controlling for concurrent high-risk maternal conditions find no association between young maternal age and the majority of obstetric complications traditionally associated with adolescent childbearing. Thus, most investigators and health care providers now believe that the majority of the medical complications associated with adolescent childbearing can be reduced or even eliminated by early, consistent, comprehensive prenatal care (Klerman, 1993; Stevens-Simon & White, 1991; Stevens-Simon, Fuller, & McAnarney, 1992).

Studies suggest that the benefits of comprehensive, multidisciplinary prenatal care could be mediated by several factors. For example, close attention to the diagnosis and treatment of cervical and vaginal infections could result in a decrease in the incidence of premature rupture of the placental membranes (McGregor et al., 1990; Heins, Nance, McCarthy, & Efird, 1990). Alternatively, improvements in maternal nutritional status and weight gain could result in a decrease in the incidence of medical complications such as anemia, induced hypertension, and intrauterine growth retardation which either culminate in preterm delivery or necessitate preterm induction of labor (Stevens-Simon & McAnarney, 1988). Finally, greater attention to the diagnosis and treatment of nonobstetric, psychosocial problems such as substance abuse and maternal stress and depression could decrease the incidence of preterm delivery of unknown causes (McAnarney & Stevens-Simon, 1990; Istvan, 1986). Comprehensive prenatal care includes both obstetric and psychosocial services, ideally in one setting. The most successful comprehensive prenatal care is provided by members of an interdisciplinary team who emphasize prenatal care, nutrition counseling, psychosocial services, and postpartum care.

A nationally recognized intervention for pregnant adolescents is the Adolescent Pregnancy Program established at the Johns Hopkins Hospital in Baltimore, Maryland, in 1974. This program enrolls between 300 and 325 adolescents under the age of 18 each year (Hardy & Zabin, 1991). It has provided high-quality standard medical care, emphasizing prevention and treatment of adolescent problems such as anemia, sexually transmitted infections, and the nutritional requirements for fetal development. In addition, comprehensive psychosocial support and health, childbirth, and parenting education have been provided.

A full-time social worker and an education specialist are part of the health care team.

The social worker screens each adolescent and, usually, her mother. Referrals are made as needed for human services, medical assistance, and nutritional supplements such as WIC and food stamps. Helping to plan for the adolescent's continued education and mental health counseling are other important social work functions. The educational specialist has responsibility for implementation of the program's education curriculum. This curriculum includes a values clarification discussion group emphasizing personal responsibility. Participation in an education group is mandatory at each prenatal visit. Fathers are encouraged to attend and to participate in the preparation-for-childbirth sessions so that they may assist the mothers during labor. The curriculum also includes a range of pregnancy nutritional, reproductive health, and infant-care issues. Two full-time obstetrical nurses work in the clinic and interview each adolescent as she leaves to ensure that she understands clinic instructions and procedures. They assist the obstetrical director in reviewing each patient's record, planning for obstetrical care, and reduce loss to follow-up among clinic staff.

In the 3-year period between 1979 and 1981, the Johns Hopkins Adolescent Pregnancy Program was effective in reducing the frequency of pregnancy complications, low birth weight, and low 5-minute Apgar scores. Specifically, the frequency of low birth weight was 9.9% compared to 16.4% for the control condition ($p < 0.0006$), and low 5-minute Apgar scores was 4.0% compared to 6.7% for the control condition ($p < 0.02$). The program's success indicates that an intervention combining medical, educational, and social services specifically directed to meet the complex needs of a young pregnant mother is highly effective.

As most published studies have not been randomized, it is still unclear to what extent the improved pregnancy outcomes of adolescents enrolled in these types of maternity programs reflect a bias toward healthier, more highly motivated young women using these services (Stevens-Simon & White, 1991; Stevens-Simon et al., 1992; Weatherley, Perlman, Levine, & Klerman, 1986; Stahler, DuCette, & McBride, 1989; Stahler & DuCette, 1991). Despite the shortcomings of these studies, the weight of the current evaluation data suggests that providing early, consistent, comprehensive prenatal care to adolescents lessens the immediate medical and social problems associated with childbearing at this age (Elster, Lamb, Tavare, & Ralston, 1987; Stevens-Simon & White, 1991; Stevens-Simon et al., 1992; Weatherley et al., 1986; Stahler et al., 1989; Stahler & DuCette, 1991).

TREATMENT OF ADOLESCENT PREGNANCY

Since the literature suggests that the rate of preterm and low-birth-weight deliveries increases with parity among adolescents, tertiary adolescent prevention programs that increase the likelihood of completing high school, having a job, and being self-supporting decreases with each additional adolescent pregnancy (tertiary adolescent prevention programs), have been extended beyond the immediate postpartum period to provide aggressive postpartum follow-up with a strong emphasis on family and career planning (Stevens-Simon & White, 1991; Card & Wise, 1978; Stevens-Simon & Reichert, 1994; Elster et al., 1987; Hardy & Zabin, 1991; Stevens-Simon, Fullar, & McAnarney, 1989; Nelson,

Key, Fletcher, Kirkpatrick, & Feinstein, 1982). These programs are based on the premise that impoverished adolescent parents require additional encouragement and support to postpone future childbearing and engage in development-promoting activities. In most cases the mother, father, and baby are seen together in an effort to decrease the complexity of obtaining preventive health care services and maximize contraceptive use (Stevens-Simon, Parsons, & Montgomery, 1986; Elster *et al.,* 1987; Hardy & Zabin, 1991; Stevens-Simon *et al.,* 1989; Nelson *et al.,* 1982). Programs that do not contain specific family planning components have been shown to be less effective at preventing recidivism and, in turn, at preventing high school drop-out and chronic welfare dependency (Polit, 1989). These findings make contraceptive agents like Norplant and Depoprovera (which have the potential to bridge the lapses in contraceptive vigilance created by the absence of a boyfriend or social pressures encouraging further childbearing) particularly attractive for adolescent parents (Stevens-Simon, Wallis, & Allen-Davis, 1995). In addition to providing consistent hospital-based medical care which is linked to community-based educational and vocational training programs, current data suggest that outreach workers who visit patients in their homes are a cost-effective way to bridge the gap between young, socially isolated families and the medical and social service systems (Olds & Kitzman, 1990).

A pregnancy can be terminated either by spontaneous or elective abortion. Abortion is a treatment for adolescent pregnancy. The number of elective abortions has steadily increased from an estimated 150,000 in 1970 to 401,128 in 1984, with a corresponding increase in rate per 1000 15- to 19-year-olds from 6 to 44 (Henshaw, 1992). Adolescents choosing abortion will benefit from discussing their feelings about the pregnancy. Careful follow-up is essential for adolescents who have had abortions. The adolescent's partner may also benefit from counseling.

Adoption is another treatment option. However, since only 3% of adolescent parents-to-be place their children with adoptive families, it is difficult to determine the effect that this management option has on the long-term sequelae associated with adolescent childbearing (Bachrach, Stolley, & London, 1992; Kalmuss, Namerow, & Cushman, 1991).

FUTURE RESEARCH CONSIDERATIONS

During the past two decades, most adolescent pregnancy studies have been observational. Although such studies have generated a wealth of correlational data, their designs preclude inferences about causality. In this chapter we have tried to highlight some of the most glaring gaps in knowledge about the antecedents and short- and long-term sequelae of adolescent pregnancy and to identify the research dilemmas and controversies that still surround many of the most important issues.

Since effective intervention requires an understanding of causal mechanisms, it is imperative that (1) future studies of adolescent pregnancy be designed to address testable hypotheses, (2) sample size calculations be performed so that erroneous conclusions are not drawn from data limited by small sample size, and (3) multivariate analytical techniques be employed so that the confounding and interactive effects can be examined.

Adolescent pregnancy is a complex problem; simple answers and solutions are unlikely. Unless rigorous research strategies are adopted, there is little hope of decreasing

CATHERINE STEVENS-SIMON and ELIZABETH R. McANARNEY

the rate of adolescent pregnancy in this country and interrupting the associated cycle of poverty.

As we move through the 1990s we need to carefully examine the validity of the assumptions on which current sex education, family planning, and adolescent pregnancy prevention programs are based. For example, while it seems unlikely that teaching young people about reproduction and contraception promotes premarital sexual activity, further studies are needed to determine if and how it is possible to simultaneously encourage abstinence and the use of contraceptives. Similarly, while it seems unlikely that young people deliberately become pregnant in order to obtain welfare benefits, studies are needed to determine if policies that guarantee young parents economic support make pregnancy and parenting less onerous and cause impoverished young people to be less diligent about preventing conceptions. Conversely, it seems that within communities where adolescent childbearing is normative, the costs of postponing pregnancy outweigh the benefits. Studies are needed to determine whether offering impoverished young people life circumstances that are comparable to those of their less disadvantaged peers (that is, providing them with positive role models, adequate schools and houses, and economic and other incentives for not bearing children) causes them to adopt pregnancy and child-bearing attitudes that are similar to their middle-class peers. As we design studies to examine these issues, it may be most expedient to focus on high-risk subgroups of adolescents, such as the siblings of teen parents, teens with negative pregnancy tests, and teens who have been pregnant before. Since the rates of pregnancy are two to three times higher within these subgroups of teenagers than they are in the teenage population as a whole, the efficacy of intervention programs can be tested more rapidly and expediently (Stevens-Simon *et al.*, 1993; Zabin *et al.*, 1991; Abrahamse *et al.*, 1988; Friede *et al.*, 1986; Cox *et al.*, 1993).

Although concern over adolescent pregnancy and parenting has generated a great deal of research over the past decade, most of the studies that have been done have concentrated on how pregnancy and parenthood affect young women and their offspring. Growing evidence of the central role that the adolescent male plays in the contraceptive decisions that antedate adolescent conceptions (Rainey *et al.*, 1993) highlights the importance of studying adolescent male attitudes toward pregnancy and parenthood. Systematic evaluations of the effects of pregnancy and parenthood on adolescent males are also a prerequisite for rational intervention (Marsiglio, 1987).

Effective treatment of the immediate morbidity associated with adolescent childbearing (e.g., prevention of the short-term sequelae listed in Table 2) requires that we learn more about the etiologic mechanisms underlying the medical risks associated with childbearing at this age. While it no longer seems likely that the nutritional requirements associated with incomplete adolescent maternal growth compete directly with those of the fetus, there is growing evidence that hormonal differences related to the immaturity of the perimenarcheal adolescent hypothalamic–pituitary–gonadal axis could increase the risk of preterm labor and delivery among young women who conceive soon after menarche by predisposing them to lower genital tract infections which have been tentatively associated with premature rupture of the placental membranes and/or by compromising the development of the uteroplacental vascular bed (Stevens-Simon, Douglas, Jamison, & McGregor, 1994; Stevens-Simon, Roghmann, & McAnarney, 1991).

Table 2. Common Medical Psychosocial Problems among Adolescent Mothers and Their Children[a]

Medical	Psychosocial
	Mother
Small size/poor weight gain	Poor education/school failure
Obesity/excessive weight gain	Limited vocational opportunities
Pregnancy-induced hypertension	Poverty
Anemia	Divorce and separation
Sexually transmitted disease	Social isolation
Cephalopelvic disproportion	Stress/depression
Peurperal complications	Substance abuse
Repeat pregnancy	Repeat pregnancy
	Child
Low birth weight	Developmental delay
Prematurity	Neglect
Sudden infant death syndrome	Behavior problems/substance use
Minor acute infections	School failure and withdrawal
Accidents	Underemployment/poverty
Neonatal and infant death	Unplanned pregnancy

[a]From Stevens-Simon, C., & White, M. (1991). Adolescent pregnancy. *Pediatric Annals, 20,* 322–331.

CONCLUSION

While it is clear that becoming pregnant as a teenager may have negative effects on the health of both the young mother and her child, it is also clear that health care alone will not have a significant effect on the problems associated with childbearing at this age. Socictal changes, including better education and employment opportunities, improved housing, and relief from poverty, are also critical.

REFERENCES

Abrahamse, A. F., Morrison, P. A., & Waite, L. J. (1988). Teenagers willing to consider single parenthood: Who is at greatest risk? *Family Planning Perspectives, 20,* 13–18.

Anderson, J. E., & Cope, L. G. (1987). The impact of family planning program activity on fertility. *Family Planning Perspectives, 19,* 152–157.

Babson, S. G., & Clarke, N. G. (1983). Relationship between infant death and maternal age: Comparison of sudden infant death incidence with other causes of infant mortality. *Journal of Pediatrics, 103,* 391–393.

Bachrach, C. A., Stolley, K. S., & London, K. A. (1992). Relinquishment of premarital births: Evidence from national survey data. *Family Planning Perspectives, 24,* 27–32.

Bongaarts, J. (1991). The KAP-gap and the unmet need for contraception. *Population and Development Review, 17,* 293–313.

Brooks-Gunn, J., & Chase-Lansdale, P. L. (1991). Children having chidren: Effects on the family system. *Pediatric Annals, 20,* 467–481.

Card, J. J., & Wise, L. L. (1978). Teenage mothers and teenage fathers: The impact of early childbearing on the parents' personal and professional lives. *Family Planning Perspectives, 10,* 199–225.

Cox, J., Emans, S. J., & Bithoney, W. (1993). Sisters of teen mothers: Increased risk for adolescent pregnancy. *Adolescent Pediatric Gynecology, 6,* 138–142.

Dolgan, J. I., & Goodman, S. M. (1989). Dollar-A-Day: Teenage Pregnancy Prevention Program. *Rocky Mountain Planned Parenthood.*

DuRant, R., & Jay, S. (1989). The adolescent heterosexual relationship and its association with the sexual and contraceptive behavior of black females. *American Journal of Disease in Children, 143,* 1467–1472.

Elkind, D. (1974). *Children and adolescents: Interpretive essays on Jean Piaget* (2nd ed.). London: Oxford University Press.

Elster, A. B., Ketterlinus, R., & Lamb, M. E. (1990). Association between parenthood and problem behavior in a national sample of adolescents. *Pediatrics, 85,* 1044–1050.

Elster, A. B., Lamb, M. E., Tavare, J., & Ralson, C. W. (1987). Medical and psychosocial impact of comprehensive care on adolescent pregnancy and parenthood. *Journal of the American Medical Association, 258,* 1187–1192.

Field, T., Widmayer, S., Greenberg, R., & Stoller, S. (1982). Effects of parent training on teenage mothers and their infants. *Pediatrics, 69,* 703–707.

Friede, A., Hogue, C. J. R., Doyle, L. L., Hammerslough, C. R., Sniezek, J. E., & Arright, R. (1986). Do sisters of childbearing teenagers have increased rates of childbearing? *American Journal of Public Health, 76,* 1221–1224.

Furstenberg, F. F. (1992). Teenage childbearing and cultural rationality: A thesis in search of evidence. *Family Relations, 41,* 239–243.

Furstenberg, F. F., Brooks-Gunn, J., & Morgan, S. P. (1987). Adolescent mothers and their children in later life. *Family Planning Perspectives, 19,* 142–151.

Gabriel, A., & McAnarney, E. R. (1983). Parenthood in two subcultures: White middle-class couples and black low-income adolescents in Rochester, New York. *Adolescence, 18,* 595–608.

Gilchrist, L. D., & Schinke, S. P. (1983). Coping with contraception: Cognitive and behavioral methods with adolescents. *Cognitive Therapy Research, 7,* 379–388.

Gross, R. T., & Duke, P. M. (1980). The effect of early versus late physical maturation on adolescent behavior. *Pediatric Clinics of North America, 27,* 71–77.

Hardy, J. B. (1991). Pregnancy and its outcome. In W. R. Hendee (Ed.), *The health of adolescents* (pp. 250–281). San Francisco: Jossey–Bass.

Hardy, J. B., & Zabin, L. S. (1991). *Adolescent pregnancy in an urban environment.* Munich: Urban & Schwarzenberg.

Hayes, C. D. (1987). *Risking the future.* Washington, DC: National Academy Press.

Heins, H. C., Nance, N. W., McCarthy, B. J., & Efird, C. M. (1990). A randomized trial of nurse-midwifery prenatal care to reduce low birth weight. *Obstetrics and Gynecology, 75,* 341–345.

Henshaw, S. K. (1992). Abortion trends in 1987 and 1988: Age and race. *Family Planning Perspectives, 24,* 85–87.

Hoffman, S. D., Foster, E. M., & Furstenberg, F. F. (1993). Reevaluating the costs of teenage childbearing. *Demography, 30,* 1–13.

Howard, M., & McCabe, J. B. (1990). Helping teenagers postpone sexual involvement. *Family Planning Perspectives, 22,* 21–26.

Istvan, J. (1986). Stress, anxiety, and birth outcomes: A critical review of the evidence. *Psychological Bulletin, 100,* 331–348.

Jessor, R. (1991). Risk behavior in adolescence: A psychosocial framework for understanding and action. *Journal of Adolescent Health, 12,* 597–605.

Kalmuss, D., Namerow, P. B., & Cushman, L. F. (1991). Adoption versus parenting among young pregnant women. *Family Planning Perspectives, 23,* 17–23.

Kelly, L., Stevens-Simon, C., Singer, D., & Cox, A. (1994). Why pregnant adolescents say they didn't use contraceptives prior to conception. *Journal of Adolescent Health, 15,* 78.

Kirby, D. (1992). School-based programs to reduce sexual risk-taking behavior. *Journal of School Health, 62,* 280–287.

Kirby, D., Waszak, C., & Ziegler, J. (1991). Six school-based clinics: Their reproductive health services and impact on sexual behavior. *Family Planning Perspectives, 23,* 6–16.

Klerman, L. V. (1993). Adolescent pregnancy and parenting controversies of the past and lessons for the future. *Journal of Adolescent Health, 14,* 553–561.

Leigh, B. C., Morrison, D. M., Trocki, K., & Temple, M. T. (1994). Sexual behavior of American adolescents: Results from a US national survey. *Journal of Adolescent Health, 15,* 117–125.

Levinson, R. (1986). Contraceptive self-efficacy: A perspective on teenage girls' contraceptive behavior. *Journal of Sex Research, 22,* 347–369.

McAnarney, E. R., & Schreider, C. (1984). *Identifying social and psychological antecedents of adolescent pregnancy: The contribution of research to concepts of prevention.* New York: William T. Grant Foundation.

McAnarney, E. R., & Hendee, W. R. (1989). The prevention of adolescent pregnancy. *JAMA, 262,* 78–82.

McAnarney, E. R., & Stevens-Simon, C. (1990). Maternal psychological stress/depression and low birth weight. *American Journal of Disease in Children, 144,* 789–792.

McGregor, J. A., French, J. I., Richter, R., Franco-Buff, A., Johnson, A., Hillier, S., Judson, F. N., & Todd, J. K. (1990). Antenatal microbiologic and maternal risk factors associated with prematurity. *American Journal of Obstetrics and Gynecology, 163,* 1465–1473.

Marsiglio, W. (1987). Adolescent fathers in the United States: Their initial living arrangements, marital experiences and educational outcomes. *Family Planning Perspectives, 19,* 240–251.

Matsuhashi, Y., Felice, M. E., Shragg, P., & Hollingsworth, D. R. (1989). Is repeat pregnancy in adolescents a "planned" affair? *Journal of Adolescent Health Care, 10,* 409–412.

Miller, B. C. (1992). Adolescent parenthood, economic issues, and social policies. *Journal of Family Economic Issues, 13,* 467–475.

Miller, B. C. (1993). Families, science, and values: Alternative views of parenting effects and adolescent pregnancy. *Journal of Marriage and the Family, 55,* 7–21.

Moore, K. A. (1988). Teenage childbearing: Unresolved issues in research/policy debate. *Family Planning Perspectives, 22,* 189–209.

Moore, K. A. (1990). *Facts at a glance.* New York: Alan Guttmacher Institute.

Moore, K. A., & Waite, L. J. (1977). Early childbearing and educational attainment. *Family Planning Perspectives, 9,* 220–225.

Nelson, K. G., Key, D., Fletcher, J. K., Kirkpatrick, E., & Feinstein, R. (1982). The teen-tot clinic: An alternative to traditional care for infants of teenaged mothers. *Journal of Adolescent Health Care, 3,* 19–23.

Newcomer, S., & Baldwin, W. (1992). Demographics of adolescent sexual behavior, contraception, pregnancy and STDs. *Journal of School Health, 62,* 265–270.

Olds, D. L., & Kitzman, H. (1990). Can home visitation improve the health of women and children at environmental risk? *Pediatrics, 86,* 108–116.

Olsen, J. A., Weed, S. E., Ritz, G. M., & Jensen, L. C. (1991). The effects of three abstinence sex education programs on student attitudes toward sexual activity. *Adolescence, 26,* 631–641.

Polit, D. F. (1989). Effects of a comprehensive program for teenage parents: Five years after project redirection. *Family Planning Perspectives, 21,* 164–169.

Rainey, D. Y., Stevens-Simon, C., & Kaplan, D. W. (1993). Self-perception of infertility among female adolescents. *American Journal of Disease in Children, 147,* 1053–1056.

Roosa, M. W., & Christopher, F. S. (1990). Evaluation of an abstinence-only adolescent pregnancy prevention program: A replication. *Family Relations, 39,* 363–367.

Shapiro, S., McCormick, M. C., Starfield, B. H., Krischer, J. P., & Bross, D. (1980). Relevance of correlates of infant death for significant morbidity at 1 year of age. *American Journal of Obstetrics and Gynecology, 136,* 363–373.

Smith, E. A., & Udry, J. R. (1985). Coital and non-coital sexual behaviors of white and black adolescents. *American Journal of Public Health, 75,* 1200–1203.

Stahler, G. J., & DuCette, J. P. (1991). Evaluating adolescent pregnancy programs: Rethinking our priorities. *Family Planning Perspectives, 23,* 129–133.

Stahler, G. J., DuCette, J. P., & McBride, D. (1989). The evaluation component in adolescent pregnancy care projects: Is it adequate? *Family Planning Perspectives, 21,* 121–126.

Stevens-Simon, C., Parsons, J., Montgomery, C. (1986). What is the relationship between postpartum withdrawal from school and repeat pregnancy among adolescent mothers? *Journal of Adolescent Health Care, 7*, 191–194.

Stevens-Simon, C. (1993) Working with the "Personal Fable." *Journal of Adolescent Health Care, 14*, 349.

Stevens-Simon, C., Beach, R., & Eagar, R. (1993). Contraception after a negative pregnancy test during adolescence. *Adolescent Pediatric Gynecology, 6*, 83–85.

Stevens-Simon, C., Douglas, J., Jamison, J., & McGregor, J. (1994). Racial differences in vaginal pH among healthy sexually active adolescents. *Sexually Transmitted Diseases, 21*, 168–172.

Stevens-Simon, C., Fullar, S. A., & McAnarney, E. R. (1989). Teenage pregnancy: Caring for adolescent mothers with their infants in pediatric settings. *Clinical Pediatrics, 28*, 282–283.

Stevens-Simon, C., Fullar, S., & McAnarney, E. R. (1992). Tangible differences between adolescent-oriented and adult-oriented prenatal care. *Journal of Adolescent Health, 13*, 298–302.

Stevens-Simon, C., & McAnarney, E. R. (1988). Adolescent maternal weight gain and infant outcome. *American Journal of Clinical Nutrition, 47*, 948–953.

Stevens-Simon, C., & Reichert, S. (1994). Child sexual abuse and adolescent pregnancy. *Archives of Pediatric Adolescent Medicine, 148*, 23–27.

Stevens-Simon, C., Roghmann, K. J., & McAnarney, E. R. (1991). First trimester vaginal bleeding and preterm delivery in pregnant adolescents. *Pediatrics, 87*, 951–952.

Stevens-Simon, C., Wallis, J., & Allen-Davis, J. (1995). Which teen mothers choose Norplant? *Journal of Adolescent Health*, in press.

Stevens-Simon, C., & White, M. (1991). Adolescent pregnancy. *Pediatric Annals, 20*, 322–331.

Stout, J. W., & Rivara, F. P. (1989). Schools and sex education: Does it work? *Pediatrics, 83*, 375–379.

Strobino, D. M., Ensminger, M. E., Nanda, J., & Young, J. K. (1992). Young motherhood and infant hospitalization during the first year of life. *Journal of Adolescent Health, 13*, 553–560.

Taylor, B., Wadsworth, J., & Butler, N. R. (1983). Teenage mothering, admission to hospital, and accidents during the first 5 years. *Archives of Disease in Childhood, 58*, 6–11.

Thiel, K. S., & McBride, D. (1992). Comments on an evaluation of an abstinence-only adolescent pregnancy prevention program. *Family Relations, 41*, 465–467.

Udry, J. R. (1988). Biological predispositions and social control in adolescent sexual behavior. *American Sociological Review, 53*, 709–722.

Upchurch, D. M., & McCarthy, J. (1990). The timing of a first birth and high school completion. *American Sociological Review, 55*, 224–234.

Vincent, M. L., Clearie, A. F., & Schluchter, M. D. (1987). Reducing adolescent pregnancy through school and community-based education. *Journal of the American Medical Association, 257*, 3382–3386

Weatherley, R. A., Perlman, S. B., Levine, M. H., & Klerman, L. V. (1986). Comprehensive programs for pregnant teenagers and teen-age parents: How successful have they been? *Family Planning Perspectives, 18*, 73–78.

Winter, L. (1988). The role of sexual self-concept in the use of contraceptives. *Family Planning Perspectives, 20*, 123–127.

Zabin, L. S., Astone, N. M., & Emerson, M. R. (1993). Do adolescents want babies? The relationship between attitudes and behavior. *Journal of Research on Adolescence, 3*, 67–86.

Zabin, L. S., & Clark, S. D. (1981). Why they delay: A study of teenage family planning clinic patients. *Family Planning Perspectives, 13*, 205–217.

Zabin, L. S., Hirsch, M. B., Smith, E. A., Streett, R., & Hardy, J. B. (1986). Evaluation of a pregnancy prevention program for urban teenagers. *Family Planning Perspectives, 18*, 119–126.

Zabin, L. S., Stark, H. A., & Emerson, M. R. (1991). Reasons for delay in contraceptive clinic utilization: Adolescent clinic and non-clinic populations compared. *Journal of Adolescent Health, 12*, 225–232.

Zellman, G. L. (1982). Public school programs for adolescent pregnancy and parenthood: An assessment. *Family Planning Perspectives, 14*, 15–21.

13

Sexually Transmitted Diseases Including Human Immunodeficiency Virus Infection

LAWRENCE J. D'ANGELO and
RALPH J. DiCLEMENTE

INTRODUCTION

The risk of acquiring a sexually transmitted disease (STD) is one of the most significant and immediate risks to the health and well-being of adolescents. From an economic and social standpoint, these infections continue to exact a significant toll on adolescents and ultimately on society. This toll can be measured in terms of projected costs of certain infections, such as chlamydia infections (Washington, 1987), and in terms of health outcomes, such as the number of ectopic pregnancies (Chow, Darling, & Greenbert, 1987) and the rate of infertility (Westrom, 1980). The real concern, however, is that in an era when a sexually transmitted infection—human immunodeficiency virus (HIV) infection—can result in a fatal illness—acquired immunodeficiency syndrome (AIDS)—we have begun to measure the impact in terms of deaths of adolescents and young adults from AIDS. For this reason, the potential impact of STDs is all the more significant and prevention of these infections an even higher priority.

LAWRENCE J. D'ANGELO • Department of Pediatrics, Adolescent/Young Adult Medicine, Children's National Medical Center, Washington, D.C. 20010.   RALPH J. DiCLEMENTE • Departments of Health Behavior and Pediatrics, University of Alabama, Birmingham, Alabama 35294.
Handbook of Adolescent Health Risk Behavior, edited by Ralph J. DiClemente, William B. Hansen, and Lynn E. Ponton. Plenum Press, New York, 1996.

Classification of Sexually Transmitted Diseases in Adolescents: By Syndromic or Specific Disease Agent

STDs in adolescents can be classified by illness syndromes or by specific disease agent. The syndromes most often seen in adolescents include urethritis (caused by *Neisseria gonorrhoeae* and *Chlamydia trachomatis*), vaginitis (caused by *Trichomonas vaginalis, C. trachomatis,* and *N. gonorrhoeae*), cervicitis (caused by *N. gonorrhoeae* and *C. trachomatis*), genital ulcers (caused by herpes simplex virus *Hemophilus ducrey'i* and *Treponema pallidum*), and, in females, pelvic inflammatory disease (*C. trachomatis* and *N. gonorrhoeae*). Also in females, cervical dysplasia and cervical carcinoma are most often the result of sexually transmitted infection with human papilloma virus. In both males and females, transmission of HIV infection can result in AIDS and transmission of human papilloma virus can result in genital warts (Table 1). The infectious agents listed as the cause of the syndromes mentioned above are the ones most prevalent in adolescents. In addition to these infections, other illnesses such as hepatitis caused by hepatitis B virus (HBV) (CDC, 1988b) and infectious mononucleosis caused by cytomegalovirus virus (CMV) (Sohn, Oh, Balcarek, Cloud, & Pass, 1991) are most likely to be sexually transmitted infections in adolescents.

Not surprisingly, the increase in both the reported number of STDs and the rates of these infections in adolescents is directly related to the decrease in the age of sexual initiation or "debut" by teenagers. The median age of first intercourse is 15.9 years for males (Sonenstein, Pleck, & Ku, 1989) and 16.9 years for females (Forrest & Singh, 1990; CDC, 1991). However, this age of sexual initiation is heavily dependent on a variety of socioeconomic (Rice, Roberts, Handsfield, & Holmes, 1991; Rosenberg, Bayona, Brown, & Specter, 1994), ethnic and racial (Halsey *et al.*, 1992; Rolfs & Nakashima, 1994), and educational factors (Huszti, Clopton, & Mason, 1989) and is also correlated with other risk behaviors such as substance use (Cox, D'Angelo, & Silber, 1992; Fullilove, Fullilove, Bowser, & Gross, 1990).

In addition to the age of sexual initiation, factors such as the number of sexual partners, the age of sexual partners, and the nature of sexual practices all influence the risk

Table 1.   Sexually Transmitted Disease Syndromes in Adolescents

Syndrome	Infectious agent
Urethritis	*Neisseria gonorrhoeae*
	Chlamydia trachomatis
Vaginitis/cervicitis	*Trichomonas vaginalis*
	N. gonorrhoeae
	C. trachomatis
Genital ulcers	Herpes simplex
Syphilis	*Treponema pallidum*
Chancroid	*Haemophilus ducreyi*
Pelvic inflammatory disease	*N. gonorrhoeae*
	C. trachomatis
HIV/AIDS	Human immunodeficiency virus

of acquiring an STD (Alan Guttmacher Institute, 1994). This chapter will review the epidemiology of STDs in adolescents, discuss ways to prevent STDs, and review diagnostic and therapeutic approaches for those adolescents who become infected.

EPIDEMIOLOGY

Defining the actual number of adolescents affected annually by STDs is difficult. The only infections for which reporting to public health authorities is mandated by law in all states are syphilis and gonorrhea. Other infections, such as chlamydia infections, are reportable in some areas. Because of this lack of uniformity, there is no way to catalogue on a national basis the number of cases of infections by organisms such *Chlamydia trachomatis* and *Trichomonas vaginalis,* felt to be the most likely organisms involved with STDs in adolescents and young adults. Similarly, there is no way to accurately estimate the rate of infection with human papilloma virus, the infectious agent linked to cervical cancer. Finally, we must realize that even the data available on reportable diseases are limited by the differences in reporting from different jurisdictions and between private and public health care providers. While data from public clinics specifically established to treat STDs are more reliable, it is heavily biased toward racial, ethnic, and socioeconomic groups that are forced to use these health services for care (Cates, 1990; Alexander-Rodriguez & Vermund, 1987).

Despite these limitations, existing data about STDs in adolescents are both informative and disturbing. For instance, while the total number of cases of gonorrhea reported nationally between 1981 and 1991 decreased from 990,864 to 620,478 cases with an accompanying decrease in the overall rate of cases to 249.5 cases/100,000 population, the rates of gonorrhea in 15- to 19-year-old males actually increased from 868.4/100,000 in 1981 to 882.6/100,000 in 1991 (Webster, Berman, & Greenspan, 1993). During this same period, while the rate in 15- to 19-year-old females fell from 1253.7/100,000 in 1981 to 1043.6/100,000, the rate remained higher in this group than in any other age and sex grouping. These rates varied both by geographic location (rates for 15- to 19-year-olds from the South were 1427.7 for females and 1378.3/100,000 for males) and by race (rates for black 15- to 19-year-olds exceeded 5000/100,000 for both males and females). For syphilis, while rates between 1981 and 1991 actually fell in males from 20.0 to 18.1/100,000, the rates in females increased from 18.4 to 35.0/100,000. Finally, for reported cases of AIDS, by the end of 1993, 1528 cases had been reported in individuals between the ages of 10 and 19 (CDC, 1994b). The majority of these cases (> 58%) were reported in minority youth and 27% of cases were reported in females, the largest percentage of cases in any age group except children less than age 5 (Table 2).

Notwithstanding the impact of the HIV epidemic on the development of one of the best surveillance systems, monitoring the evolving HIV epidemic has proven challenging because of the reliance on surveillance data that emphasize a clinical endpoint, namely, AIDS. The number of clinical AIDS cases among adolescents severely underestimates the threat posed by HIV infection and provides insufficient information for the allocation of health care and prevention resources. Another, more precise gauge of the threat of HIV for adolescents is based on findings from HIV seroprevalence studies.

Table 2. AIDS Cases in U.S. Adolescents, Ages 13–19:
By Gender, Ethnicity (through 12/31/93)

Ethnicity	M (%)	F (%)	Total
Caucasian	499 (32.7)	104 (6.8)	603 (39.5)
African-American	329 (21.5)	295 (19.3)	624 (40.8)
Hispanic	202 (13.2)	74 (4.8)	276 (18.1)
Other	21 (1.4)	3 (0.1)	24 (1.6)
Total	1051 (68.8)	477 (31.2)	1528 (100)

Currently, however, there are no representative population-based studies for estimat-ing HIV seroprevalence among adolescents. The absence of population-based data limits assessing the magnitude of risk for adolescents and reduces the capability to monitor changes in infection rates over time. Much of the HIV seroprevalence data are derived from selected segments of the adolescent population; for example, studies of applicants for military service or active-duty military personnel. Other studies have focused on disadvantaged youth receiving training in the Job Corps, homeless youth, adolescents seeking treatment in STD clinics, and adolescents seeking medical care. HIV se-roprevalence data from a variety of adolescent surveys are shown in Table 3 (DiClemente, 1992a). Overall, the results from a number of serosurveys conducted with selected adoles-cent populations indicate that African-American adolescents have, with few exceptions, markedly higher seroprevalence rates.

Table 3. Prevalence of HIV Infection per 1000 Population
for Selected Surveys: By Race/Ethnicity[a]

Study	Sample or site	Race/ethnicity		
		Black	Latino	White
Burke et al. (1990)	Military applicants	1.0	0.29	0.17
Kelley et al. (1990)	Active-duty military[b]	5.1	4.0	1.25
St. Louis et al. (1991)	Job Corps entrants	5.3	2.6	1.2
St. Louis et al. (1990)	General hospital	8.3	4.9	2.7
Stricof et al. (1991)	Homeless shelter	46	68	60
D'Angelo et al. (1991)	Ambulatory clinics[c]	3.7	—	—
Ilegbodu et al. (1994)	HIV test sites	12.9	5.2	6.2
Young et al. (1992)	STD clinic	4.5	—	1.3
Lemp et al. (1994)	Gay/bisexual youth[d]	212	95	81

[a]All findings have been converted and are presented as rate of seropositive adolescents per 1000 to permit comparability with other surveys.
[b]Sample of active-duty military personnel is not exclusively comprised of adolescents.
[c]This survey does not report ethnic comparisons. More than 88% of the sample was African-American, while 12% was defined as "other" ethnic groups. Attributable to their small proportion in the sample, comparisons with "other" ethnic groups would not be informative.
[d]Adolescents ranged in age from 17 to 22.

Of particular importance are data derived from HIV seroprevalence surveys conducted in inner-city STD clinics. Results from one such survey indicated that the seroprevalence of HIV infection among adolescents ages 15–19 seen in STD clinics is 2.2%; the gender-specific rates are 2.5% for females and 2% for males. In this patient population, 28% of all seropositive women were 19 years of age or younger (Quinn et al., 1988). Likewise, in a review of seroprevalence studies conducted at STD clinics in the United States, the median seroprevalence rate for persons less than 20 years of age was 1.1% with rates ranging from 0 to 2%. Persons between 20 and 29, however, show a substantially higher median seroprevalence of 4.5%; with a range from 0.5 to 7.5% (Cannon, Schmid, Moore, & Pappaioanou, 1989). These findings are of importance given the association between having genital ulcers and increased likelihood of HIV infection which strongly indicates that having an active STD may be an independent risk factor strongly associated with HIV seropositive status (Wasserheit, 1992). Thus, adolescent clients attending STD clinics are a population at increased risk for new STDs and HIV infection (Quinn, Groseclose, Spence, Provost, & Hook, 1992).

While trend data are limited, recent findings from the continuing HIV serosurvey of Job Corps training program applicants have identified marked changes in infection rates between 1988 and 1992 with African-American female applicants revealing a twofold increase in seroprevalence rates, from 3.2 per 1000 to 6.6 per 1000. In 1992, African-American females had seroprevalence rates that not only exceeded rates for white and Hispanic women, but also exceeded HIV seroprevalence rates for African-American males (Conway et al., 1993). We recommend caution in interpreting these rates. While these subpopulation studies provide an assessment of the impact of HIV on adolescents, their utility for assessing temporal trends in seroprevalence is limited and the findings not generalizable to the adolescent population-at-large.

Because syphilis and gonorrhea are reportable infections, they represent the most easily quantifiable of the STDs. Other infections, such as those caused by C. trachomatis and HPV, may actually be of greater overall economic and long-term medical importance but are not reportable diseases in all states (Blythe et al., 1992). We are therefore left guessing at the actual prevalence of these infections based on surveys in adolescent health clinics (Fraser, Rettig, & Kaplan, 1983; Sweeney et al., 1995) and studies of university student health centers (MacDonald et al., 1990). Best estimates give the prevalence of infection in asymptomatic females as between 5 and 12% for chlamydia (Hammerschlage, 1989) and between 18 and 35% for HPV (Martinez et al., 1990). Rates of both of these infections in males are even harder to establish, but studies of asymptomatic males put the infection rate for chlamydia at about 8% (Stamm & Cole, 1986). Data are unavailable for rates of HPV infection in males.

Factors Associated with STD Acquisition in Adolescents

A variety of epidemiologic factors determine the actual risk of an adolescent acquiring an STD. As mentioned earlier, age of first intercourse is correlated with an overall increased risk of infection (Rosenthal, Baro, Succop, Cohen, & Stanberry, 1994). However, it must be acknowledged that this observation may actually be an indirect measure of adolescents who have more sexual partners. The earlier an adolescent initiates intercourse, the longer is the interval in adolescence during which the adolescent can be exposed to more partners. Women who initiate intercourse by age 15 are four times as likely to have ten or more lifetime partners as women who initiate intercourse at age 20 (Cates, 1990). Subfactors that appear to contribute to an earlier age of sexual initiation include earlier onset of puberty and menarche, maternal education, religious affiliation, and family stability.

Biological Vulnerability

Age, as a key variable for the acquisition of STDs, is also a reflection of basic biologic differences in adolescents that relate directly to the risk of STDs. In adolescent females, for up to 3 to 4 years after menarche, columnar epithelium is the cell type that covers the outer surface of the cervix. Under the influence of estrogen and ultimately progesterone, this cell type is eventually replaced by stratified squamous epithelium, but in the interim the adolescent is more susceptible to infection by both *N. gonorrhoeae* and *C. trachomatis* because these pathogens more readily adhere to the surface of columnar epithelial cells (Harrison, 1985).

Gender Differences in STD Rates

As opposed to older age groups, the usual ratio of males to females for STDs is reversed in adolescents. Cases of the reportable STDs, gonorrhea and syphilis, are more prevalent in females than in males (Webster *et al.*, 1993). While AIDS cases are more common in adolescent males than in adolescent females, the fact that the incubation period from infection to actual clinical or immunologic manifestation of an AIDS defining condition is a median of 8 to 12 years, cases of AIDS in adolescents may be a poor surrogate marker for the overall rate of HIV infection in teenagers (Bacchetti & Moss, 1989). A variety of blinded seroprevalence studies including those run by the military and Job Corps indicate that the rate of infection with HIV may well be higher in females than in males (Burke *et al.*, 1990; Conway *et al.*, 1993). Data from adolescent pregnancy studies may provide an explanation for this phenomenon. The fathers of many children born to adolescent mothers are themselves not adolescents. Similarly, for many adolescent women who acquire STDs, their partners are not adolescent males, but rather older males. In a study of age of mothers and age of partners, 30% of 15-year-old mothers bore children of fathers 6 or more years older (Alan Guttmacher Institute, 1994). It is likely that this sort of observation would extend to females with STDs.

Geographic Differences in STD Rates

While it is difficult to establish any verifiable difference in STDs by geographic area, data from reported cases of gonorrhea allow us to demonstrate some differences (Table 4). The data show a higher risk of STDs in 15- to 19-year-olds from the South and Midwest as compared to adolescents from the Northeast and West (Webster *et al.*, 1993). This finding, comprehensive as it is, still excludes certain municipalities (New York) and must therefore be considered to be of limited value. Moreover, recent findings from within the same city

Table 4. Gonorrhea Rates for 15- to 19-Year-Olds: By Geographic Region

Region	Rates/100,000 population	
	Male	Female
Northeast	516.3	701.1
South	1378.3	1426.7
Midwest	897.6	1149.6
West	365.0	485.3

indicate that black adolescents living in public housing developments had rates of chlamydia and gonorrhea three- and fourfold greater than black adolescents living in other neighborhoods in San Francisco.

Racial Differences in STD Rates

Establishing racial differences for STDs in adolescents is again heavily dependent on data concerning the reportable STDs. The rate of gonorrhea in black male and female adolescents is 44 and 16 times higher, respectively, than the rate of infection in their white counterparts (Webster *et al.*, 1993). Hispanic adolescents exceed the rates of reported infection in whites but show rates that are still substantially lower than for black adolescents. This may be a reflection of the theory of an urban core of infection in a relatively defined group of economically deprived minority adolescents who are exposed to an environment of concurrent risk-taking behavior, particularly the use of illicit drugs (Yorke, 1978).

Behavioral Factors

In addition to the traditional epidemiologic factors that can be analyzed with regard to the overall risk of STDs, a variety of behavioral factors influence the likelihood of acquiring a STD. We have already discussed age of sexual initiation and number of sexual partners. Other issues such as history of condom use and concurrent use of illicit drugs influence the risk of STD. Many of these are significantly interrelated. For instance, condom use or nonuse is a complex combination of basic knowledge of what the adolescent might gain by using a condom, the ability to plan for a future event (purchase condom, have it available prior to intercourse, etc.), and the ability to discuss the need to use a condom with one's sexual partner (Wilson, Kastrinakis, D'Angelo, & Getson, 1994). In view of this cascade of requirements, it is not surprising that sorting out whether or not adolescents have improved their behaviors with regard to condom use has not been easy (Kegeles, Adler, & Irwin, 1988; Hausser & Michaud, 1994). It does now seem, however, that condom use is increasing and it is hoped that a decrease in STDs will follow (Sonenstein *et al.*, 1989).

Drug use does appear to be related to the risk of having had an STD. This may be the result of the drug altering the decision-making skills of an individual acutely intoxicated by one or many drugs (Jemmott, & Jemmott, 1993), altering sex drive, or may be the result of adolescents trading sex for drugs which in turn may expose the adolescent to multiple sex partners (Fullilove, Fullilove, Bowser, & Gross, 1990; Fullilove *et al.*, 1993; Shafer *et al.*, 1993a). Finally, although adolescents are not frequent injection drug users, those who do use injection drugs could obtain one of the bloodborne STDs such as HIV or HBV via the use of contaminated drug paraphernalia or by exposing themselves to drug-using peers who might infect them sexually.

PREVENTION

The STD/HIV Epidemic as Psychosocial and Cultural Phenomenon

The STD/HIV epidemic is not only a biomedical phenomenon, but also a psychosocial and cultural phenomenon in which an individual's behavior, more specifically, the lack of appropriate preventive behavior, propels the epidemic. The persistence of STDs as a major public health problem (Yankauer, 1986, 1994) indicates that the presence of an effective medical treatment alone is not sufficient to control the epidemic. Thus, to control the STD/HIV epidemic we must reduce the prevalence of STD/HIV-associated risk behaviors which result in exposure and infection. Much of the behavior associated with STD/HIV exposure is of an interpersonal nature resulting from intimate sexual interaction. And precisely because STD/HIV infection links sexuality with disease, it is inextricably a psychosocial and cultural phenomenon. To most effectively meet the challenges posed by the HIV epidemic, it is important to reconceptualize the epidemic as a psychosocial–biomedical phenomenon and confront it from an interdisciplinary perspective (DiClemente & Peterson, 1994).

Primary Prevention of STD/HIV

Sexual abstinence is clearly the most effective strategy for prevention of STD/HIV infection. However, a substantial proportion of adolescents (Hein, 1992; Kann *et al.*, 1991; DiClemente, 1991; Anderson *et al.*, 1990) do not adopt this preventive practice. Indeed, the expectation that sexually active adolescents will routinely adopt sexual abstinence as an STD/HIV prevention strategy is unrealistic. For sexually active individuals, appropriate and consistent use of latex condoms represents the most effective strategy for preventing transmission of viral pathogens, including HIV (Cates & Stone, 1992; Van de Perre, Jacobs, & Sprecher, 1987); their effectiveness as a risk-reduction strategy is dependent on appropriate and consistent use (Hein, 1993; Roper, Peterson, & Curran, 1993).

Evidence derived from prospective epidemiologic studies of HIV-discordant couples indicates that consistent condom use is a highly effective prevention strategy (DeVincenzi, 1994; Sacco *et al.*, 1993; Laurian, Peynet, & Verroust, 1989). The recent findings from the European Study Group on Heterosexual Transmission of HIV (DeVincenzi, 1994) identified a markedly higher seroconversion rate among the seronegative partner of HIV-discordant couples who used condoms inconsistently relative to couples who used condoms consistently. Among couples who reported inconsistent condom use, a seroconversion rate of 4.8 per 100 person years was observed. Conversely, among couples who used condoms consistently, no seroconversions were observed. The data suggest that condoms can be an effective STD/HIV prevention strategy; however, a high degree of individual compliance is necessary to ensure that condoms are used consistently during sexual intercourse.

Modifying Adolescents' Use of Condoms

Changing adolescents' sexual behavior so that condoms are used consistently during sexual intercourse is a formidable challenge. Condom use represents the behavioral endpoint of a decision-making process which weighs relevant internal and external influences: interpersonal, social, economic, psychological influences within a cultural context that are superimposed over traditions, values, and patterns of social organization. Such a complex decision-making process is not likely to be understood in unidimensional or simplistic terms. Unfortunately, sexual behavior, though complex, remains one of the least studied human behaviors.

A myriad of factors—psychological, social, interpersonal, developmental, and cultural—have been hypothesized to play prominent and interactive roles in influencing an adolescent's decision to use condoms. Consequently, understanding the influences underlying an adolescent's decision to use condoms has been difficult, in large part, because many of these factors are not easily defined, isolated, or quantified. While challenging, identifying and understanding the interrelationships between the determinants of condom use, within the context of the STD/HIV epidemic, is of paramount importance if we are to develop more efficacious risk-reduction programs. While an exhaustive review is beyond the scope of this chapter, the following section summarizes empirical findings describing factors affecting adolescents' use of condoms during sexual intercourse.

Factors Associated with Adolescents' Use of Condoms

Though there is considerable variation in the constructs assessed, the adolescent populations studied, and research methodologies utilized, reviews of the factors influencing adolescents' use of condoms (Joffe, 1993; DiClemente, 1992b; Wight, 1992) have identified some potentially important variables associated with condom use which warrant further investigative inquiry. With respect to demographic characteristics, males, white race, and younger adolescents were more likely to be consistent condom users. With respect to ethnic/racial differences, the findings suggest that perhaps cultural factors, not assessed, may be of critical importance in understanding condom use among multicultural adolescent populations. Moreover, the finding that male gender is associated with condom use may reflect inappropriate phrasing of the questions included in interviews and self-administered measures. Younger age, on the other hand, may suggest that these adolescents may have less opportunity to demonstrate a failure to use condoms because they have fewer sex partners or a lower cumulative frequency of sexual episodes.

Behavioral variables also demonstrate predictive capability. Having a sex partner more than 5 years older, smoking, and greater number of lifetime sex partners or risk behaviors were all associated with less condom use. Interestingly, earlier onset of sexuality was not associated with less condom use. Psychosocial constructs have a substantial impact on condom use. In particular, communication about AIDS, condom self-efficacy, and the perception of peer norms supporting condom use were strongly associated with consistent use. Another construct, negative attitudes toward condoms or the perceived costs associated with condom use (e.g., embarrassing, reduce sexual pleasure), was strongly predictive of infrequent condom use. Conversely, enjoyment of condoms and a positive attitude (low costs of use) was highly associated with condom use. Other factors that emerged as potentially important determinants were: perceived condom efficacy to prevent AIDS/HIV infection and, to a lesser extent, perceived susceptibility/worry about AIDS. Other factors were also significant predictors of condom use; however, they were usually isolated findings that were not corroborated by other studies. In some cases, a particular factor was examined in only one study; thus, this factor may be important but, because it lacks confirmation from other studies, it was not emphasized in this summary. More recent surveys, however, have corroborated the importance of many of the factors highlighted in our review above, in particular the effect of peer norms as a potential key mediator of adolescents' sexual decision-making (Romer et al., 1994; Walter et al., 1992).

The studies reviewed are not without limitations. Foremost, the findings cited above are often derived from studies utilizing a cross-sectional research design. Cross-sectional surveys, while informative, are limited in their capacity to delineate the temporal order (causality) between antecedent factors (determinants) and outcomes (condom use). Further, cross-sectional research designs are limited by potential response or recall biases in which adolescents may inaccurately recall past behavior or actively bias their responses. There are, unfortunately, few longitudinal studies available to evaluate the significance and the stability of identified determinants to predict consistent condom use over time.

Findings from Longitudinal Studies

Recently, findings from longitudinal studies of adolescents' sexual behavior have become available. One prospective study was conducted among black adolescents between 12 and 21 years of age residing in two public housing developments in San Francisco (DiClemente et al., 1996). In this study, adolescents were recruited through street outreach and asked to complete a theoretically derived research interview assessing sexual risk behavior, prevention attitudes, and beliefs. Six months later, adolescents completed a follow-up interview similar to the baseline measure.

Among adolescents reporting sexual activity in the 6 months prior to completing the baseline interview ($N = 116$), logistic regression analysis evaluated the influence of demographic, psychosocial, and behavioral factors on frequency of condom use. Adolescents with high assertive self-efficacy to demand condom use, who perceived peer norms as supporting condom use, who had greater impulse control, were male, and were younger were 11, 4.2, 3.7, 4.7, and 2.9 times, respectively, more likely to report consistent condom use. Frequency of sexual intercourse was inversely related to condom use; adolescents with a higher number of sexual episodes were less likely to use condoms consistently.

Prospective analyses identified baseline level of condom use as the best predictor of condom use at 6 month follow-up. Adolescents who were consistent condom users at baseline were 7.4 times as likely to be consistent condom users during the follow-up period. Unfortunately, this study also identified changes in condom use patterns over time. Specifically, of those adolescents changing their frequency of condom use over the follow-up interval, significantly more engaged in risky behavior as 33.3% changed from consistent to inconsistent condom use while 20.6% changed from inconsistent to consistent use (odds ratio = 1.6; $p = 0.0004$). Further longitudinal studies, with longer follow-up periods, are necessary to monitor the stability of psychosocial, behavioral, and demographic factors to explain and predict condom use at subsequent time points.

In general, the findings strongly suggest that effective sexual communication and negotiation skills, the self-efficacy to request condom use, and the perception of HIV-preventive social norms are key factors associated with condom use. In conjunction with more favorable attitudes toward condom use, these factors suggest that HIV prevention efforts for promoting the adoption and maintenance of condom use should strive to incorporate program elements that directly target these critical skills, beliefs, and attitudes.

DESIGN AND EVALUATION OF EFFECTIVE SEXUAL BEHAVIOR MODIFICATION INTERVENTIONS

There is an overriding urgency to develop and implement behavioral interventions that motivate adolescents to adopt and/or maintain STD/HIV prevention practices, particularly condom use, which reduce and/or eliminate the risk of infection. Behavioral change interventions have attempted to reduce or eliminate adolescents' STD/HIV-related risk behaviors. And, admittedly, while modifying adolescents' sexual behavior has been a challenge, there is accumulating data suggesting that increasing adolescents' condom use is an achievable goal.

There is, fortunately, a growing body of prevention interventions that have demonstrated an ability, though modest, to change adolescents' STD/HIV-related sexual risk behaviors. These findings are summarized below. However, it is important to note that adolescents are not a homogeneous population, but rather a mosaic of subgroups, each with differing subcultural values and norms. Thus, the prevention interventions described below, while broadly applicable for changing adolescents' sexual risk behaviors, should be tailored to the needs of specific adolescent subgroups to be maximally effective.

To facilitate a description of prevention interventions, we have elected to provide site-specific analyses which may be useful for interventionists operating in a particular setting. Thus, the following section will be divided into intervention studies conducted in schools, community settings, and clinics. In addition, we will provide an overarching summary delineating commonalities between these interventions and offer suggestions for enhancing the design and implementation of future prevention interventions.

School-Based STD/HIV Prevention Programs

Schools, primarily in response to the growing threat of HIV, are implementing STD/HIV prevention programs in many districts in the United States as the primary strategy for educating adolescents about STDs and HIV (Kenney, Guardado, & Brown, 1989). Initially, programs focused on enhancing adolescents' knowledge of STD/HIV, particularly the identified routes of disease transmission. These programs were based on the explicit assumption that increased knowledge of STD/HIV transmission would result in changes in risk behavior. Unfortunately, many school districts do not rigorously evaluate their programs.

Many of the limited program evaluations indicate no significant behavioral changes, although most suggest increased adolescent knowledge about HIV disease and, to a lesser degree, modification of attitudes. Unfortunately, many of these program evaluations did not or could not measure sexual risk behavior, and thus, there is no evidence of effectiveness in modifying behaviors that increase adolescents' risk for STD/HIV (Office of Technology Assessment, 1988).

Recently, a school-based STD/HIV prevention program has demonstrated a statistically significant effect in reducing adolescents' sexual risk behaviors (Walter & Vaughan, 1993). There are a number of key elements that contribute to the intervention's success. The prevention curriculum is based on established psychological models of behavioral change. Moreover, the investigators were able to target key psychosocial constructs which directly affect adolescents' decision-making and sexual risk-taking based on a needs assessment and recent empirical data. In particular, the prevention curriculum emphasized risk information, self-efficacy and sexual negotiation skills, beliefs about perceived susceptibility, barriers and benefits to engaging in preventive behaviors, and perceptions of the acceptability and norms for involvement in preventive behaviors. Finally, teacher inservice was provided to familiarize teachers with the curriculum.

Based on a 3-month follow-up, the findings indicate that the intervention was most effective in increasing knowledge, changing adolescents' beliefs, enhancing self-efficacy, and, most importantly, reducing high-risk sexual behaviors. Adolescents in the intervention group reported a lower frequency of sexual intercourse with high-risk partners, decreased number of sex partners, and an increase in consistent condom use relative to their peers in the control group.

In another, more recent report, Main and her colleagues (1994) developed a 15-session skills-based HIV prevention curriculum implemented by trained teachers. Using a nonrandomized research design, students in ten schools received the intervention curriculum while students in seven schools were assigned to a comparison condition. Students completed baseline and 6-month follow-up questionnaires designed to assess changes in adolescents' knowledge, attitudes, and sexual behaviors. However, to preserve anonymity, the investigators matched baseline and follow-up questionnaires on the basis of demographic characteristics. This procedure yielded 979 students with both a baseline and follow-up questionnaire.

Results indicate that students receiving the intervention exhibited greater knowledge about HIV and greater intent to engage in safer sex practices than students in the comparison schools. Among sexually active students at the 6-month follow-up assessment, intervention students reported fewer sexual partners within the 2 months prior to assessment ($p = 0.046$), greater frequency of condom use ($p = 0.048$), and greater intentions to engage in sexual intercourse less frequently ($p = 0.017$) and to use condoms when having sexual intercourse ($p = 0.039$). This intervention, however, neither delayed the onset nor decreased the frequency of sexual intercourse and the frequency of alcohol and other drug use before sex.

Clearly, these studies may provide the impetus for the development of a new generation of school-based HIV prevention programs: those that are theoretically based, empirically driven, emphasize social competency skills acquisition, and are systematically evaluated. And although the findings are encouraging, the small effect sizes observed suggest that other innovative and effective strategies are urgently needed to increase the proportion of adolescents who use STD/HIV preventive behaviors (DiClemente, 1993). For instance, in a recent review of school-based prevention programs, several key elements were identified which may enhance program effectiveness (Kirby & DiClemente, 1994). These critical elements include: (1) using social learning theories as a foundation for program development (e.g., social learning theory, cognitive behavioral theory, social influence theory), (2) maintaining a narrow focus on reducing sexual risk-taking behaviors, (3) using active learning methods of instruction, (4) including activities that address the social and/or media influences and pressures to have sex, (5) focusing on and reinforcing clear and appropriate values against unprotected sex (i.e., postponing sex, avoiding unprotected intercourse, avoiding high-risk partners), and (6) providing modeling and practice of communication or negotiation skills. Furthermore, to maximize program effectiveness, HIV/AIDS prevention programs must also be tailored to be developmentally appropriate and culturally relevant.

Community-Based STD/HIV Prevention Programs

Schools offer a great deal of promise for developing and implementing adolescent HIV prevention interventions. However, the impact of schools as agents of change, promoting the adoption and/or maintenance of HIV preventive behaviors, should not be exaggerated. Schools alone will not achieve maximal effectiveness if adolescents live in environments that counteract newly acquired HIV-prevention knowledge and skills. There is ample evidence, for instance, that adolescents who do not attend school are at disproportionately greater risk for HIV infection (CDC, 1993). Thus, community-based HIV prevention interventions may be better able to access this hard-to-reach adolescent population.

Studies conducted with non-school-based adolescent populations indicate that increasing health-promoting behavioral change is possible when skills training is incorporated into prevention curricula. A recent study by Jemmott, Jemmott, and Fong (1992) tested the effectiveness of a sexual risk-reduction intervention for black male adolescents. One hundred and fifty-seven black male adolescents were recruited from a local medical center, community-based organizations, and a local high school and assigned randomly to an HIV risk-reduction condition or a control condition on career opportunities and to a small group of about six boys led by a specially trained black male or female facilitator.

Adolescents in the HIV risk-reduction condition received a 5-hour intervention involving videotapes, games, and exercises aimed at increasing AIDS-related knowledge, weakening problematic beliefs and attitudes toward HIV risk-associated sexual behavior, and increasing skill at negotiating safer sex. Adolescents randomly assigned to the control condition also received a 5-hour intervention. Structurally similar to the HIV risk-reduction intervention, it involved culturally and developmentally appropriate videotapes, exercises, and games, but regarding career opportunities.

Analyses of covariance, controlling for preintervention measures, revealed that adolescents who received the HIV risk-reduction intervention subsequently had greater AIDS knowledge, less favorable attitudes toward risky sexual behavior, and reduced intentions for such behavior compared with adolescents in the control condition. At 3-month follow-up, adolescents in the HIV risk-reduction condition reported less risky sexual behavior in the 3 months postintervention than did those in the control condition. For instance, they reported having coitus less frequently and with fewer women, reported using condoms more consistently during coitus, and fewer of them reported engaging in heterosexual anal intercourse. In summarizing their community-based research, Jemmott and Jemmott (1994) emphasize the need for further methodologically rigorous research design which incorporates social psychological theory in the selection of variables to be assessed and in guiding the development of the behavioral change intervention.

Similarly, a recent study by St. Lawrence and her colleagues (1995) randomly assigned 246 African-American adolescents to an educational program or a social cognitive-behavioral skills intervention in which health educators provided training in correct condom use, sexual assertion, refusal, self-management, problem-solving strategies, and risk recognition. Six- and twelve-month follow-up showed that the behavioral-skills training participants reported a greater percentage of condom-protected intercourse and were more skillful at handling high-risk sexual situations than control participants.

In another community-based prevention program, Rotheram-Borus and her associates (Rotheram-Borus, Koopman, Haignere, & Davies, 1991; Rotheram-Borus, Feldman, Rosario, & Dunne, 1994) developed and evaluated sexual risk-reduction programs for high-risk runaway and homeless adolescents. Over a 2-year period (from 1988 to 1990), consecutive recruitment of adolescents at two residential shelters in New York City (one designated the nonintervention site and the other the intervention site) resulted in 79 and 188 runaways available for enrollment in the program at the intervention and nonintervention sites, respectively. After attrition, the final sample was comprised of 78 adolescents in the intervention condition and 67 adolescents in the nonintervention condition.

Runaways participating in the risk-reduction program were exposed to a multiple-session intervention administered by skilled trainers. The program addressed the following: general knowledge about HIV/AIDS, coping skills, access to health care and other resources, and individual barriers to use of safer sex practices. General HIV knowledge was addressed by having adolescents participate in video and art workshops and review commercial AIDS/HIV videos. Coping skills training addressed runaways' unrealistic expectations regarding emotional and behavioral responses in high-risk situations. Additional medical and mental health care and other resources were made available to address specific individual health concerns. Individual barriers to adopting and maintaining safer sex practices were reviewed in private counseling sessions. Participants in the nonintervention condition were exposed to individual counseling from staff; but this counseling did not specifically address HIV prevention. Condoms were available and staff members, on an unsystematic basis, discussed condom use.

Runaways in the risk-reduction program demonstrated a significant and dramatic increase in consistent condom use and less frequently reported engaging in a high-risk

SEXUALLY TRANSMITTED DISEASES

pattern of HIV-associated behaviors over 6 months. A high-risk pattern of sexual behavior was defined as consistent condom use occurring in fewer than 50% of sexual encounters, ten or more sexual encounters, and/or three or more sexual partners. A greater proportion of adolescents (22%) in the control group reported this high-risk pattern of sexual behavior compared to those adolescents (9%) who received between 10 and 14 intervention sessions and those (0%) who received 15 or more intervention sessions. Reports of consistent condom use increased from about 32% of runaways at initiation of the project to 62% 6 months after receiving more than 15 intervention sessions. A 2-year follow-up of the same sample continued to show significant reductions in risk acts among those who received the intervention.

Clinic-Based STD/HIV Prevention Programs

While school and community-based prevention efforts are undoubtedly important in disseminating HIV prevention information, another critical, but underutilized, access point for educating adolescents about STD/HIV is during the provision of health care. Physicians, in particular pediatricians and adolescent medicine specialists, are most likely to be engaged in treating adolescents during the time of their onset of sexual and drug behaviors. Thus, clinical interactions between the pediatrician and adolescent patient become an opportunity to assess the prevalence of sexual and drug risk behaviors, evaluate the adolescent's physical and psychological maturation, and provide developmentally appropriate HIV prevention information (DiClemente & Brown, 1994).

In one recent report, the effects of physicians' assessment of adolescents' risk behaviors and counseling about HIV risks and prevention were evaluated in an inner-city hospital-based adolescent clinic (Mansfield, Conroy, Emans, & Woods, 1993). Ninety adolescents (mean age 17.6 years) seeking care were randomly assigned to one of two groups: a standard care group in which physicians interviewed adolescents about high-risk behaviors related to HIV disease and a counseling group in which physicians provided discussion of HIV risks and prevention. At follow-up, approximately 2 months after baseline assessments and randomization, 25% of patients reported less sexual activity, 32 and 18%, respectively, of the standard care and counseling group reported less sexual activity. Consistent use of condoms also significantly increased among adolescents in both groups (standard care, $p = 0.03$; counseling, $p = 0.02$). Use of condoms at last intercourse increased in the counseling group from 37% to 42% ($p = 0.03$).

Another adolescent clinic-based intervention implemented a peer educator risk-reduction program targeting multiethnic females 12–19 years of age (Slap, Plotkin, Khalid, Michelman, & Forke, 1991). This study used a single group pretest–posttest research design to evaluate an intervention consisting of a single counseling session of HIV education and condom skills administered by peer educators using observational learning techniques (i.e., videos and brochures). At follow-up, 2–6 weeks after baseline assessment, adolescents demonstrated increased HIV knowledge ($p < 0.05$), decreased frequency of sexual intercourse ($p < 0.05$), and decreased frequency of times adolescents reported "never using condoms" during sexual intercourse from 22% at baseline to 11% at follow-up ($p < 0.05$).

Overall, the findings from school, community, and hospital-based studies suggest that behavioral change, while difficult, is attainable. Significant reductions in adolescents' risk behaviors over a brief and less often, extended follow-up period, have been reported. Thus, while much more remains to be learned, these findings are promising and suggest key intervention constructs that may enhance the efficacy of prevention interventions.

Components Critical to the Success of STD/HIV Prevention Interventions

There are several key theoretical and implementation features that appear to be associated with changing adolescents' sexual risk behavior. Foremost, programs need to be tailored to meet the specific needs of different adolescent populations. "Tailoring" would include ensuring that the intervention was culturally sensitive, developmentally appropriate, and gender-relevant (Wingood & DiClemente, 1992, 1995; Airhihenbuwa, DiClemente, Wingood, & Lowe, 1992; Fullilove, Fullilove, Bowser, & Gross, 1990).

Second, utilizing a theoretical model on which to base the intervention, one that addresses the interplay between the adolescents' cognitions, attitudes, and beliefs, their behavior and environmental influences, improves the likelihood of programmatic efficacy. This is a critical consideration. Sexual behavior, in particular, takes place within a social-cultural context. Understanding the contextual nature of adolescents' behavior, the factors that promote the adoption of preventive behaviors, and those countervailing influences that reinforce risk-taking behavior, is programmatically important. One model that is particularly useful as a foundation for developing sexual risk-reduction behavioral change interventions, especially for adolescents and multicultural populations, is Social Cognitive Theory (Bandura, 1992, 1994). The cornerstones of this model include the provision of timely and accurate information, developing and mastering social competency skills through observational learning techniques (e.g., social modeling) and active learning techniques (e.g., role playing, preferably a series of graded-intensity high-risk situations), enhancing self-efficacy to communicate assertively and effectively with sex partners, and developing a supportive peer network to reinforce the maintenance of safer sex behaviors. Many of the effective prevention interventions reviewed earlier were based on this model.

Another key component is maintaining a narrow focus on reducing sexual risk-taking behaviors. Thus, each sexual risk behavior targeted for change, whether it enhances condom use, reduces the number of sexual partners, or even postpones sexual intercourse, should be clearly specified with appropriate strategies designed to directly address them. This is of critical importance, for too often prevention programs have targeted a broad spectrum of risk behaviors for change without including behavior-specific change strategies in the program. An example will help to illustrate this key concept. For instance, designing a prevention intervention to enhance adolescents' self-efficacy to reduce their number of sexual partners is an important and appropriate endpoint. However, the behavior-specific strategies and techniques used to enhance their self-efficacy may not generalize to increasing self-efficacy to assert that sex partners use condoms. Thus, while there may be generalized effects attributable to participation in a prevention program, in general, the techniques and strategies should be narrowly focused rather than assuming that these skills and knowledge will be translated by the adolescent to other behaviors or situations. Programs designed to reduce the number of sex partners and increase condom use are addressing two important, but qualitatively different, risk behaviors. To be maximally effective, each risk behavior, the underlying psychosocial factors that reinforce these behaviors, and the strategies and skills needed to achieve behavioral change must be adequately addressed.

Finally, there are specific psychosocial constructs that have been identified as associated with condom use. Interventions that are tailored to emphasize these constructs are more likely to be effective in modifying adolescents' behavior. Key constructs include: (1) providing specific skills training in sexual communication, negotiation, and assertiveness skills; (2) enhancing adolescents' perceptions of peer norms as supporting safer sex behavior; (3) enhancing self-efficacy to avoid high-risk situations and refuse high-risk sex; (4) increasing adolescents' awareness of the effects of alcohol and drug use on their sexual behavior, and (5) providing condom use skills and increasing the availability of condoms.

Though we have identified core components of prevention interventions that have yielded promising results, given the magnitude of observed behavioral changes reported and the limited follow-up periods for evaluating the stability of treatment effects, new and innovative intervention approaches are needed. One approach, used by Slap *et al.* (1991), is to utilize peer educators to implement prevention intervention. Peer-based interventions represent an underutilized implementation strategy that may be particularly effective for promoting adolescents' adoption of safer sex behaviors.

Peer Involvement: An Implementation Strategy That May Enhance Program Efficacy

Theoretically, peer involvement offers a number of advantages over traditional, didactic, STD/HIV prevention programs. Derived from Social Cognitive Theory, and based in developmental theory, peer-facilitated interventions recruit and train peers indigenous to a large target population to serve as leaders, educators, and counselors. Peer involvement targets two theoretically important psychosocial constructs related to consistent condom use: communication between sex partners and peer norms (DiClemente, 1992b; Joffe, 1993; Wight, 1992). For instance, research findings indicate that even high-risk incarcerated adolescents are influenced by these factors. In a study of incarcerated adolescents in San Francisco, adolescents who report discussing HIV with their sex partners and those who perceived peer norms to be supportive of condom use were approximately 15 and 7 times, respectively, more likely to report being consistent condom users (DiClemente, 1991).

Peer-facilitated interventions have been used with adolescents to address a variety of health behavior problems. Peer interventions with adolescents have successfully delayed onset of smoking, decreased alcohol use, and reduced initiation and prevalence rates of marijuana use (Botvin, 1986; Perry & Grant, 1988; Robinson *et al.*, 1987; Telch *et al.*, 1990; Hansen & Graham, 1991; Klepp, Halper, & Perry, 1986). Overall, the data suggest that peer-assisted programs are more effective than didactic programs without peer involvement in modifying health-risk behaviors.

Peer interventions offer a number of advantages over adult-led programs when working with adolescents. Peers may be more effective teachers of social skills, more influential models of health-promoting behavior, and can serve as credible role models because they are members of the adolescents' social milieu. Peers can also help to change normative expectations about the frequency of the targeted behavior in the peer group. Finally, peers can offer social support for performance of desired behaviors and for avoidance of health-damaging behaviors. These advantages are particularly important when educating adolescents in inner-city environments where social networks are limited and social norms, which may encourage and support risk-taking behavior, are highly influential (DiClemente & Houston-Hamilton, 1989).

Several studies have successfully used peer-based models for reducing high-risk sexual behavior in adult populations (Kelly *et al.*, 1991). However, peer interventions, such as the one developed by Slap *et al.* (1991), are just now being evaluated with adolescents. Perry and Sieving (1993) describe promising peer-led programs designed to reach especially high-risk and hard-to-access populations of homeless and out-of-school adolescents. Although not yet published, available data indicate that peer leaders were positively perceived by other youth and were effective at communicating sexual risk-reduction messages and dispelling perceptions of high-risk sexual behavior as normative. Clearly, peer involvement in the implementation of STD/HIV prevention interventions warrants further consideration as one strategy for enhancing programmatic efficacy.

Development of STD/HIV Prevention Curricula

To be effective, STD/HIV prevention curricula must (1) include the most recent medical information about the cause, transmission, and prevention of HIV disease; (2) identify and discuss known risk factors; and (3) clearly and unequivocally dispel myths and misconceptions about HIV acquisition, especially the myth of casual contagion of HIV disease.

Adolescents who harbor misconceptions about casual contact have reported unnecessarily high and at times debilitating levels of fear and anxiety regarding their personal susceptibility to HIV infection. Dispelling such misconceptions may therefore reduce unnecessary fear and anxiety and the potential for stigmatization of segments of the population most adversely affected by the STD/AIDS epidemic.

STD/HIV prevention curricula, whether used in school, community, or clinical settings, need to go beyond didactic presentation of information about signs and symptoms of disease. Curricula should employ interactive learning techniques that emphasize development of social competency skills, especially communication and negotiation about sex, assertiveness, resistance and insistence, and recognition of supportive peer norms. Skills in communication and negotiation about safer sex help adolescents avoid risk situations and increase the likelihood of condom use. Resistance to negative peer pressure to engage in risky behaviors and assertiveness training are also important. In general, the objective of the curriculum is to enhance adolescents' decision-making skills about unsafe or drug practices and to provide effective coping strategies that permit a "range of options" for risk management, while not isolating them from their friends or alienating adolescents from their peers.

Specific strategies useful for enhancing adolescents' social skills include the following: (1) decision-making exercises, (2) rehearsal of communication skills such as asking partners to use condoms, (3) learning techniques of resistance to negative peer pressure through guided role-play scenarios, (4) group discussions to modify adolescents' attitudes and values toward condom use, and (5) behavioral training to increase adolescents' confidence to use newly acquired information and skills gained in role-play scenarios in real-life risk situations (Flora and Thoresen, 1989).

It is not necessary to develop STD/HIV prevention curricula. The CDC's AIDS Health Education Subfile provides curricula that incorporate many of these recommendations. In addition to the curriculum components described above, STD/HIV prevention curricula should also be (1) tailored to the maturational level of the target audience, (2) culturally sensitive, and (3) structured so that those administering the curricula will feel comfortable in using them.

Future Directions in STD/HIV Prevention

In general, promising STD/HIV prevention programs have been developed and evaluated. This does not mean, however, that these programs cannot be improved. While demonstrating the ability to significantly enhance adolescents' adoption and use of STD/HIV prevention strategies, the magnitude of effects has been generally modest. Future programs must be developed and evaluated on an ongoing basis to monitor programmatic efficacy. Programs must be modified according to evaluation feedback. And, finally, programs that are evaluated and identified as effective should be widely disseminated to encourage their adoption and use.

TREATMENT

Diagnosis and Treatment of STDs in Adolescents

Despite the best prevention efforts of patients, their health care providers, and public health officials, adolescents will continue to develop STDs. Although specific biologic organisms are responsible for STD syndromes in adolescents as well as in adults, clinical presentations for diagnostic and therapeutic purposes will be on the basis of presenting complaints and immediate physical and laboratory findings. For this reason, we will group the specific STDs by syndrome and comment on the most efficient diagnostic approaches and therapeutic regimens for use in adolescent patients.

General Principles

Adolescents will often not seek medical care until they are very symptomatic. Moreover, they may not return for follow-up evaluation and often do not adhere to medication regimens. Finally, adolescents may or may not be able to effectively communicate with their sex partners and inform them of their own infection and the possibility that either they were infected by or transmitted their infection to their partners. Given these concerns, certain approaches that simplify the diagnostic and therapeutic process are warranted in adolescents (Table 5). These principles include the following.

1. *Treat patients on the basis of history and epidemiology of disease syndromes.* Patients may present with a history of symptoms that are not immediately verifiable. Other patients will present with a history of an STD exposure and no symptoms what-

Table 5.   General Principles of Treating Sexually Transmitted Diseases
in Adolescents

Principle 1. Treat on basis of history of exposure and epidemiology of disease
Principle 2. If possible, treat at time of evaluation
Principle 3. Use simple (preferably single dose) regimens
Principle 4. Remember that multiple infections are likely
Principle 5. Females suspected of having an STD should be screened for possible pregnancy
Principle 6. Patients suspected of having an STD are candidates for HIV testing

soever. Rather than waiting for definitive diagnostic information, health care providers are
urged to plan treatment of adolescents on the basis of their histories and to use physical
and laboratory findings to modify the therapeutic approach. This means treating asymptomatic males on the basis of history of exposure to a partner or partners with an STD.
This can be challenging, making it necessary for providers to sometimes decide therapy
on the basis of what condition or conditions might be most common in a particular patient
or group of patients. For instance, the male patient exposed to a female with a vaginal
discharge should be treated for *both N. gonorrhoeae* and *C. trachomatis.*

2. *Diagnosis and treatment should take place in the same office session.* While
diagnostic tests that take more time than a single office session are appropriate to defini-
tively diagnose a syndrome and provide crucial epidemiologic information, patients
strongly suspected on the basis of history of physical findings to have a sexually transmitted infection should receive treatment. This will hopefully lessen the likelihood that an
untreated infection will be spread to others, and will make a return visit, while *highly*
desirable, not an absolute necessity. If this is not practical, possible, or desirable, every
effort must be made to ensure that the patient will be able to be contacted and informed of
the testing results. In an effort to maintain confidentially for this information, a special
"call back" time or method of contacting the patient will be necessary.

3. *Treatment regimens should be as simple as possible and administered in the
context of the diagnostic office visit if possible.* This approach would emphasize the use of
single-dose medications, such as a unit dose of azithromycin instead of multidose doxycycline to treat chlamydia infection. While the latter therapy is cheaper and may even be
more efficacious in eradicating infection in those who actually take the medication as
prescribed, the higher cost and slight reduction in therapeutic response of the single-dose
treatment are certainly justifiable on the basis of being able to provide immediate therapy
and eliminate the need for the patient to have to take medication multiple times daily for 7
to 10 days.

4. *Remember that multiple infections may be present in a single patient.* Suspecting
or confirming a diagnosis of one STD should not preclude the practitioner from considering and looking for other possible infections. When treatment is initiated, regimens that
may actually treat several pathogens at once should be favored if at all possible.

5. *Adolescent female patients who present for evaluation of an STD should always be
screened for possible pregnancy.* This should also include patients who are using a reliable
form of contraception (birth control pills, injectable medroxyprogesterone, subdermal
levonorgesterol) on a regular basis to account for possible human or method failure. This

test should then be used to plan what form of therapy will be utilized since certain medications should not be used in pregnancy.

6. *Patients at risk of any STD are at risk of HIV infection as well.* Special care must be employed in identifying patients at even greater risk (injection drug users; patients who have traded sex for drugs, money, or shelter; males who have had sex with other males; males or females with a past or current history of syphilis; males with hemophilia who have received factor therapy; anyone who received a blood transfusion prior to 1985). HIV testing should be available and offered to those at risk of HIV infection. Regular HIV testing needs to be done in patients who continue to be at risk of infection.

Diagnosis and Treatment of Specific Infections

Urethritis

This infection, an inflammation of the anterior urethra, is more commonly related to a sexually transmitted pathogen in men than in women. While such urethral infections can be asymptomatic, patients will usually complain of burning and stinging on urination and a urethral discharge. Back pain, fever, pelvic pain (in women), perirectal pain, and pain during ejaculation (in men) suggest upper urinary tract or genital organ (adnexa, prostate) involvement.

The most common organisms causing asymptomatic urethritis are *C. trachomatis* and *N. gonorrhoeae*. A variety of other pathogens (e.g., *Ureaplasma urealyticum, Trichomonas vaginalis, Staphylococcus epidermidis*) are often grouped with chlamydia infections under the category "nongonococcal urethritis" (NGU). In the United States, NGU is more commonly the cause of urethritis than is *N. gonorrhoeae*. In economically disadvantaged communities, the reverse is often true (Rice *et al.*, 1991; Zimmerman *et al.*, 1990). There is great overlap in the clinical syndromes produced by these different organisms.

Diagnosis. For asymptomatic males, screening a first void urine with the use of a leukocyte esterase dipstick may identify up to 80% of males with urethritis (Sadof, Woods, & Emans, 1987; Shafer *et al.*, 1993b). Those with symptoms can bypass this screening test and have a specimen of urethral discharge obtained via Dacron swab from the anterior urethra. While culture for *N. gonorrhoeae* on special microbiologic media and testing for *C. trachomatis* by means of direct immunofluorescent antibody test (DFA) or enzyme-linked immunoassay (EIA) are the diagnostic standard in many clinical settings, in male patients, simple Gram stain of the urethral discharge will allow reliable differentiation between gonococcal and nongonococcal urethritis and produce a remarkable overall cost savings (D'Angelo, Mohla, & Sneed, 1987). On Gram stain, patients with gonorrhea will have gram-negative diplococci embedded in polymorphonuclear leukocytes. The absence of these bacteria suggests a diagnosis of NGU.

Treatment. While it is of value to distinguish the type pathogen causing a patient's symptoms, the initial treatment of urethritis is the same for patients with gonococcal or nongonococcal urethritis (Table 6). The antibiotic of choice according to the Centers for Disease Control and Prevention (CDC, 1993) is doxycycline, 100 mg orally twice daily. If

Table 6.   Treatment of Sexually Transmitted Disease Syndromes in Adolescents

Syndrome/infection	Treatment regimen(s)

Urethritis	a. Unknown pathogen
	    • Doxycycline* 100 mg po BID × 7 days
	b. GC confirmed
	    • Cefixime 400 mg po × 1 dose or
	    • Ceftriaxone 125 mg IM × 1 dose or
	    • Cefpodoxime 200 mg po × 1 dose
	c. Chlamydia confirmed
	    • Azithromycin 1 g po × 1 dose

Vaginitis/cervicitis	a. Unknown pathogen
	    • Cefpodoxime 200 mg po × 1 dose plus doxycycline[a]
	     100 mg po BID × 7 days or
	    • Azithromycin 1 g po × 1 dose 100 mg po BID × 7 days
	b. GC confirmed
	    • Ceftriaxone 250 mg IM × 1 dose
	c. Chlamydia confirmed
	    • Doxycycline[a] 100 mg po BID × 7 days or
	    • Azithromycin 1 g po × 1 dose or
	    • Erythromycin base 500 mg po QID × 7 days or
	    • Erythromycin ethylsuccinate 800 mg po QID × 7 days

Genital ulcer syndrome	a. HSV suspected or confirmed
	    • Acyclovir* 200 mg 5×/day × 7 days (first episode)
	    • Acyclovir* 200 mg 5×/day × 5 days (subsequent episodes)
	b. Syphilis suspected or confirmed early
	    • Benzathine penicillin G, 2.4 million units IM in single dose
	    • Doxycycline* 100 mg BID × 14 days
	c. Syphilis suspected or confirmed late
	    • Benzathine penicillin G, 7.2 million units IM in 3 weekly
	     doses of 2.4 million units
	d. Chancroid, suspected or confirmed
	    • Azithromycin 1 g po × 1 dose or
	    • Ceftriaxone 250 mg IM × 1 dose or
	    • Erythromycin base 500 mg po QID × 7 days

Genital warts/human
  papilloma virus
	• Cryotherapy with liquid nitrogen or cryoprobe weekly
	  × 6 weeks
	• Podophyllin* 10–25% applied once weekly × 6 weeks;
	  wash off in 1–4 hr
	• Trichloroacetic acid applied once weekly × 6 weeks

Pelvic inflammatory disease	a. Outpatient regimen
	    • Ceftriaxone 250 mg IM × 1 dose plus doxycycline[a]
	     100 mg po BID × 14 days
	b. Inpatient regimen
	    • Cefoxitin 2 g IV q 6 hr × 4–7 days plus doxycycline[a]
	     100 mg po q 12 hr × 14 days
	    • Clindamycin 900 mg IV q 8 hr plus gentamicin 80 mg
	     (1.5 mg/kg) IV q 8 hr. [Complete 14 days of therapy
	     with doxycycline 100 mg po BID]

[a]Contraindicated in pregnancy.

the diagnosis of gonococcal urethritis is certain, ceftriaxone 125 mg in a single IM dose, cefixime 400 mg orally in a single dose, cefpodoxime 200 mg orally in a single dose are acceptable antibiotics to use in adolescents. If the diagnosis of chlamydia is certain, azithromycin 1 g orally in a single dose is an acceptable albeit more expensive alternative approach to therapy. Since compliance for a full 7 days of therapy with an antibiotic will be challenging for most adolescents, we recommend treating with a combination of acceptable single-dose regimes (i.e., azithromycin and an IM or po cephalosporin).

Follow-up. Patients with suspected or proven *N. gonorrhoeae* infection should have a urethral culture for a "test-of-cure" in 7 to 10 days. Retesting for chlamydia is usually not necessary in patients with urethritis.

Vaginitis/Cervicitis

The majority of vaginal and lower genital tract infections in women are *not* sexually transmitted. Infections caused by various fungal species as well as infections caused by anaerobic bacteria can be seen in women who are not sexually active. A variety of pathogens that can be transmitted person-to-person via sexual intercourse can also cause infection and inflammation of the lower genital tract. Among the most common of these is infection with the parasite *Trichomonas vaginalis.* Up to 25% of women with this infection will be asymptomatic. The rest will have some combination of vaginal symptoms including vaginal discharge and vulvovaginal irritation. The other common sexually transmitted pathogens, *Chlamydia* and *N. gonorrhoeae,* cause infection of the cervix. As mentioned earlier, the fact that columnar epithelium covers a larger portion of the cervix in adolescents than in adults makes adolescents more susceptible to cervical infections, particularly those caused by *C. trachomatis* and *N. gonorrhoeae.*

Infections of the vaginal mucosa are more likely to present with vaginal and vulvar itching and irritation as well as vaginal discharge. Cervical infections frequently have less overt irritation externally, but may have associated abdominal and pelvic pain and tenderness, particularly if the infection has extended upward into the uterine endometrium and Fallopian tubes. Irritation and friability of the cervical os as well as discharge directly from the os are highly suggestive of cervical infection with either *C. trachomatis* or *N. gonorrhoeae.*

Diagnosis. Similar to the evaluation of patients with urethritis, physical exam should confirm the presence of a discharge, attempt to localize its source, then be directed to ensuring the lack of associated infections such as condyloma accuminata (genital warts), genital ulcers, or upper genital tract infection (Biro *et al.,* 1994). In order to accomplish this, the care provider will need to perform a full pelvic exam. This should include a speculum exam and a bimanual exam. It is also desirable to examine a sampling of vaginal discharge or secretions by mixing with a drop of saline and viewing this under the microscope. An increased number of white blood cells (> 1 WBC/epithelial cell) suggests ongoing infection or inflammation. The discharge should also be tested with pH indicator paper. A pH above 4.5 suggests some sort of active infection. Cultures for *N.*

gonorrhoeae and rapid diagnostic tests for *C. trachomatis* should be obtained on all patients. Unlike male patients with urethritis, Gram stain of vaginal or cervical discharge is not usually diagnostic.

   Treatment.   Therapy of vaginal and cervical infections with *C. trachomatis* and *N. gonorrhoeae* infections are similar to the regimens suggested for urethritis (Table 6). Because of the high frequency of dual infections with both of these organisms, a combination of medications that will treat both organisms is strongly recommended. An example of such a regimen would be cefpodoxime 200 mg orally in a single dose and doxycycline 100 mg twice daily for 7 days. Alternatively, azithromycin 1 g orally in a single dose could be used instead of doxycycline if cost is not a major issue and there is concern over possible lack of compliance. Since pregnancy obviates the use of doxycyline or other tetracycline antibiotics, for pregnant females who are suspected or proven to have gonococcal or chlamydia cervicitis, IM ceftriaxone (250 mg) and oral erythromycin (500 mg 4 times daily for 7 days or 250 mg 4 times daily for 14 days of base preparation or 800 or 400 mg 4 times daily for 7 or 14 days, respectively, of the ethylsuccinate preparation) are recommended. The intramuscular higher dose of ceftriaxone is preferred because of the greater concern for endometrial infection in pregnant patients. Although azithromycin appears to be safe, it is not yet approved for use in pregnant patients.

   Vaginal or cervical infections with trichomonas should be treated with a single 2-g dose of metronidazole orally. If this cannot be tolerated as a single dose, 500 mg orally twice daily should be given for 7 days. Metronidazole cannot be used in pregnant patients within the first trimester. After that interval, standard doses of the drug can be utilized.

   Follow-up.   Because of the high percentage of patients who can harbor vaginal or cervical infections without symptoms, test or cure cultures for gonococcal cervicitis at 7–10 days after completing therapy and repeat diagnostic testing for chlamydia 21–28 days are strongly recommended. No repeat testing is recommended in follow-up of trichomonas infections.

Genital Ulcer Syndrome

   In adolescents and young adults, herpes simplex virus infection is the leading cause of genital ulcer syndrome. Syphilis is the next most likely cause in this age group. Chancroid, caused by the bacterium *Haemophilus ducreyi,* is a distant third (Silber, 1986). While chancroid is a severe infection that can cause much discomfort, it will usually resolve on its own, even without treatment. In contrast, both herpes and syphilis have the potential to be chronic infections of significant morbidity. They differ in that the spirochete that causes syphilis, *Treponema pallidum,* responds dramatically to treatment with penicillin while the chronic relapsing course of herpes infection is not altered by treatment with the antiviral drug acyclovir, even though this treatment shortens the course of infection. All three infections have the added complication of placing victims at increased risk of HIV infection.

   While each of these infections is characterized by ulcers, they are distinctly different in their presentations. Genital herpes infection is initially characterized by groups of small vesicles on an erythematous base. These rupture leaving tender, shallow-based ulcers with sharp margins. The primary lesion of both chancroid and syphilis is a painless papule that then breaks down to an expanding ulcer. The ulcer of syphilis, the chancre, is usually deep with "heaped up" margins but is remarkably painless. On the other hand, the ulcer of chancroid is deep but painful. The chancre of syphilis is characteristically a single lesion while chancroid ulcers often occur as multiple lesions.

Syphilis is unique in that the primary infection and ulceration will heal without therapy, but the organism will remain viable in the host. It can then reappear in 4 to 26 weeks as a systemic illness characterized by fever, rash, and sore throat. This "secondary syphilis" may also be accompanied by genital ulceration, with the ulcers less well defined than in the primary infection. Herpes infection may also recur with characteristic genital lesions appearing on a variable basis for years after the primary infection.

Diagnosis.   While physical examination and history are highly suggestive, laboratory diagnostic testing can provide useful corroborating information on patients with genital ulcers. For herpes simplex infections, viral cultures can be obtained by swabbing the base of the ulcer. For chancroid, special nutritive media are necessary but can allow for growth of the somewhat fastidious bacterium. For syphilis, direct observation of material swabbed from the base of the ulcer under a special darkfield microscope can reveal the characteristic motile spirochetes. Alternatively, a blood test for antibodies stimulated by the presence of the spirochete can be obtained. Sometimes the blood test will not be positive for several weeks to months after infection takes place.

Treatment.   The antiviral drug acyclovir in a dose of 200 mg orally taken 5 times a day for 7–10 days will shorten the course of a primary or reactivation case of herpes (Table 6). Unfortunately, it does not appear that the drug alters the likelihood of experiencing a recurrence of the genital ulcerations at a later date. For chancroid, azithromycin in a single 1-g oral dose or ceftriaxone in a single 250-mg IM injection are usually curative. Alternative regimens with other antibiotics have the disadvantage of requiring multiple doses for 3 to 7 days (erythromycin base, 500 mg orally 4 times daily for 7 days; amoxicillin 500 mg plus clavulanic acid 125 mg orally 3 times daily for 7 days; ciprofloxacin 500 mg orally 2 times daily for 3 days). Primary and secondary syphilis can be treated with a single dose of long-acting benzathine penicillin, 2.4 million units IM. In patients with severe penicillin allergies, doxycycline 100 mg orally twice daily for 14 days is an appropriate alternative treatment regimen. In patients who have blood tests positive for antibodies with no history of prior infection ("latent syphilis of unknown duration"), three weekly injections of benzathine penicillin, 2.4 million units IM is the recommended course of therapy.

Follow-up.   No follow-up is recommended for either chancroid or herpes genital ulceration. For syphilis, assessing the response to treatment is difficult. The titer of antibodies will usually fall, but over a variable time period. It is recommended that patients be reexamined clinically and by repeat blood test 3 months after treatment.

Genital Warts/Human Papilloma Virus Infection

The exophytic, warty-appearing lesions on the external genitalia are an indication of infection with the human papilloma virus. Many types of this virus can produce wart lesions, with types 6 and 11 being the most common and also being the least likely to be associated with dysplasia and carcinoma (linked with types 16, 18, 33, and 35). Most infections with this virus will not cause overt symptoms, however, and the actual prevalence of infection with HPV in adolescents is *much* higher than the prevalence of observable genital warts in this age group (Becker *et al.,* 1987).

Diagnosis. The external lesion of genital warts, known as condyloma accuminata, is a polyploid mass of tissue with a fissured and irregular surface often described as "cauliflower" in appearance. Flatter white plaques are usually seen on mucosal surfaces, including the uterine cervix. On mucosal surfaces, these lesions will turn intensely white when 5% acetic acid is applied. In women, the Papanicolaou smear (Pap smear), a cytologic examination of cells scraped from the surface of the cervix, may show changes suggestive of HPV infection. This test is only a screen, however, for women who need more definitive diagnostic techniques such as culposcopy and biopsy. Even this more invasive testing will show changes in the host but will not necessarily define actual viral infection. Sophisticated molecular genetic techniques can identify DNA from the virus, but at this time these tests are of little practical value.

Treatment. The purpose of treating genital warts is to remove the external manifestations of HPV infection or to treat cellular changes induced by the virus (Table 6). At this time there is no therapy available that can actually eradicate the virus. Cryotherapy with liquid nitrogen or via a cryoprobe is effective in three out of four cases in removing external lesions. Similar results can be achieved by using one of several caustic chemicals that must be applied by a health care provider, including podophyllin (10–25%) and trichloroacetic acid. A new regimen that the patient can apply utilizes podofilox, a chemical agent similar in structure to podophyllin. Both podophyllin and podofilox must be avoided in pregnancy. Cryotherapy is also the treatment of choice for intravaginal or cervical lesions.

Follow-up. While no special follow-up is necessary once the warts have responded to therapy, women with abnormal cytologic exams should be seen every 6 months. Patients with external lesions should be made aware that they are contagious to others. In both males and females who have had genital warts, the regular use of condoms should be emphasized.

Pelvic Inflammatory Disease

This syndrome, commonly referred to as PID, is actually an array of infectious disorders of the upper genital tract in women, including endometritis, salpingitis, tuboovarian abscess, and pelvic peritonitis. Sexually transmitted infections, and in particular infection by *N. gonorrhoeae* and/or *C. trachomatis,* are the most likely causes of this syndrome. However, other pathogens such as *Mycoplasma hominis* and *Ureaplasma urealyticum* have also been mentioned as potential etiologic agents.

Diagnosis. The diagnosis of PID is based on physical findings including abdominal pain, cervical motion tenderness, and adnexal tenderness. Evaluating a patient for these findings necessitates a pelvic examination with appropriate cultures and/or rapid diagnostic tests for *N. gonorrhoeae* and *C. trachomatis*. However, the decision to treat patients with PID should not await the results of these tests, since many individuals with PID will have negative microbiologic results despite ample clinical evidence of infection.

Despite this approach, since symptoms may not be severe enough to prompt women to seek medical care, many cases of PID are probably undetected. When the diagnosis is not made, or when inadequate therapy is received, complications such as scarring of the Fallopian tubes can ultimately result in severe consequences such as ectopic pregnancy. For this reason, health care providers are urged to have a high index of suspicion for this diagnosis and treat women aggressively even when the actual diagnosis may not be 100% certain. In women at increased risk of tuboovarian abscesses (adolescents, those with prior PID, those who are pregnant), a sonogram (transabdominal and/or transvaginal) should be performed.

Treatment. The medication regimens for PID must be broad enough to cover the array of potential pathogens (Table 6). While many patients can be given medication as outpatients, hospitalization is recommended for those women in whom the diagnosis is uncertain, a pelvic abscess is suspected, there is concurrent HIV infection, the patient is unable (nausea and vomiting) or unwilling to take oral medication, the patient is pregnant, or, according to some, merely if the patient is an adolescent. The regimen for outpatients is 250 mg of ceftriaxone IM plus 100 mg of doxycycline orally twice daily for 14 days. For inpatients the regimen is cefoxitin 2 g IV every 6 hours and doxycycline 100 mg orally every 12 hours. An alternative inpatient regimen utilizes clindamycin 900 mg IV every 8 hours plus gentamicin 1.5 mg/kg IV every 8 hours (after an initial loading dose of 2 mg/kg).

Follow-up. In addition to the patient, the sex partner(s) of the patient should be empirically treated for gonorrhea and chlamydia infections. Women who have been admitted to the hospital can be discharged 48 hours after substantial clinical improvement (usually 4–7 days after initiating therapy) and should be seen within 7–10 days to assess overall clinical status. Those women treated as outpatients must be reevaluated within 72 hours and if not substantially improved, should be admitted for inpatient therapy.

HIV Infection/AIDS

Adolescents who are sexually active and at risk of other STDs are also at risk of HIV infection. While adolescents who have participated in acknowledged high-risk behaviors are more likely to be exposed to HIV infection, the majority of teens carrying the virus either have other exposure and transmission experiences not captured in most behavioral surveys done in HIV-infected adolescents or are not giving an accurate history of their risk behaviors (Stiffman & Earls, 1990).

Because of the long time from infection to actual manifestation of signs and symptoms of chronic HIV infection, most adolescents who are infected are asymptomatic. However, at the time of diagnosis a surprising number show significant evidence of immunosuppression. At this time there is insufficient information concerning the natural history of HIV infection in adolescents as compared with adults and children. Early studies that followed adolescent hemophiliacs implied that individuals in this age group might be more resilient in maintaining their health status, but anecdotal observations in other HIV-infected populations point to a more rapid course of illness.

Concurrent sexually transmitted infections, and ulcerogenital infections in particular, appear to increase the risk of acquiring HIV infection. Other risk factors include the number of sexual partners, nature of sexual practices, and the use of injection drugs.

Diagnosis.   Since the majority of adolescent patients with HIV infection will be asymptomatic, the diagnosis of infection is most often the result of screening an individual with some risk behavior for the presence of antibodies in the blood. Since it may take up to 6 months after acute infection to develop these antibodies, serial testing is often necessary, particularly if an adolescent is involved in ongoing risk behaviors. The procedure is a two-step process with the blood first screened for the presence of antibodies by means of an enzyme-linked immunosorbant assay (EIA). Positive specimens are then confirmed by means of a sophisticated electrophoretic assay, the Western blot test.

While any sexually active adolescent is at risk of HIV infection, the following appear to be the cohorts of patients for whom HIV testing should be particularly recommended: male teens who have had sex with other males; females or males who have used injection drugs; females or males who have had sex with injection drug users; females or males with a history of other STDs (particularly genital ulcer diseases); females or males who have engaged in the exchange of sex for drugs, money, shelter, or goods; females or males who have received blood or blood component transfusions; and females or males with a history of four or more sexual partners or partners who are 2 or more years older. Most adolescent care providers recommend confidential as opposed to anonymous testing because the former will allow for immediate linkage to support and care services.

Patients with concomitant opportunistic infections or profound immunosuppression (CD_4 lymphocyte count < 200 cells/mm^3) are currently classified as having AIDS. It is apparent that for the most part this is a distinction of little consequence other than as a means to better surveillance.

Treatment.   Treatment with antiretroviral drugs or drugs meant to provide protection against opportunistic infections is currently based on level of immunosuppression, as determined by quantifying the absolute number of lymphocytes with CD_4 surface markers (Table 7). It is currently recommended that zidovudine 200 mg orally every 8 hours be initiated in patients whose CD_4 count has dropped below 500 cells/mm^3 (normal = 1200–1400 cells/mm^3). Patients who have CD_4 counts of < 200 cells/mm^3 should be offered prophylaxis against the ubiquitous parasitic pathogen, *Pneumocystis carinii* (trimethoprim/sulfamethoxasole, 1 double-strength tablet daily), a common cause of pneumonia in immunosuppressed patients. Patients with CD_4 counts < 100 cells/mm^3 should

Table 7. Asymptomatic/Prophylactic Treatment of HIV Infection

Syndrome/infection		Treatment regimen(s)
CD$_4$ count > 500	HIV	Regular follow-up
CD$_4$ count 200–500	HIV	Zidovudine 200 mg TID or DDI 200 mg BID or DDC 0.75 mg TID
CD$_4$ count 100–200	HIV	Continued antiretroviral therapy
	PCP	Trimethoprim–sulfamethoxasole 1 DS tab 3×/week
CD$_4$ count < 100	HIV	Continued antiretroviral therapy
	PCP	Continued TMP/SMX or aerosolized pentamidine 300 mg q 4 weeks
	MAI	Rifabutin 300 mg po Q D

receive prophylaxis against *Mycobacterium avium intracellulare* (Rifabutin 300 mg orally daily) and *Candida albicans* (difluconazole 100 mg orally daily).

Specific treatment of concurrent infections seen in patients with HIV infection is determined by the nature of the identified pathogen. Supportive care for nutritional and psychosocial aspects of an HIV-infected individual's life circumstances is also important.

Follow-up. Patients with HIV infection should be seen regularly. Those with CD$_4$ counts of > 600 cells/mm^3 should be seen every 6 months. Those with CD$_4$ counts of > 200 cells/mm^3 but < 600 cells/mm^3 should be seen every 3 months. Finally, those with CD$_4$ counts of < 200 cells/mm^3 should be seen monthly.

All patients should be urged to inform sexual partners or drug-injecting partners of their HIV status so that they can also be tested. Patients who continue to be sexually active should be aggressively counseled to adopt low-risk behaviors that do not involve the actual or potential exchange of bodily fluids. Condoms are of help, but are no substitute for abstinence or behavioral change.

CONCLUSION

Adolescents are at greater risk of STDs than any other age group. The reasons for this are a complex mix of biologic, behavioral, and psychosocial factors. While the health implications of these infections have always been of considerable importance, in an era when as severe an infection as that caused by HIV exists, adolescents must change their attitudes and their behaviors to avoid potentially fatal consequences.

Communicating an appropriate prevention message to adolescents is a challenge. Those providing care to adolescents need knowledge of the best counseling and treatment approaches in an effort to help them in the formidable task ahead.

REFERENCES

Airhihenbuwa, C. O., DiClemente, R. J., Wingood, G. M., & Lowe, A. (1992). HIV/AIDS education and prevention among African-Americans: A focus on culture. *Journal of AIDS Education & Prevention, 4,* 251–260.

Alan Guttmacher Institute. (1994). *Sex and America's teenagers* (pp. 1–86). New York.

Alexander-Rodriguez, T., & Vermund, S. H. (1987). Gonorrhea and syphilis in incarcerated urban adolescents: Prevalence and physical signs. *Pediatrics, 80,* 561–564.

Anderson, J. E., Kann, L., Holtzman, D., Arday, S., Truman, B., & Kolbe, L. (1990). HIV/AIDS knowledge and sexual behavior among high school students. *Family Planning Perspectives, 22,* 252–255.

Bacchetti, P., & Moss, A. R. (1989). Incubation period of AIDS in San Francisco. *Nature, 338,* 251–253.

Bandura, A. (1992). A social cognitive approach to the exercise of control over AIDS infection. In R. J. DiClemente (Ed.), *Adolescents and AIDS: A generation in jeopardy* (pp. 89–116). Newbury Park, CA: Sage Publications.

Bandura, A. (1994). Social cognitive theory and exercise of control over HIV infection. In R. J. DiClemente & J. Peterson (Eds.), *Preventing AIDS: Theories and methods of behavioral interventions* (pp. 25–59). New York: Plenum Press.

Becker, T. M., Stone, K. M., & Alexander, E. R. (1987). Genital papillomavirus infection: A growing concern. *Obstetric and Gynecologic Clinics of North America, 14,* 389–396.

Biro, F. M., Reising, S. F., Doughman, J. A., Kollar, L. M., & Rosenthal, S. L. (1994). A comparison of diagnostic methods in adolescent girls with and without symptoms of Chlamydia urogenital infection. *Pediatrics, 93,* 476–479.

Blythe, J. J., Katz, B. D., Batteiger, B. E., Ganser, J. A., & Jones, R. B. (1992). Recurrent genitourinary chlamydial infections in sexually active female adolescents. *Journal of Pediatrics, 121,* 487–493.

Botvin, G. (1986). Substance abuse prevention research: Recent developments and future directions. *Journal of School Health, 56,* 369–373.

Burke, D. S., Brundage, J. D., Goldenbaum, M. S., Gardner, L. I., Peterson, M., Visintine, R., Redfield, R. R., and the Walter Reed Retrovirus Research Group. (1990). Human immunodeficiency virus infections in teenagers: Seroprevalence among applicants for U.S. Military Service. *Journal of the American Medical Association, 263,* 2074–2077.

Cannon, R. O., Schmid, G. P., Moore, P. S., & Pappaioanou, M. (1989). Human immunodeficiency virus (HIV) seroprevalence in persons attending STD clinics in the United States, 1985–1987. *Sexually Transmitted Diseases, 16,* 184–189.

Cates, W. (1990). The epidemiology and control of sexually transmitted diseases in adolescents. *Adolescent Medicine State of the Art Review, 1,* 409–427.

Cates, W., & Stone, K. M. (1992). Family planning, sexually transmitted diseases and contraceptive choice: A literature update—part I. *Family Planning Perspectives, 24,* 75–84.

Centers for Disease Control. (1988a). Number of sex partners and potential risk of sexual exposure to HIV. *Morbidity and Mortality Weekly Report, 37,* 565–568.

Centers for Disease Control. (1988b). Changing patterns of groups at high risk for hepatitis B in the United States. *Morbidity and Mortality Weekly Report, 37,* 429–431.

Centers for Disease Control. (1991). Premarital sexual experience among adolescent women—United States, 1970–1988. *Morbidity and Mortality Weekly Report, 39,* 929–932.

Centers for Disease Control and Prevention. (1993). 1993 sexually transmitted diseases treatment guidelines. *Morbidity and Mortality Weekly Report, 42,* 47–75.

Centers for Disease Control and Prevention. (1994a). Health risk behaviors among adolescents who do and do not attend school—United States, 1992. *Morbidity and Mortality Weekly Report, 43,* 129–132.

Centers for Disease Control and Prevention. (1994b). *HIV/AIDS Surveillance Report, 5,* 1–33.

Chow, W. H., Darling, J. R., & Greenbert, R. S. (1987). The epidemiology of ectopic pregnancy. *Epidemiology Review, 9,* 70–94.

Conway, G. A., Epstein, M. R., Hayman, C. R., Miller, C. A., Wendell, D. A., Gwinn, M., Karon, V. M., & Petersen, L. R. (1993). Trends in HIV prevalence among disadvantaged youth: Survey results from a national job training program 1988 through 1992. *Journal of the American Medical Association, 269,* 2887–2889.

Cox, J. M., D'Angelo, L. J., & Silber, T. J. (1992). Substance abuse and syphilis in urban adolescents: A new risk factor for an old disease. *Journal of Adolescent Health, 13,* 483–486.

D'Angelo, L. J., Getson, P. R., Luban, N. L. C., & Gayle, H. D. (1991). Human immunodeficiency virus infection in urban adolescents: Can we predict who is at risk? *Pediatrics, 88,* 982–986.

D'Angelo, L. J., Mohla, C., & Sneed, J. (1987). Diagnosing gonorrhea: A comparison of standard and rapid techniques. *Journal of Adolescent Health Care, 8,* 344–348.

De Vincenzi, I. (1994). A longitudinal study of human immunodeficiency virus transmission by heterosexual partners. *New England Journal of Medicine, 331,* 341–346.

DiClemente R. J. (1990). The emergence of adolescents as a risk group for human immunodeficiency virus infection. *Journal of Adolescent Research, 5,* 7–17.

DiClemente, R. J. (1991). Predictors of HIV-preventive sexual behavior in a high-risk adolescent population: The influence of perceived peer norms and sexual communication on incarcerated adolescents' consistent use of condoms. *Journal of Adolescent Health, 12,* 385–390.

DiClemente, R. J. (1992a). Epidemiology of AIDS, HIV seroprevalence and HIV incidence among adolescents. *Journal of School Health, 62,* 325–330.

DiClemente, R. J. (1992b). Psychosocial determinants of condom use among adolescents. In R. J. DiClemente, (Ed.), *Adolescents and AIDS: A generation in jeopardy* (pp. 34–51). Newbury Park, CA: Sage Publications.

DiClemente, R. J. (1993). Preventing HIV/AIDS among adolescents: Schools as agents of change. *Journal of the American Medical Association, 270,* 760–762.

DiClemente, R. J., & Brown, L. K. (1994). Expanding the pediatrician's role in HIV prevention for adolescents. *Clinical Pediatrics, 32,* 1–6.

DiClemente, R. J., & Houston-Hamilton, A. (1989). Strategies for prevention of human immunodeficiency virus infection among minority adolescents. *Health Education, 20,* 39–43.

DiClemente, R. J., Lodico, M., Grinstead, O. A., Harper, G., Rickman, R. L., Evans, P. E., & Coates, T. J. (1996). African-American adolescents residing in high-risk urban environments do use condoms: Correlates and predictors of condom use among adolescents in public housing developments. *Pediatrics,* in press.

DiClemente, R. J., & Peterson, J. (1994). Changing HIV/AIDS risk behaviors: The role of behavioral interventions. In R. J. DiClemente & J. Peterson (Eds.), *Preventing AIDS: Theories and methods of behavioral interventions* (pp. 1–4). New York: Plenum Press.

Flora, J. A., & Thoresen, C. E. (1989). Components of a comprehensive strategy for reducing the risk of AIDS in adolescents. In V. M. Mays, G. W. Albee, & S. F. Schneider (Eds.), *Primary prevention of AIDS* (pp. 374–389). Newbury Park, CA: Sage Publications.

Forrest, J. D., & Singh, S. (1990). The sexual and reproductive behavior of American women, 1982–1988. *Family Planning Perspectives, 22,* 206–214.

Fraser, J. J., Rettig, P. J., & Kaplan, D. W. (1983). Prevalence of cervical Chlamydia trachomatis and Neisseria gonorrhoeae in female adolescents. *Pediatrics, 71,* 333–336.

Fullilove, M. T., Fullilove, R., Bowser, B. P., Haynes, K., & Gross, S. A. (1990). Black women and AIDS: Gender rules. *Journal of Sex Research, 27,* 47–64.

Fullilove, M. T., Golden, E., Fullilove, R. E., Lennon, R., Porterfield, D., Schwarcz, S. K., & Bolan, G. (1993). Crack cocaine use and high-risk behaviors among sexually active black adolescents. *Journal of Adolescent Health, 14,* 295–300.

Fullilove, R. E., Fullilove, J. T., Bowser, B. P., & Gross, S. A. (1990). Risk of sexually transmitted disease among black adolescent crack users in Oakland and San Francisco, Calif. *Journal of the American Medical Association, 263,* 851–855.

Halsey, N. A., Coberly, J. S., Holt, E., *et al.* (1992). Sexual behavior, smoking, and HIV-1 infection in Haitian women. *Journal of the American Medical Association, 267,* 2062–2066.

Hammerschlage, M. R. (1989). Chlamydia infections. *Journal of Pediatrics, 114,* 727–734.

Hansen, W. B., & Graham, J. W. (1991). Preventing alcohol, marijuana and cigarette use among adolescents: Peer pressure resistance training versus establishing conservative norms. *Preventive Medicine, 20,* 414–430.

Harrison, H. R., Phil, D., & Costin, M. (1985). Cervical *Chlamydia trachomatis* infection in university women: relationship of history of contraception, ectopy, and cervicitis, *American Journal of Obstetrics and Gynecology, 153,* 244–251.

Hausser, D., & Michaud, P. A. (1994). Does a condom-promoting strategy (the Swill STOP-AIDS Campaign) modify sexual behavior among adolescents? *Pediatrics, 93,* 580–585.

Hein, K. (1992). Adolescents at risk for HIV infection. In R. J. DiClemente (Ed.), *Adolescents and AIDS: A generation in jeopardy* (pp. 3–16). Newbury Park, CA: Sage Publications.

Hein, K. (1993). "Getting real" about HIV in adolescents. *American Journal of Public Health, 83,* 492–494.

Huszti, H. C., Clopton, J. R., & Mason, P. J. (1989). Acquired immunodeficiency syndrome educational program: Effects on adolescents' knowledge and attitudes. *Pediatrics, 84,* 986–994.

Ilegbodu, A. E., Frank, M. L., Poindexter, A. N., & Johnson, D. (1994). Characteristics of teens tested for HIV in a metropolitan area. *Journal of Adolescent Health, 15,* 479–484.

Jemmott, J. B., & Jemmott, L. S. (1993). Alcohol and drug use during sexual activity. Predicting the HIV-risk related behaviors of inner-city black male adolescents. *Journal of Adolescent Research, 8,* 41–57.

Jemmott, J. B., & Jemmott, L. S. (1994). Interventions for adolescents in community settings. In R. J. DiClemente & J. Peterson (Eds.), *Preventing AIDS: Theories and methods of behavioral interventions* (pp. 141–174). New York: Plenum Press.

Jemmott, J. B., Jemmott, L. S., & Fong, G. T. (1992). Reductions in HIV risk-associated sexual behaviors among black male adolescents: Effects of an AIDS prevention intervention. *American Journal of Public Health, 82,* 372–377.

Joffe, A. (1993). Adolescents and condom use. *American Journal of Diseases of Children, 147,* 746–754.

Kann, L., Anderson, J. E., Holtzman, D., Ross, J., Truman, B. I., Collins, J., & Kolbe, L. J. (1991). HIV-related knowledge, beliefs, and behaviors among high school students in the United States: Results from a national survey. *Journal of School Health, 61,* 397–401.

Kegeles, S. M., Adler, N. E., & Irwin, C. E. (1988). Sexually active adolescents and condoms: Changes over one year in knowledge, attitudes, and use. *American Journal of Public Health, 78,* 460–461.

Kelley, P. W., Miller, R. N., Pomerantz, R., Wann, F., Brundage, J. F., & Burke, D. S. (1990). Human immunodeficiency virus seropositivity among members of the active duty US Army 85–89. *American Journal of Public Health, 80,* 405–410.

Kelly, J. A., St. Lawrence, J. S., Diaz, Y. E., Stevenson, L. Y., Hauth, A. C., Brasfield, T. L., Kalichman, S. C., Smith, J. E., & Andrew, M. E. (1991). HIV risk behavior reduction following intervention with key opinion leaders of population: An experimental analysis. *American Journal of Public Health, 81*(2), 168–171.

Kenney, A. M., Guardado, S., & Brown, L. (1989). Sex education and AIDS education in the schools: What states and large school districts are doing. *Family Planning Perspectives, 21,* 56–64.

Kirby, D., & DiClemente, R. J. (1994). School-based interventions to prevent unprotected sex and HIV among adolescents. In R. J. DiClemente & J. Peterson (Eds.), *Preventing AIDS: Theories and methods of behavioral interventions* (pp. 141–174). New York: Plenum Press.

Klepp, K. I., Halper, A., & Perry, C. L. (1986). The efficacy of peer leaders in drug abuse prevention. *Journal of School Health, 56,* 407–411.

Laurian, Y., Peynet, J., & Verroust, F. (1989). HIV infection in sexual partners of HIV seropositive patients with hemophilia. *New England Journal of Medicine, 320,* 183.

Lemp, G. F., Hirozawa, A. M., Givertz, D., Nieri, G. N., Anderson, L., Lindegren, M. L., Janssen, R. S., & Katz, M. (1994). Seroprevalence of HIV and risk behaviors among young homosexual and bisexual men. *Journal of the American Medical Association, 272,* 449–454.

MacDonald, N. E., Wells, G. A., Fisher, W. A., Warren, W. K., King, M. A., Doherty, J. A., & Bowie, W. R. (1990). High-risk STD/HIV behavior among college students. *Journal of the American Medical Association, 263,* 3155–3159.

Main, D. S., Iverson, D. C., McGloin, J., Banspach, S. W., Collins, J. L., Rugg, D. L., & Kolbe, L. J. (1994). Preventing HIV infection among adolescents: Evaluation of school-based education program. *Preventive Medicine, 23,* 409–417.

Mansfield, C. J., Conroy, M. E., Emans, S. J., & Woods, E. R. (1993). A pilot study of AIDS education and counseling of high-risk adolescents in an office setting. *Journal of Adolescent Health, 14,* 115–119.

Martinez, J., Smith, R., Farmer, M., Resau, J., Alger, L., Daniel, R., Gupta, J., & Sharh, K. (1988). High prevalence of genital tract papilloma virus infection in female adolescents. *Pediatrics, 82,* 604–608.

Office of Technology Assessment. (1988). *How effective is AIDS education?* Washington, DC: U.S. Congress.

Perry, C. L., & Grant, M. (1988). Comparing peer-led to teacher-led youth alcohol education in four countries. *Alcohol Health Research World, 12,* 322–326.

Perry, C. L., & Sieving, R. (1993). *Peer involvement in global AIDS prevention among adolescents.* Report prepared for the World Health Organization. Genevea, Switzerland: WHO.

Quinn, T. C., Glasser, D., Cannon, R. O., Matuszak, D. L., Dunning, R. W., Kline, R. L., Campbell, C. H., Israel, E., Fauci, A. S., & Hook, E. W. (1988). Human immunodeficiency virus infection among patients attending clinics for sexually transmitted diseases. *New England Journal of Medicine, 318,* 197–203.

Quinn, T. C., Groseclose, S. L., Spence, M., Provost, V., & Hook, E. W. (1992). Evolution of the human immunodeficiency virus epidemic among patients attending sexually transmitted disease clinics: A decade of experience. *Journal of Infectious Diseases, 165,* 541–544.

Rice, R. J., Roberts, P. L., Handsfield, H. H., & Holmes, K. K. (1991). Sociodemographic distribution of gonorrhea incidence: Implications for prevention and behavioral research. *American Journal of Public Health, 81,* 1252–1288.

Robinson, T. N., Killen, J. D., Taylor, C. B., Telch, M. J., Bryson, S. W., Saylor, K. E., Maron, D. J., Maccoby, N., & Farquahar, V. W. (1987). Perspectives on adolescent substance abuse. *Journal of the American Medical Association, 258,* 2072–2076.

Rolfs, R. T., & Nakashima, A. K. (1990). Epidemiology of primary and secondary syphilis in the United States, 1981 through 1989. *Journal of the American Medical Association, 264,* 1432–1437.

Romer, D., Black, M., Ricardo, I., Feigelman, S., Kaljee, L., Galbraith, J., Nesbit, R., Hornik, R. C., & Stanton, B. (1994). Social influences on the sexual behavior of youth at risk for HIV exposure. *American Journal of Public Health, 84,* 977–985.

Roper, W. L., Peterson, H. B., & Curran, J. W. (1993). Commentary: Condoms and HIV/STD prevention— clarifying the message. *American Journal of Public Health, 83,* 501–503.

Rosenberg, E. I., Bayona, M., Brown, H., & Specter, S. (1994). Epidemiologic factors correlated with multiple sexual partners among women receiving prenatal care. *Annals of Epidemiology, 4,* 472–479.

Rosenthal, S. L., Baro, F. M., Succop, P. A., Cohen, S. S., & Stanberry, L. R. (1994). Age of first intercourse and risk of sexually transmitted disease. *Adolescent Pediatric Gynecology, 7,* 210–213.

Rotheram-Borus, M. J., Feldman, J., Rosario, M., & Dunne, E. (1994). Preventing HIV among runaways: Victims and victimization. In R. J. DiClemente & J. Peterson (Eds.), *Preventing AIDS: Theories and methods of behavioral interventions* (pp. 175–188). New York: Plenum Press.

Rotheram-Borus, M. J., Koopman, C., Haignere, C., & Davies, M. (1991). Reducing HIV sexual risk behaviors among runaway adolescents. *Journal of the American Medical Association, 266,* 1237–1241.

Sadof, M. D., Woods, E. R., & Emans, S. J. (1987). Dipstick leukocyte esterase activity in first-catch urine specimens. *Journal of the American Medical Association, 258,* 1932–1934.

Saracco, A., Musicco, M., Nicolosi, A., Angarano, G., Arici, C., Gavazzeni, G., Costigliola, P., Gafa, S., Gervasoni, C., Luzzati, R., Piccinino, F., Puppo, F., Salassa, B., Sinicco, A., Stellini, R., Tirelli, U., Turbessi, G., Vigevani, G. M., Visco, G., Zerboni, R., & Lazzarin, A. (1993). Man-to-woman sexual transmission of HIV: Longitudinal study of 343 steady partners of infected men. *Journal of Acquired Immune Deficiency Syndromes, 6,* 497–502.

Shafer, M. A., Hilton, J. F., Ekstrand, M., Keogh, J., Gee, L., DiGiorgio-Haag, L., Shalwitx, J., & Schachter, J. (1993a). Relationship between drug use and sexual behaviors and occurrence of sexually transmitted diseases among high-risk male youth. *Sexually Transmitted Diseases, 20,* 307–313.

Shafer, M. A., Schachter, J., Moncada, J., Keogh, J., Pantell, R., Gourlay, L., Eyre, S., & Boyer, C. B. (1993b). Evaluation of urine-based screening strategies to detect Chlamydia trachomatis among sexually active asymptomatic young males. *Journal of the American Medical Association, 270,* 2065–2070.

Silber, T. J. (1986). Genital ulcer syndrome. *Seminars in Adolescent Medicine, 2,* 155–162.

Slap, G. B., Plotkin, S. L., Khalid, N., Michelman, D. F., & Forke, C. M. (1991). A human immunodeficiency virus peer education program for adolescent females. *Journal of Adolescent Health, 12,* 434–442.

Sohn, Y. M., Oh, M. K., Balcarek, K. B., Cloud, G. A., & Pass, R. F. (1991). Cytomegalovirus infection in sexually active adolescents. *Journal of Infectious Diseases, 163,* 460–463.

Sonenstein, F. L., Pleck, J. H., & Ku, L. C. (1989). Sexual activity, condom use and AIDS awareness among adolescent males. *Family Planning Perspectives, 21,* 152–158.

Stamm, W. E., & Cole, B. (1986). Asymptomatic Chlamydia trachomatis urethritis in men. *Sexually Transmitted Diseases, 13,* 163–165.

Stiffman, A. R., & Earls, F. (1990). Behavioral risks for human immunodeficiency virus infection in adolescent medical patients. *Pediatrics, 85,* 303–310.

St. Lawrence, J. S., Brasfield, T. L., Jefferson, K. W., Alleyne, E., O'Bannon, R. E., & Shirley, A. (1995). Cognitive-behavioral intervention to reduce African-American adolescents' risk for HIV-infection. *Journal of Consulting and Clinical Psychology, 63,* 221–237.

St. Louis, M. E., Conway, G. A., Hayman, C. R., Miller, C., Petersen, L. R., & Dondero, T. J. (1991). Human immunodeficiency virus infection in disadvantaged adolescents. *Journal of the American Medical Association, 266,* 2387–2391.

St. Louis, M. E., Rauch, K. J., Petersen, L. R., Anderson, J. E., Schable, C. A., Dondero, T. J., & Sentinel Hospital Surveillance Group. (1990). Seroprevalence rates of human immunodeficiency virus infection at sentinel hospitals in the United States. *New England Journal of Medicine, 323,* 213–218.

Stricof, R. L., Kennedy, J. T., Nattell, T. C., Weisfuse, I. B., & Novick, L. F. (1991). HIV seroprevalence in a facility for runaway and homeless adolescents. *American Journal of Public Health, (Suppl.) 81,* 50–53.

Sweeney, P., Lindegren, M. L., Buehler, J. W., Onorato, I. M., & Hanssen, R. S. (1995). Teenagers at risk of human immunodeficiency virus type I infection: results from seroprevalence surveys in the United States, *Archives of Pediatric and Adolescent Medicine, 149,* 521–528.

Telch, M. J., Miller, L. M., Killen, J. D., Cooke, S., & Maccoby, N. (1990). Social influences approach to smoking prevention: The effects of videotape delivery with and without same-age peer leader participation. *Addictive Behavior, 15,* 21–28.

Van de Perre, P., Jacobs, D., & Sprecher-Goldberger, S. (1987). The latex condom, an efficient barrier against sexual transmission of AIDS-related viruses. *AIDS, 1,* 49–52.

Walter, H. J., & Vaughan, R. D. (1993). AIDS risk reduction among multiethnic urban high school students. *Journal of the American Medical Association, 270,* 725–730.

Walter, H. J., Vaughan, R. D., Gladis, M. M., Ragin, D. F., Kasen, S., & Covall, A. T. (1992). Factors associated with AIDS risk behaviors among high school students in an AIDS epicenter. *American Journal of Public Health, 82,* 528–532.

Washington, A. E., Johnson, R. E., Sanders, L. L. (1987). *Chlamydia trachomatis* infections in the United States: what are they costing us? *Journal of the American Medical Association, 257,* 2070–2072.

Wasserheit, J. (1992). Epidemiological synergy: Interrelationships between human immunodeficiency virus infection and other sexually transmitted diseases. *Sexually Transmitted Diseases, 9,* 61–77.

Webster, L. A., Berman, S. M., & Greenspan, J. R. (1993). Surveillance for gonorrhea and primary and secondary syphilis among adolescents, United States. 1981–1991. *Morbidity and Mortality Weekly Report, 42,* 1–11.

Westrom, L. (1980). Incidence, prevalence, and trends of acute pelvic inflammatory disease and its consequences in industrialized countries. *American Journal of Obstetrics & Gynecology, 238,* 882.

Wight, D. (1992). Impediments to safer heterosexual sex: A review of research with young people. *AIDS Care, 4,*(1), 11–21.

Wilson, M. D., Kastrinakis, M., D'Angelo, L. J., & Getson, P. (1994). Attitudes, knowledge, and behavior regarding condom use in urban black adolescent males. *Adolescence, 113,* 13–26.

Wingood, G. M., & DiClemente, R. J. (1992). Cultural, gender and psychosocial influences on HIV-related behavior of African-American female adolescents: Implications for the development of tailored prevention programs. *Ethnicity & Disease, 2,* 381–388.

Wingood, G. M., DiClemente, R. J. (1995). Understanding the role of gender relations in HIV prevention research. *American Journal of Public Health, 85,* 592.

Yankauer, A. (1986). The persistence of public health problems: SF, STD and AIDS. *American Journal of Public Health, 76,* 494–495.

Yankauer, A. (1994). Sexually transmitted diseases: A neglected public health priority. *American Journal of Public Health, 84,* 1894–1897.

Yorke, J. A., Hethcote, H. W., & Nold, A. (1978). Dynamics and control of the transmission of gonorrhea, *Sexually Transmitted Diseases, 5,* 51–56.

Young, R. A., Feldman, S., Bracklin, B. T., & Thompson, E. (1992). Seroprevalence of human immunodeficiency virus among adolescent attendees of Mississippi sexually transmitted disease clinics: A rural epidemic. *Southern Journal of Medicine, 85,* 460–463.

Zimmerman, H. D., Potterat, J. J., Dukes, R. L., Muth, J. B., Zimmerman, H. P., Fogle, J. S., & Pratts, C. I. (1990). Epidemiologic differences between chlamydia and gonorrhea. *American Journal of Public Health, 80,* 1338–1342.

14

Runaway and Homeless Youths

MARY JANE ROTHERAM-BORUS,
MICHELLE PARRA,
COLEEN CANTWELL,
MARYA GWADZ, and
DEBRA A. MURPHY

INTRODUCTION

The number of youths who run away or are forced from their homes and become homeless is a growing and significant problem. Many of these young people have left or been forced from dysfunctional or abusive families only to face a life on the streets that can bring a variety of negative outcomes: poverty, substance abuse, physical and sexual assault, pregnancy, injury or illness, HIV infection, psychological and emotional problems, and suicide (Kennedy, 1991; Rotheram-Borus, Rosario, & Koopman, 1991; Rotheram-Borus & McDermott, 1995). Furthermore, their prospects for a healthy and productive adulthood are reduced by the health risks they face and the lack of educational and employment opportunities for homeless youths. Over the last 10 years, researchers have documented the breadth of these problems. The goals of this chapter are: to examine the extent and course of homelessness; to describe the health status of homeless youths; to identify the risk factors and potential strategies for prevention of the consequences of homelessness; to describe a model program for homeless youths; and to identify structural barriers to effective implementation of health care for homeless youths.

MARY JANE ROTHERAM-BORUS, MICHELLE PARRA, COLEEN CANTWELL, MARYA GWADZ, and DEBRA A. MURPHY • Division of Social and Community Psychiatry, Department of Psychiatry, University of California, Los Angeles, Los Angeles, California 90024.
Handbook of Adolescent Health Risk Behavior, edited by Ralph J. DiClemente, William B. Hansen, and Lynn E. Ponton. Plenum Press, New York, 1996.

THE EPIDEMIOLOGY OF HOMELESSNESS

Estimates of the Number of Homeless Youths

Homelessness is primarily a problem in developing countries, although it is a substantial and increasing problem in the United States (Robertson, 1991b). Conservative estimates are that 100 million youths are homeless worldwide (United Nations Children's Fund (UNICEF), 1989). Economic, political, and social problems are the primary determinants of homelessness. In Africa, many youths are homeless because their parents have died of AIDS-related illnesses. In Kagara, Tanzania, 22,000 children have been orphaned by the AIDS pandemic (Rutayuga, 1992). The United States Agency for International Development predicts that by 2015, the disease could be responsible for 16 million children becoming orphans in Africa (Rutayuga, 1992). However, extreme poverty, often associated with the breakdown in extended and nuclear families, is the primary determinant of homelessness (Luna & Rotheram-Borus, 1992). For example, in Brazil two-thirds of the country's 140 million people live below the poverty level (Meyers, 1989). Many Brazilian children are abandoned or forced to leave their homes because their parents cannot support them. In Brazil, as in other developing countries, homelessness is a way of life rather than a temporary status.

There have been no comprehensive studies of the number of homeless youths in the United States. In 1975, it was estimated that there were 519,500 to 635,000 homeless youths in the United States based on an estimate from the Opinion Research Center that 1.7% of adolescents are homeless (Brennen, Huizinga, & Elliot, 1979). By 1982, the estimate rose to 733,000 to 1.3 million (Children's Defense Fund, 1988; Chelimsky, 1982). In 1987, the United States Conference of Mayors estimated that youths represented 4% of homeless persons (United States Conference of Mayors, 1987). In 1987, about 330,000 youths were served in federally funded shelters (Robertson, 1991b). Given the early estimates, it appears that homelessness among youths is an increasing problem. However, a 1988–1989 survey by the Justice Department of about 10,000 households and 127 institutions indicated that about 500,000 youths under the age of 18 run away each year (Barden, 1990).

The most comprehensive surveys of homeless youths have been conducted at the city level. In 1984, Shaffer and Caton conducted an epidemiological survey of the number of homeless youths in New York City. Their estimate included youths in shelters, on the streets, and in institutional settings (e.g., emergency overnight housing by foster care services). Given their exhaustive strategies for estimating the number of homeless youths, it was estimated that 2000 youths were homeless in New York City on any one night. Using a less comprehensive sampling, Luna (1987) estimated that there were 5000 homeless youths in San Francisco. In Los Angeles, the estimate was at least 34,800 each year (Pennbridge, Yates, David, & MacKenzie, 1990).

Given the variability in these estimates, it is clear that homelessness for youths is a substantial problem, but the exact scope of the problem is difficult to estimate. It is unclear whether the problem is increasing or the estimates in 1975 and 1982 were too high. Yates (1988) hypothesized that the number of homeless youths is underestimated because there is no way to estimate the number of youths who are not receiving services. However, it may be that the number of homeless youths is inflated. Estimating homelessness has political implications: categorical funding for homeless youths is often contingent on the number of youths needing service; therefore, service providers may be motivated to inflate the extent of the problem. While it is not clear whether the number of homeless youths is increasing, there are data indicating that the youths served at shelters appear to be increasingly more troubled (i.e., having more stressful lives prior to running away), are younger, and are more likely to have multiple problems (Rothman & David, 1985).

Defining Homeless Youths

The conceptualization and current methods of classifying homeless youths have hampered the development of effective strategies for addressing their physical- and mental-health problems. Many systems for categorizing have been suggested for homeless youths (Robertson, 1991b). Bucy (1987) classified youths without homes as homeless, throwaways (expelled from the home), runaways, victims, and system kids. These categories, however, cannot be considered exclusive, for often a youth will belong to more than one classification. For example, a homeless youth could have run away from home and have been a victim of sexual abuse. The National Network of Runaway and Youth Services, Inc. (1985) distinguishes *runaways* as those who choose to leave home while *homeless youths* have been thrown out of their homes. Choice, access, and time away from home are dimensions that distinguish subgroups of youths under the age of 18 who are not living with their parents (Robertson, 1991b).

Within the international homeless youth political movement, distinctions are made between *children on the street* and *children of the street* (Bond, Jiminez, & Mazin, 1992). Children working at a very young age who have adult supervision available nearby would be considered *on the street*. *Children of the street* are independent from familial adult attachments. These youths often band together to "squat," or live communally, and provide for each other's basic survival needs. In this chapter, we will refer to all youths who have spent at least 2 nights in a shelter away from home or living on the streets as *homeless*.

Characteristics of Homeless Youths

There are some living situations that are associated with increased risk for homelessness. Teenage parents may represent a sizable subgroup of homeless youths (Robertson, 1991a). For example, in 1985 it was estimated that one-third of the 21,000 homeless adolescents in Illinois were teen mothers or pregnant (Hemmens & Luecke, 1988). Towber (1985) found that 11.3% of a sample of families ($N=77$) in shelters in New York City were teenage parents. In a subsequent survey, Towber (1986) found that 4% of the homeless parents at the Martinique Hotel and 12% at a city shelter were under the age of 21.

The demographic profile of homeless youths varies by subpopulations. It has been estimated that the ethnic profile of homeless youths reflects the social demographics of the general population of the United States (General Accounting Office (GAO), 1989). According to some reports, runaways are equally likely to be males or females (Upshur, 1986; GAO, 1989). However, other studies indicate there are more females in shelters (Robertson, 1991b). Youths living on the streets are more likely to be male and older than those in shelters (Shaffer & Caton, 1984; GAO, 1989). About one-half of the youths who have run away have been in foster care and appear to be attempting to leave a poor placement, and 12% were in foster care immediately prior to receiving shelter (GAO, 1989). To be provided shelter, youths must be between the ages of 12 and 17; at the age of 18, youths are referred to the adult shelter system.

According to studies, most homeless youths remain in their local area, but many migrate to large, urban areas, especially, it seems, on the West Coast. Shaffer and Caton (1984) found that more than 90% of homeless youths in New York City were from New York City. Chelimsky (1982) reported that, in a national survey, 72% of homeless youths remained in their local area. However, Kennedy (1991) reported that 78% of the youths served at the Larkin Street Youth Center in San Francisco were from outside of the city area, with 38% from outside of California. By 1994, one-fifth were Latinos from outside the country (M. Kennedy, personal communication, January 25, 1995). Many youths who are gay, lesbian, or bisexual, or suspect that they are, are attracted to San Francisco because it has been identified as a "gay town" (Rotheram-Borus, Luna, Marotta, & Kelly, 1994). About one-fifth of the youths served by the Larkin Street Center identified themselves as gay, lesbian, bisexual, or undecided (Kennedy, 1991). In Los Angeles County, Robertson (1990) found that 52% of the homeless adolescents studied had moved to the county in the 6 months prior to being interviewed. Pennbridge *et al.* (1990) found that about 38% of the youths in shelters in Los Angeles County and 75% of the youths served by outreach/drop-in agencies were from outside the county.

Factors Leading Youths to Become Homeless

Homeless youths frequently report stressful life events, but the lack of a supportive and functional family is the most common factor associated with homelessness (GAO, 1989; Rotheram-Borus, 1993). Adolescents living within dysfunctional families may be better off leaving these homes than attempting to resolve possibly unsolvable problems with limited resources (Bucy & Obolensky, 1990). Among the domain of family stressors, 30% of runaways reported that a family member had died in the previous 3 months, 11% had parents who lost their jobs, and 28% had parents who had separated or divorced in the previous 3 months. The National Network of Runaway and Youth Services reports that as many as 70% of the runaways at emergency shelters have been severely physically abused or sexually assaulted (Kennedy, 1991). Besides family problems, among a cohort of 103 runaway youths (Rotheram-Borus, Rosario, & Koopman, 1991), many reported frequent problems with school and peers. For example, 32% had changed schools in the previous 3 months, 40% had failed a grade, 40% had trouble with a specific teacher, and 23% had been expelled from school. These high rates lead us to hypothesize a strong relationship between stressful events in young people's home and/or school life and their running away.

Risk Factors and Behaviors of Homeless Youths

Researchers have documented the breadth and scope of risk acts that homeless youths experience (e.g., Rotheram-Borus, Koopman, & Ehrhardt, 1991; Robertson, 1991b). The stress experienced by homeless youths is exhibited in multiple problem behaviors that place these youths at risk for a variety of negative long-term outcomes (Rotheram-Borus & Koopman, 1991; Rotheram-Borus et al., 1992). However, many of these behaviors can be viewed in terms of youths' strategies for survival while living on the streets (e.g., trading sex for food or shelter).

In many cases, these youths have difficulty satisfying even the most basic needs for shelter, food, and health care. About half have difficulty obtaining adequate food and clothing (Robertson, 1990). Many cannot obtain shelter, even in public facilities, which are often filled to capacity (Pennbridge et al., 1990). The majority of youths resort to improvised shelter, sites that are often regarded as illegal by law enforcement officials (Greenblatt & Robertson, 1993). In the 3 months prior to seeking shelter at an agency in New York City, approximately 1 in 5 youths was physically assaulted, 1 in 5 was raped or sexually assaulted, and 1 in 5 was robbed or burglarized (Rotheram-Borus, Rosario, & Koopman, 1991).

Serious health problems occur more frequently in adolescent runaway populations than among nonrunaways (Yates, MacKenzie, Pennbridge, & Cohen, 1988). In a recent study, approximately 30% of homeless youths reported a recent major illness or injury (Rotheram-Borus, Rosario, & Koopman, 1991), yet only one-third studied by Robertson (1990) had any kind of health coverage. About one-fifth believed that their health deteriorated after they became homeless, and about one-fifth reported an untreated health problem in the year prior to being interviewed (Robertson, 1990).

The HIV pandemic exacerbates the health-care needs of homeless adolescents. Approximately 4% were estimated to be HIV-infected (Stricof, Novick, & Kennedy, 1990), with estimates as high as 8% in San Francisco (Shalwitz, Goulart, Dunnigan, & Flannery, 1990). These rates emerge because of the high frequency of risk acts in this population, as well as the level of HIV seropositivity among their sexual partners (Rotheram-Borus, Koopman, & Bradley, 1989). About half of these youths reported at least one instance of high-risk behavior for HIV exposure (Robertson, 1990). Sexual risk behaviors are more common among homeless than among nonhomeless adolescents. Homeless youths are more likely to engage in survival sex. Twenty-six percent of runaways in Los Angeles engaged in survival sex whereas only 0.2% of nonrunaways reported the same (Yates et al., 1988). In a New York City study, 13% of males and 7% of females engaged in survival sex (Rotheram-Borus et al., 1992). Among predominantly African-American and Hispanic runaways in New York City, the mean age for any genital or anal sex was 12.9 years (Rotheram-Borus et al., 1992). Having multiple sex partners was another characteristic of this adolescent subgroup. Among runaways in New York City, 47% of males and 16% of females reported having ten or more opposite-sex partners (Rotheram-Borus et al., 1992). One of the most alarming findings among homeless youths was their inconsistent use of condoms. Only 14% of male and 18% of female street runaways in New York City reported consistent condom use with opposite-sex partners. Among the same group, condoms were rarely or never used by 38% of both males and females (Rotheram-Borus et al., 1992). Although Greenblatt and Robertson (1993) found that the majority of sexually active homeless youths did use some form of birth control during the most recent sexual encounter, little more than half used a condom in that encounter. In addition to risk of HIV exposure, the sexual behaviors of these youth put them at greater risk for other sexually transmitted diseases and pregnancy. Between 50 and 71% of street youths reported having a sexually transmitted disease (Shalwitz et al., 1990). In New

York City, 25% of female runaways reported a pregnancy within the previous 3 months (Rotheram-Borus, Rosario, & Koopman, 1991).

In conjunction with the risky sexual behaviors of these youths are high rates of substance abuse. Just over half of the male homeless youths in Los Angeles were on drugs more than half of the time during survival sex, and 32% were on drugs more than half of the time during recreational sex (Pennbridge, Freese, & MacKenzie, 1992). Running away in early adolescence is positively correlated with drug and alcohol use (Windle, 1989). Robertson (1989b) found that almost 40% of runaway youths studied met the *Diagnostic and Statistical Manual of Mental Disorders–III* (1980) criteria for drug abuse, which is five times higher than the rate found in their age peers who have homes (Stiffman, Felton, Powell, & Robins, 1987). In New York City, 19% of runaways reported having used cocaine/crack, 43% marijuana, and 71% alcohol (Koopman, Rosario, & Rotheram-Borus, 1994).

Comorbidity of drug and alcohol abuse is high with this population. One-quarter of homeless youths studied by Robertson (1989a) met dual diagnostic criteria for both drug and alcohol abuse. About half of the runaways in New York City had at least one symptom of alcohol abuse (Koopman *et al.*, 1994). Homeless youths with alcohol problems start drinking at a younger age, have greater social impairment as a result of their drinking, and drink more frequently than nonhomeless adolescents (Robertson, 1989a,b). Those with alcohol problems are also more likely than their homeless peers to have histories of abuse or neglect, including being removed from their home by authorities, and, thus, tend to be more estranged from their families. They also tend to have more chronic histories with homelessness, spend more time in institutional settings, have more difficulty meeting basic survival needs, and generate more of their income illegally.

The relationship between stress and mental health problems has been well documented (Dohrenwend & Dohrenwend, 1974). Given the overwhelming stress in these adolescents' lives, it is not surprising that they are at increased risk for multiple mental health problems. Englander (1984) found that female runaways had significantly lower self-esteem than nonrunaways and were more likely to attribute socially undesirable traits to themselves. Female runaways also perceived their families as being less supportive than did male runaways. Although homeless youths appeared similar to nonhomeless youths in terms of their goals and aspirations, they were more likely than their nonhomeless peers to report being lonely, having less in common with their peers, and feeling that no one cares. Compared with their nonrunaway peer group, runaways are three times more likely to meet DSM-III criteria for a mental disorder (Robertson, 1992). Mundy, Robertson, Robertson, and Greenblatt (1990) found that 30% of homeless youths reported psychotic symptoms. These youths often exhibit high rates of depression and suicidal behavior (Powers, Eckenrode, & Jaklitsch, 1990; Robertson, 1990; Rotheram-Borus, 1993). In New York City, 16% of runaway youths reported current suicidality, and almost 40% had attempted suicide at least once. Among attempters, 44% had made the attempt within the month prior to being interviewed (Rotheram-Borus, 1993). Robertson (1989b) found that 24% of youths had been hospitalized overnight for mental health or emotional problems; about two-thirds of these hospitalizations were for suicide attempts.

Runaways report high rates of conduct problems (Robertson, 1989b; Rotheram-Borus, 1993) and very often experience trouble with school. About half of the runaways studied in New York City had dropped out of school and almost a quarter had been expelled (Rotheram-Borus, 1993). Runaways who do attend school tend to be below average in their academic performance. In Los Angeles, 25% had repeated at least one grade, and another quarter had been placed in special education classes (Robertson, 1989b). The difficulties that these youths encounter with the educational system can be anticipated given their unstable living situations.

Life on the streets also places many homeless youths in conflict with the criminal justice system. In New York City, 21% of runaways studied had spent time in jail within the previous 3 months (Rotheram-Borus, Koopman, & Ehrhardt, 1991); in Los Angeles, 56% of youths had spent time in a detention facility (Robertson, 1990). Many of the behaviors that put youths in conflict with the criminal justice system can be viewed as adaptive responses to meet basic needs (e.g., stealing clothing to keep warm). Work is not a ready solution because many are not of legal working age. Although a slight majority of youths in Los Angeles reported their main source of income in the previous 3 months as coming from legal sources (e.g., job or family), almost 40% reported that their income was gained through illegal activities; 22% reported trading sex for food or shelter (Robertson, 1990). Lack of education and contact with the criminal justice system may make it less likely that these youths will find gainful legal employment at any time in their lives.

Exploration of social roles, identity formation, and experimentation with sex, drugs, and other risky behaviors are characteristics of the adolescent period. Placed in the uncompromising street environment, these youths are challenged to survive in a manner inconsistent with their developmental stage. They are burdened with adult responsibilities and must provide for their own food, shelter, and security with little or no social support systems.

Homeless youths have become victims of a society that provides neither support nor caretaking and are forced to place their lives at risk in order to survive. This victimization affects not only their self-esteem and self-worth, but also their outlook on the future. Many perceive the world as "out to get them" and that their lives are insignificant (Luna, 1991). Some homeless youths continue the cycle by victimizing others, as petty theft and drug dealing are among the few options for unskilled, isolated adolescents to secure food and shelter. As a result of this, many in the mainstream hold negative sentiments toward these youths, who are sometimes viewed as hustlers taking advantage of the public (Luna & Rotheram-Borus, 1992).

YOUTHS' EXPERIENCE OF HOMELESSNESS: CASE STUDIES

To help youths establish a stable living pattern that is characterized by consistent positive daily interactions (Gallimore, Goldenberg, & Weisner, 1993), it is key to understand youths' experience of living on the streets. Rather than focusing on youths' lives within a set time period, it is perhaps more useful to delineate trajectories that describe an adolescent's status over time. The life paths of male and female youths who have been homeless vary (Rotheram-Borus, Koopman, & Ehrhardt, 1991), but there are at least six primary constellations of homeless youths. These are: (1) those who have lost parents through death or divorce, (2) those who are gay or lesbian, (3) those who have long-standing mental health problems, (4) those who are expelled from home by their family, (5) those who are sexually abused, and (6) those who have substance-abuse problems. As mentioned previously, often youths fall into many of these categories, which can be seen in several of the following case studies illustrating these constellations. These case studies are taken from transcripts of life histories collected during an intervention study with 300 homeless youths seeking shelter in New York City from 1988 to 1990. At the beginning of the interview process, the youths ranged in age from 12 to 17, and were followed longitudinally over 2- to 6-year periods (Rotheram-Borus *et al.*, 1994). These vignettes are not from atypical children, but rather reflect common stories of homeless youths' lives.

Parental Loss through Death or Divorce

Youths who, at any early age, lose a parent or parents through death or divorce appear to leave home at a relatively early age, and it is not feasible to anticipate that their families will ever be stable settings for them. If stable living placements are found for these youths, their lives can and do stabilize. Often, however, a group home placement is problematic. The staff may have unrealistic expectations regarding an individual adolescent's ability to adhere to house regulations and, thus, not individually tailor their expectations for the youth. Therefore, the life paths of these youngsters may continue to be problematic.

Janice's story typifies this pathway. Janice's mother died when she was 10 years old. Her aunt told her she had 2 months to "get over it." By the time she was 15, she began to have grave misgivings about her future. She bounced among family members and ended up living with her favorite aunt, Stephanie. Despite Stephanie's caring and concern, Janice began skipping school and stealing money from her. Janice thought, "I'm just gonna make them mad, just like I'm mad." She and Stephanie agreed that the best thing to do would be to place her in a residential school.

At the school, Janice was torn: she liked the school but was lonely and upset about not getting visitors. Feeling angry one day, she impulsively left the grounds and hitchhiked toward New York City, then took a bus into the large central terminal. There, she met a group of young people surviving on the streets by "hustling," or trading sex for money, and selling drugs. She said, "When I got there, I just watched and I picked up on my own. I wasn't trying to be with pimps and things like that, I did it all by myself."

She started using crack cocaine during this time. She said, "Everybody was doing it, and they just kept saying, 'Come on, do it, it ain't gonna hurt you.' The first day I did cocaine, to me, it didn't bother me. It just kept me up. I was able to go and make my money all night long instead of getting sleepy. But right as soon as I found out I was pregnant, I said, the baby or the drugs. And I chose the baby."

Janice stayed on the streets while pregnant until a social worker from a nearby group home for pregnant girls convinced her to go there. This began a long series of institutional placements, including group homes, runaway shelters, and welfare apartments. During her teenage years she was hospitalized twice for "nervous breakdowns." She described herself as having been an alcoholic at one point, but not addicted to drugs, although she used them for about a year.

Most recently, Janice lived with her two young daughters and her boyfriend in a one-bedroom apartment. She also has two older daughters who have been legally adopted by another family. She lost custody of her oldest daughter after her boyfriend was incarcerated and she became homeless. She lost custody of her second when she became homeless again and went to a shelter. The shelter staff checked her records, noted previous custody problems, and took the child.

Janice is an example of a runaway who later became homeless and then a system kid. Currently she plans to retake the high school equivalency exam and train to be a medical technician, but for now her children take up her time. Both of her daughters suffer from asthma and she is frequently at the hospital with them. Her life is relatively stable and she considers herself lucky, but she has a long way to go to meet her goals. She is thankful that she has continued to test HIV-negative despite years of risky sexual behavior while on the streets.

Gay and Lesbian Youths

A second group of youths leaves or is forced from home because their sexual and/or love interests include, or are exclusively for, members of their same sex. Youths who may be gay or lesbian recognize that they are different from the majority of their peers and often fear disclosure or discovery by others, particularly family members. Indeed, if the adolescent discloses his or her suspected or confirmed sexual orientation, many are ejected from their family (Hunter & Schaecher, 1990).

Bob had been in foster care since he was 3 years old. He was fortunate to be in a loving family who had taken in both Bob and his sister and provided a comfortable, stable life for them. Bob was doing well in school, had a large friendship network, and was leading a relatively "normal" childhood. At about age 13, Bob realized that his sexual orientation was homosexual: he was attracted to boys in his classes, he bought magazines with pictures of gay adults, and he started frequenting places where members of the gay community were likely to be found. He did not experiment sexually, but he felt he was gay. When the family decided to adopt Bob and his sister, Bob felt he "owed" it to his parents to share with them his sexual orientation. When he was 14 years old, he disclosed his feelings to his parents. His parents were highly religious and a gay lifestyle was unacceptable to them. Bob was immediately ejected from the family. He was also expelled from the religious school he attended after his parents informed the school of his orientation. His clothes, books, and eyeglasses were thrown onto the front yard by the family. Bob became homeless and lived in alleys for 2 or 3 nights. He sought help from a gay-identified social service agency and was placed, after 2 to 3 months, with a gay couple in foster care in another town. He was able to resume a relatively stable adolescence. He did not spontaneously disclose his sexual orientation to his peers at his new school and became far less social until early adulthood.

Youths with Long-Standing Mental Health Problems

Adolescents who have a history of psychiatric problems and conduct problems also may run away or be forced from their home. William's life course represents the pathway of a *throwaway* whose pattern of conduct problems at an early age contributed to a path of homelessness. When William was 10, he started skipping school, acting up in class, stealing from stores, and smoking cigarettes. His mother, a single parent who also had three younger children, said she was unable to control him. She began to use more and more physical punishment against William, which did not result in improved behavior. As William's conduct problems increased, his mother became more frustrated. When he was 13, she told him that she could no longer handle him and that he had to leave the apartment. That night, when he returned to ask for another chance, she had changed the locks.

William spent his first night out on the street, then heard about a runaway shelter from young people he met. He arrived, was admitted, and lived there for nearly a year. During this time, he had limited contact with his mother. In family therapy sessions, she expressed an unwillingness to take him back, saying, "I've spent too much of my time trying to control William. I've got my younger kids to consider now." She said she felt overwhelmed and scared. William had little to say about how this affected him.

William spent much of his time on the corner near the shelter, hanging out with neighborhood boys and shelter residents. Shelter staff believed that local drug dealers recruited from that corner, and that such youths often became socialized into criminal activity. At age 14, William was picked up by the police for acting as a lookout for the drug dealers. He said that he felt pressured to have money and possessions with which to impress girls. He was placed briefly in a juvenile detention center, then released to a group home.

Over the next several years, William moved through a variety of institutional placements, as he either ran away from them or was discharged because of behavior problems or lack of space. He continued to be involved with the drug trade. He dropped out of school around this time. At 17, he was arrested again, pleaded guilty to possession of an illegal substance, and was incarcerated in an adult facility for several years. Jail was difficult for him; although he was tall and strong, he was frequently the victim of violence. He also hinted about the sexual assaults that occur in prison.

When he was released from jail at age 20, he was reunited with his family. He had a strong desire to stay out of jail but also a pessimistic, though perhaps realistic, outlook. He said, "For a black man with no education, there are only two options: get a shit job or be on the streets." William started looking for a job and began dating. He did not use condoms because he felt it wasn't a masculine thing to do, that it meant he was implying his partner was unclean, and that protection was a woman's responsibility.

William did not remember the last time he had a medical checkup. He had not been and did not want to be tested for HIV. He said, "I couldn't handle knowing, so I just better not find out." Nor did he remember being tested for other sexually transmitted diseases, hepatitis, or tuberculosis. William is a young man at risk for negative outcomes in multiple ways. He may become the victim of violence because of the neighborhood in which he lives. He is unlikely to get a job because of the high unemployment rate in his community, and there is the possibility that he will again become involved in the drug trade, which is the only "job" he has held. He may experience psychiatric distress (e.g., depression, suicide) and many of the health problems noted above, as well as future incarceration. He is a throwaway who became a "system kid," runaway, and then a criminal.

Family-Precipitated Homelessness

A large group of youths become homeless because their family lacks the personal resources to provide for the basic necessities of life (shelter, food, medical care) during the child's adolescence. The adolescent is prematurely left to provide these resources for him- or herself. The increasing problem of family homelessness contributes to the problem of adolescent homelessness. While this is not the dominant route to adolescent homelessness in the United States, some cases are a result of this pattern. The case of Shaun typifies this pattern.

When Shaun's mother, Lizette, lost the family apartment, they packed up everything they owned into suitcases and went to a homeless shelter. Shelter policy dictated that small children, but not teenagers, could be admitted. Shelter staff gave Shaun subway fare and the address of a youth runaway shelter located about an hour's train ride away. Shaun attempted to maintain contact with his family from the shelter and expected that his mother soon would obtain another apartment, at which point they would be reunited. However, maintaining contact was difficult because his mother did not have easy access to a phone and was moved periodically to other shelters. His counselor recommended placement in a group home, and Shaun began a series of institutional placements, including adult homeless shelters.

Shaun dropped out of school at 16 and found life "boring." In the shelters he started "hanging out" and smoking crack with his friends. He quickly realized that crack was problematic for him: when he hit his postuse lows, he felt he would do anything for the next hit. He found that in the shelters, men would exchange sex for drugs. He started to do the same to support his drug habit. Around this time he began a romantic relationship with Brenda, who was staying in the woman's shelter. Brenda and Shaun became inseparable, and several months later Brenda became pregnant. They were thrilled, and Brenda increased her efforts to obtain "Section 8" (welfare) housing. That summer, an apartment was awarded to her and they moved in. Brenda was 8 months pregnant.

Not long after the birth of her son, Brenda became pregnant again. Shaun and Brenda devoted their time to raising their sons. They had occasional contact with her family, who did not like Shaun. Shaun's doctor suggested that he be tested for HIV as part of a physical. His test came back positive.

Brenda became desperate and suicidal on hearing the news. The idea that she and Shaun would die and leave their sons orphaned was overwhelming to her. That all four of them would die of AIDS was even worse. She was seen at an emergency room and hospitalized overnight. She then saw a counselor to make decisions about HIV testing for herself and her sons and what to do next. Two weeks later she learned that she and her sons were HIV-negative. However, Brenda felt depressed and hopeless, particularly about protecting herself during sexual intercourse. She said, "I don't use condoms because they don't work. They can fall off and get stuck up inside you." Shaun and Brenda were both fairly knowledgeable about HIV transmission and safer sex; however, they continued to have unprotected intercourse. Shaun said, "I know I have it, but it doesn't seem real."

The counselor set them up with a couple's support group, medical care, and safer-sex counseling, all of which they did not attend. In part, their care was problematic because services were located all over the city in unfamiliar neighborhoods. Brenda stated that raising her two sons was overwhelming enough, and that she did not want to talk or think about HIV. A year later she contacted the counselor again, still HIV-negative. She and Shaun were more willing to focus on how to stay healthy and safe. However, around this time they lost their apartment and went back into the shelter system. This disruption resulted in their putting off obtaining care for another long period of time.

Shaun became homeless when his family became homeless, and then lived in shelters until Brenda obtained an apartment. Without adequate mental and physical health care, he is unlikely to have a stable living situation or be employed.

Sexual Abuse

Sexual abuse has often been identified as a primary precipitant of homelessness among adolescent girls (Bucy, 1987). The extent of this problem is unclear. Estimates on the number of homeless youths, male or female, who were sexually abused before leaving home has ranged from 23 to 70% (Rotheram-Borus, Koopman, & Ehrhardt, 1991). This is a huge range. Therefore, it is not clear that the rate of sexual abuse of youths who become homeless is any higher than that among other subpopulations of youths living in stressful situations (e.g., those living in the inner city or who are gay or lesbian). The case history of LaShell typifies the life story of adolescents whose homelessness is associated with early victimization. LaShell saw her childhood as one abusive episode after another. When she was 12, she ran away from home after experiencing what she called "the last straw": her mother's new husband sexually abused her and when LaShell told her mother, she was beaten by her for "lying." LaShell arrived at the runaway shelter depressed and angry. Over time, LaShell and her mother reconciled and she moved back into the home. Although her stepfather never sexually approached her again, she had nightmares about the incident and felt perpetually wary.

LaShell experienced periods of depression during which she was preoccupied with suicide and found it difficult to leave the house. On one occasion, her friends convinced her to attend a party with them. They were dancing and drinking and LaShell went up on the roof to get some air and look around. There, she was raped by a young man. She blamed herself, and her depression worsened. She attempted suicide and was psychiatrically hospitalized, then placed in a residential treatment center. She felt confined and trapped there and ran away to the youth shelter. Her mother offered her the opportunity to return home, but LaShell refused. She stayed at the shelter for as long as she could while she applied for a welfare apartment.

During this time she became pregnant. She was 17 at the time. Her relationship with her boyfriend became violent, as he blamed her for the pregnancy. LaShell felt trapped and confused. When she obtained her apartment, he moved in with her and, she said, "watched and controlled her every move." She was torn between her desire for her baby to know her father and her growing feeling that the relationship should end. She found it difficult to get out of bed in the morning.

After seeing the baby's father treat the infant roughly, she fled to her mother's apartment. When the baby was a year old, she entered a community college program sponsored by public assistance. She was placed in remedial courses so that she could obtain a high school equivalency degree, and was given help with child care. Around the time she began school, her mother died after a long struggle with AIDS. LaShell was devastated, but remained somewhat hopeful for her, and her child's, future. She hoped to major in business and be a role model for her child so that she does not suffer the way LaShell has.

Substance Abuse

Rarely is substance abuse alone the route into homelessness. In the case below, sexual abuse led the adolescent to leave her home, but once "in the culture" of homelessness, substance abuse was difficult to escape.

Martina's is a typical life story of a sexually abused homeless adolescent. Martina was a 16-year-old, Hispanic female living at a runaway shelter in New York City after having been picked up on the street for prostitution. She expressed concern about her possible HIV status but was resistant to talk about it. Her uneasiness seems to have been increased by the AIDS education she received at the shelter because it made her aware of her past high-risk behaviors. She complained of being tired all the time and did not want to go to school or do her chores around the shelter.

Martina had been physically abused by her father for as long as she could remember. At age 9, he began sexually abusing her. At age 10, she became pregnant and gave the baby up for adoption. She first came to the attention of the Child Welfare Administration at age 13. A chaotic life followed, with her moving among foster and group homes. When she was 14, she began living on the street. She used "all kinds of drugs" including crack and LSD. She said she had never injected drugs. At 15, she started prostituting herself and sleeping with her pimp, who was an intravenous drug user. She said she always used condoms with her "johns" but not with her pimp. She became very depressed about her life, attempted suicide, and was hospitalized in a psychiatric ward in a New York City hospital for several months. After being released from the hospital, she was encouraged to see a psychologist at the shelter but refused.

At the time of the interview, she had had a boyfriend for 1 month. She said that she really loved him and did not use condoms because that would make him seem like a "john." Although he has never done so before, she was concerned that he might become abusive if she were to suggest they use condoms because he might think she was "fooling around" with other men. She seemed very dependent on this relationship. She kept saying that she's not going to "blow this one. He doesn't 'diss' me but really treats me right!" At other times, she expressed interest in becoming more self-reliant, saying she wanted to get her high school equivalency degree and go to college.

Not all youths who have abused substances face negative outcomes, however. The case of Carol demonstrates a positive trajectory. Carol was a 20-year-old Hispanic woman working as a practical nurse and saving for college. Carol had been homeless for 5 years and supported a drug habit for much of the time as a prostitute. However, 3 years ago she entered drug rehabilitation and subsequently began a career as a political activist. She worked with groups who lobby for drug rehabilitation facilities, had been on television several times, and met with the city's mayor often. She was bright, well-spoken, and clear in her direction and goals. A year before being interviewed, she tested HIV-negative, despite her past high-risk behavior and has used condoms consistently since. Safer sex is as much a crusade for her as finding funding for drug rehabilitation programs.

Carol planned to be in college within a year to study nursing while continuing to be a political activist. Her goal was to work with runaway and homeless youths, whom, she felt, need a great deal of help. Carol described herself as having been part of the "dregs of society," yet she was optimistic about her future.

The cases described above are not meant to be exhaustive nor empirically derived. Yet these youths' stories reflect the range and diversity of both the initial challenges that lead youths to become homeless and the diversity of their life paths after they become homeless. As research accumulates on the longitudinal life paths of these youths, true pattern analysis of the paths of homelessness can be conducted.

SOCIAL SERVICES FOR HOMELESS YOUTHS

Social Service Needs

The United States has endorsed the dictates of the United Nations on the basic rights of children to food, shelter, and health care in a safe environment up to the age of 18 (United Nations Convention on the Rights of the Child, 1991). However, there has not been a concerted effort to meet these goals in this country. There is a wide gap between the estimates of the number of homeless youths in the United States and the number of shelter beds and social services available for these youths (National Academy of Sciences, 1988). Even more disturbing is that transitioning these youths to long-term placements is problematic. The number of temporary housing placements far exceeds the number of potentially stable, long-term group home or foster-care placements. Furthermore, the existing system of social services assumes that most homeless youths are magically able to care for themselves at age 18. There are only a few programs for "independent living" (i.e., transitional living programs that provide partial support to youths up to the age of 21).

Statistics from New York City illustrate the lack of stable and transitional housing for youths. Shaffer and Caton (1984) estimated that there were 9000 to 12,000 homeless youths in New York City. According to mid-1980s' police estimates, the number was 20,000 in any year at that time (M. Hirsch, Empire State Coalition of Runaway and Homeless Youths, personal communication, January 25, 1995). More than 85% of these New York City youths will never return to their homes to live (Rotheram-Borus, Koopman, & Ehrhardt, 1991). A phone survey of the Empire State Coalition of Runaway and Homeless Youths and the New York Child Welfare Administration conducted in the spring of 1993 revealed the following statistics: In 1991 in New York City, there were 285 short-term residential beds (30-day crisis care); approximately 80 transitional residential beds (up to 1-year placements); 5600 foster-care group home placements that were predominantly filled by youths who were removed from their homes because of neglect or abuse; and 120 placements for independent living situations for youths from 18 to 21 years old. These data indicate that there were at least 3000 runaway and homeless youths for whom no stable placement was available (conservatively estimating that all runaway and homeless youths were occupying the foster-care beds). This scenario is not unique to New York City but is a problem that is repeated in every major urban center. For example, in Los Angeles, Rothman and David (1985) estimated that returning home was a realistic possibility for only about 19% of youths in shelters.

Temporary crisis shelter is one type of social service needed by homeless youths. However, there is a need for services from a variety of sectors, given the pervasiveness of the types of problems experienced by them. For example, among a cohort of 300 runaways (Rotheram-Borus, 1992), 25% of males and 34% of females had experienced foster care within a 3-year time frame following an overnight stay in a runaway shelter. Foster care in New York City costs approximately $585 per month in a family setting and $3548 per month in congregate care. About 16% of the females and 8% of the males had been hospitalized in a psychiatric hospital with an average cost of care in New York being $9382 per month for a mean of 2.4 months each. Over 3 years, about 26% of the males and 11% of the females had been in jail at an average cost of $4860 per month. Thus, in reviewing just three other sectors (juvenile justice, mental health, and foster care), it is clear that there is substantial use of social services other than that of the runaway services, and that consideration of any preventive services requires integration of care across service sectors.

The specific types of problems experienced by homeless youths also lead to the need for targeted services. For example, the high rate of unprotected sex among homeless youths led to relatively high rates of sexually transmitted diseases (10%), pregnancies (24%), and abortions (14%) over a 2-year period (Rotheram-Borus, Reid, Rosario, & Gwadz, 1993). The cost of reproductive health care for female runaways, given these base rates and the cost of services for these conditions in New York City, yielded an estimated $242,485 over 2 years for 148 female runaways (Rotheram-Borus et al., 1993). These data again suggest the need for coordinated, comprehensive care among adolescents.

Thus, there is a continuum of care that is necessary to address the needs of homeless youths. There are at least six types of services for homeless youths (Robertson, 1991b) that should be, at the least, continued, and ideally, improved on and enlarged. They are:

1. *Short-term emergency shelter.* As a result of the Runaway and Homeless Youth Act passed by Congress in 1974, a national network of short-term residential shelters was established to serve an estimated 300,000 youths per year. While service providers have argued that the number of homeless youths has increased, funding has diminished. For example, in a 12-month period in Los Angeles, 65% of 4500 requests for shelter were denied because of lack of space (Pennbridge et al., 1990). This deficit of services leads to a screening and selection of homeless youths as to who receives emergency shelter. Youths must be 12 to 17 years old, a requirement that sometimes leads youths to lie about their age when they are over 18 years old. Most programs are designed to triage youths to a more permanent setting within 2 to 4 weeks. However, often there are no permanent placements available for youths, so many live in the temporary emergency shelters for longer periods. In temporary shelters there is typically a social worker who is attempting

to reunite a youth with his or her family, adult child-care workers to provide 24-hour-per-day supervision, and housekeeping staff (e.g., a cook). The youths typically have a daily routine that includes a "house meeting" and are assigned tasks to facilitate their permanent placement (e.g., go to school). In the past, shelters were funded as "full-service" agencies, offering more comprehensive services (health care, mental health care, vocational and educational planning) than those above (McCoard, 1987; Kennedy, 1991). Few agencies provide full services today.

2. *Tailored programs and treatment services.* There are many subpopulations of homeless youths who have needs for specific programs and services. Tailored programs have been developed for youths living in each of the following life circumstances: those coping with substance-abuse addictions; those living at home, but who are in danger of out-of-home placement; those who have been sexually abused; those who are or may be gay or lesbian; those who have been battered by boyfriends; teenage parents; those who are seropositive for HIV infection; those who are involved in prostitution; and those who are political refugees or victims of war.

3. *Comprehensive service approaches.* Whenever the goal is to provide comprehensive care, case management will be a central issue of the program. Homeless youths have multiple needs; identification and coordination of different services among a network of providers is key to the success of establishing a treatment plan with positive outcomes.

There are two issues embedded in the definition of a comprehensive service approach. First is the notion of a holistic approach to the adolescent. This has sometimes been translated as "one-stop shopping" for adolescent health, mental health, and social services (e.g., *The Door* in New York City). Most agencies, however, cannot provide all of the social service needs of an individual; therefore, effective agencies that attempt to provide a holistic approach are well networked into their community and are part of a community-planning process that identifies the types of problems and situations that staff at each agency are best equipped to handle. Service providers can refer and effectively link youths to care at other sites. A second meaning of the term *comprehensive* is that there is continuity of care so as to provide stability in the life of the adolescent. Both a holistic approach and continuity of care are critical in evaluating adolescent care.

4. *Special education systems.* Youths who have a history of running away often have problems in a typical school and are more likely to have been in special education programs (Rotheram-Borus, Rosario, & Koopman, 1991). An example of educational systems adapting to the needs of homeless youths is the locating of schools within emergency shelters (Zucker, 1994). More often, school districts sponsor alternative high schools for youths who have difficulties adjusting to the structured routine of the typical classroom environment. These schools typically have less structure, give class credit for employment activities, have relaxed dress codes, and have fast-track timetables for early graduation.

5. *Stable residential placements.* Many homeless youths have left poor foster care placements, as well as difficult home environments. It is not feasible for these youths to return home. Residential placements, either in foster homes or group homes, must be found for these youths, but it is often difficult to place adolescents, particularly males and any youths with a history of conduct problems or substance abuse. If foster-care parents are found for a youth, it is critical that they be highly skilled and effective managers of problem behaviors. However, foster parents generally have not had the training to effec-

tively deal with multiple-problem youths. Therefore, group home settings, whose staff often are better trained and more experienced in dealing with these youths, are the desirable placement for homeless youths. Unfortunately, however, many group home settings can be problematic in other ways. If youths who are violent are admitted to a group home, the residence is unlikely to provide safety to the other youths in the shelter. Adolescents who have run away from poor home environments do not hesitate to run away from poor group-home environments. It is key to recognize that setting limits with difficult adolescents is an evolving process in which the adolescent and the caretaker negotiate rules and expectations. If the rules are too rigid, it is unlikely that the adolescent will be able to meet the demands. Sophisticated developmental patterning of rules and behavioral codes for shelters is difficult to design and consistently implement on a daily basis. Such skills are needed, however, to conduct an effective program.

6. *Transitional, independent living options for youths aged 18 to 21 years.* Most youths with multiple problems and those who are in foster care do not magically become adults with stable employment and housing on their 18th birthday. However, youths who turn 18 years old often become ineligible for most social services. Psychologists have recognized that there is a special risk associated with developmental transitions. Therefore, there is a need for transitional services for youths aged 18 to 23, who are making the transition to early adulthood. Transitional services usually consist of a home in a low-income neighborhood that houses eight to ten adolescents. There are live-in parents in the home who are specially trained to work with high-risk youths. The rules of the house are set by the residents and the adult supervisors. Youths must maintain good conduct while living in these residences and must progress toward the goal of independent living. The number of programs that serve youths aged 18 to 23 are very limited and underfunded. However, the costs associated with not making a successful transition to an employed adult are high for society. It is critical that we begin to conduct cost/benefit analyses of youths receiving services through this developmental transition.

Larkin Street Youth Center: A Model Program for Homeless Youths

There are many positive models of agencies serving homeless youths. An example of one outstanding program is the Larkin Street Youth Center in San Francisco. Reviewing the outlines of the program at Larkin Street offers an understanding of the challenges facing those attempting to provide a continuum of care. Where to locate a service agency is the first decision facing providers. If programs are located in "nice" neighborhoods, the agency will not attract the youths in greatest need. Homeless youths are often drawn into neighborhoods that are the center of substance use and prostitution. However, placing runaway shelters in dangerous and/or undesirable neighborhoods increases youths' exposure to violence and crime. Larkin Street is located in the Tenderloin district of San Francisco, a poor community inhabited by injecting drug users and where frequent male and female prostitution occurs.

The mission of Larkin Street is to create a network of communities that inspire youths to move beyond the streets. The agency has pieced together funding from a variety of sources, as well as networked extensively in its local community. Larkin Street offers numerous services: an emergency, short-term shelter; a drop-in service that provides food, clothing, showers, social relationships, and group settings; outreach services by child-care workers who walk the streets to provide services; educational programs; a health-care center; special programs for HIV-seropositive youths; short-term housing for youths in independent living settings; counseling and case management services; programs for Latino immigrants; and a drug detox program (Kennedy, 1991). Each of these programs emerges from the agency's mission and values statement. Without the multiple foci of the program, it would be unlikely that youths' lives could become stable across time.

A study conducted at Larkin Street in 1988–1989 found that of the more than 1000 youths (average age 16.3 years) served by the program, more than 60% were female (Kennedy, 1991). About one-fifth had been in special education classes. More than 50% had contact with other social service agencies prior to coming to Larkin Street. Almost two-thirds had been victims of some type of familial abuse; 50% had been placed outside their home prior to coming to Larkin Street. About one-third had been psychiatrically hospitalized at some point for at least a day, typically for a suicide attempt. Substance use was high: 81% used alcohol or drugs routinely; 15% used heroin; 42% used cocaine and 37% used crack; 72% used marijuana; and 40% used speed. These are youths with multiple problems who will need long-term support in order to become productive, happy, and healthy adults.

The staff at Larkin Street spans the spectrum of professionals, paraprofessionals, and volunteers. The agency has a highly trained, stable staff that has been a key to the long-term success of the agency. Most community-based agencies that serve low-income, minority youths pay poorly, recruit primarily untrained personnel, and have an extremely high turnover rate. The values of the mission statement apply to the treatment of staff, as well as youth. Therefore, there are many training opportunities, salaries are competitive, and benefits are relatively generous for a small agency. Such policies benefit both the youth and the agency. Because the staff is stable, the same staff interact repeatedly with the police. Therefore, the police have confidence in the ability of staff members to accurately report on a youth's status. When youths have been exploited, the staff has worked with the police to help them leave abusive relationships.

Not only has Larkin Street been able to integrate funding to provide a full-service agency, the agency has initiated two particularly innovative programs: (1) a for-profit business that employs adolescents, helping them on the road to adult employment, and (2) an international focus with a special relationship with agencies in India and Africa that provides training options to staff from both countries. While relatively new, the first business enterprise initiated by Larkin Street (a Ben & Jerry's Ice Cream store) is aimed at providing funding to the agency independent of the government, and providing independence to youths. The success of this strategy will be tested over the next few years. The second innovative strategy, linking to international partner agencies, also may be useful in identifying and analyzing cultural differences in attitudes toward homeless youths.

SUMMARY AND CONCLUSIONS

The review outlined above points to at least five potential strategies for reducing the number of homeless youths and reducing long-term negative consequences related to homelessness.

1. *Alternatives to categorical funding for youth programs must be considered.* Pro-

grams for homeless youths are generally supported by categorical funding, i.e., there is a set amount of money set aside by Congress to provide for a certain type of need. Therefore, each of the ten types of services is often competing with the others for support. For example, short-term emergency shelters compete for categorical funding with providers serving youths in congregate settings (e.g., group homes) and with programs for long-term care (e.g., mental health). Service providers are not rewarded for triaging and linking youths to long-term stable placements. The amount of funding available to short-term crisis centers is dependent on the number of youths on the street. If the number of homeless youths decreases because youths are stabilized in foster care, funding for programs serving street youths is decreased. There is no incentive for crisis shelters to decrease the number of youths they serve. The incentives are for maintaining high numbers of disenfranchised, homeless youths. If programs were reimbursed for the number of youths that they were able to stabilize over a 6-month period rather than for providing short-term relief, the configuration of services would shift dramatically. There has been little attention to the coordination of care across funding streams. Legislative mandates and local political action committees could change these practices.

2. *Innovative funding strategies are needed to finance social services.* Social service programs are generally funded by governmental funds: federal, state, county, and city. This places social service agencies at the mercy of shifting political and economic policies. Not only do levels and types of funding shift constantly, but the beliefs about the desirable intervention strategies also shift. Intervention programs are trendy. Recently, the funding of peer programs was a high priority; now, three investigators are publishing papers indicating the drawbacks of peer-led HIV interventions (Luna & Rotheram-Borus, 1995). Funding is often available for establishing new programs, but not for maintenance of noninnovative programs that provide basic care. Initiation of innovative programs and maintenance of ongoing, nontrendy programs is difficult within such shifting political climates. In particular, after agencies have become stabilized and raised their level of competence in service-delivery, they sometimes become ineligible for continued funding, the reasoning being that they are supposed to be self-sufficient and not require ongoing funds. It is critical that agencies establish endowments to maintain basic programs and to initiate programs that may not be solicited by the government. However, this is a difficult task.

It is critical that nonprofit agencies recognize the strengths of for-profit management and funding strategies. By adopting such policies, a stable funding base may be established. As discussed earlier, Larkin Street's Ben & Jerry's Ice Cream franchise will provide employment and training for homeless youths and will provide profits that can be used by the nonprofit agency to provide programs for youths. Another example of an innovative funding strategy can be found at the Venice Family Clinic in Los Angeles, California, which has established an annual fund-raising event: the Venice Art Walk. Within a few years, this event has become a focus point for innovative artists to sell their paintings and sculptures, and it raises substantial funds for the agency. These are only two examples of the types of programs that could be used to generate a stable funding base for nonprofit agencies.

3. *Longitudinal research on the outcomes of homelessness is vital.* A recent publication (Link *et al.*, 1994) indicated that there appears to be significantly more homeless persons than previously believed. Robertson's (1991b) review of homeless adolescents indicates that these youths may be the next generation of homeless adults. In order to stop

the establishment of a cycle of homelessness, it is critical that we implement systematic observations of the paths into and out of homelessness. To develop positive intervention models, it is critical to identify factors associated with positively stabilizing the lives of homeless youths. To date, there has been very little longitudinal research. Longitudinal studies must be initiated if solutions are to be found for the negative consequences of homelessness.

4. *Alternative treatment models must be developed that are tailored to adolescents.* Many of the programs provided to youths have been modeled on adult services. This is particularly true in the area of substance abuse and substance-abuse treatment. Adolescent substance abuse appears to be quite different from that of adults. Most adolescent treatment is based on Alcoholics Anonymous; self-help groups are provided that are grounded in a spiritual framework. Also, detox services are not typically available to adolescents, the role of peer groups in adolescent abuse is underrecognized, and services for adolescents are incorporated into ongoing adult groups. Each of these characteristics is likely to decrease the potential effectiveness of an intervention program for adolescents. The programs are not tailored to the pattern of use by adolescents. Nor have the existing intervention programs been able to resolve the complex ethical and legal issues involved in attempting to provide social and medical services to adolescents. These issues must be addressed directly by networks of service providers attempting to cope with homeless adolescents.

5. *An emphasis on group and community values must be fostered to increase recognition of the rights of and responsibilities toward children and adolescents.* It is relatively easy to attract charitable contributions for homeless youths; the largest agencies serving homeless youths in the United States are sponsored by the Catholic Church (i.e., Covenant House in New York City; Houston, Texas; Los Angeles; Newark, New Jersey; and Toronto, Canada). Having been labeled as a "charity" cause, it is difficult to place the needs of these youths on the public agenda. Children are the responsibility of their parents; the usurping of parents' rights is not undertaken without considerable reflection and repeated demonstration that the parents are incapable. With increasing numbers of homeless youths, it is critical that we reexamine community values regarding communal responsibility toward children. Only by recognizing that all children have a basic right to food, shelter, health care, and education will we be able to adequately care for the next generation. With sustained, strategic attention on these issues, the delivery of services and treatment of homeless youths will be fundamentally modified.

ACKNOWLEDGMENT.   Preparation of this chapter was funded by grant No. R01DA07903 from the National Institute on Drug Abuse to Mary Jane Rotheram-Borus, Ph.D.

REFERENCES

American Psychiatric Association. (1980). *Diagnostic and statistical manual of mental disorders* (3rd ed.). Washington, DC: Author.

Barden, J. C. (1990, February 5). Strife in families swells tide of homeless youths. *The New York Times*, pp. A1, B8.

Bond, L. S., Jiminez, M. V., & Mazin, R. (1992). Street kids and AIDS. *AIDS Education and Prevention, (Fall Suppl.)*, 14–23.

Brennen, T., Huizinga, D., & Elliot, D. S. (1979). *The social psychology of runaways*. Lexington, MA: Lexington Books.

Bucy, J. (1987). Prepared statement of June Bucy, Executive Director, the National Network of Runaway and Youth Services, Washington, DC. In *The crisis in homelessness: Effects on children and families*. Hearing before the Select Committee on Children, Youth, and Families, House of Representatives. Washington, DC: U.S. Government Printing Office.

Bucy, J., & Obolensky, N. (1990). Runaways and homeless youths. In M. J. Rotheram-Borus, J. Bradley, & N. Obolensky (Eds.), *Planning to live: Evaluating and treating suicidal teens in community settings* (pp. 333–353). Tulsa: University of Oklahoma Press.

Chelimsky, E. (1982). The problem of runaway and homeless youth. In *Oversight hearing on runaway and homeless youth program*. House of Representatives, Subcommittee on Human Resources, Committee on Education and Labor, Washington, DC.

Children's Defense Fund. (1988). *A children's defense budget Fiscal Year 1989: An analysis of our nation's investment in children*. Washington, DC: Author.

Cohen, P. (1985). *Homeless children in New York City*. Grand Rounds, New York State Psychiatric Institute, Columbia University, New York.

Dohrenwend, B. P., & Dohrenwend, B. S. (1974). Overviews and prospects for research on stressful life events. In B. S. Dohrenwend & B. P. Dohrenwend (Eds.), *Stressful life events: Their nature and effects* (pp. 313–331). New York: Wiley.

Englander, S. W. (1984). Some self-reported correlates of runaway behavior in adolescent females. *Journal of Consulting & Clinical Psychology, 52,* 484–485.

Gallimore, R., Goldenberg, C. N., & Weisner, T. S. (1993). The social construction and subjective reality of activity settings: Implications for community psychology. *American Journal of Community Psychology, 21*(4), 537–559.

General Accounting Office. (1989). *Homelessness: Homeless and runaway youth receiving services at federally funded shelters*. Washington, DC: Author.

Greenblatt, M., & Robertson, M. J. (1993). Life-styles, adaptive strategies, and sexual behaviors of homeless adolescents. *Hospital and Community Psychiatry, 44*(12), 1177–1180.

Hemmens, K. C., Luecke, M. R. (1988). *Sheltering homeless youths: A guide to Illinois law and programs*. Chicago: The Chicago Law Enforcement Study Group.

Hunter, J., & Schaecher, R. (1990). Teenage suicide: Lesbian and gay youth. In M. J. Rotheram-Borus, J. Bradley, & N. Obolensky (Eds.), *Planning to live: Evaluating and treating suicidal teens in community settings* (pp. 297–316). Tulsa: University of Oklahoma Press.

Kennedy, M. R. (1991). Homeless and runaway youth mental issues: No access to the system. *Journal of Adolescent Health, 12*(7), 576–579.

Koopman, C., Rosario, M., & Rotheram-Borus, M. J. (1994). Alcohol and drug use and sexual behaviors placing runaways at risk for HIV infection. *Addictive Behaviors, 19,* 95–103.

Link, B. G., Susser, E., Stueve, A., Phelan, J., Moore, R. E., & Struening, E. (1994). Lifetime and five-year prevalence of homelessness in the United States. *American Journal of Public Health, 84*(12), 1907–1912.

Luna, G. C. (1987). HIV and homeless youth. *Focus: A Review of AIDS Research, 2,* 10.

Luna, G. C. (1991). Street youth: Adaptation and survival in the AIDS decade. *Journal of Adolescent Health, 12,* 511–514.

Luna, G. C., & Rotheram-Borus, M. J. (1992). Street youth and the AIDS pandemic. *AIDS Education and Prevention (Fall Suppl.),* 1–13.

Luna, G. C., & Rotheram-Borus, M. J. (1995). The limitations of empowerment programs for young people living with HIV. Manuscript submitted for publication.

McCoard, W. D. (1987). A crisis intervention model. In M. J. Rotheram-Borus, J. Bradley, & N. Obolensky (Eds.), *Planning to live: Evaluating and treating suicidal teens in community settings* (pp. 195–209). Tulsa: University of Oklahoma Press.

Meyers, H. (1989). Poverty and bias: Enemies in Brazil AIDS fight. *American Medical News, 32*(9), 33–35.

Mundy, P., Robertson, M., Robertson, J., & Greenblatt, M. (1990). The prevalence of psychotic symptoms in homeless adolescents. *Journal of the American Academy of Child and Adolescent Psychiatry, 29*(5), 724–731.

National Academy of Sciences, Institute of Medicine, Committee on Health Care for Homeless People. (1988). *Homelessness, health, and human needs*. Washington, DC: National Academy Press.

National Network of Runaway and Youth Services, Inc. (1985). *To whom do they belong?* Washington, DC: Author.

Pennbridge, J. N., Freese, T. E., & MacKenzie, R. G. (1992). High-risk behaviors among male street youth in Hollywood, California. *AIDS Education & Prevention, (Fall Suppl.)*, 24–33.

Pennbridge, J. N., Yates, G. L., David, T. G., & MacKenzie, R. G. (1990). Runaway and homeless youth in Los Angeles County, California. *Journal of Adolescent Health Care, 11*(2), 159–165.

Powers, J. L., Eckenrode, J., & Jaklitsch, B. (1990). Maltreatment among runaway and homeless youth. *Child Abuse and Neglect, 14*(1), 87–98.

Robertson, M. J. (1989a). Alcohol use and abuse among homeless adolescents in Hollywood. *Contemporary Drug Problems, 16*, 415–452.

Robertson, M. J. (1989b). *Homeless youth in Hollywood: Patterns of alcohol use*. A report to the National Institute on Alcohol Abuse and Alcoholism. Berkeley, CA: Alcohol Research Group.

Robertson, M. J. (1990, August 11). *Characteristics and circumstances of homeless adolescents in Hollywood*. Paper presented at the annual meeting of the American Psychological Association, Boston.

Robertson, M. J. (1991a). Homeless women with children: The role of alcohol and other drug abuse. *American Psychologist, 46*(11), 1198–1204.

Robertson, M. J. (1991b). Homeless youth: An overview of recent literature. In J. H. Kryder-Coe, L. M. Salamon, & J. M. Molnar (Eds.), *Homeless children and youth* (pp. 33–68). New Brunswick, NJ: Transaction Publishers.

Robertson, M. J. (1992). The prevalence of mental disorder among homeless people. In R. I. Jahiel (Ed.), *Homelessness: A prevention oriented approach* (pp. 57–86). Baltimore: Johns Hopkins University Press.

Rotheram-Borus, M. J. (1992). *HIV prevention with high risk youths*. Presented at a working meeting on HIV Related Change and Prevention. National Institute of Mental Health, Washington, DC.

Rotheram-Borus, M. J. (1993). Suicidal behavior and risk factors among runaway youths. *American Journal of Psychiatry, 150*, 103–107.

Rotheram-Borus, M. J., & Koopman, C. (1991). Sexual risk behaviors, AIDS knowledge, and beliefs about AIDS among runaways. *American Journal of Public Health, 81*(2), 208–210.

Rotheram-Borus, M. J., Koopman, C., & Bradley, J. (1989). Barriers to successful AIDS prevention programs with runaway youth. In J. O. Woodruff, D. Doherty, & J. Garrison Athey (Eds.), *Troubled adolescents and HIV infection: Issues in prevention and treatment* (pp. 37–55). Washington, DC: Janis Press.

Rotheram-Borus, M. J., Koopman, C., & Ehrhardt, A. A. (1991). Homeless youths and HIV infection. *American Psychologist, 46*(11), 1188–1197.

Rotheram-Borus, M. J., Luna, G. C., Marotta, T., & Kelly, H. (1994). Going nowhere fast: Methamphetamine use and HIV infection. In R. Battjes, Z. Sloboda, & W. Grace (Eds.), *The context of HIV risk among drug users and their sexual partners* (National Institute on Drug Abuse Monograph No. 143, pp. 155–183). Rockville, MD: U.S. Department of Health and Human Services.

Rotheram-Borus, M. J., & McDermott, R. (1995). Mental health needs of homeless youths. In N. Alessi (Ed.), *The basic handbook of child and adolescent psychiatry*. New York: Wiley.

Rotheram-Borus, M. J., Meyer-Bahlburg, H. F. L., Koopman, C., Rosario, M., Exner, T. M., Henderson, R., Matthieu, M., & Gruen, R. (1992). Lifetime sexual behaviors among runaway males and females. *The Journal of Sex Research, 29*(1), 15–29.

Rotheram-Borus, M. J., Reid, H. M., Rosario, M. R., & Gwadz, M. (1993, June). Effectiveness of HIV prevention with homeless youth over 2 years. In *Abstracts of the IXth International Conference on AIDS* (WS-C13-3). Berlin, Germany.

Rotheram-Borus, M. J., Rosario, M., & Koopman, C. (1991). Minority youths at high risk: Gay males and runaways. In S. Gore & M. E. Colton (Eds.), *Adolescent stress: Courses and consequences* (pp. 181–200). New York: Aldine de Gruyter.

Rothman, J., & David, T. (1985). *Status offenders in Los Angeles County: Focus on runaway and homeless youth: A study and policy recommendations*. School of Social Welfare, University of California at Los Angeles.

Rutayuga, J. B. K. (1992). Assistance to AIDS orphans within the family/kinship system and local institutions: A program for East Africa. *AIDS Education and Prevention: HIV and Street Youth, (Fall Suppl.),* 57–68.

Shaffer, D., & Caton, C. (1984). *Runaway and homeless youth in New York City. A report to the Ittleson Foundation.* New York: Division of Child Psychiatry, New York State Psychiatric Institute and Columbia University College of Physicians and Surgeons.

Shalwitz, J. C., Goulart, M., Dunnigan, K., & Flannery, D. (1990, June). *Prevalence of sexually transmitted diseases (STD) and HIV in a homeless youth medical clinic in San Francisco.* Presentation at the Sixth Annual International Conference on AIDS, San Francisco, CA.

Stiffman, A. R., Felton, E., Powell, J., & Robins, L. N. (1987). Correlates of alcohol and illicit drug use in adolescent medical patients. *Contemporary Drug Problems, 14,* 295–314.

Stricof, R., Novick, L. F., & Kennedy, J. (1990, June). *HIV-1 seroprevalence in facilities for runaway and homeless adolescents in four states: Florida, Texas, Louisiana, and New York.* Paper presented at the Fourth Annual International Conference on AIDS, San Francisco, CA.

Towber, R. I. (1985). *Characteristics of homeless families: December, 1985.* New York: Human Resources Administration, Office of Program Evaluation. Unpublished manuscript.

Towber, R. I. (1986). *Summary of findings of a one-day survey of homeless families housed at the Martinique Hotel and Forbell Street Shelter.* New York: Human Resources Administration, Office of Program Evaluation.

United Nations Children's Fund (UNICEF). (1989). Annual report, New York: Author.

United Nations Convention on the Rights of the Child: Unofficial summary of articles. (1991). *American Psychologist, 46,* 50–52.

United States Conference of Mayors. (1987). *The continued growth of hunger, homelessness and poverty in America's cities in 1986.* Washington, DC: Author.

Upshur, C. C. (1986). Research Report: The Bridge, Inc., Independent Living Demonstration. In *Amendments to the Foster Care and Adoption Assistance Program.* Hearing before the Subcommittee on Public Assistance and Unemployment Compensation of the Committee on Ways and Means, House of Representatives, Ninety-Ninth Congress (September 19, 1985) (Serial 99–54). Washington, DC.

Windle, M. (1989). Substance use and abuse among adolescent runaways: A four-year follow-up study. *Journal of Youth and Adolescence, 18,* 331–334.

Yates, G. L. (1988, December). *The service delivery system for runaway/homeless youth in Los Angeles County.* Paper presented at the Olive View Medical Center Research Conference on "Homeless Adolescents: A Population in Crisis." Sylmar, CA.

Yates, G., MacKenzie, R., Pennbridge, J., & Cohen, E. (1988). A risk profile comparison of runaway and non-runaway youth. *American Journal of Public Health, 78,* 820–821.

Zucker, J. (Executive Producer). (1994, December 18). *Today Show.* New York: National Broadcasting Corporation.

15

Academic Underachievement and School Refusal

JOHN B. SIKORSKI

INTRODUCTION

That the spectrum of behaviors from subtle academic underachievement to blatant school refusal and drop-out are considered serious health risks in adolescence is no surprise to concerned parents, teachers, professionals, and the American public at the end of the 20th century. This century was proclaimed to be "The Century of the Child" in the first White House Conference on Children in 1909 (Beck, 1974), wherein the national consciousness and governmental policy was to be mobilized to improve the care, education, and welfare of the nation's children.

While pronouncements to the effect that "children are our most valuable resources" have become part of our conventional wisdom, concerned parents and professionals have long known that academic underachievement and school failure have become the arena in which we see the greatest loss of potential, was well as high risk for adverse consequences and co-morbidities in later life development, especially in the areas of mental and physical illness, teen pregnancy, substance abuse, conduct disorder and delinquency, and adult criminal behavior and unemployability. Thus, school refusal and academic underachievement are part of a spectrum of risk behaviors that include psychiatric as well as psychosocial consequences.

The scope and severity of school failure as both a risk behavior and a national crisis were brought to the nation's attention a decade ago with the publication of *A Nation at Risk* (National Commission on Excellence in Education, 1983). The political and econo-

JOHN B. SIKORSKI • Child and Adolescent Psychiatry, University of California, San Francisco, San Francisco, California 94143.

Handbook of Adolescent Health Risk Behavior, edited by Ralph J. DiClemente, William B. Hansen, and Lynn E. Ponton. Plenum Press, New York, 1996.

mic implications of school failure and a call for higher academic achievement were
spurred on by the business community (Committee for Economic Development, 1987),
underscoring our country's critical need for an educated work force to stay competitive in
the global economy of the 21st century. To further the public debate, various historical,
societal, home and family, and school-based factors that contribute to a student's academic underachievement and/or school failure were summarized and published in *Educational Reforms and Students at Risk: A Review of the Current State of the Art* (Office of
Educational Research and Improvement, 1993a). The recognition and mobilization of
these trends culminated in the passage of Public Law 103–227 (Goals 2000: Educate
America Act, 1994), which serves as the national framework for restructuring the U.S.
educational system for *all* children through the framing of goals and implementing processes, including high academic achievement as measured through periodic achievement
assessments; a safe, disciplined environment conducive to learning; and increased parental involvement and participation in children's educational process.

These lofty goals, articulated in the federal statute, highlight some of the identifiable
individual, family, environmental, school-based, and systematic risk factors involved in
academic underachievement and school failure. The goals also provide a formidable
challenge to students, parents, communities, concerned professionals, school districts,
and taxpayers to resolve the impediments that interfere with each student's ability to
realize her or his individual potential.

Academic underachievement and school refusal have become a grave concern not
only to contemporary Americans and not only to industrialized nations, but to all nations
challenged by the optimal development of their human potential and threatened by the
waste of their human resources.

Why Children Reject School: Views from Seven Countries

A yearbook of the International Association for Child and Adolescent Psychiatry and
Allied Professions (Chiland & Young, 1990) highlights the magnitude of this problem and
views the phenomena from the contemporary experiences of seven different countries.
These perspectives on school refusal are not only informed by the particular historical and
sociocultural influences and expectations in each country, but also explore the individual
developmental psychopathology, family and community influences, and structural or
systemic forces within each country.

Two examples from different countries serve to highlight the sociocultural, developmental, and structural factors that affect this risk behavior. In Japan, 92% of school-
age children graduate from high school (Horio & Sabouret, 1990). Nevertheless, there
is increasing concern about the nature of rigid expectations and curriculum, and the
increasing numbers of youth who cannot or will not avail themselves of the educational
opportunities that are present. Thus, school rejection is seen to have a complex etiology, with multiple factors including structural features of the educational system (Horio
& Sabouret, 1990), the interaction of individual developmental factors (Nakane, 1990),
and sociocultural and familial factors (Murase, 1990) which include maternal overin-
volvement with the child, inadequate paternal involvement with the family, and external factors such as undue pressure from peers and authority figures, and outright bully-

ing. In this context, the symptoms of school refusal can be understood as a symptomatic regression in the service of diminishing the intensity of internal and external conflicts the child experiences within a specific structural context. This formulation also lends itself to specific individual, family, and school-based or institutional interventions and treatment strategies.

In a developing country like Brazil, where the vast majority of the population is poor, there are limited opportunities for economic advancement, and where the social structure is rather stratified, only 27% of children remain in school into the fourth grade, and only 6.4% of children complete their third year of secondary education (Celia, 1990). While Celia (1990) notes that there are "some cases of classic school refusal with an elaborate symptomatology similar to those described in the developing world," particularly in children from more privileged backgrounds, he observes that in the majority of Brazilian children, "school refusal is caused by a pathogenic, sociopolitical structure that nurtures such symptoms as loss of self-esteem, insecurity, and anti-social behavior . . . as well as school drop-out." From this etiological perspective, structural changes in the sociocultural context of the schools, as well as more school-based group interventions are critical ingredients in intervention and treatment strategies.

As U.S. society becomes increasingly diverse in its racial and ethnic composition, it also becomes necessary to include and integrate the various ethnic and cultural components of our population into our public and private educational systems. In this regard, we have much to learn (and then apply to our schools), not only about the particular influences of culture and environment on family and individual motivation and values, but also about the universality of the human condition in terms of parental desires for safety, security, and opportunities for achievement for their children.

EPIDEMIOLOGY

The core problem in the study of the academic underachievement and school refusal arena is that of definitions, especially in light of the underlying data bases, implied etiologies, symptomatic manifestations, and consequent intervention and treatment strategies involved with the use of each particular term.

Definition of Academic Underachievement and School Refusal

Consider, for example, the phrase *academic underachievement*. It is conventionally meant to imply that an individual has functioned or performed at some level or standard below which he or she was expected (by self or others) to perform on some task or area of function within the academic setting. An academic test resulting in a specific number or grade equivalent can tell us the actual achievement or performance on that particular test, but it tells us nothing about the expectations or the student's capacity or capability for information acquisition beyond that specific performance.

In *The Condition of Education* (Office of Educational Research and Improvement, 1993b), the U.S. Department of Education does not refer to the term *underachievement*, but, rather, uses the term *achievement*, providing data on student proficiency in the areas of reading, writing, science, and mathematics, as measured by the National Assessment of Educational Progress (NAEP) programs.

The Diagnostic and Statistical Manual of Mental Disorders, Fourth Edition (American Psychiatric Association, 1994), refers to *underachievement* only in the context of V62.3, Academic Problem:

> This category can be used when the focus of clinical attention is an academic problem that is not due to a mental disorder or, if due to a mental disorder, is sufficiently severe to warrant independent clinical attention. An example is a pattern of failing grades or of significant underachievement in a person with adequate intellectual capacity in the absence of a learning or communication disorder or any other mental disorder that would account for the problem.

Specific *learning disabilities,* as defined and used by school districts, were first formulated by the U.S. Office of Education in 1968 and in 1975 were included in the handicapping conditions covered by Public Law 94-142, the Education for the Handicapped Act (EHA) (legal citation: 20 U.S.C. 1400 *et seq.*) (McGee & Sikorski, 1986). This landmark federal legislation provided for a free, appropriate, public education for all handicapped children within the least restrictive environment, based on an Individualized Educational Program (IEP) with related services and due process safeguards.

This federal legislation, with its implementing regulations and subsequent amendments, including the name change in 1990 to *Individuals with Disabilities Education Act* (IDEA) (Public Law 101-476) (legal citation: 20 U.S.C. 1401 *et seq.*), provides the legal basis and partial funding mechanisms for all of the special education programs and services in the public school systems that receive any federal funding and fall within the jurisdiction of federal courts.

The U.S. Department of Education, through the Office of Special Education Programs, is required to transmit an annual report to Congress which "describes progress being made in the implementation of the Act" (15th Annual Report to Congress, 1993). This report compiles the nature and scope of programs and services within the 12 designated disability categories by State and other demographic characteristics, and provides data on other aspects such as early intervention and effectiveness of programs and services.

While the federal government has mandated this complex system of programs and services for all handicapped or disabled students in the public school systems throughout the nation, the overall federal revenue contribution to the local school districts to implement these and other school programs averages about 6%, while state governments contribute about 47%, with the local tax base being responsible to provide the remaining 47% of the total costs of public education services (Snyder, 1993). This revenue discrepancy, along with the far-reaching federal mandates, provides much of the fuel for the incendiary battles that are being fought between regular and special education proponents under the current banner of "inclusion," that is, providing all services within the regular classroom, with additional support services and accommodations for those disabled students available in the regular classroom setting.

Consider now the various terms used to describe nonattendance at school, including *school avoidance, school phobia, truancy, school refusal, separation anxiety disorder,* and *drop-out*. In a review article on school avoidance, school phobia, and truancy (Berg, 1991), definitional and characteristic features of these terms within a historical, developmental, and treatment context are articulated. Berg (1991) notes that in the United Kingdom, 10% of all school children are out of school at any given time and that lower socioeconomic status, lack of parental interest in education, and specific adverse factors related to the school are related to school avoidance.

The term *school phobia* (Johnson, Felstein, Szurek, & Svendsen, 1941) was introduced in the American literature to "recognize a type of emotional disturbance in children associated with great anxiety that leads to serious absence from school." There was considerable work in the subsequent decades developing the psychodynamic considerations, family interactions, and treatment strategies for this condition.

Berg (1991) notes that "in Britain, an alternative term, school refusal, was more generally employed for similar problems." He describes the following features associated with school refusal: The child remains at home with the knowledge of the parents; there is absence of severe antisocial behavior; parents make reasonable attempts to secure the child's attendance at school; there is emotional upset at the prospect of having to go to school.

In an earlier review of school refusal, Hersov (1985) distinguishes between school refusal and truancy, noting that the word *truant* carries a pejorative connotation, deriving from an old French word meaning "an assemblage of beggars." The current concept of truancy connotes a voluntary absence from school without parental knowledge or permission, is estimated to be between 3 and 8% of school children, is more common in older grades than younger grades, is more common in boys than in girls by about 3 to 1, and is associated with punitive discipline, low socioeconomic family status, negative peer group influences, and conduct disorders and Juvenile Court involvement.

Concerning the prevalence of *school refusal,* Hersov (1985) suggested that a reasonable estimate would be 5% of all children with psychiatric disorders, but with peak periods around the beginning of school, at about ages 5 to 7 (probably associated with separation anxiety), and again at age 11 and again at age 14 or older (associated with other psychiatric disorders or depressive states). The association of school refusal with separation anxiety disorder (Last & Strauss, 1989) or other primary or comorbid disorders such as social phobia, simple phobia, panic disorder, and depressive disorders (Tisher, 1985) has been demonstrated and is thought to be highly correlated with pathogenic family functioning (Bernstein, Svingen, & Garfinkel, 1989).

DSM-IV (APA, 1994) makes no specific reference to "school phobia" in the general section on anxiety disorders, which include phobic disorders. However, under diagnosis number 309.21, Separation Anxiety Disorder, "persistent reluctance or refusal to go to school or elsewhere because of fear of separation" is listed as one of the criteria by which the diagnosis is made. It must be noted that the formal diagnostic criteria require evidence of three or more criteria of developmentally inappropriate or excessive anxiety concerning separation from home or from those to whom the individual is attached, of which refusal or reluctance to go to school is but one. In addition, the diagnostic criteria require that the duration of disturbance is at least 4 weeks, the age of onset is before 18 years, the disturbance causes clinically significant distress or impairment in social, academic, or other important areas of functioning, and that the disturbance is not better accounted for by other, presumably more severe, psychiatric disorders.

Concerning the term *truancy,* it is mentioned in *DSM-IV* (APA, 1994) only as one of the 15 diagnostic criteria, of which three are required for the diagnosis of 312.8, Conduct Disorder. The diagnostic phrase reads, "is often truant from school beginning before age 13 years," and it must be noted that three or more diagnostic criteria must be manifest in the past 12 months with at least one criterion present for the past 6 months.

The term *drop-out* is not used in *DSM-IV* as a diagnostic or descriptive term. It is, however, used within school systems and is defined by the Department of Education (Office of Educational Research and Improvement, 1993) as follows:

> Drop-out: The term is used both to describe an event—leaving school before graduating—and a status—an individual who is not in school and is not a graduate. . . . Measures to describe these often complicated behaviors include the event drop-out rate (or the closely related school persistence rate), the status drop-out rate, and the high school completion rate.

It is clear that definitional problems have clouded this field, but recent studies are beginning to clarify the problem.

Gender and Ethnic Differences

With these definitional and statistical differences in mind, the National Center for Education Statistics (1993) publishes reports that shed some light on the nature and scope of the academic underachievement and school refusal problem. These data reveal that, for example, concerning school enrollment in the year ending October 1991, 96% of all 14- to 17-year-olds attended some type of school or educational program. Concerning the issue of school dropouts, however, the Youth Indicator data revealed that for the year ending October 1991, 12.5% of 16- to 24-year-olds had dropped out of school. This figure compares to 17% of 16- to 24-year-olds who had dropped out of school in the year 1967. The 1991 figures, broken down for gender and ethnicity, reveal the dropout rate of males to be 13%, of females to be 11.9%, and by race and ethnicity, whites 8.9%, blacks 13.6%, and Hispanic 35.3%. Also, 1991 data reveal that among the age group of 20- to 29-year-olds, 14.6% had not completed high school by 1991.

Thus, the specific incidence and prevalence of these conditions are dependent on the particular definition of the condition and sample of population under study. It is clear, however, that over 12% of youth fail to complete high school.

Analysis of these data reflects that the percentage of high school students from lower-income families dropping out of school is considerably higher than that from higher-income families. In 1991, 11% of low-income family students dropped out of high school, compared to 1% of higher-income families in that same year. Similarly, concerning high school graduates who enroll in college, 40% of high school graduates from low-income families enroll in college, compared to 78% of high school graduates from high-income families. Of those high school graduates who do not enroll in college, 49% from low-income families are employed the year after graduating, compared to 78% from higher-income families. Other data about the high school dropout rate according to socioeconomic and income background reveal that of high school dropouts, in the year following dropping out, 27% from low-income families are employed, compared to 42% from middle-income families. It is clear that low socioeconomic status, plus dropping out of high school, predispose to higher rates of unemployability.

Concerning measures of academic achievement, the Youth Indicator (National Center for Education Statistics, 1993) data are reflected in indices compiled by the National Assessment of Educational Progress (NAEP) on a scale ranging from 0 to 500 points, and the proficiency ratings in the areas of reading, math, and science. During the 1990 academic year, 17-year-olds were tested in the reading proficiency scale, with the national average being 290. Breakdown according to gender and ethnicity is as follows: males 284, females 297, whites 297, blacks 267, Hispanics 275. On the mathematics proficiency scale in 1990, the national average for 17-year-olds was 305. Breakdown according to gender and ethnicity revealed: females 303, males 306, whites 310, blacks 289, Hispanics 284.

The science proficiency examination in 1990 revealed a national average of 290, with breakdown according to gender and ethnicity: females 297, males 314, whites 301, blacks 253, Hispanics 262. In comparison with previous years, Youth Indicator (National Center for Education Statistics, 1993) data reveal that the gap between achievement scores for minorities is narrowing substantially in the past two decades, with black students improving faster than Hispanics relative to whites.

In terms of international comparisons on mathematics and science assessments, American 13-year-olds in the school year 1991 scored 55%, ranking 13th among nations in mathematics, and 67% in science, ranking 12th among nations. On the same examination, 13-year-olds from Korea, Taiwan, Switzerland, and the former Soviet Union averaged 70% or above in both science and mathematics.

Youth Indicators (National Center for Education Statistics, 1993) also sampled the TV watching habits of sophomore students in the school year 1991. It was noted that over 9% of students reported watching five or more hours of television per school night, and the higher number of hours of television watching correlated with lower socioeconomic status families and lowest test performance by the students.

In addition to these factors, there is considerable evidence (DeBaryshe, Patterson, & Kapaldi, 1993) that additional family risk factors, such as lower parental academic achievement and aspirations, adversely affect the child's academic achievement. This adverse consequence can come about by providing sometimes not-so-subtle role modeling and approval for the child's academic underachievement, as well as through fostering derisive attitudes toward educational achievement, which lessens the child's engagement in the academic process. There is also evidence (DeBaryshe et al., 1993) that a more ineffective, inconsistent, and punitive parental discipline style, more frequently utilized by lower-achieving parents, correlates with a child's diminished engagement in the school and academic process, lower academic achievement, and higher rates of antisocial behaviors.

On the other hand, parental styles that correlate with a child's higher probability for academic success reflect a rather authoritative parenting style, which is both knowledgeable and involved, and which encourages the child in a context of warmth and communication within the parent–child relationship (Steinberg, Lamborn, Dornbasch, & Darling, 1992).

Other than the types of gender or ethnic categorical data referred to above, a more specific delineation of gender or ethnic differences or trends is difficult to cull from the educational literature which tends to focus on age and grade parameters rather than highlight other student differences.

PREVENTION

Epidemiological data outline parameters of identifiable risk factors and behaviors, which are certainly multicausal and multifactorial (from the perspectives of developmental psychopathology), that may increase the likelihood of negative outcomes in the spectrum from academic underachievement to school dropout. It also suggests identifiable individual, family, community, and systemic school-based protective factors (Rutter, 1980), as well as preventive intervention venues and strategies which may not only minimize negative outcomes, but may produce more positive results through enhancing resilience factors.

From the traditional public health perspectives (Sameroff & Fiese, 1989), primary prevention attempts to elucidate the biological causes of the disease. Secondary prevention identifies and prevents the disease or pathological condition before it causes suffering or impairment, and tertiary prevention attempts to treat the manifested diseased condition and prevent further disability. In the areas of psychiatric disorders and psychosocial pathological behaviors, at our present state of knowledge, primary prevention of inherent biological factors may account for only a small percentage of prevention efforts, albeit in some of the more severe cases of mental and emotional illnesses, while tertiary prevention or treatment of the disability condition has been the traditional mainstay of clinical practice.

Secondary Prevention

It is in this area of secondary prevention that interventions at the earliest identifiable developmental stage, particularly with identifiable high-risk individuals, within the transactional model context (Sameroff & Fiese, 1989) provide opportunities for diminishing negative outcomes while at the same time enhance more positive achievement and prosocial behaviors. By definition, secondary prevention, which intervenes and aims to prevent the development of school failure behaviors before they become enmeshed in personality patterns, is both necessary and cost-effective in terms of diminishing suffering and enhancing human potential.

Early childhood education and intervention programs such as Head Start are invaluable to a discussion of prevention, as they demonstrate the efficacy of early intervention strategies utilizing specialized curriculum and focusing on higher-risk populations. The Head Start program (Zigler & Trickett, 1978), while not maintaining the initial robust intellectual and academic gains that were expected, did demonstrate some measurable gains in academic achievement and prosocial behaviors, while at the same time showing reduced rates of special education program utilization and reduced rates of school failure in adolescence.

The single largest constellation of programs of preventive intervention for academic underachievement and school failure developed in the United States are the special education programs, initially authorized and funded in part through Public Law 94-142, The Education for the Handicapped Act (EHA) in 1975 (McGee & Sikorski, 1986). These special education identification, remediation, and related service programs were reauthorized and expanded in the Individuals with Disabilities Education Act (IDEA), Public Law 101-476, in 1990, to provide that "all children have available to them . . . a free appropriate public education which emphasizes special education and related services designated to meet their unique needs" (Fifteenth Annual Report to Congress on IDEA, 1993).

This Fifteenth Annual Report (1993) defined disability categories and provided data on the number and percent of children and youth served within the special education programs in the public school system during the 1991–1992 school year (Table 1).

There are approximately 181,000 additional school-age disabled children who are served through separate legislation and cared for in various state-operated programs, bringing the total of school-age children and youth (ages 6–21) with all disabilities covered by existing federal law and programs to 4,505,448 in the 1991–1992 school year. This figure of 4.5 million constitutes approximately 11% of all children and youth attending public schools in the United States.

It is beyond the scope of this chapter to discuss the changing definitions, incidence of various conditions, and changes in educational and intervention strategies contained in each of these disability categories in the years since Public Law 94-142 was enacted in 1975. Suffice it to say that 94.2% of all children with disabilities fall within the four categories of Specific Learning Disabilities, Speech and Language Impairments, Mental Retardation, and Serious Emotional Disturbance, with Learning Disabilities being the fastest growing and largest diagnostic category.

Once eligibility is defined based on measured academic underachievement and the existence of a specifically designated handicapping or disabling condition as the cause of that underachievement, an Individualized Education Plan (IEP) is developed to provide

Table 1. Number and Percent of Children with Disabilities[a]

Disability category	Number of children	Percent
Specific learning disabilities	2,218,948	51.3
Speech or language impairments	990,016	22.9
Mental retardation	500,986	11.6
Serious emotional disturbance	363,877	8.4
Multiple disabilities	80,655	1.9
Hearing impairments	43,690	1.0
Orthopedic impairments	46,333	1.1
Other health impairments	46,401	1.3
Visual impairments	18,296	0.4
Deaf-blindness	773	<0.1
Autism	3,555	<0.1
Traumatic brain injury	285	<0.1

[a]From Fifteenth Annual Report to Congress on IDEA (1993).

the specific intervention, support, and/or accommodation services, within the structure of special education program services.

Some schools, at their own option and expense, may provide additional tutorial or support services to children whose academic underachievement is not caused by a federally designated handicapping condition. No comprehensive data on these voluntary services are available on a national level.

While these federally mandated special education programs were initially focused on early assessment and remedial programs, along with supplementary services such as counseling or accommodation services, it became apparent that handicapped and disabled students were having a more difficult time in high school programs and were also having a more difficult time than their nonhandicapped peers in successfully making the transition from the teenage years of high school to adult life of more independent living and working.

To further evaluate this area of adolescent transitional difficulty, Congress authorized the Department of Education, as part of the 1983 Amendments to the Education for Handicapped Act (EHA), to conduct a national study of the nature and scope of the transitional problems of disabled youth who had been receiving special education services. This massive study has become known as the National Longitudinal Transition Study of Special Education Students, conducted by SRI International under contract with the Office of Special Education (Wagner *et al.,* 1991). This study consisted of a sample of over 8000 students ages 15 to 23 who participated in special education programs in 1985. The data were collected between 1987 and 1990 from the subsamples of students, school records, parent interviews, and surveys of teachers and school administrators.

This National Longitudinal Transition Study of Special Education Students, while focusing on student experience and outcome, reflects some information about the nature and results of the special education program interventions, as well as the demographic and educational characteristics of students already served in the existing special education program interventions. It should also be noted here that effectiveness or outcome studies of such large sample size and national scope are extremely rare in the educational literature.

In terms of specific school-based special education programs (Wagner, 1993), 92% of disabled students attended regular high school and approximately one-fourth of them had attended extra classes in terms of summer schools or an extra semester. Less than 5% of disabled students who dropped out of high school subsequently graduated 3 to 5 years after dropping out.

In terms of vocational preparation, 89% of high school students with disabilities took some vocational education classes, and one-third of those disabled students participated in work experience programs while in high school. Disabled students spent approximately 70% of their time in regular education classrooms supported by accommodation procedures, behavioral management programs, and other individualized instruction with teacher consultation. Approximately 30% of their time was spent in specific special education settings. Despite these accommodations and support for teachers and students, special education students in regular classrooms were more likely to fail courses than their nonspecial education peers. Support services included transition planning for up to 80% of disabled students, and life skills training for approximately 43% of disabled students. Support services, including physical therapy, personal counseling, and speech therapy, were utilized by approximately 20% of disabled students.

A partial summary of the salient features of the initial report of the National Longitudinal Transition Study relevant to adolescent risk characteristics and behaviors reflects the following data (Wagner *et al.*, 1991): 68.3% of disabled youth came from households with incomes less than $25,000 per year, 41% from households whose head is not a high school graduate, and 36.8% from single-parent homes. Average days absent from school is about 15 per year, and approximately 31% received at least one failing grade in the most recent school year. High school dropout rates for the four major categories of disability were 49.5% for emotionally disturbed, 32.2% for learning disabled, 29.9% for the mentally retarded, and 28.3% for the speech impaired. The percentage of dropout by ethnic classification was: whites, 24.9%; blacks, 38.5%; Hispanics, 33.7%.

Associated risk behaviors for these special education students include arrest rates for all conditions, which average 9% while still in school and about 30% 3 to 5 years out of school. Rates of arrest were highest for emotionally disturbed students, varying from 19.9% while still in school to 57.6% 3 to 5 years out of school. The percentage of these youth living independently of parents or extended family 2 years out of school averaged 11.2%, and 37.4% 3 to 5 years out of school. Forty-four percent of the learning disabled students attained independent living 3 to 5 years out of school.

Gender differences for this population indicate that one-fourth of disabled women dropped out of school for reason of pregnancy, and rates of parenting for youth out of school 3 to 5 years was 16.5% for males and 40.6% for females, whereas the rate of parenting for women in the general population 3 to 5 years out of school is 26%. In terms of postschool employment, 39.8% of dropouts with disabilities were employed, whereas 55% of high school graduates with disabilities were employed 2 years out of school. In summarizing these data, Wagner, Blackorby, and Hebbeler (1993) conclude that high-risk personal characteristics, along with high rates of school absenteeism and course failure, predispose to school dropout and higher rates of arrest, pregnancy, unemployability, and failure at independent living.

Adverse characteristics of the school setting such as large, less personal, and affiliative school size and structure, and low-income student body, along with poverty and disability, place an individual at higher risk for school failure. Poverty alone renders one less likely to receive family and community support services and to spend more time in special education classes than similarly disabled but not poor peers.

There is still much to be accomplished in terms of early identification of high-risk students, greater administrative efficiency in developing and coordinating programs, and more effective utilization of basic science in clinical research in the development of innovative special education programs, as well as more focused in-service training for regular education teachers in working with handicapped and disabled students in the regular ("mainstream" or "inclusion") classroom settings. Nevertheless, there is a nationwide system firmly in place in the public schools and available to all students who meet specific eligibility criteria for special education remedial and related supportive services. The data from the National Longitudinal Transition Study of Special Education Students (cited above) clearly highlight the extensive special needs and additional efforts that are required to enable these high-risk, high-need students to succeed in life after their teenage and school years.

In addition to the preventive intervention (essentially remedially based) programs available to all students in the public school systems, several kinds of smaller prevention programs utilizing private clinics, community-based assessment, early intervention, and specific intervention programs have been developed. These more limited programs focus on specific etiological factors, particular risk characteristics, or have developed a particular context for the intervention.

An example of one of the more comprehensive interventions that integrated school, family, and community factors into an effective intervention program was developed in conjunction with the Yale University Child Study Center (Comer, 1988) and has become known as the Yale–New Haven Prevention Project (YNHPP) (Comer, 1985), successfully replicated in many schools throughout the country. In his analysis of the academic underachievement and school failure of the largely African-American and poor population of the inner-city schools that were studied, Comer (1988) suggested that "the key to academic achievement is to promote psychological development in the student which encourages bonding to the school. Doing so requires fostering positive interaction between parents and school staff, a task for which most staff people are not trained." Components of this intervention program include a comprehensive school plan, developed by the governance and management team, which consists of principal, parents, teachers, and a mental health worker. This comprehensive school plan covers a range of academic, social activities, and special programs at the school. The program includes parent involvement and family participation in a broad array of activities and governance in the schools. It also enables the participation of mental health team members to assist in working with individual students; to consult with parents, teachers, and administrators; and to function within the school in ways to foster changes in procedures to prevent behavioral problems, improve relationships between parents and school personnel, and promote program changes that create a school climate conducive to learning. Internal feedback and assessment factors are usually built into this model. A more comprehensive long-term outcome evaluation compared to other massive intervention strategies is yet to be completed.

While it takes several years of dedicated and persistent work to transform the culture of a school, the Comer program provides a replicable model of dealing with individual, family, sociocultural, and school-based risk factors. Such a model enhances the probability of academic achievement, school- and family-based affiliation, and outcome success.

Another example of a school-based clinic program focusing on school avoidance behavior underscores the motivational basis for school avoidance and attempts to develop intervention strategies based on differential motivational characteristics (Taylor & Adelman, 1990). This type of program focuses on "student attempts to act in ways that make them feel in control, competent, and connected to significant others" (Taylor & Adelman, 1990). Intervention strategies include individual assessment of the motivational characteristics of the student, consultation with parents and teachers, and counseling or psychotherapy with students and families, with treatment efforts directed toward amelioration of the underlying motivational issues by mobilizing the student's intrinsic motivation for competence and self-determination.

A model of early intervention with truants based in a community youth clinic study (Levine, Metzendorf, & Van Boskirk, 1986) proposes the reduction of "runaway," "throwaway," and "homeless" youth, i.e., youth who are under 18 years of age and are voluntarily away from home, usually without parental permission, for significant periods of time. At the time of self-report of being a runaway, 60% had been truant for six or more school days, 44.7% reported being suspended from school, and 29% reported failing two or more grades. School failure and truancy are seen as high-risk behaviors for runaway status. Preventive intervention strategies to reduce truancy, such as school-based counseling programs, school-initiated conferences with parents, and timely and judicious referral to Juvenile Court or Protective Service Agencies, are sometimes necessary to both protect and contain a troubled youth. A coordinated effort between community-based youth service workers and specifically designated school-based personnel is a critical ingredient in the functioning of this model (McGee & Sikorski, 1986).

The demarcation between secondary prevention and tertiary treatment can be as imperceptible as the difference between late adolescence and young adulthood. Preventive intervention focuses on the earlier or less symptomatic forms of potentially dysfunctional behaviors, which, in turn, may develop into more fully manifested forms of similar or other more dysfunctional behavior that then require more robust and direct treatment efforts. More comprehensive systematic research along interdisciplinary lines and with prospective studies in these arenas of prevention and treatment for adolescents at risk have started to come of age in the past decade (Kazdin, 1993; Jessor, 1993; Sameroff & Fiese, 1989). Research studies have become more vigorous in definition and methodologically more broadly focused on multifactorial components and interactive contextual factors, including both subjective experience and objective behavior, in a more developmental and longitudinal perspective. In the arenas of academic underachievement and risk for school failure, the National Longitudinal Transition Study is a current example of a complex study including gender, racial and ethnic, and personal characteristic differences in programmatic effectiveness and outcome. Specialized programs utilizing these and other data relevant to selected high-risk populations are being developed (Office of Educational Research and Improvement, 1993a).

Future research will be necessary to delineate the emerging knowledge of biogenetic vulnerabilities and predispositions to such conditions as learning disabilities, speech and language disorders, and other forms of mental and emotional disorders, along with their environmental and experiential contexts that result in academic underachievement and school failure. The specific resilience and protective factors that mitigate against vulnerabilities to academic underachievement and school failure have begun to be identified (Garmezy, 1993; Keogh & Weisner, 1993), but need further delineation in terms of mechanisms of interaction and influence, as well as strategies for their enhancement. Research priorities must also be extended to fully include underserved and high-risk populations, as well as differential methodologies for effective interventions among diverse populations.

TREATMENT

Treatment of clinical dysfunctions and behavioral disorders associated with this risk behavior of academic underachievement and school refusal begins where preventive intervention has not been implemented or has not been successful in mobilizing protective factors, minimizing risk factors, and preventing the development of clinical symptomatic behavior.

At the point of referral to the clinical practitioner, it is sometimes difficult to engage the child and family in the diagnostic and treatment planning process. Members of many distressed families still view the psychiatric clinic as a place to be stigmatized and therefore avoided, rather than as a place of support, understanding, and problem-solving. In our clinical experience with both school-age children and rebellious adolescents, especially from the perspective of school consultation and collaboration (American Psychiatric Association, 1992; Comer, 1989), the manner of referral and procedure for obtaining psychoeducational assessment and/or psychiatric evaluation is critical to the ultimate goal of obtaining assistance for the troubled child.

One useful strategy to combat these problems includes the development of student study teams, as in the San Francisco Unified School District. These teams can facilitate this process by engaging the troubled youth and the parents in an initial school-based conference, with school-based interventions and with teachers and counselors known to the student and family. This process facilitates the development of a cooperative, problem-solving attitude, as well as the development of concern and trust among the participants. This student study team can then recommend and facilitate the process of outside referral for further specialized evaluation when local, school-based interventions are insufficient. Specialized psychoeducational and/or psychiatric evaluation may be requested to delineate the differential diagnosis, which may include separation anxiety disorder, phobia, other anxiety conditions, depression, conduct disorder, adjustment disorder, or psychosis, along with other comorbid conditions such as learning disabilities, attention-deficit hyperactivity disorder, and substance abuse. Such an evaluation sometimes requires more confidential information about complex family histories of these conditions, which may be difficult or impossible to obtain, particularly in a school-based setting, and especially with children in unconventional or substance-abusing families.

There are multiple psychosocial stressors on children in poor, underserved, deprived, or neglected family circumstances, exacerbating a multiplicity of intrinsic factors that may result in their sense of depression, alienation, and subsequent refusal to show up for school at the appointed time and place in order to participate in the learning process. For these reasons, treatment cannot be implemented without an appropriate clinical evaluation that takes into consideration at least the relevant family history of the child, the psychosocial and developmental experience of the child, the course of the symptomatic manifestations of dysfunctional conditions, and the results of previous attempts at intervention. Optimally, these comprehensive data are developed into a biopsychosocial dynamic formulation (Shapiro, 1989) which then informs the treatment plan and infuses the course of treatment with the knowledge of the child's strengths and weaknesses, risk and resilience factors, and historical patterns of defenses, vulnerabilities, and achievements.

Only after completing a comprehensive evaluation is the course of appropriate treatment formulated and implemented. This treatment plan may include individual or highly selected small-group remedial therapy for specific learning disabilities or speech and language disorders. In the case of specific learning disabilities, the strategy and methodology for remedial treatment (Lerner, 1988) are derived from a task analysis evaluation of the student's information processing through language use and auditory, visual, and motor modalities. Individualized remedial treatment interventions are then directed to the areas of information processing deficiency (i.e., teach to the weakness) or are directed to the cognitive and information processing strengths, circumventing or compensating for the deficiency by teaching to the child's inherent effective learning pathways and styles.

In the case of the diagnosis of one or more mental or emotional disorders, the appropriate treatment plan derived from the biopsychosocial formulation may include individual, group, or family psychotherapy, collateral individual work with parents or other family members, as well as consultation with school, social service, juvenile court, or other community agencies if appropriate to facilitate the achievement of the treatment goals.

Psychoactive medication may be helpful and used for specific indications and target symptoms. As with all licensed treatment with minors, the informed consent of the parent or legal guardian, as well as the assent or cooperation of the minor is required, unless the minor meets the requirements of state laws to provide for their own informed consent or emergency treatment (California Physicians' Legal Handbook, 1993).

Children and youth with school refusal behaviors may present to the clinician a complex picture of anxious (Last & Strauss, 1989), phobic (Last, Francis, Herson, Kazdin, & Strauss, 1987), avoidant and depressive (Kearney, 1993) symptoms, along with learning disabilities and language disorders (Naylor, Staskowski, Kenney, & King, 1994), confounding family and environmental stressors. These stressors may in turn serve to reinforce or mitigate against school refusal risk behavior. The School Refusal Assessment Scale (Kearney & Silverman, 1993) is a clinically useful tool which distinguishes functional characteristics, identifies positive and negative reinforcement factors, and assists in differentiating diagnostic clusters.

The principles of treatment of school refusal include making every reasonable effort to return the child to school as soon as possible (Hersov, 1985; Kearney & Beasley, 1994). This usually requires careful collaboration with school authorities and close involvement and cooperation with the child's family. Behavior modification techniques, cognitive behavioral psychotherapy, and various desensitization techniques (Mansdorf & Lukens, 1987), as well as more traditional psychodynamically oriented psychotherapy with children, are the commonly used therapeutic approaches (Berg, 1991; Hersov, 1985).

Separation anxiety-disordered school refusers usually present a reluctance to go to school in order to stay with their attachment figure or stay at home until that person's return. This is usually seen in the context of other relevant family psychopathology and other symptomatic complaints in the child, such as excessive worry about harm coming to the attachment figure or to the self when separated, clinging behavior with the attachment figure, or physical or somatic complaints out of proportion to the physical findings or without physiologic basis.

Separation anxiety and phobic disorder can be differentiated on a phenomenological and contextual basis (Last et al., 1987; Last & Strauss, 1989), with phobic-disordered children showing excessive fears about some aspect of the school setting. In contrast, separation anxiety-disordered children seem to be younger, more likely to be female and from lower socioeconomic status families, and more likely to have mothers with affective disorders, thus rendering these children to be vulnerable to greater psychopathological severity of symptoms than children with phobic diagnosis.

Comprehensive treatment efforts must be aimed at both the alleviation of dysfunctional symptoms and the resolution of underlying biogenetic and psychodynamic etiological factors wherever possible. In this regard, psychopharmacologic treatment of school refusers (Bernstein, Garfinkel, & Borchardt, 1989) has had mixed reviews depending on the parameter of the samples and the nature of the studies (Klein, Koplewicz, & Kanner, 1992). Tricyclic antidepressants, used on an empirical basis for target symptoms of separation anxiety and/or depression, seem to be the psychopharmacologic agents of choice in research studies and clinical practice thus far, though there is increasing anecdotal reference to the use of serotonin reuptake inhibitors in the past few years.

Concerning treatment research, definitional and criteria problems, age, stage of development, intensity, and severity and duration of symptoms, as well as modality of treatment intervention, including characteristics of the therapist and treatment setting, are confounding variables which need coordinated study (Kazdin, 1993; Sameroff & Fiese, 1989). The longer-term impact of various treatment techniques must be validated with appropriately defined outcome criteria. Research should also focus on developing variations and adaptations of reliable treatment processes in different population subsets so as to be more efficacious with the various high-risk populations. Reliable data on the possible variations and differential results of treatment techniques from academic research to clinical practice settings should also be developed.

SUMMARY

Academic underachievement and school failure are seen as adolescent risk behaviors within the school domain. Demographic studies indicate that in the United States, over 12.5% of older teenagers and young adults have dropped out of school, and that minority status and poverty increase the probability of failing to complete high school. These risk factors and associated risk behaviors increase the probability of antisocial behavior and higher arrest rates, as well as increase the likelihood of unemployment, welfare dependency, and failure at independent living.

These risk behaviors result from a complex developmental interaction of individual biogenetic substrates, interaction with ongoing accumulating psychosocial and environmental experiences, and with the particular cognitive style and personality features that are experienced by the individual at their particular stage in individual development. Specific cultural historical contexts and systemic institutional factors impinge on the individual and group psychological processes, resulting in risk behaviors which, in turn, increase the probability of risk outcomes.

Further research delineating these biogenetic, contextual, interactive, and pathogenic developmental risk factors, as well as protective and resilience factors which may buffer the risk factors and enhance the development of more prosocial behavior, must be pursued. Salient features of this research effort need to be extended to the understanding of, and intelligent, humane intervention with, high-risk youth in both school and community settings (Office of Educational Research and Improvement, 1993a).

REFERENCES

American Psychiatric Association. (1992). *Psychiatric consultation in schools*. Washington, DC: Author.

American Psychiatric Association. (1994). *Diagnostic and statistical manual of mental disorders* (4th ed.). Washington, DC: Author.

Beck, R. (1974). The White House Conference on Children: An historical perspective. The rights of children. *Harvard Educational Review,* Reprint Series No. 9.

Berg, I. (1991). School avoidance, school phobia, and truancy. In M. Lewis (Ed.), *Child and adolescent psychiatry: A comprehensive textbook* (pp. 1092–1098). Baltimore: Williams & Wilkins.

Bernstein, G. A., Garfinkel, B. D., & Borchardt, C. M., (1989). Comparative studies of pharmacotherapy for school refusal. *Journal of the American Academy of Child and Adolescent Psychiatry, 29*(5) 774–781.

Bernstein, G. A., Svingen, P. H., & Garfinkel, B. D. (1989). School phobia: Patterns of Family Functioning, *Journal of the American Academy of Child and Adolescent Psychiatry, 29,*(1) 24–30.

California Medical Association. (1993). *California Physicians' Legal Handbook*. San Francisco: Sutter Publications.

Celia, S. (1990). School refusal and school problems in Brazil. In C. Chiland, & J. G. Young (Eds.), *Why children reject school: Views from seven countries* (pp. 152–159). New Haven: Yale University Press.

Chiland, C., & Young, J. G. (Eds.). (1990). *Why children reject school: Views from seven countries*. New Haven: Yale University Press.

Comer, J. P. (1985). The Yale–New Haven Primary Prevention Project: A follow-up study. *Journal of the American Academy of Child Psychiatry, 24,*(2) 154–160.

Comer, J. P. (1988). Educating poor minority children. *Scientific American, 259*(5), 42–48.

Comer, J. P. (1989). School consultation. In R. Michaels (Ed.), *Psychiatry,* V2 (70), 1–10. Philadelphia: Lippincott.

Committee for Economic Development. (1987). *Children in need: Investment strategies for the educationally disadvantaged*. New York: Research and Policy Committee for the Committee for Economic Development.

DeBaryshe, B. D., Patterson, G. R., & Kapaldi, D. M. (1993). A performance model for academic achievement in early adolescent boys. *Developmental Psychology, 29*(5), 795–804.

Fifteenth Annual Report to Congress on the Implementation of the Individuals with Disabilities Education Act. (1993). Office of Special Education Programs, U.S. Department of Education. Washington, DC: U.S. Government Printing Office.

Garmezy, N. (1993). Children in poverty: Resilience despite risk. *Psychiatry, 56,* 127–136.

Goals 2000: Educate America Act. (1994). Washington, DC: U.S. Government Printing Office.

Hersov, L. (1985). School avoidance. In M. Rutter & L. Hersov (Eds.), *Child and adolescent psychiatry: Modern approaches* (pp. 382–389). Oxford: Blackwell Scientific Publications.

Horio, T., & Sabouret, J. F. (1990). Education in Japan: The issues at stake at the dawn of the twenty-first century. In C. Chiland & J. G. Young (Eds.), *Why children reject school: Views from seven countries* (pp. 45–61). New Haven: Yale University Press.

Jessor, R. (1993). Successful adolescent development among youth in high risk settings. *American Psychologist, 48*(2), 117–126.

Johnson, A. M., Felstein, E. I., Szurek, S. A., & Svendsen, M. (1941). School phobia. *American Journal of Orthopsychiatry, 11,* 702–708.

Kazdin, A. E. (1993). Adolescent mental health: Prevention and treatment programs. *American Psychologist, 48*(2), 127–141.

Kearney, C. A. (1993). Depression and school refusal behavior: A review with comments on classification and treatment. *Journal of School Psychology, 31,* 267–279.

Kearney, C. A., & Beasley, J. F. (1994). The clinical treatment of school refusal behavior: A survey of referral and practice characteristics. *Psychology in the Schools, 31*(4), 128–132.

Kearney, C. A., & Silverman, W. K. (1993). Measuring the function of school refusal behavior: The school refusal assessment scale. *Journal of Clinical Child Psychology, 22*(1), 85–96.

Keogh, B. K., & Weisner, T. (1993). An ecocultural perspective on risk and protective factors in children's development: Implications for learning disabilities. *Learning Disabilities Research and Practice, 8,* 3–10.

Klein, R. G., Koplewicz, H. S., Kanner, A. (1992). Imipramine treatment of children with separation anxiety disorder. *Journal of the American Academy of Child and Adolescent Psychiatry, 31*(1) 21–28.

Last, C. G., Francis, G. Herson, M. Kazdin, A. E., & Strauss, C. C. (1987). Separation anxiety and school phobia: A comparison using *DSM-III* criteria. *American Journal of Psychiatry, 144*(5), 653–657.

Last, C. G., & Strauss, C. C. (1989). School refusal in anxiety-disordered children and adolescents. *Journal of the American Academy of Child and Adolescent Psychiatry, 29,* 31–35.

Lerner, J. W. (1988). Educational interventions in learning disabilities. *Journal of the American Academy of Child and Adolescent Psychiatry, 28,* 326–331.

Levine, R. S., Metzendorf, D., & Van Boskirk, K. A. (1986). Runaway and throwaway youth: A case for early intervention with truants. *Social Work in Education, 8,*(2), 93–106.

McGee, T., & Sikorski, J. B. (1986). Learning disabilities and the juvenile justice system. *Juvenile and Family Court Journal, 37*(3). Reno, Nevada: National Council of Juvenile and Family Court Justices.

Mansdorf, I. J., & Lukens, E. (1987). Cognitive behavioral psychotherapy for separation anxious children exhibiting school phobia. *Journal of the American Academy of Child and Adolescent Psychiatry, 26*(2), 222–225.

Murase, K. (1990). School refusal and family pathology: A multifactorial approach. In C. Chiland & J. G. Young (Eds.), *Why children reject school: Views from seven countries* (pp. 73–87). New Haven: Yale University Press.

Nakane, A. (1990). School refusal: Psychopathology and natural history. In C. Chiland & J. G. Young (Eds.), *Why children reject school: Views from seven countries* (pp. 62–72). New Haven: Yale University Press.

National Center for Education Statistics, Office of Educational Research and Improvement. (1993). *Youth indicators: Trends in the wellbeing of American youth.* U.S. Department of Education. Washington, DC: U.S. Government Printing Office.

National Commission on Excellence in Education. (1983). *A nation at risk: The imperative for education reform.* Washington, DC: U.S. Government Printing Office.

Naylor, M. W., Staskowski, M., Kenney, M. C., & King, C. A. (1994). Language disorders and learning disabilities in school-refusing adolescents. *Journal of the American Academy of Child and Adolescent Psychiatry, 33*(9), 1331–1337.

Office of Educational Research and Improvement. (1993a). *Educational reforms and students at risk: A review of the current state of the art.* Washington, DC: U.S. Department of Education.

Office of Educational Research and Improvement. (1993b). *The condition of education.* U.S. Department of Education. Washington, DC: U.S. Government Printing Office.

Rutter, M. (1980). School influences on children's behavior and development. *Pediatrics, 65,* 208–220.

Sameroff, A. J., & Fiese, B. H. (1989). Conceptual issues in prevention. In D. Shaffer, I. Philips, & N. Enzer (Eds.), *Prevention of mental disorders, alcohol and other drug use in children and adolescents* (pp. 23–53). Rockville, MD: Office of Substance Abuse Prevention.

Shapiro, T. (1989). The psychodynamic formulation in child and adolescent psychiatry. *Journal of the American Academy of Child and Adolescent Psychiatry, 28,* 675–680.

Snyder, T. D. (1993). *120 years of American education: A statistical portrait.* National Center for Education Statistics, U.S. Department of Education. Washington, DC: U.S. Government Printing Office.

Steinberg, L., Lamborn, S. D., Dornbasch, S. M., & Darling, N. (1992). Impact of parenting on adolescent achievement: Authoritative parenting, school involvement, and encouragement to succeed. *Child Development, 63,* 1266–1281.

Taylor, L., & Adelman, H. S. (1990). School avoidance behavior: Motivational bases and implications for intervention. *Child Psychiatry and Human Development, 20*(4), 219–233.

Tisher, M. (1985). School refusal: A depressive equivalent. In I. H. Berkowitz & J. S. Selinger (Eds.),

Expanding mental health interventions in schools (pp. 109–115). Dubuque, IA: Kendall/Hunt Publishing Company.

Wagner, M. (1993). *The secondary school programs of students with disabilities.* The Office of Special Education Programs, U.S. Department of Education. Menlo Park, CA: SRI International.

Wagner, M. Blackorby, J., & Hebbeler, K. (1993). *Beyond the report card: The multiple dimensions of secondary school performance of students with disabilities.* The Office of Special Education Programs, U.S. Department of Education. Menlo Park, CA: SRI International.

Wagner, M., Newman, L., D'Amico, R., Jay, E. D., Butler-Nalin, P., Marder, C., & Cox, R. (1991). *The First Comprehensive Report from the National Longitudinal Transaction Study of Special Education Students.* For the Office of Special Education Programs, U.S. Department of Education. Menlo Park, CA: SRI International.

Zigler, E., & Trickett, P. K. (1978). I.Q., social competence, and evaluation of early childhood prevention programs. *American Psychologist, 33,* 789–799.

16

New Directions for Adolescent Risk Prevention and Health Promotion Research and Interventions

RALPH J. DiCLEMENTE, LYNN E. PONTON, and WILLIAM B. HANSEN

INTRODUCTION

The lessons learned from research on individual adolescent health risk behaviors show that all of these behaviors have similar patterns of development and etiologic roots, and may respond to similar prevention and treatment programs. Surprisingly, research on each of these areas has proceeded relatively independently, yet similar findings are emerging. There are, of course, important differences across risk behaviors as well. Understanding the similarities and differences across risk behaviors expands the options for prevention and treatment.

Among the lessons learned from the epidemiologic research is that each risk behavior is tied to both a developmental sequence and a pattern of etiology that is similar. Use of tobacco, alcohol, marijuana, inhalants; unsafe sexual behavior; violence; and delinquency

RALPH J. DiCLEMENTE • Departments of Health Behavior and Pediatrics, University of Alabama, Birmingham, Alabama 35294.   LYNN E. PONTON • Langley Porter Psychiatric Institute, Division of Child and Adolescent Psychiatry, University of California, San Francisco, San Francisco, California 94117. WILLIAM B. HANSEN • Department of Public Health Sciences, Bowman Gray School of Medicine, Winston-Salem, North Carolina 27157.

Handbook of Adolescent Health Risk Behavior, edited by Ralph J. DiClemente, William B. Hansen, and Lynn E. Ponton. Plenum Press, New York, 1996.

follow a trajectory of increasing prevalence and intensity during adolescence. Substance use and sexual activity follow patterns of predictable increasing involvement whereas early involvement with milder behaviors seems to act as a gateway for more intense involvement in later years.

The common etiologic themes that emerge have their roots in personality and social relations. Adolescents vulnerable to high-risk behaviors have problems in multiple arenas. They also tend to belong to social networks that foster the development of these high-risk patterns of behavior and reinforce the continuation of risk behaviors. A component of this process appears to be the communication and transfer of group norms to vulnerable individuals.

These findings highlight the importance of targeting multiple risk behaviors simultaneously. At a minimum, ignoring co-occurring risk behaviors may lead to ineffective interventions and, in some cases, may even be counterproductive. It also suggests that, in addition to intervening with the individual, interventions need to extend to the family, the peer group, and the community. Changing the context within which the behaviors are studied will be at least as important as addressing the individual issues that cause or maintain those behaviors (Millstein, Nightingale, Petersen, Mortimer, & Hamburg, 1993).

The bulk of current research represents an extremely ambitious effort on the part of many investigators. Launching and evaluating programmatic interventions requires considerable expenditure of funds. Unfortunately, the bulk of funding designed to prevent and treat problem behaviors has been allocated to non-research-linked programs. In the drug prevention field for instance, approximately $1.5 billion in federal funds is allocated for prevention activities. Of this, only about $14 million directly funds prevention research. Most of the prevention and treatment programming that federal, philanthropic, and insurance sources support has not had the benefit of an assessment component which would provide a solid research base. Diverting some of the funds from providing hasty responses to social problems and earmarking them specifically to plan methodologically rigorous program evaluations will, in the end, be a worthwhile investment to the development of effective interventions.

The current funding zeitgeist requires increased accountability coinciding with reduced budgets. In such an environment, the use of well-planned and carefully assessed studies is of even greater importance. The cost of longitudinal field studies and clinical trials has been high. Nonetheless, the past 20 years have seen the emergence of robust and productive methods and a science-based technology of treatment and prevention. No single study controls for all threats to validity. However, methodologies for achieving and gauging the effectiveness of programs and for gathering essential knowledge for making interventions more effective have progressed substantially and are now well established. The prognosis for a combined approach that includes future epidemiologic studies and carefully assessed treatment and prevention efforts to answer problems of human behavior has never been better.

GROWING INTEREST IN ADOLESCENT RISK BEHAVIORS

In recent years, there has been an increased focus on adolescent risk behaviors. First, in stark contrast to previous decades where infectious diseases were the major cause of illness and death, specific risk behaviors (e.g., violence, unintentional injury, and suicide) now have been recognized as major contributors to morbidity and mortality among young people. Investigation of adolescent risk behavior has also indicated that Westernized cultures, and most specifically the United States, which places a high premium on broad and nondirective choices for youth, have higher overall rates of adolescent risk behavior. Cultures with structured, adult-sanctioned, supervised challenges for youth, and which emphasize a narrower socialization, with promotion of developing adult roles in the early teenage years (e.g., early marriage, apprenticeship programs), have lower overall rates of risk behavior (Arnett, 1992; Arnett & Taber, 1994). Finally, improved methodology and statistical techniques have been developed and have also spurred on investigation in this field. For example, Feisher, Ziervogal, Chalton, Leger, and Robertson (1993) underscore the importance of using a multivariate model and methodology for research, a technique that allows relationships between forms of behavior to surface.

MODELS AND THEORETICAL CONSIDERATIONS

Theoretical frameworks of risk-taking behavior are helpful both to researchers interpreting empirical findings and to clinicians trying to understand the behaviors of their patients. One of the key models conceptualizes adolescent risk-taking as interrelated domains of risk and protective factors affecting both individual adolescents and groups of adolescents (Jessor, 1990). This model effectively countered the early proclivity in the field to attach global meaning to a single variable, exemplified by the noteworthy "Just Say No" public awareness campaign against drugs, which was single-focused and failed to take into account the complexity of behavioral patterns and the multiplicity of influences on behavior.

Jessor's model divides the factors that contribute to adolescent risk behaviors into five areas: *biological or genetic* contributions; the *social environment,* which includes factors like poverty and quality of schools; an area called *perceived environment,* which is defined as how the adolescent sees his or her own environment and includes contributions to a teen's behavior from environmental models for both abnormal and conventional behavior; *individual personality factors,* which include self-esteem, the way a teenager visualizes or fails to visualize his or her own future, his or her propensity for risk-taking, and his or her values related to achievement and health; and, finally, *behavioral factors,* such as school attendance and drinking. Also emphasized are the importance of protective factors, which are those factors that protect or buffer an adolescent against participation in risk behavior.

A second model underscores the importance of life-styles in adolescent risk-taking, and emphasizes the interrelated nature of behavior. Using this approach, specific behaviors are understood to be embedded in general styles of adaptation which are maintained by complex networks of social and cultural reinforcement (Nutbeam, Aar, & Catford, 1989). This model has obvious clinical applications indicating that individual, clinical, and larger-scale prevention programs should attempt to influence the life-style in which a particular behavior is embedded versus focusing on specific forms of behavior.

Igra and Irwin (in this volume) underscore the importance of utilizing a biopsychosocial perspective when explaining adolescent risk behavior. They characterize contributors to risk-taking behavior from the biological sphere as genetic predispositions, direct hormonal influences, and the interplay of hormones and the developmental period of puberty. Psychological contributors include an adolescent's cognitive ability and dispositional personality traits. Social or environmental aspects of risk-taking include the roles of peers, parents, family structure, and social institutions. All of these components are woven into the biopsychosocial model, including an evaluation of cultural factors.

The biopsychosocial model proposed by Igra and Irwin attempts to define the current perceptions of the complex interrelationships between the various adolescent risk behaviors using the broad term "covariation of risk factors" to encompass multiple meanings. They refer to at least three theoretical approaches which attempt to explain the connections. One approach focuses on how individual behaviors influence others. Substance abuse and its associated progression of risk behaviors (see Hansen & O'Malley, this volume) offers a good example of this perspective. A second model proposes that risk-taking behaviors can be seen as alternative manifestations of a general tendency. Nutbeam *et al.* (1989) proposed a "life-styles" model largely reflecting this perspective. The third theoretical model proposed by Igra and Irwin to explain the connections proposes that a finite constellation of factors are responsible for multiple risk-taking behaviors. Jessor's model utilizes this third approach with respect to covariant risk behavior, highlighting underlying factors which enhance adolescents' vulnerability or protection.

All of the risk behaviors that our authors examined are currently conceptualized as the result of a complex interaction of factors. The authors of the chapters on disordered eating and suicidal behavior use a modified biopsychosocial model. The authors of the chapter on teen pregnancy theorize a life options approach paralleling Nutbeam and colleagues' idea of life-styles and modes of adaptation. The authors of the chapter on unintentional injury acknowledge that the work in their field initially took an accident-management perspective, but that current work appreciates a greater complexity of contributors. The author of the chapter on academic underachievement and school refusal utilizes an early identification and detection model which also evaluates and includes a number of factors. Several chapters referred to earlier theoretical perspectives which regarded risk behaviors from a more restricted perspective. Stiffman and colleagues' chapter on adolescent violence utilizes a chain of events model which looks at vulnerabilities and protective factors across an adolescent's lifetime and describes how several theories of adolescent violence omit environmental factors. The exclusion has had far-reaching consequences, directly affecting prevention and treatment efforts. The authors' recognition of the importance of the exclusion of environmental factors in the causation of violence is an important contribution to this area.

COMMON ETIOLOGIC ROOTS

The chapters on tobacco, alcohol, and drug abuse clearly demonstrate similar epidemiologic and etiologic patterns for all substances and reveal numerous similarities in treatment and prevention approaches to these problems. While each substance has its clear specific domain, and the consequences of tobacco use, alcohol abuse, and drug abuse are different in nature, there are, nonetheless, remarkable similarities in observed developmental patterns. For example, social influences have been clearly documented as a major force that promotes experimentation, increased use and maintenance of use of all substances. This is true despite the obvious differences in pharmacologic effects that are associated with specific substances.

The recent increase in illegal substance use underscores the need for the development of effective programs. Of particular interest is the recent increase in inhalant use, a problem heretofore not observed. The challenge in such reversals in substance use trends is that the availability of programs and establishment of policies are often reactive and politically motivated. The research literature on all areas of substance abuse supports a systematic, science-based, planned approach as opposed to a reactionary, ideology-based, political approach. The literature reviewed in these chapters provides a clear vision that etiologically informed treatment and prevention interventions are not only effective, but make sound strategic social problem-solving sense. Furthermore, the history of research demonstrates the need to actively seek transference from one domain of investigation to the next. What was learned in tobacco prevention and treatment benefitted alcohol prevention and treatment, and has the potential to benefit drug abuse prevention and treatment. Similarly, STD/HIV prevention, violence and delinquency prevention, teen pregnancy prevention, and the yet-to-be-identified problems of the next century will all benefit from our understanding of the epidemiology, etiology, prevention, and treatment of contemporary risk behaviors.

CONNECTIONS AND CONTRIBUTIONS: THE ASSOCIATIONS AMONG RISK BEHAVIORS

Across the spectrum of risk behaviors we found both striking similarities and important differences. We discovered that each of the individual areas of risk behavior investigation can make important contributions to others as well as adding to a more complex understanding of the overall process. The risk behavior of teenage pregnancy as described by Stevens-Simon and McAnarney (this volume) serves as a prime example. Because it has been recognized as an adolescent risk behavior for decades, it has been targeted by multiple generations of intervention efforts. Although assessment of individual interventions has been flawed, each generation of intervention has contributed knowledge to the next about how teenage pregnancy can be prevented most effectively. Current interventions are at the fourth generation, spanning almost 40 years. The knowledge gained within this field can be applied by newly recognized or developed risk behaviors such as HIV-related risk behavior and disordered eating. Prevention programs that address these new behaviors have only been developed in the past 10 years, but can incorporate knowledge from the older areas. The early work on teenage pregnancy prevention illustrated this. Early programs that focused on providing knowledge about biology and contraception to teens resulted in increased knowledge and changed attitudes, but did not significantly alter teen behavior. Later generations of prevention efforts yielded other necessary information such as the importance of early interventions which target elementary and middle school children with prevention efforts designed to reach the children before their ideas and intentions about their future behaviors are fully formed, perhaps even before attitudes about a behavior have been established. The type of "progressive learning" which has accumulated from multiple generations of teenage pregnancy prevention programs is both time-consuming and expensive, and should be shared by the entire field of adolescent risk behaviors.

It is also important to look at the field as a whole because the behaviors themselves have many complex connections. There are clusters of risk behaviors that occur together, for example, alcohol and substance abuse and unintentional injury as described by Lescohier and Gallagher (this volume). Behaviors such as school refusal (i.e., dropping out) and teenage pregnancy frequently co-occur. Until recently it was believed that teenage pregnancy preceded dropping out of school. It is now recognized (Sikorski, this volume; Stevens-Simon & McAnarney, this volume) that a whole spectrum of school-related risk behaviors—poor performance or school failure which ultimately results in school refusal—may precede a girl's decision to become pregnant. Sikorski's chapter, which offers an in-depth examination of a spectrum of risk behaviors, including school failure and refusal, which often begin early in a child's life, indicates that the early presence of these risk behaviors develops a fertile ground for the presence of others later in life. Understanding an association such as the one observed between teenage pregnancy and school refusal not only increases theoretical knowledge but allows for the development of more effective interventions.

UNDERSTANDING AND UTILIZING RESILIENCY IN DEVELOPING HEALTH-PROMOTING INTERVENTIONS

The concept of an inherent resiliency in youth is an idea developed by Garmezy (1991), Rutter (1979), and others who identify resiliency as an internal strength observable in all youth, but perhaps most important to vulnerable youth in high-risk environments. Garmezy defines resiliency as "the evaluative awareness of a difficult reality combined with a commitment to struggle, to conquer the obstacle, and to achieve one's goals despite the negative circumstances to which one has been exposed" (Garmezy, 1991). Understood in this way, resiliency can be appreciated as the capacity to confront hardships, or even traumas, rather than merely enduring them, and to conquer and succeed rather than merely survive. Such a concept is valuable particularly with respect to developing interventions that address risk behaviors.

Adolescents have to confront challenges to develop a sense of self-efficacy and empowerment. Youth from high-risk backgrounds are confronted with even greater challenges. They have to develop a keen ability to assess risk at the same time that they take on challenges to avoid being a victim. Specific interventions need to address the aspect of healthy, even mandated, risk-taking at the same time that they sharpen a youth's skills about unacceptable risks.

Resiliency can also be a dangerous concept applied to youth by a society unwilling to provide the fiscal resources to develop and implement much needed preventive and treatment interventions. All youth are not "resilient," certainly not against the incredible obstacles that they currently face in contemporary culture. It is, however, a concept that can be worked toward, incorporated into treatment and prevention programs, and encouraged and fostered in all of our youth.

DESIGNING INNOVATIVE PROGRAMS: THE INTEGRATION OF EPIDEMIOLOGY, TREATMENT, AND PREVENTION

This volume has included sections on epidemiology, treatment, and prevention for each risk behavior in order to promote integrative approaches to prevention and treatment. To illustrate, we use disordered eating as an example. As noted (see Ponton, this volume), recent epidemiological investigations have shown that adolescent girls are at highest risk; this finding encourages a careful investigation of treatment and prevention efforts targeted to this age group. The chapters have repeatedly indicated the importance of linking prevention and treatment efforts, as adolescents who utilize treatment are generally at high risk to reengage in the risk behavior, and are in need of targeted intervention efforts. Programs that combine treatment and prevention efforts ensure that teens do not lose out while being referred from one type of program to another. This type of sharing can work both ways. A prevention program can identify teens in need of treatment and refer them in that direction. Likewise, a treatment program can attach and assess a prevention component which reduces the risk that the targeted population will reengage in the focus risk behavior or engage in other related or nonrelated risk behaviors in the future.

All of the chapters make recommendations for prevention. Almost all recommend utilizing a comprehensive prevention approach which is developmentally and culturally appropriate, including targeted interventions for high-risk groups, and almost all highlight the importance of attached assessment. As described earlier, prevention programs addressing teenage pregnancy and substance abuse prevention appear to be the most sophisticated in terms of theoretical approach and curriculum, having had several generations of programs to learn from. The current fourth generation of pregnancy prevention programs attempts to target children and adolescents early and utilizes a "life options" approach which underscores adolescent opportunities, choice, and postponing child-rearing. Programs that combine alcohol, tobacco, and drug use prevention have addressed specific theoretical issues related to intervening on known psychological and sociological mediating mechanisms that account for use. These programs have expanded to include comprehensive individual, school, family, and community elements.

Attaching prevention efforts to sites where adolescents are being treated for a severe consequence of a risk behavior, such as a hospital emergency room postsuicide attempt or a psychiatric clinic or hospital after treatment for an eating disorder, is another recommended innovation. Such linkages ensure that high-risk groups which formerly fell through the cracks will not be forgotten only to surface again in acute need of care.

SOCIAL CONTEXT AS AN IMPORTANT DETERMINANT OF RISK BEHAVIORS

Increasingly we see that strategic intervention planning is being called for. Efforts that target individuals and at-risk groups are being coordinated within a framework of communitywide interventions. These broader intervention approaches acknowledge the importance of social context. Clearly, to understand and effectively intervene with adolescents, we must not only examine and understand the context of internal psychological factors which may influence the initiation and continuance of risk behaviors; we also need to understand how the influences of social networks and the culture of the larger society in general affect behavior. The challenge of developing such comprehensive and coordinated strategies of intervention requires extensive understanding of the multilevel processes which are amenable to intervention.

CONCLUSION

To avert further increases in adolescent risk behaviors and the adverse health and social consequences that accompany these behaviors, development of effective prevention and treatment interventions is urgently needed. To facilitate this research effort, a comprehensive and coordinated infrastructure is critical to conceptualize, stimulate, and support the continuum of intervention research. One clear advantage of this systematic approach is that it avoids development of isolated prevention and treatment programs which have impeded cross-fertilization of information and the sharing of new and effective prevention and treatment strategies between investigators and practitioners working with different risk behaviors. Furthermore, this approach would also permit more rapid integration of findings derived from longitudinal cohort studies focused on identifying the determinants of specific risk behaviors to be consolidated into existing and planned prevention and treatment programs. And, finally, a systematic approach encourages continued rigorous evaluation of prevention and treatment programs as one mechanism of identifying efficacious programs and eliminating ineffective approaches. Without a defined, structured response to the problem of adolescent risk behaviors, many adolescents will experience the pain and suffering that are often the consequence of these behaviors.

REFERENCES

Arnett, J. J. (1992). Reckless behavior in adolescence: A development perspective. *Development Review, 12,* 339–373.

Arnett, J. J., & Taber, S. (1994). Adolescence terminable and interminable: When does adolescence end? *Journal of Youth and Adolescence, 23*(5), 517–537.

Feisher, A. J., Ziervogal, C. F., Chalton, D. O., Leger, P. H., & Robertson, B. A. (1993). *Risk-taking behavior of South African high school students: A multi-variate analysis.* Presented at the 40th annual meeting of the American Academy of Child and Adolescent Psychiatry, San Antonio, TX, October 26–31.

Garmezy, N. (1991). Resilience in children's adaptation to the negative life events and stressed environments. *Pediatric Annals, 20,* 9.

Jessor, R. (1990). Risk behavior in adolescence: A psychosocial framework for understanding. In D. Rogers & E. Ginzberg (Eds.), *Adolescents at risk: Medical and social perspectives.* San Francisco: Westview Press.

Millstein, S. G., Nightingale, E. O., Petersen, A. C., Mortimer, A. M., & Hamburg, D. A. (1993). Promoting the healthy development of adolescents. *Journal of the American Medical Association, 269,* 1413–1415.

Nutbeam, D., Aar, L., & Catford, J. (1989). Understanding children's health behavior: The implications for health promotion for young people. *Social Science and Medicine, 29,* 317–325.

Rutter, M. (1979). Protective factors in children's responses to stress and disadvantage. In M. W. Kent & J. E. Rolf (Eds.), *Primary prevention of psychopathology: Vol. III. Social competence in children* (pp. 49–74). Hanover, NH: University Press of New England.

Index

Obesity
  in American Indians, 93
  definition, 85
  sociocultural attitudes towards, 91
  treatment, 105–106
Ombudsman program, 181
Opiates, endogenous, in anorexia nervosa, 102
Opiates use, etiologic research in, 174
Opportunity model, of adolescent violence, 300
Oppositional defiant disorder, 27
Oregon Social Learning Center, delinquency preven-
      tion program, 271–272
Organization development methods, use in delin-
      quency prevention, 275
Outdoor experience training, 136, 280, 305
Outpatient treatment, of alcohol abusers, 147
Outward Bound, 280, 305

Pacific Islander adolescents, sexually-transmitted
      diseases in, 19
Panic disorder, comorbidity with school refusal, 397
Parasuicide, 194
Parental factors
  in alcohol use, 26, 27, 132, 142–143
  in drug abuse, 26, 27, 175
  in risk-taking behavior, 43–44
  in smoking, 62
Parent Communication Project, 131
Parenting programs
  for alcohol-related problems prevention, 131, 133
  for delinquency prevention, 271–272, 273
  for violence prevention, 303
Parenting style
  academic achievement and, 399
  as delinquency risk factor, 267–268
    interventions for, 271–272, 282
  as risk-taking behavior risk factor, 43–44
  as violence risk factor, 299
Parents
  alcohol use by, 26, 27, 132, 142–143
  death of, as homelessness cause, 376–377
  drug abuse by, 26, 27, 175
  involvement in substance abuse prevention and
      treatment programs, 182–183, 186–187
  smoking by, 62
Passive smoking, 73
Pedestrians, motor vehicle-related injuries, 235–
      236
Pediatricians, suicidal behavior diagnosis by, 204
Peer-based prevention programs
  for alcohol use, 134
  for alcohol-related problems, 138–139
  for eating disorders, 95
  for sexual high-risk behavior, 349–350
Peer cluster theory, of substance abuse, 172, 173

Peer factors
  in alcohol use, 125, 142
  in condom use, 342, 349
  in delinquency, 266, 268–269
    interventions for, 272, 273–274
  in drug abuse, 175
  in risk-taking behavior, 44, 45, 46
  in school refusal, 394–395
  in smokeless tobacco use, 63–64
  in smoking, 61–62
  in violence, 299–300
Peer mediation program, 273–274
Peers, suicide by, 200
Pelvic inflammatory disease, 334, 354, 358–359
Penile cancer, 19
Pennsylvania Substance Abuse System, 151
People of color, adolescent
  population trends, 5, 6
  poverty, 7
  See also specific ethnic and racial groups
Periactin, as eating disorder therapy, 104, 105
Peritonitis, pelvic, 358
Personality disorders, as suicide risk factor, 200
Personality factors
  in drug abuse, 175
  in risk-taking behavior, 414, 415
Phenelzine, as bulimia nervosa therapy, 104
Phenothiazines, as eating disorder therapy, 104, 105
Phobias, school refusal-associated, 397, 407–408
Physical abuse, 25
  of homeless and runaway adolescents, 372
    treatment programs for, 384
  as suicide risk factor, 202
Physical fitness, effect of smoking on, 55
Physicians, prevention program involvement of
  for alcohol-related problems, 139
  for alcohol use, 132
  for sexually-transmitted diseases/HIV, 347–348
  suicidal behavior diagnosis by, 204
Pimazide, as eating disorder therapy, 105
Poisoning, 9
  as mortality cause, 232
  as suicide method, 194, 196, 197, 198
Police
  adolescent substance abuse program involve-
      ment, 181
  delinquency control involvement, 260
  violence by, 309
Polydrug abuse, 60, 145
Postponing Sexual Involvement program, 322
Posttraumatic stress disorder, as violence risk fac-
      tor, 297, 298
Poverty
  of adolescent mothers, 20–21
  as injury-related mortality risk factor, 234

Quadriplegia, football-related, 244–245
Quality of later life, 2–3
Quest Skills for Living program, 180, 181

Racism, as violence risk factor, 296
Rape
  of homeless adolescents, 373
  reported rates, 292
Reasoned action theory, of substance abuse, 171,
    172, 173
Reasoning, 41
Reducing the Risk, 322
Referrals, for psychoeducational assessment, 406
Rehabilitation, of injured patients, 239, 249, 251–252
Religion, as suicide prevention factor, 197
Remove Intoxicated Drivers (RID), 242
Reproductive counseling
  at school health clinics, 186
  See also Family planning
Reproductive health care costs, of female runaway
    adolescents, 383
Residential facilities, student assistance programs
    in, 184–185
Residential treatment
  for alcohol abuse, 146, 149, 151–152
  of homeless and runaway adolescents, 382–383,
    384–385
  for substance abuse, 188
  for violence, 306
Resiliency, of adolescents, 418
Resistance skills programs, for substance abuse pre-
    vention, 177
Risk, definition, 35, 226
Risk estimators, 226
Risk exposure, 226–227
Risk perception, 40–41, 45, 46
Risk-taking behavior
  "clusters" of, 418
  common etiologic causes, 413–414, 416–417
  continuum, 413–414
  cost, 3
  definition, 35
  deviant, 225–226
  as epidemic, 3–4
  excessive, 225–226
  as health risk, 225–226
  of homeless and runaway adolescents, 372–375
  interrelatedness, 3, 417–418
  interventions for, 414, 418–420
  negative consequences, 35
  as nonnormative behavior, 36
  as normative behavior, 36
  predisposing factors, 45, 47
  protective factors, 47
  quality of later life and, 2–3

Risk-taking behavior (*cont.*)
  research in, 414–415
    federal funding of, 414
  smoking and, 62, 73
  theories of, 35–51, 415–416
    biological theories, 38, 39–40, 48, 415–416
    biopsychosocial theories, 38, 45–47, 48, 415–416
    cognitive theories, 38, 40–42
    covariation theories, 36, 37–38, 416
    developmental theories, 36–37
    psychological theories, 38, 40–42, 48
    social/environmental theories, 38, 42–45, 48
  trends, 2
Robbery, 11
Role-model programs, 308
Role models, influence on risk-taking behavior, 4
Runaway adolescents, 25–26, 369
  differentiated from homeless adolescents, 371
  as homeless adolescents, 371
  school problems, 372
  sexual behavior, 373
  sexual risk-reduction programs for, 346–347
  suicide
    attempts, 202
    prevention interventions for, 204
  truancy interventions with, 405
Runaway and Homeless Youth Act, 383
Russia, academic achievement levels in, 399

Safety belts, 9, 232–233, 240, 243–244
Salpingitis, 358
San Francisco, homeless and runaway youth in,
    370, 372
  Larkin Street Youth Center for, 385–386, 387
San Francisco Unified School District, 406
Schizophrenia, as suicide risk factor, 200
School avoidance, 396–397
  prevention programs, 404–405
  See also School refusal
School-based clinics
  reproductive health services, 321
  See also Clinic/hospital-based prevention pro-
    grams
School-based prevention programs
  for alcohol-related problems, 138–139
  for alcohol use, 130, 132, 134–135, 137, 143, 144
    treatment component of, 147
  for delinquency, 270–271, 275
  for sexually-transmitted diseases/HIV, 343–345
  for smoking, 69
  for substance abuse, 175, 176–184
    classification, 178–179
    curriculum effectiveness, 179–184
  for suicide, 208–209
  for violence, 303

ISBN 0-306-45147-6
90000

9 780306 451478